FROM THE PUBLISHER

I have had the opportunity to work with Oklahoma physicians recently and I've never enjoyed working with a group of people more than these doctors. The doctors and staff of the Tulsa County Medical Society have been a delight to work with. I dedicate this book to all of you with special thanks to Dr. Wally Hooser for his recognition of past TCMS Executive Directors and current director Mona Whitmire. I'll always remember my good friend, Dr. Bill Simcoe, a true patriot and dedicated physician who typifies the selflessness of Tulsa physicians.

John Compton
Publisher

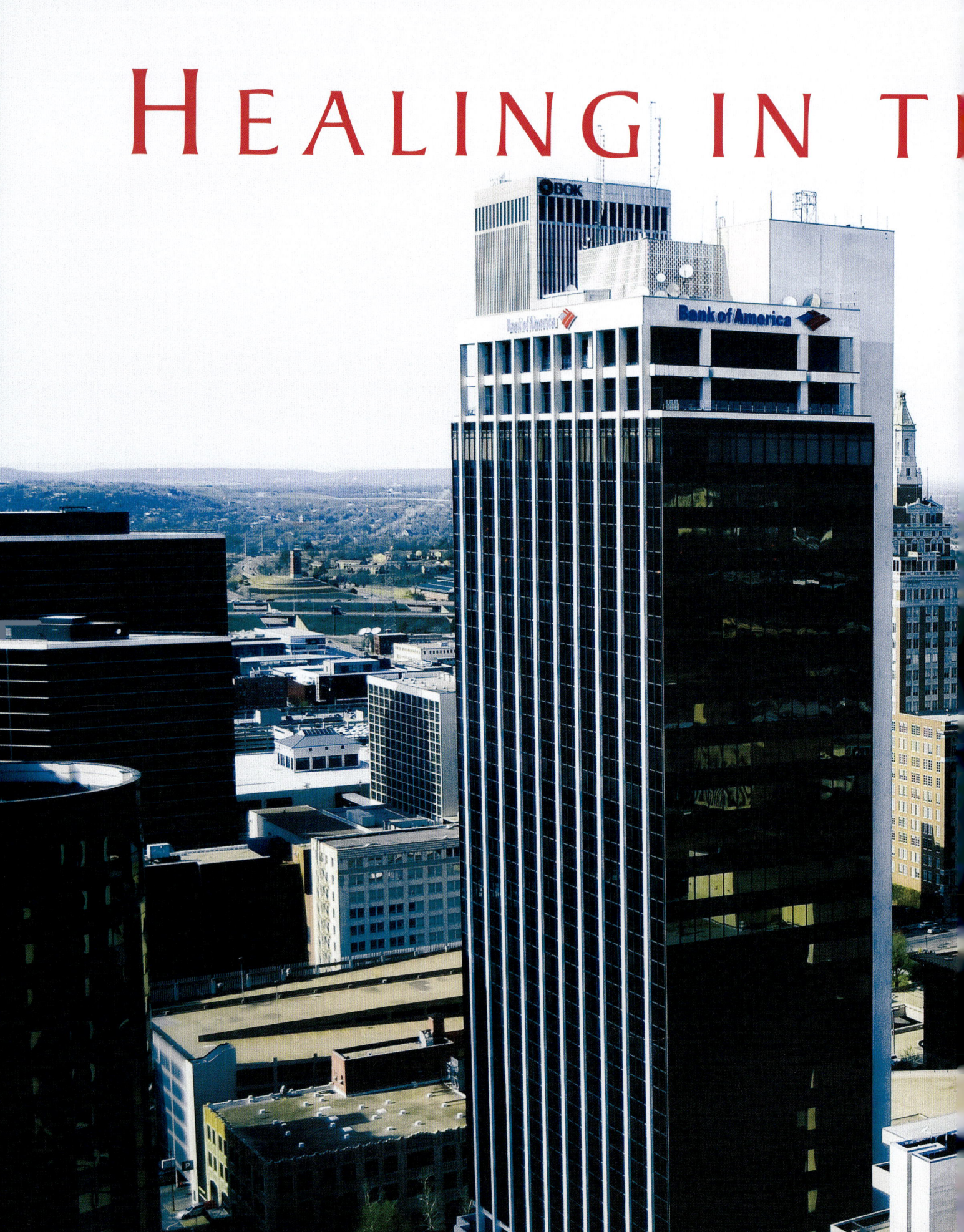
Healing in t

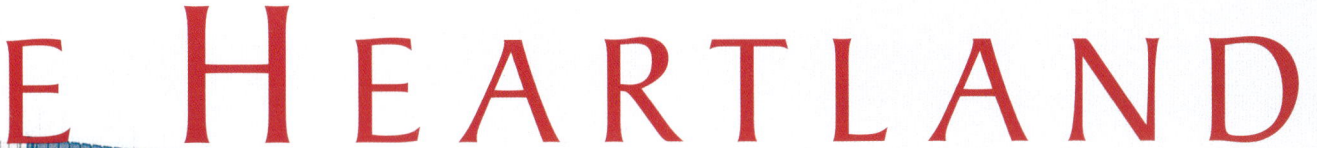

e Heartland

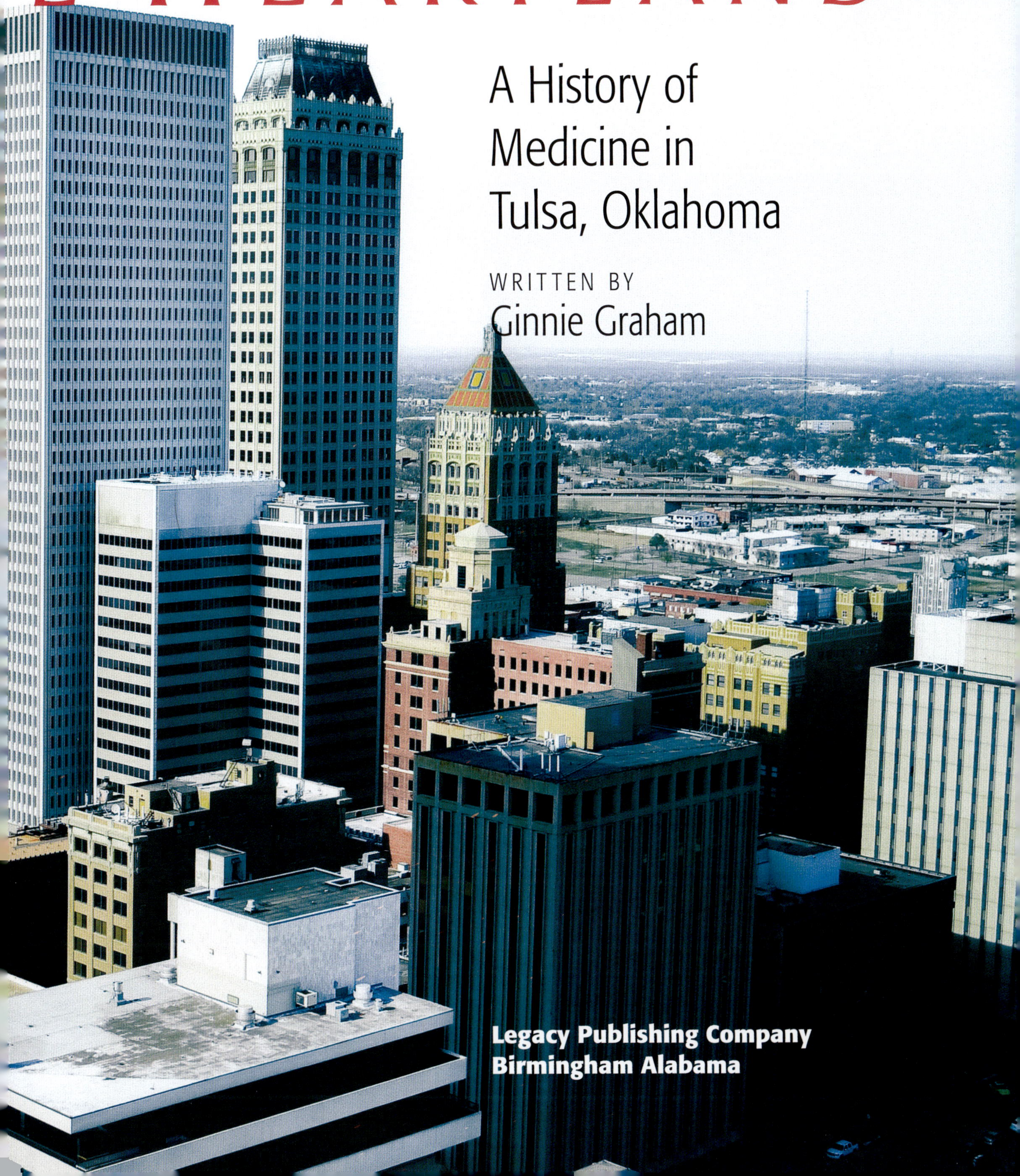

A History of
Medicine in
Tulsa, Oklahoma

WRITTEN BY
Ginnie Graham

Legacy Publishing Company
Birmingham Alabama

HEALING IN THE HEARTLAND
A HISTORY OF MEDICINE IN TULSA, OKLAHOMA

Published By
Legacy Publishing Company
100 Oxmoor Road, Suite 110, Birmingham, Alabama 35209 • (205) 941-4623

Publisher
John Compton

Published with the cooperation and assistance of
The Tulsa County Medical Society
Mona Whitmire, Executive Director

Author
Ginnie Graham

Medical History Writers
Debra Laizure
Sarah Soon
Brenda Wilson

Graphic Design
John Cruncleton

Photo Editor
Sarah Soon

Index
Ginnie Graham

COYRIGHT 2017 BY LEGACY PUBLISHING CO.
All Rights Reserved. Published 2017

Printed in the United States of America yy
Balfour Publishing Company, Dallas, Texas

FIRST EDITION

ISBN 978-0-9843095-4-2
Library of Congress Control Number: 2017938662

TABLE OF CONTENTS

From the Publisher	III
Foreword	VIII
Early Medicine	1
Chapter 1 • through 1910 • Founding of a City	5
Chapter 2 • 1910 - 1919 • Building a Foundation	17
Chapter 3 • 1920 - 1929 • Bustling City	27
Chapter 4 • 1930 - 1939 • Digging Out From the Depression	41
Chapter 5 • 1940 - 1949 • Advancing Medicine in War-Time	51
Chapter 6 • 1950 - 1959 • Modernizing Medicine	67
Chapter 7 • 1960 - 1969 • Constructing New Heights in Care	89
Chapter 8 • 1970 - 1979 • Emerging Schools and Treatments	111
Chapter 9 • 1980 - 1989 • Changing Health Practices	139
Chapter 10 • 1990 - 1999 • Transforming Health Care	167
Chapter 11 • 2000 - 2016 • Moving into a New Era of Medicine	193
Chapter 12 • Epilogue • The Future • Forecasting the Future of Medical Care	215
Tulsa County Medical Profiles	219
Patrons	308
In Memoriam	309
Bibliography	313
Photo Credits	320
Index	321

FORE

For physicians, the love of neighbors, friends, and patients propel us to put our undivided and committed attention on caring for patients above all else during our medical careers. As students and residents rotate through my office, it matters not that medicine is changing; young physicians' desire to care for patients remains the same.

Oklahoma has a rich heritage of innovation to improve the health of Oklahomans and challenges looking to the future will certainly remain. Buyer beware! Those ignorant of the past are likely to repeat its mistakes and shortcomings. Understanding the history of medicine in Oklahoma has thus become the cornerstone for enhancing the same excellence of care to future generations.

Tulsa has now become a significant provider of health services in Oklahoma: we owe our futures success to the dedication and pledge of those physicians you'll read about in the chapters on Tulsa's medical pioneers that probably had no idea of their future impact. What were these colleagues thinking when daring to dream about a downtown hospital complex? As medical care has changed over the past three decades, who had the courage to move forward despite significant challenges that hospitals and medical clinics alike were forced to swallow?

Answers are to be uncovered in this excellent book, *Healing in the Heartland*. Our motivation must be strong for the task of caring for our community. I hope you find the adventure will bring you the satisfaction of knowing you can help write the next chapter in the legacy of compassion for all Oklahomans.

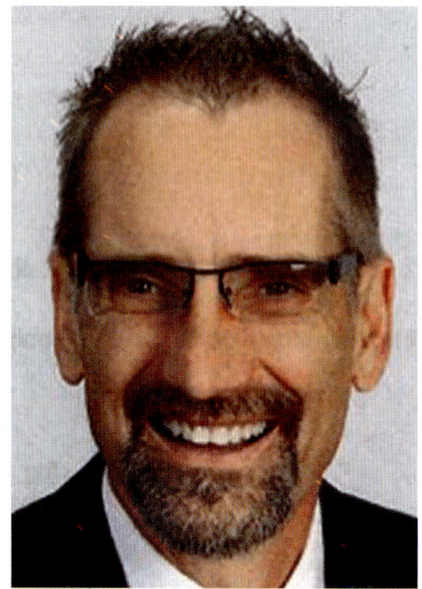

LYNN A. WIENS, M.D.
2015 TCMS PRESIDENT

It is a privilege to serve as the President of Tulsa County Medical Society. I am honored to follow 109 Presidents whose vision and insight have guided this organization since our beginning in 1907. Our goal of improving the health of our neighbors in and around Tulsa County has been the impetus for our many physician-led initiatives over the years.

I am excited TCMS has the opportunity to share *Healing in the Heartland* which will give readers a snapshot of medicine from statehood through today. Ours is a vivid history of challenges, progress and growth. Individually and collectively, our physician community is innovative and driven by the greater good as we advocate for patients and the practice of medicine. You will meet many of the pioneers of medicine in Tulsa on these pages. This book represents the body of work from men and women who were determined to address local healthcare issues and improve access to high quality medical care for all.

Public Health continues to be an important outreach of Tulsa County Medical Society and our TCMS Foundation. We also support and mentor medical students and residents… 100 years from now their experience and stories will be the sequel to *Healing in the Heartland*.

Thank you to John Compton, Publisher, and Ginnie Graham, Author, of *Healing in the Heartland*.

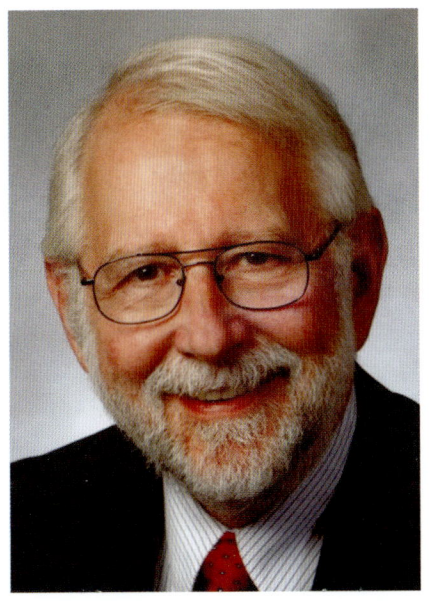

MICHAEL A. WEISZ, M.D.
2017 TCMS PRESIDENT

Early Medicine

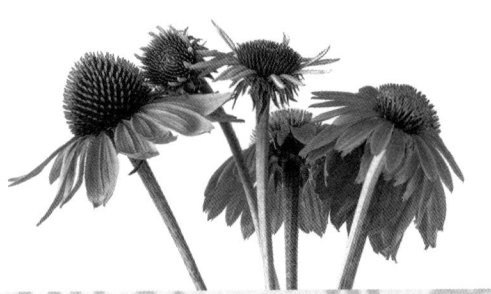

Tulsa was founded along a wild Arkansas River as a Creek Nation town in Indian Territory by tribal members and pioneers seeking an independent state to pursue prosperity. Medical practices came with the settlers, remedies passed down from ancestors coupled with emerging knowledge. The earliest physicians took a chance on the budding town, working in conditions without plumbing and electricity, to form the foundation of public health.

Purple Cone Flower: A medicinal plant still widely used.

Just prior to statehood, medical associations formed to guide the growing profession as the state and cities flourished. Tulsa doctors led the way in establishing standards and continuing education for the state and joined with business leaders to build hospitals and systems of care. Many physicians volunteered their time in city affairs as elected officials, board members for nonprofits and activists for social issues.

Tulsa evolved into a major medical hub for the region. Health care currently provides 64,000 direct jobs in an 11-county region with a $3.8 billion impact. When adding in a multiplier effect, other related jobs created and health-experts, the impact is closer to $7.3 billion, resulting in about $240 million in local tax collection.

Tulsa is a hub to four major hospital systems — St. John Medical Center, Hillcrest Medical Center, Oklahoma State University Medical Center and Saint Francis Medical Center. Also, the city is home to the University of Oklahoma-University of Tulsa School of Community Medicine and Oklahoma State University College of Osteopathic Medicine.

To understand how the medical community grew from unregulated herbalists and doctors to a billion-dollar industry, the story must begin with the earliest medical practices.

Ancient Medicine

The ancient world — Egypt, Greece and Rome — may have adopted beliefs steeped in mythology and legend, but historians say the people had knowledge of human anatomy and treatments.

In Egypt, hieroglyphics and papyruses indicate sicknesses were treated by people referred to as physicians and doctors, not magicians or medicine men. Imphotep was the physician to King Zozer in about 2,600 BC who later was worshipped as a god of healing. The tomb of Irj, who lived around 1,500 BC, described him as a "palace doctor." Archeologists found an Egyptian papyrus with knowledge about heart rates, blood and air flows through bodies as well as names to organs. Texts show about 200 diseases were identified with treatments. Only when physicians could no longer find a reason for an illness would the treatment turn to spells or potions to drive out bad spirits.

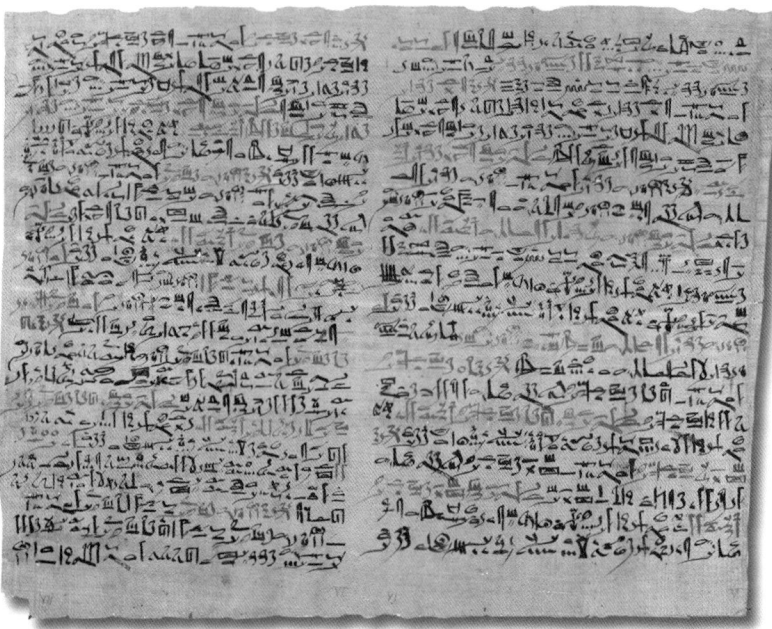

The Edwin Smith papyrus: The only surviving copy of an ancient Egyptian textbook on trauma surgery, written around 1600 BC.

Hippocrates is considered a founder of medicine though most of his work was performed about 430 years before the birth of Christ. An oath in his name — the Hippocratic Oath — was historically invoked by physicians to uphold specific ethical standards. The original version was written in Ionic Greek and sworn by several gods in the Greek and Roman cultures. That oath evolved through the generations as a rite of passage for physicians. Greek doctors separated themselves from religious leaders, emphasizing the power of observing a patient to find a natural cause for illness. Greece became a province of the Roman Empire by 27 BC.

Roman society emphasized infrastructure such as aqueducts and sewers to promote healthier living. The people held beliefs that a strong mind led to a strong body and keeping fit was imperative to fight sickness. Public health was a priority with programs of draining marshes, acquiring a clean water supply and draining used water. Personal hygiene was emphasized with regular bathing and flushable toilets.

Claudius Galen developed a method of clinical observation and dissected animals to study anatomy. He was a Greek surgeon of the gladiators until he moved to Rome in 161 AD. He used treatments to restore the "four humors" with opposites. If a person had a fever, he recommended cold remedies. Or, if a person felt weak, Galen suggested exercise to build strength.

Middle Ages

Time stood still in medical knowledge after the ancient civilizations were destroyed. The main advances were from medical schools differentiating diseases, such as smallpox and chickenpox. While students debated Hippocrates and Galen, the Roman Catholic Church held the power. The church dictated medical knowledge, and anything contradictory was heresy. The church standard was that sinning brought the onset of illness. This is what led to people inflicting pain upon themselves during sickness or eras of plague. They believed the pain would be a sign to God of their repentance and devotion.

Planets, stars and the status of the moon played a part in diagnosis. A physician would confer with a patient's astrological sign to determine a course of action. Blood letting was a popular treatment. Too much blood in the body was considered the root of many problems, so physicians either cut into a vein or used leeches to remove small amounts.

THE TIDE TURNS

The 17th century brought about a change in medical thinking, shifting from speculation to experimentation. This century introduced tools such as the microscope and thermometer. Andreas Vesalius offered great contributions in his work with human anatomy, correcting mistakes made by ancient texts.

Belgium Anatomist, Andreas Vesalius: An illustration of the base of the brain from Vesalius's, De humani corporis fabrica.

During the next century, the biggest threats were smallpox, yellow fever and diphtheria. English doctor Edward Jenner discovered an inoculation for smallpox, which started the development of vaccinations.

The 19th century advances eliminated the mysterious humors and treatments of purgings and bleedings. In 1846, anesthesia became widely available and expanded options for surgery. The most popular first surgeries were to remove tumors. In 1867, British surgeon Joseph Lister began the promotion of surgical cleanliness with his publication of the antiseptic principle. With his techniques, infections plummeted. In 1881, Louis Pasteur and George Miller isolated and grew the pneumococcus organism. The first successful appendectomy was performed in Iowa in 1885, and the mastectomy was developed as a breast cancer treatment. By 1890, medical practitioners were using chemical agents to minimize germs, including the use of carbolic acid on incisions which cut down the incidence of infections.

This century brought out the professionalization of medical care. In 1847, Dr. Nathan Davis founded the American Medical Association in Philadelphia to create professional standards for physicians and establish educational requirements.

Permanent settlement of Oklahoma and Tulsa occurred during this century, with statehood just around the corner. ■

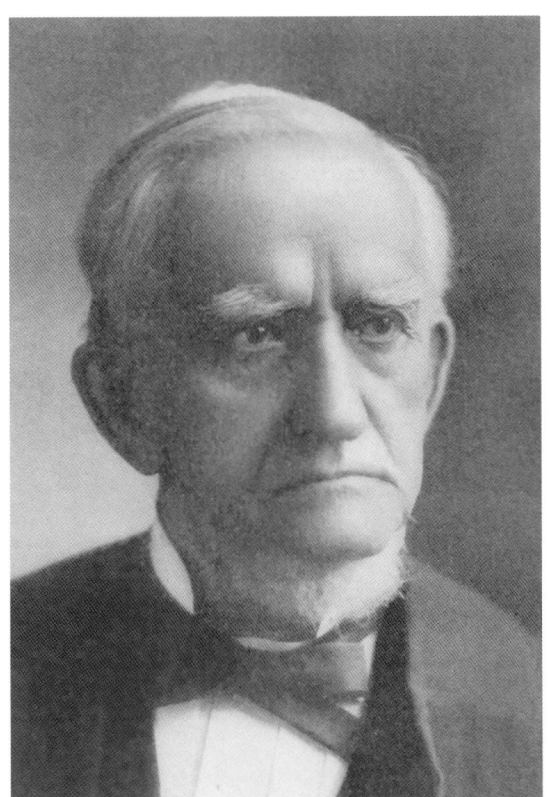

Dr. Nathan S. Davis

Dr. E.N. (Eliphalet Nott) Wright

In an impassioned speech to his fellow physicians in June 1904, Dr. E.N. (Eliphalet Nott) Wright, foresaw Oklahoma's statehood and called for unity among medical practitioners to set high standards. He cited Dr. Benjamin Rush, a signer of the U.S. Declaration of Independence, to bolster his plea for the doctors in different territories to merge with one vision.

"We must lay aside all personal feelings, political and others, and get to work to secure such laws in relation to the practice of medicine that will protect our people from quackery and elevate our professional standard that all others states may point to us with pride," he said.

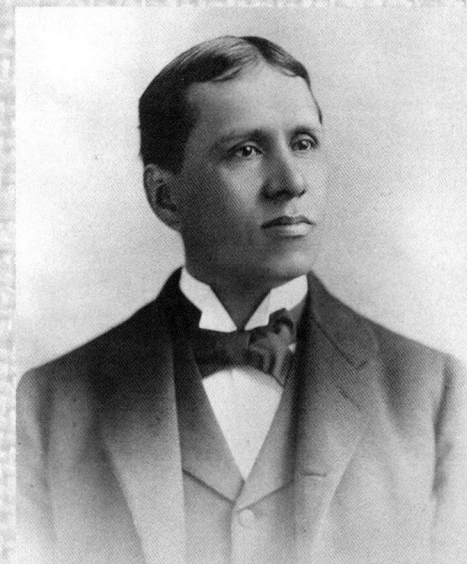

Dr. Wright was born on April 3, 1858, as the oldest son of the Rev. Allen and Harriet (Mitchell) Wright. His father was a member of the Choctaw Nation who led the Presbyterian Church at Boggy Depot, a village near Atoka that once served as the tribe's capital and trade center. After completing medical courses in 1884 at Albany Medical College in New York, he was employed as chief surgeon and physician for the Missouri-Pacific Coal Mines at Lehigh in the Choctaw Nation. In 1894, he spent a year in post-graduate work at the College of Physicians and Surgeons in New York City. He returned to the Boggy Depot area to start a private practice because his tribal people did not have access to many trained physicians.

Among his first actions was advocating for a law governing the regulation of medical practitioners within the Choctaw Nation. Dr. Wright was placed on the first tribal board of medical examiners and found some claiming to be medical professionals had never "seen a college" and had an "appalling" level of ignorance. He crafted the law passed by the tribe credited for driving out quack practitioners and supporting efforts of the Indian Territory Medical Association.

Dr. Wright developed the reputation as a talented diagnostician and skilled surgeon. Among his other interests was development of oil within tribal lands. He was elected the first president of the Choctaw Oil and Refining Company, which included the names of many tribal leaders of that time. Dr. Wright's work led to the first drilling test for oil within the boundaries of Oklahoma.

Dr. Wright was involved in the production and contracts for the tribe regarding resources such as coal, stone and timber, and oversight of railroad construction. He had a hand in politics including as a tribal delegate to the convention of the Five Civilized Tribes as it met with the Dawes Commission.

"Those were the days of the pioneer in this country when a person with his ability and training could not devote himself to one pursuit alone. The hour of the specialist in a chosen field had not yet arrived. As a leader in the van of progress, versatility was demanded of him. To have refused a call in any line of endeavor would have been tantamount to a lack of intelligence, vision, and courage," wrote Muriel Wright, his daughter.

Sometimes, those talents merged. While on a trip near Avery, Texas, in pursuit of a new oil field, an influenza epidemic hit during 1918-1919.

"Even though he was not at Avery in the capacity of his profession, nearly 1,000 persons throughout that community, including doctors and nurses, came to know him as the trained physician through the advice and care that he freely gave them. It was that way throughout his life, when the need arose, he was instantly the trained physician," wrote Muriel Wright.

Dr. Wright married Ida Bell Richards in April 1888, and the couple had two daughters, Muriel Hazel and Gertrude Ideala. One son, Eliphalet Nott Wright Jr., died in infancy. Muriel had a noted career as an historian and is in the Oklahoma Hall of Fame and one of the first inducted in the Oklahoma Historians Hall of Fame.

He died on January 10, 1932, and is buried in a family plot in Old Boggy Depot. ■

CHAPTER 1
(through 1910)

Founding of a City

Early Tulsa physician:
S.G. Kennedy, M.D.

Oklahoma Origins

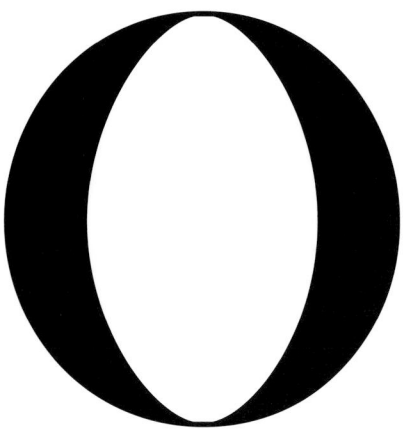

Oklahoma and Indian territories were originally a portion of the Mississippi Valley known as the Louisiana Territory. The first known inhabitants of the state were from many different Native American tribes including the Osage, Quapaw, Caddo, Wichita, Waco, Tawakony, Kiowa, Comanche and the Apache of the Plains. Spanish explorers are considered the first white men to have crossed into the area.

Four survivors of the Cabeca de Vaca expedition were alleged to have been captured by an Indian tribe between 1528 and 1536 and taken across Oklahoma. In 1541, Francisco Vasquez de Coronado led his group from Mexico, across western Oklahoma and into Kansas. That same year, eastern Oklahoma is believed to have been traversed by survivors of Hernando de Soto and Luis de Moscoso parties. Following was Antonio de Bonilla in 1549, Juan de Oñate in 1601 and Don Dego Del Castillo in 1650.

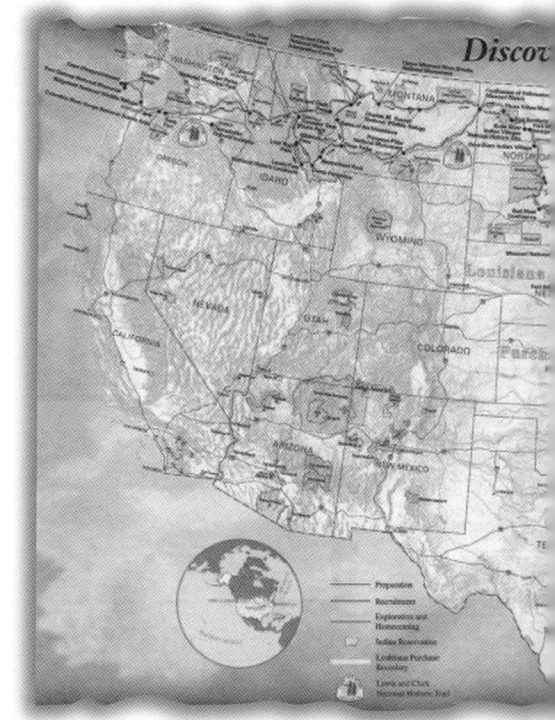

Eventually, the area became home to French and Creole trappers and traders. The region was explored between 1678 and 1682 by Robert de la Salle as he claimed all land drained by the Mississippi River and its tributaries for the King of France, naming it Louisiana. It led to a string of missionaries and frontiersmen passing through what is now Oklahoma.

After President Thomas Jefferson made the purchase of the land in 1803, more expeditions were sent to survey the landscape and its native peoples.

Early Native American Medical Practices

The William Clark and Meriwether Lewis Expedition took extensive notes on the medical remedies used by indigenous peoples during its trek across the west from 1804-1806. The exploring party came into contact with at least 50 different tribes and found Native American health practices equal or more advanced than the white settlers. Tribal members used similar techniques of observation and experience rather than strict scientific experiments, according to documents held at the University of Virginia.

Native Americans used bloodletting, purging, induced sweating and vomiting as treatments, mingled with mysticism and ritual. The expedition led to tribal members adding at least 59 drugs to the pharmacopeia of the day including quinine, ipecac, cocaine and witch hazel. Medications were taken by chewing roots or through decoctions imbibed in teas or inhaled in steam. Wounds were treated with poultices, heat, washing and draining; abscesses drained; and fractures healed with splints and traction.

Tribal healers had a strong understanding of obstetrics and gynecology, using plants for pregnancy prevention and speeding delivery. The native guide Sacagawea was given several rattles of rattlesnakes during her pregnancy to accelerate delivery. Lewis noted she gave birth within 10 minutes of taking the rattle, but he wasn't convinced of its effectiveness.

Malaria, known as the "ague" in the 19th century, was the most common disease in the U.S. Dr. Benjamin Rush, a prominent physician and signer of the Declaration of Independence, believed, as other doctors, that it was caused by bad air coming from swamps. He never made the connection to the swamp-dwelling mosquito. Historian Stephen Ambrose wrote in his book about the expedition that malaria was "so inescapable that many refused to regard it as a disease; like hard work, it was just part of life." As a treatment, Native Americans used quinine, which halts the growth and reproduction of malaria-causing parasites in red blood cells.

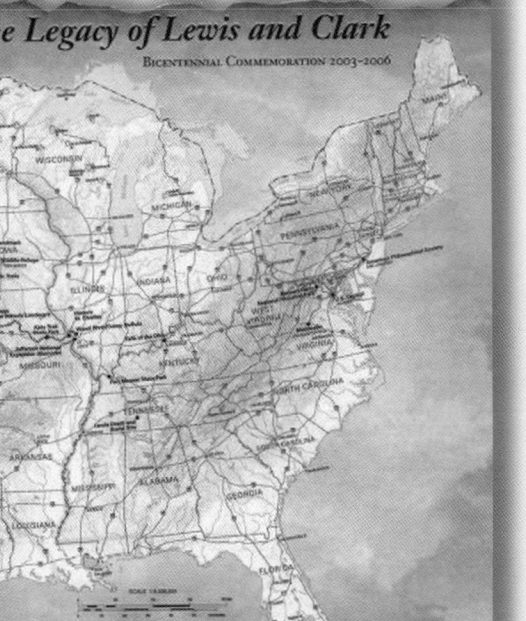

TULSA SETTLEMENT

The city was settled as a Creek tribal town, one of three "Tallasee" towns in the Muscogee Nation west of the Mississippi River. Histories differ on how the city got its name. One states the government published it as a contraction of the Indian word "Talsi" (also spelled "Tallasi")," which is derived from "Tallasi" or "Tallahassee" (also spelled "Tullahassee.") The meaning of the word is "old town." However, a former Creek Nation Chief, the Hon. Legust Perryman, gave an interview in 1921 stating the name came from the tribal word "Tulwa," meaning a town or group of people.

In 1879, a post office was established on the pony-mail route going through Indian Territory. In January 1882, the foundation stone was laid with the building of the railroad. The first building in Tulsa was the Frisco Depot and first permanent home was built that year by Bob Childers. The population was 200 people. By the time it was incorporated as a town in January 1898, there were 1,100 in residence. A couple of years later, it rose to 1,390 people. Then, the oil was discovered at Red Fork in 1901 followed by the Glenn Pool oil boom in 1905. By 1910, Tulsa's population soared to nearly 20,000.

THE FIRST DOCTOR

Dr. W.P. Booker was the city's first physician and opened a tent as his office and home west of what is now First Street, where it crosses the railroad near Main Street. In 1882, once the town attracted more settlers, Dr. Booker moved his tent between Main Street and Boulder Avenue, which was a location desired by H.C. Hall. Hall was the contractor who built the railroad and was considered one of the city's founders. Dr. Booker was given $10 to move his tent south to between First and Second streets.

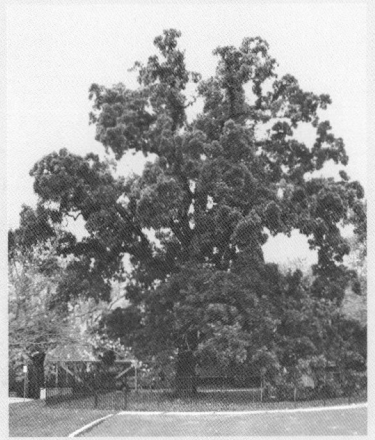

The Creek Council Oak Tree: An historic landmark representing the founding of Tulsa by the Lochapoka Clan of the Creek Nation. They settled here after they were forced to leave their homeland in the southeastern United States and travel across the Mississippi River, where the U.S. Government had granted them land in Indian Territory. After their arrival In 1836, the Lochapokas chose this burr oak tree on top of a hill overlooking the Arkansas River as the site of their council ground.

7

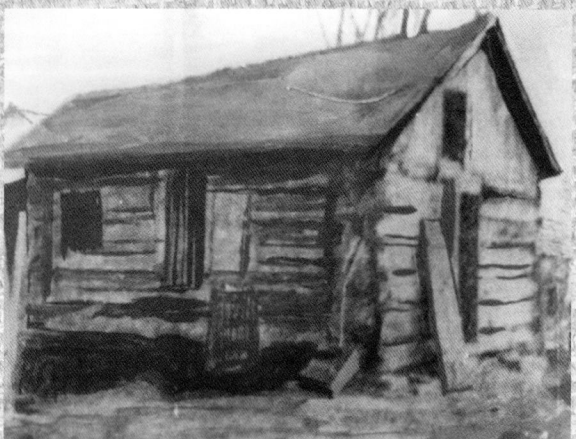
Tulsa's first post office: Opened March 1879, located on what's now 31st, west of Lewis.

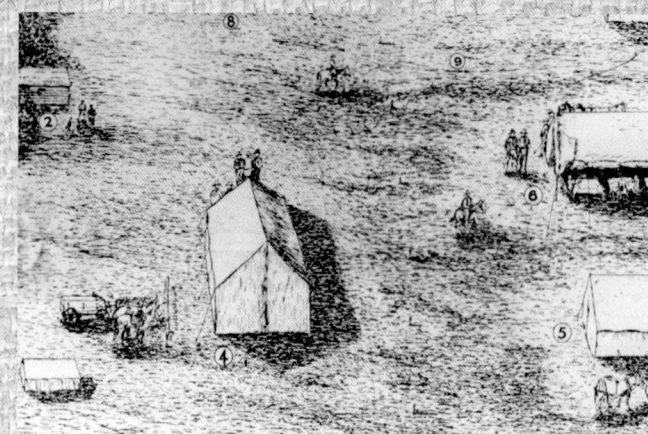
Sketch of the tent city Tulsa in 1882.

Accounts differ on whether payment was made by Hall or his younger brother, James Monroe, known as J.M. Years later, Dr. Booker moved to Caney, Kansas, where he died.

It is apparent J.M. Hall and Dr. Booker were friends. The two — along with the wife of a carpenter named Mrs. Slater — established Tulsa's first Sunday School in 1881, moving from various tents and residences. It was an interesting arrangement, with Hall a Presbyterian, Slater a Congregationalist and Booker a Baptist.

THE FIRST BABIES

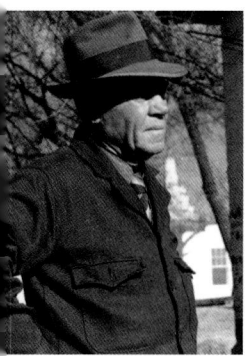
Robert Besser: born in Tulsa in 1883.

Obviously babies had been born in Indian Territory since its establishment. The first baby born in Tulsa after 1882 has been credited to John Carr and his wife. Their baby was born in January 1883 in a tent near an elm tree, not far from Dr. Booker. Carr was a carpenter working on the railroad in Tulsa and later in private construction. The couple named the child Ord, and the family moved about six or seven years later. However, for years, Dr. and Mrs. James T. Besser, who lived near the site, believed they had the first child born in the city, which was on April 18, 1883, with their son Robert. The first baby claim was also made by the family of Joe Patrick, who eventually settled in Keystone, and by another woman in Michigan.

INDIAN TERRITORY MEDICAL ASSOCIATION

Before statehood in 1907, two medical associations were created for the Indian and Oklahoma territories. Tulsa fell within the jurisdiction of Indian Territory and based its association activities in Muskogee. Dr. Fred S. Clinton, a noted early physician in Tulsa, was part of the Indian Territory Medical Association and preserved most of the historical records on the founding of the city's medical profession.

"Many pioneer physicians and surgeons in the Indian Territory were well-qualified, professional, and endowed with good nature, courage, intelligence, industry and humanity. Without benefit of roads, bridges, automobiles or comfortable means of transportation, hospitals, electric or gas lights, laboratories, trained nurses, and at times with no shelter for their patients, they carried on, rendering a fine, constructive service by providing or securing relief. These conscientious and understanding physicians came to this new world determined to develop it and perform their part as God-fearing, home-loving, patriotic citizens," — Dr. Fred Clinton.

The organization formed on April 18, 1881, in Muskogee, with Dr. Benjamin F. Fortner of Claremore elected president. The following year, Dr. Fortner moved to Fayetteville, Arkansas, to

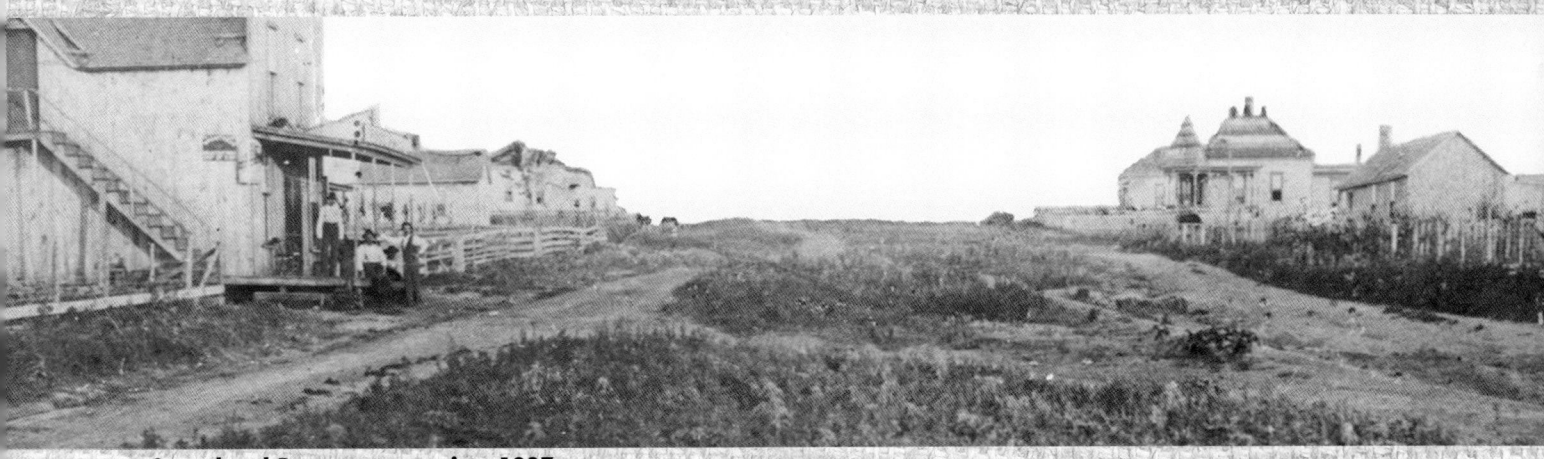
Second and Boston streets circa 1897.

practice for two years before relocating to Vinita. During his absence, the association was inactive. It was revived by Dr. Fortner in either 1888 or 1889 with 23 members.

When the group met on Dec. 8, 1891, the program discussed malarial fever and "ovarian hyperaemia and haemorrhage." McAlester's Dr. H.B. Smith spoke of "a few errors of country surgeons," and the group accepted papers contributed by request on obscure abdominal abscesses, pleurisy with effusion, abscess of the middle ear and peritonitis after the amputation of a thigh.

The association also sought legislation, such as agreeing on Dec. 4, 1900, to secure congressional approval to establish "some modern methods of caring for the insane and feeble-minded and for dealing with tuberculosis." That same year, a committee was sent to advocate for an "insane asylum" to be built in Indian Territory and to establish a system of public records. The following year, the association adopted reforms aligning itself with the American Medical Association guidelines. Dr. Clinton made that proposal and wrote this about the moment:

"This is an opportunity to pay homage to a few of the rugged pioneers who blazed the trail in this new empire of first impressions. These sturdy men of medicine, braved all inclement weather over bad roads, or lonesome trails, day or night, to personally examine and minister to their patients. They had no thought for their individual convenience, comfort or fear of exposure or fatigue when called to render professional service to one in need. These men were leaders. They had training, improvement, and refinement of mind, morals, and taste. This enlightenment could be and usually was a blessing and friendly helper in whatever community one of these distinguished doctors resided." — Dr. Fred Clinton.

Associations Merge

The Indian Territory Medical Association elected Dr. Eliphalet Nott Wright as its president at the annual meeting on June 7, 1904. He was a member of the Choctaw Nation and a well-known physician practicing near Atoka. The following year, Dr. Wright acknowledged the impending establishment of statehood and encouraged a cordial consolidation of the two medical associations. In a speech,

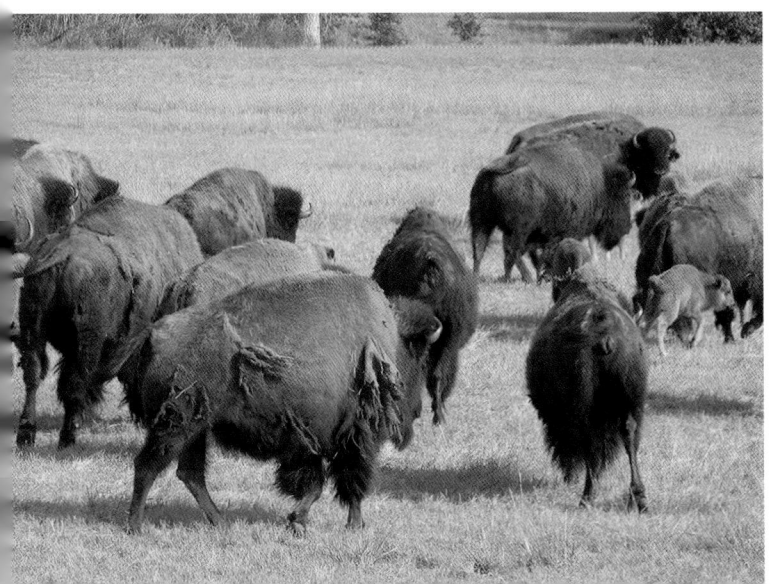
Oklahoma Bison.

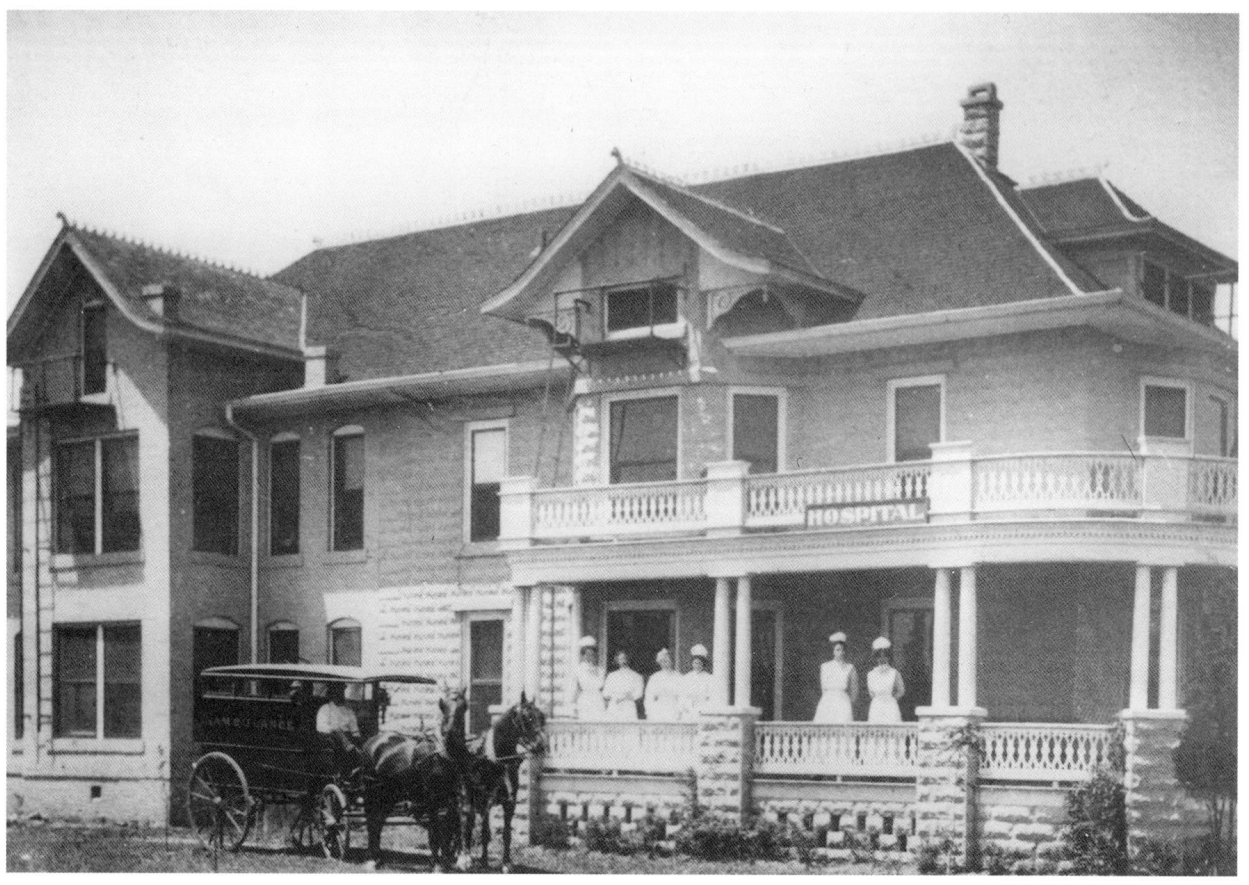

Tulsa Hospital: Tulsa's first hospital.

he criticized the laws regarding the practice of medicine in both territories and stressed finding lawmakers willing to strengthen standards for practitioners.

"As laws of both territories are inadequate, it will be well to take time by the forelock and draw up such laws as will be required for the new state, and urge the election of such legislators as will favor such laws, regardless of political party." — Dr. Eliphalet Nott Wright.

The groups met in May 1906 to form the Oklahoma State Medical Association. The officers of the newly formed professional organization were a mix of leaders from the former associations. Dr. Fortner was elected president, and Dr. Clinton was one of the first delegates to the AMA. This move made Dr. Clinton the AMA's last delegate from Indian Territory and the first from the Oklahoma State Medical Association.

An editorial in the *Oklahoma Medical News-Journal* in June 1906 complimented the union: "Oklahoma and Indian Territory are to be congratulated upon the harmonious and successful amalgamation of the two societies in to one compact and powerful association, which was accomplished at the last meeting of the two societies in Oklahoma City. In accordance with the law of evolution, which is but another name for progress, the general tendency has always been from the simple to the complex, from individualism to association, and from the smaller unit to the larger.

"When we work in harmony with this idea, we align ourselves with the forces of nature and success is sure to be the outcome... There is no doubt that the recent meeting was one of the most important, if

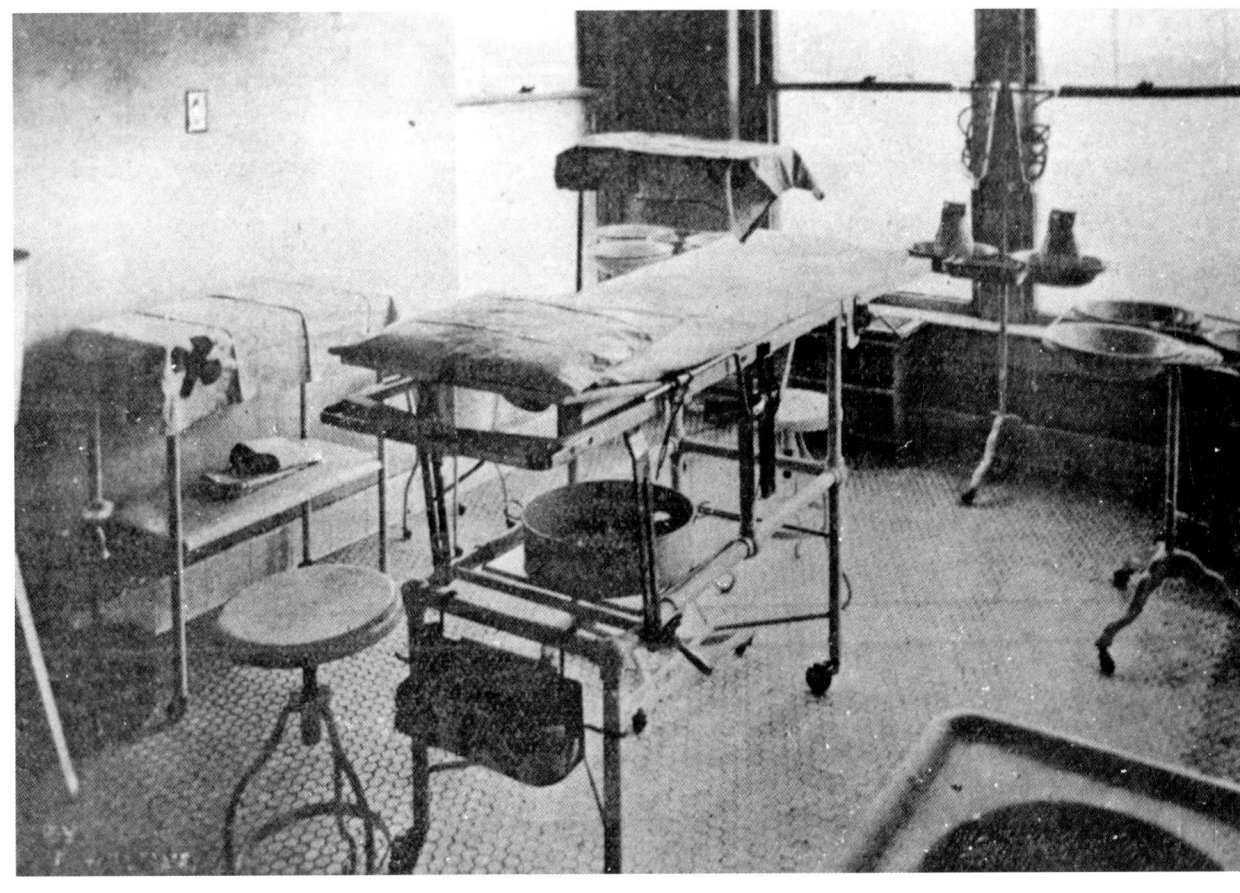

Operating Room: Tulsa Hospital.

not the most important, that has ever been held in these two territories. It has marked an epoch in the history of medicine in the new state that is to be."

THE APPLE ORCHARD HOSPITAL

In 1900, a smallpox epidemic raged in the Tulsa section of Indian Territory, no hospitals were available for treatment and few homes were large enough to isolate a patient from other family members. Dr. Clinton organized the first hospital to segregate people with contagious diseases from the population. The building was a six-room cottage in an apple orchard near Greenwood and Archer avenue.

Membership of the hospital's organization was by invitation, stressing immunization to smallpox as a requirement. Businessman Sam P. McBirney handled the finances, and Jenks Ramsey, who was an African American, managed the building and kitchen. The first patient was Erick Albert, who recovered from smallpox to later enter the oil business in Texas.

FIRST INCORPORATED HOSPITAL

The hospital was discontinued in 1901, but Dr. Clinton persisted in finding a permanent hospital. In a memoir about this venture, he wrote about the process:

"The general practice of medicine and surgery without benefit of hospital and nurses became more wearisome as the number of patients increased and the scope of service extended," —Dr. Fred Clinton.

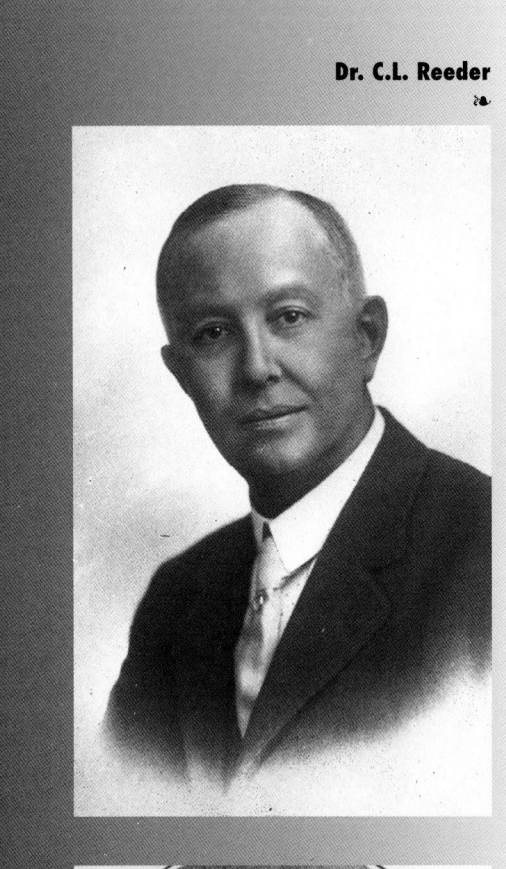

Dr. C.L. Reeder

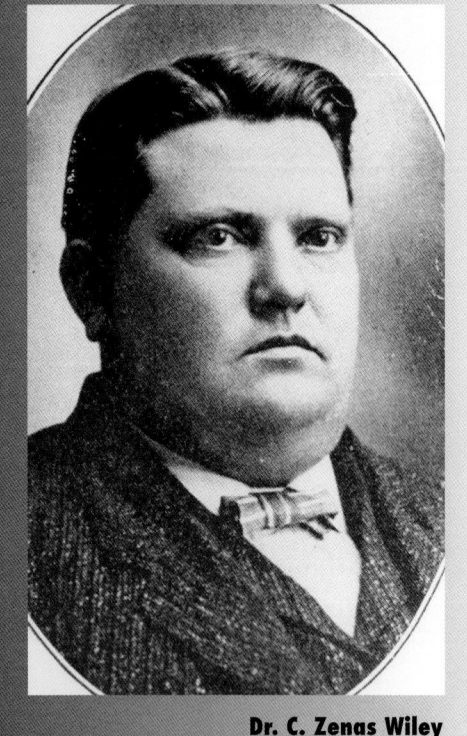

Dr. C. Zenas Wiley

In November 1906, Dr. Clinton invited Dr. C.L. Reeder and Dr. C. Zenas Wiley to his office in the First National Bank Building and presented them with a hospital proposal. Before leaving that afternoon, articles of agreement were signed to establish the Tulsa Hospital Association. The charter was issued by Perry Freeman, clerk of the U.S. Court of Appeals in Indian Territory in South McAlester.

While incorporated as a hospital and training school for nurses, the group still needed funding for a facility.

"Since the health of a people is the greatest resource and wealth of a nation, the challenge to provide means and facilities to preserve this natural capital advantage is the responsibility of every progressive and forward-looking person to develop the proficiency in this field and make it available to all the sick. It is important to realize that the hospital is a cross section of the community, and a medical and surgical clearing house where the doctor may obtain his proper rating, when high standards are maintained." — Dr. Fred Clinton.

An unfinished 10-room residence located at west Fifth Street and Lawton Avenue owned by R.S. and Ora Waddell was purchased for $5,000 on Nov. 20, 1906. There were no sidewalks, pavement, electricity, sewer or streetcars. While the construction was ongoing, a temporary location was established on north Cheyenne Street. The interim location may have been better accommodations but it lacked a water supply. Dr. Clinton, as president of the association, was tasked with pumping water by hand from a nearby well to an attic storage tank. Typhoid fever cases required a great deal of water, and residents were drinking bottled water for safety. By January 1907, the association moved into a section of the new hospital and hired Henrietta C.C. Ziegler as its superintendent.

First Nurses

Indian Territory had few educated physicians and possibly fewer trained nurses. This lack of professional staff led to the Tulsa Hospital's other mission — a school for nurses. Superintendent Ziegler oversaw the direction of the curriculum, which focused on practical nursing through lectures and experience. A register was created of the graduates to help physicians acquire medically educated nurses.

The first class of graduates in 1907 consisted of students with some training elsewhere but finished their education in Tulsa. They were Kate B. Scott, Etta McAllister, Sallie Birnie and Irene Richards.

Scott became an active member in professional organizations, attending the first meeting of the Oklahoma State Nurses Association in 1908 in Guthrie. She attended national nursing conventions as a delegate, served as president of the state association, recruited nurses for the National Red Cross and became superintendent of nurses for the Tulsa Hospital in 1920. McAllister worked in several areas of nursing in private practice including operating room supervisor, anesthetist and surgical assistant. It is unknown what became of Birnie and Richards. ■

Calamities and Casualties

The emerging city full of manufacturing, railroad and oil workers brought major accidents, according to Dr. Clinton's memoirs. Some cases he recorded came from other medical practices. Those include:

■ A 22-year-old Deputy U.S. Marshal was shot twice in the abdomen while making an arrest in May 1904. The bullets from a 45-caliber revolver pierced the intestines. Surgery took place under a gasoline light in a room at the Alcorn Hotel. The man recovered.

■ A 17-year-old housekeeper was shot twice by a jealous lover with a revolver in November 1904. Bullets passed through her arm into her small intestine. Two doctors performed surgery in the woman's tent, which was by the Arkansas River, with a dirt floor. Drs. S.G. Kennedy and L.A. O'Brien provided much of the equipment used. They had light through the tent flap, heat from a small stove and chloroform for anesthesia. The patient survived.

■ A farmer had a knife wound to the back of his hand with muscles and tendons supplying use to four fingers slashed to nearly severed. He had been trying to staunch the bleeding for 24 hours with chewed tobacco, soot and spider webs. Dr. Clinton was called as a specialist and used an anesthesia while he reconstructed the hand through cleansing, suturing, splinting and dressing. The hand was saved.

■ On July 4, 1912, a train wreck near a Sand Springs park killed three people and injured 48. All were brought to the Tulsa Hospital for treatment. Philanthropist Charles Page was moved by the event and stated: "I am sorry because of this unpredictable tragedy, and I will assume and pay all necessary expenses."

■ A tornado in 1912 at Bigheart transported a train full of injured people to the Tulsa Hospital. The physicians worked on patients in an emergency capacity for 24 hours.

■ It is not necessary to multiply the reports of cases to justify the need for a good hospital service to care for ill or injured," Dr. Clinton wrote.

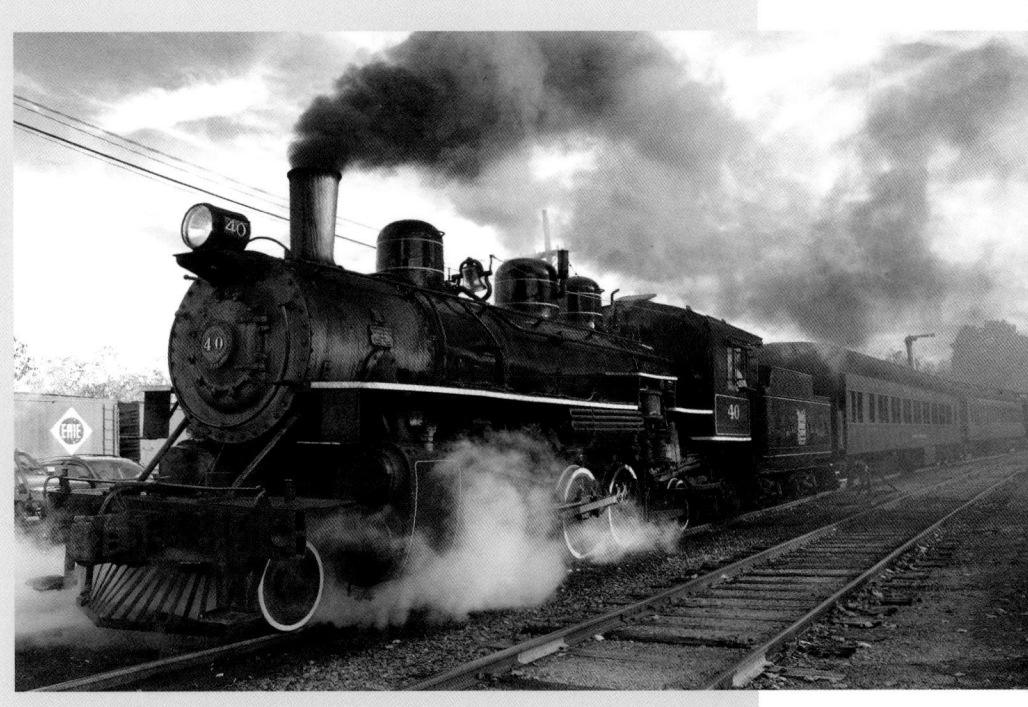

Steam locomotion: In the height of rail travel, up to 36 passenger trains a day visited Tulsa.

Dr. Fred Severs Clinton and Jane (Heard) Clinton

Among the earliest founders and physicians, Dr. Fred Clinton stands out as an entrepreneur, businessman and prolific author of the city's history. He documented some of the most-cited works on the establishment of Tulsa and medical practices from before statehood through the 1940s. He served as the only delegate to the American Medical Association representing both the Indian Territory and state of Oklahoma, co-established the first Tulsa hospital and other medical systems. His wife, Jane (Heard) Clinton, was so influential, she was called "a pioneer in building the soul of the city," at her funeral.

Dr. Clinton was born in April 1874 near Okmulgee in the Creek Nation of Indian Territory to Charles and Louise (Atkins) Clinton. His father was among the first white settlers into the territory, where he married an educated woman, who was a member of the Creek Nation. Charles Clinton shaped the cattle industry in the territory and became an early advocate in the mineral resources and wealth within the Creek lands. They sent their son to the top schools within the Creek Nation before continuing his education at the St. Francis Institute at Osage and then Drury College in Springfield, Missouri. Charles Clinton died in 1888 and Louise Clinton died in 1920.

Clinton's path to the medical field started at the Gem City Business College in Quincy, Illinois, Young Harris College of Georgia and in the Kansas City College of Pharmacy, where he graduated with honors in 1896. While pursuing his pharmaceutical credential, he was also studying at the University Medical College of Kansas City, graduating in 1897. After receiving his medical degree, he returned home and established a practice in Red Fork. Soon, he moved and planted roots in Tulsa. During this time, he rose as a prominent member of the Indian Territory Medical Association, pushing for high medical standards and ongoing professional development. In the territorial medical association, Dr. Clinton served in every elected office and represented Indian Territory at the national conference in 1906 in Boston. After Oklahoma was admitted to the union and the medical associations merged into one, Dr. Clinton represented the state organization at a national conference in 1908 in Washington, D.C.

In 1900, Dr. Clinton organized a hospital in a six-room cottage in Tulsa near Greenwood Avenue and Archer Street primarily for smallpox patients. Recognizing the need for a larger facility and training program for nurses, Dr. Clinton organized the Tulsa Hospital Association and served as its first president in 1906. The association oversaw the Tulsa Hospital located at the west end of Fifth Street. He didn't stop there. In 1915, he organized the Oklahoma Hospital, the city's first fire-proof medical facility, and served as president and chief surgeon. In 1919, he created and served as president of the Council of Hospitals in Tulsa and the Oklahoma State Hospital Association. Also, he worked as the chief surgeon for the Sand Springs railroad, Tulsa railway, Sapulpa and Oil Fields railroad. He was a surgeon for about four other rail systems as well and was a member of the American Association of Railway Surgeons.

He served as a surgeon or medical officer for various accident and insurance companies and had a hand in starting the Oklahoma branch of the American Red Cross.

Finance, energy and community service were other interests. He co-founded the Clinton Investment Company, which erected an eight-story building. Dr. Clinton went into partnership with Dr. J.C.W. Bland in completing the first oil well near Red Fork. This effort is credited for bringing other investments into Oklahoma leading to an oil boom.

"They successfully promoted the drilling of the first well in the Tulsa district and this attracted to the field eventually some of the most experienced oil men from the older fields and resulted in the opening of what is probably the greatest oil-producing territory in the world. The remarkable development of these natural resources, including the operations of the Glenn Pool, maybe said to have originated with the work of those doctors. Dr. Clinton is one of the leaders among the men of enterprise and initiative and constructive ability who have made Tulsa one of the most important centers of the oil and gas industry in the United States. There are few men who have more wisely improved their opportunities or more fully met their obligations in citizenship and all relations to their fellowmen." – writer C.B. Douglass, 1921.

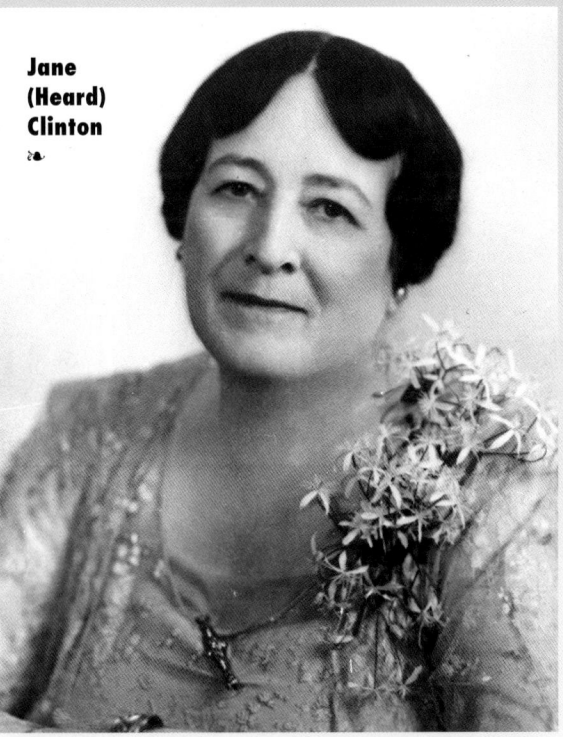

Jane (Heard) Clinton

Dr. Clinton is the author of several pieces about the early days including "First Hospitals in Tulsa" and "Tulsa, Oklahoma."

Equally influential was Dr. Clinton's wife, Jane Heard, whom he married in 1897 in Elberton, Georgia. Heard was the daughter of James Lawrence Heard, who was an infantry colonel in the Confederate Army and member of the Georgia legislature. Her mother had been one of the first graduates of Wesleyan Female College at Macon, Georgia. The couple raised their daughter to be a patron of the arts, becoming a talented pianist. She graduated with honors from the Elberton Collegiate Institute and was socially popular, traveling among elite groups in Washington, D.C. and St. Louis. In 1897, her photo was published in the magazine *Munsey's Magazine*, portraying

Continued on following page

15

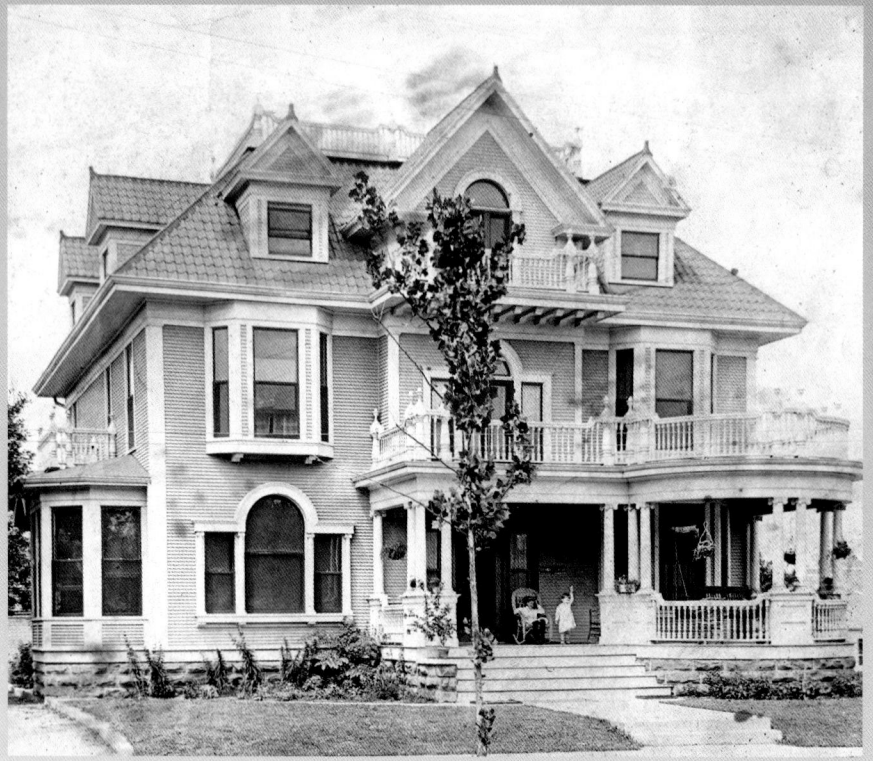

The Clintons' residence on the southwest corner of West 5th Street and South Cheyenne Avenue.

her as a "Southern woman of personal charm and outstanding musical ability."

The couple were members of the Methodist Episcopal Church South. Dr. Clinton served on three consecutive capital campaigns as the congregation grew. It eventually became Boston Avenue United Methodist Church. Jane Clinton secured the first pipe organ for the church and volunteered as organist. For years, she taught young girls in a Sunday school class known as the "Clintonian Class." In 1907, she and other women founded a mission to support international projects, which became known as the Women's Society of Christian Service. She served as president for many years and hosted meetings in her home.

Jane Clinton was a known hostess in early Tulsa, holding dinners and parties at the couple's home often welcoming newcomers. Their home at the corner of Fifth Street and Cheyenne Avenue was considered a showcase.

Her list as a founder, member and supporter of civic organizations is extensive and includes being a charter member of the Tulsa Art Association, Tulsa Garden Club, Children's Day Nursery, Parent-Teacher Association, Philbrook Art Center and Tulsa Civic Music Association. Her greatest accomplishment was likely the Hyechka Club. It was founded with 10 other musicians in 1904. The name is the Creek word for "music" and has a mission to promote music throughout the community. Jane Clinton was president for 17 years and then made president for life. The Hyechka Club is credited for bringing national performers to the budding city, which led to a dedication to the arts and construction of the Convention Hall. It was such a force that when Louisiana, Arkansas, Missouri and Oklahoma formed a district of the National Federation of Music Clubs, it adopted the name "Hyechka District."

"For while she was great as an individual, she was greatest of all as a wife. She and her husband complemented each other so perfectly that any estimate of one without the other is a mere fragment. When she left her sheltered Georgia home to join the young Indian Territory doctor in shaping the swirling tides of frontier society, she gave herself with naturalness and simplicity to her new environment. And where except in Oklahoma of the past half century could two joined lives yield such dividends of creative achievement." — Historian Angie Debo.

Dr. Fred Clinton died at age 81 on April 25, 1955, and Jane Clinton died at age 70 on Nov. 8, 1945.

CHAPTER 2
(1910 - 1919)

Building a Foundation

Mary Penn No. 1:
One of many gushers during Tulsa's oil boom.

The Booming City

By 1910, Tulsa's population was not slowing down, having grown from 1,390 to 25,240 in just a decade. The surge of the oil industry would continue to attract residents and, with it, the need for trained physicians and medical facilities. The infrastructure was in its infancy. Much of the water supply was either from dug or bored wells, and some companies harnessed nearby mineral springs for bottled water. The sewage system ran about 14 miles with 17 miles in storm sewer drainage.

Oil and gas were at the start of a major boom, and Tulsa was the center of the Mid-Continent field. The area included the Glenn Pool, Bird Creek district, the Red Fork, Taneha and Sapulpa. The Mounds and Twin Hills districts were in the Creek Nation, but also part of the Tulsa area. These fields contained between 2,500 to 3,000 oil wells and 100 gas wells. The crude oil well produced about 90,000 barrels a day, which was about half of the Mid-Continent field's yield.

With World War I came a surge in demand for petroleum products as industries changed from coal-based energy to oil. Up to 20 percent of the oil that powered the Allied armies passed through Tulsa's pipeline terminals, refineries and rail yards. About $36 million in building permits were issued from 1917 to 1921, including Central High School, the Exchange National Bank, City Hall and the Atlas Life Building.

Neighborhoods were established north along the Arkansas River away from the drilling fields. A bridge was built in 1904 for oil workers to travel and supplies and food to be transported to the city. Public schools were established in 1905, and the first school bond — $230,000 — was passed in 1904 to build more schools. By 1910, Tulsa had 10 public school buildings. Four major railways served the city: St. Louis and San Francisco; Atchison, Topeka and Santa Fe; Missouri, Kansas and Texas; and Midland Valley Railroad.

Birth of Public Health System

Dr. W.E. Wright served as the city's superintendent of health, who served as a clearinghouse in a system of data collection. Using his reports, city officials backed projects such as an incinerator plant,

Arkansas River Bridges, 1905: Toll bridge on right, built in 1903. Building is where toll collector lived. Far left is Frisco Railroad Bridge built in 1886.

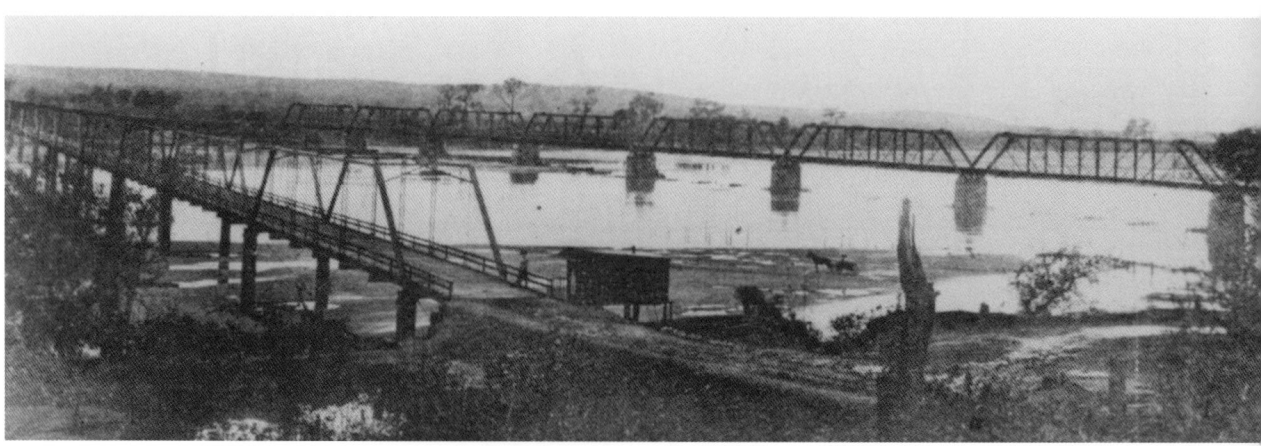

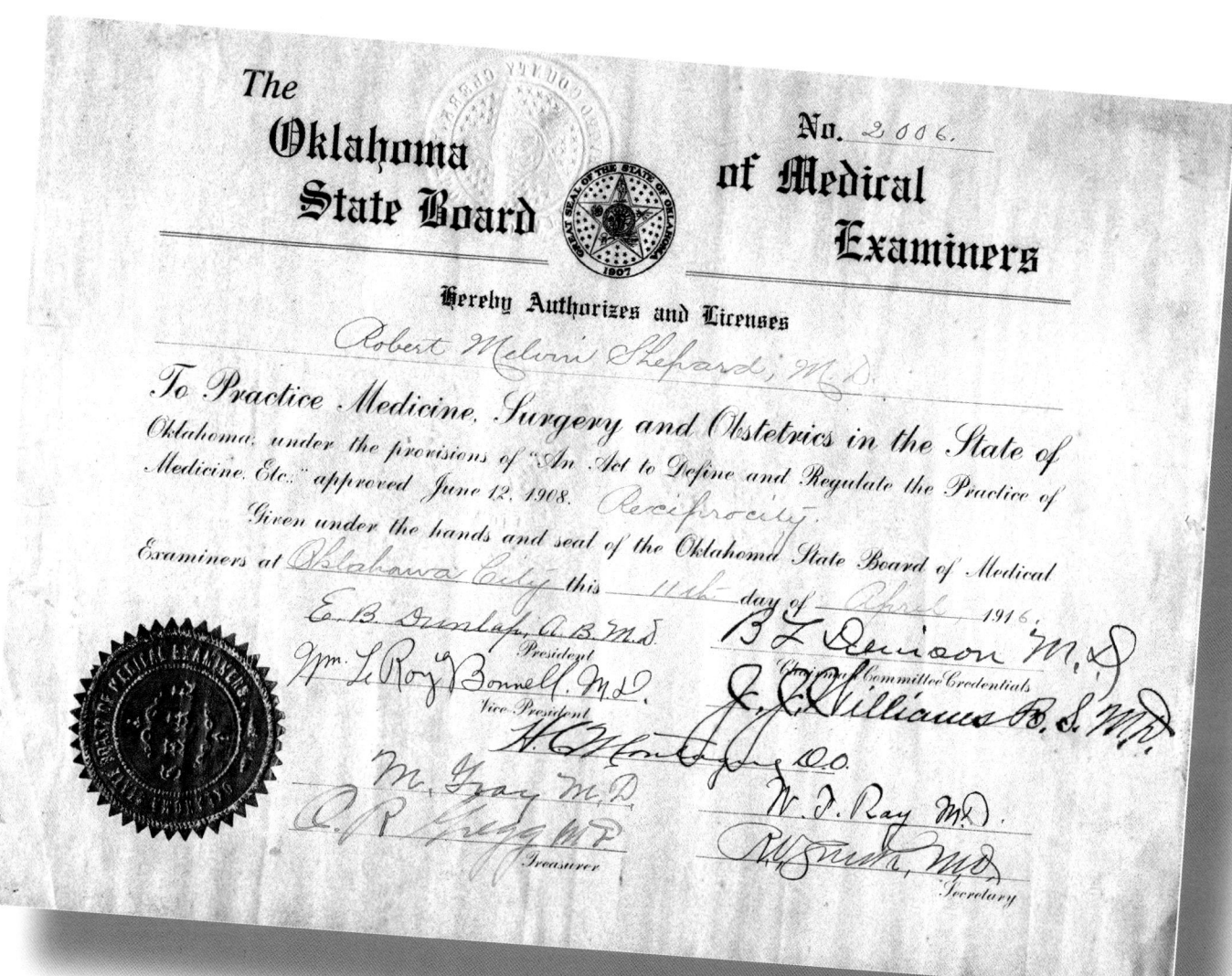

Certification #2006: Medical license from 1916.

which was considered the most modern method of garbage disposal. Tulsa's Department of Health had three divisions. The first collected reports on births, deaths and contagious diseases and helped in establishing protocols, such as quarantines and sanitary regulations. The second oversaw the inspection of bakeries, dairies, hotels, restaurants and other establishments where food was sold. It also inspected food stuffs and livestock shipped to the city. The third division provided for the collection and disposal of garbage, trash, dead animals and surface waste.

The health department's work led to several systemic changes and improved sanitary conditions. The facility inspections of food handling operations led to consistent sterilization of utensils and properly constructed dairies and barns. Garbage collection was made daily by the city and required each household to have a covered can. In the previous two years, 68 cases of smallpox were handled in the "contagious hospital" with only two deaths reported.

"The building of a city such as Tulsa, though in the midst of a vast and resourceful empire, has not been free from struggle, but the threatening clouds that gathered about the human landscape have always parted at the right time, and through the rift has shone with resplendent glory, the sparkling stars of hope. Tulsa today, though full of magnificent achievement, is only prophetic of a greater des-

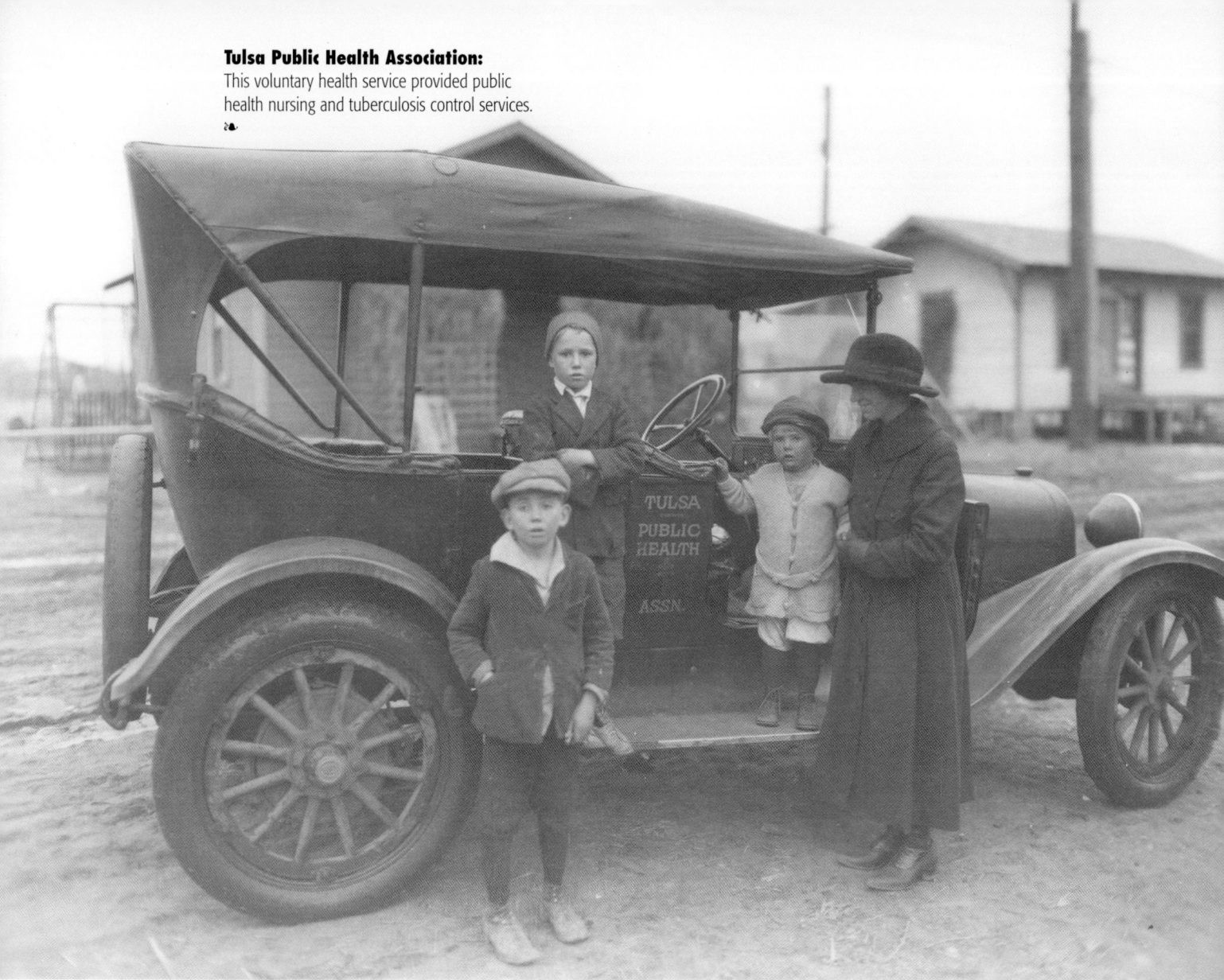

Tulsa Public Health Association:
This voluntary health service provided public health nursing and tuberculosis control services.

tiny. Over her homes now floats Old Glory, and a free people with local self-government, exultantly raise his emblem of progress so that the breezes of the North, South, East and West may kiss it and the sun of all the earth reflect it." — Dr. Fred Clinton, 1910.

When Dr. Clinton described the overall health of Tulsans, he said epidemics of acute diseases such as scarlet fever, diphtheria and typhoid fever "appear much milder" than in northern states. He attributed this to the 220 days of sunshine, ample rainfall, drainage system and improved sanitary conditions.

Modernizing Hospitals

Moving into the decade, the Tulsa Hospital remained the leading facility with a 40-bed capacity at the west end of Fifth Street, which served as the emergency room for the railroads. An advertisement in *The Journal of the Oklahoma State Medical Association* in 1910 stated the facility had "sunlight and air in every room, silent signal system, modernly planned and equipped." It retained an ambulance, which was a clapboard wagon pulled by two horses. Also, amenities included long-distance telephone and a location on the horse-drawn line. Dr. Clinton led the hospital as president until 1915. It closed soon after the Great War.

After its closing, Dr. Clinton turned his attention to building the Oklahoma Hospital at west Ninth Street and Jackson Street in the Riverview neighborhood. The war caused a shortage in construction materials, delaying the facility's opening until June 1916 with a 50-bed capacity. It was a brick building featuring a three-room surgery area, x-ray equipment and a first-floor laboratory. It overlooked the city but was within a 10-minute walk to the center of the business district. The modern facility was meant to encourage an integrated approach to care.

"The taking of case records on the dictaphone and finally placing them in the private record of the patient, encourages study, diagnosis, care and treatment of the patient." — Dr. Fred Clinton.

Nurses were housed on the fourth floor. The head of the nursing program, Mrs. Henrietta Ziegler, followed Dr. Clinton to establish a school of nursing at the hospital. She came to Tulsa after graduating from the University of Pennsylvania Training School for Nurses. She was considered a "gold medal pupil of her class" and had served as superintendent of the country branch of Rush Hospital in Malvern, Pennsylvania. Originally from the Netherlands, she spoke four languages and was considered a good musician.

Oklahoma Hospital: Tulsa's first fireproof hospital.

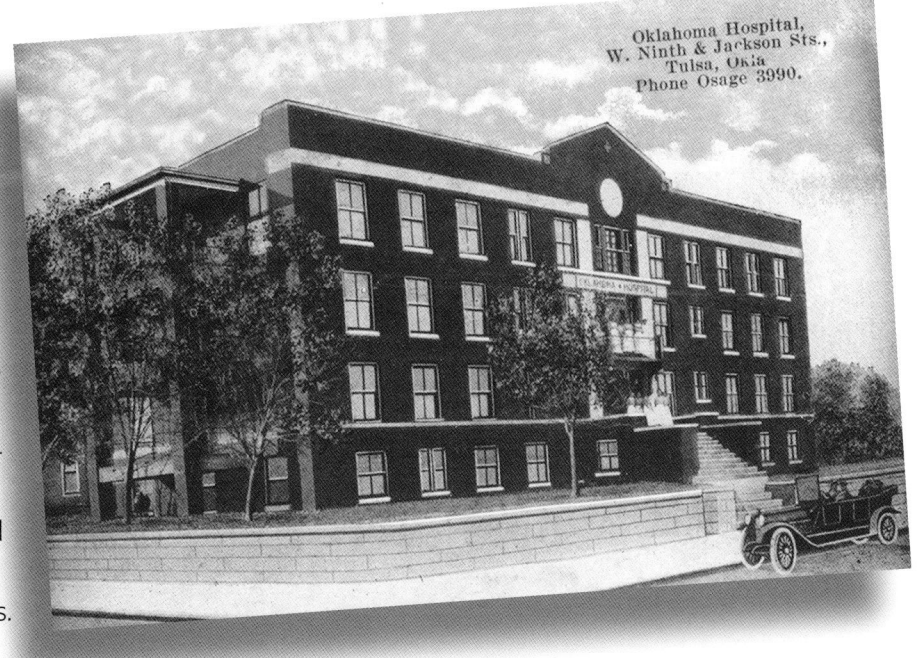

"During all those years when thousands of patients were cared for and the institution gradually grew and extended its usefulness, none deserves greater praise for self-sacrifice and eternal application through her never-ending duties than Miss Ziegler, the superintendent. This community will forever owe a debt of gratitude to her for the service rendered in aiding in this pioneer hospital work; in guiding it, through her intelligence, integrity and industry from the shoals of financial disaster." — Author Clarence Douglass.

GREAT INFLUENZA OUTBREAK OF 1918

A worldwide pandemic made its way into Tulsa, causing local officials to shut down nearly all public life and quarantine a significant amount of the population. Reports say the wave may have killed up to 30 million people internationally, with about 550,000 American deaths.

History refers to it as the "Spanish flu," but it originated in the United States. The first case was reported on March 4, 1918, near Fort Riley, Kansas. An Army cook reported having a headache, sore throat, fever and pain in the muscles and joints. U.S. service members carried the disease on troop ships to Europe, where World War I was still being fought.

Continued on page 23

Dr. Ross Grosshart

After spending his youth as a manual laborer, Dr. Ross Grosshart eventually went back to school and became a prominent surgeon in Tulsa by 1920. He was born in Papinsville, Missouri, to Dr. Joel Emory and Anna Grosshart. His father died just four years after finishing medical school. Dr. Grosshart was 1 when his father passed and spent much of his childhood on a stepfather's farm. He went to school until age 13, when he then began working as a coal miner and later as a "cowpuncher" in Dodge City, Kansas. He made his way to New Mexico and eventually Indian Territory, working as a farmer for a few years.

Dr. Grosshart returned to Missouri to complete his education. After graduating from the Normal School at Chillicothe, Missouri, he went to the Kansas City Medical College. He worked as a nurse and administered anesthetics to pay for medical school. After obtaining his degree in 1899, he practiced in Rockville, Missouri, for five years. Then, he entered a post-graduate program in the New York Post Graduate Medical School to specialize in surgery. On June 11, 1905, Dr. Grosshart moved to Tulsa to open a practice. He established the Grosshart Sanitarium, which merged with the Physicians and Surgeons Hospital. He stayed on staff as a surgeon.

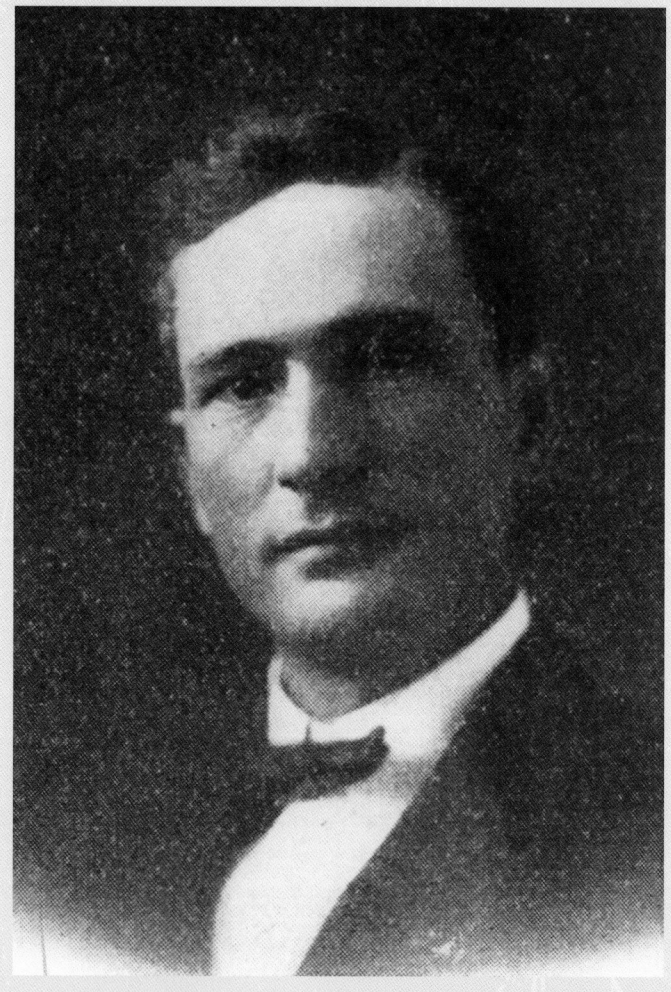

Farming never left Dr. Grosshart's life. He maintained a ranch near Alsuma and is considered among the first in the country to import full-blooded Holstein cattle to create a herd. His ranch was known to have the most modern agricultural tools to apply new research. He was married to Emma Staley, and they had four children. Dr. Grosshart was known as an outdoorsman, a lover of dogs, fishing and hunting. He was president of the Tulsa County Medical Society in 1913 and was affiliated with the state and national medical associations as well. Like many professional men of the time, he was a member of fraternal organizations such as the Elks Lodge, Mason and Akdar Temple of the Mystic Shrine.

"The experiences of his early life were varied and there were many hardships to be overcome or endured, but with resolute spirit Dr. Grosshart has worked his way upward, actuated at all times by a laudable ambition and what he has accomplished indicates the force of his character and his ready adaptability," said writer Clarence Douglass.

Before the pandemic, physicians and scientists believed the flu was caused by bacteria, not a virus. As autopsies were conducted on victims, the theory was attacked after not finding bacillus. Because of limited understanding of the cause, treatments were often ineffective. Popular were patent medicines, which were trademarked with secret ingredients. These included Vicks Vap-Rub and atropine (belladonna) capsules. Prevention became the prevailing method of containing the influenza.

In Oklahoma, about 7,350 people died of influenza and related illnesses between Oct. 1, 1918, and April 1, 1919. In October alone, 200 Tulsans died, according to a story in the *Tulsa Democrat*. During this outbreak, doctors were required to report all cases so patients could be quarantined. This was usually a sign on the front door and a fumigation of the home by the health department.

"The influenza seemed to be no respecter of persons, some of the most important and best known citizens of Tulsa, as well as those in moderate circumstances being numbered among the victims." — *Tulsa Spirit*, November 1918.

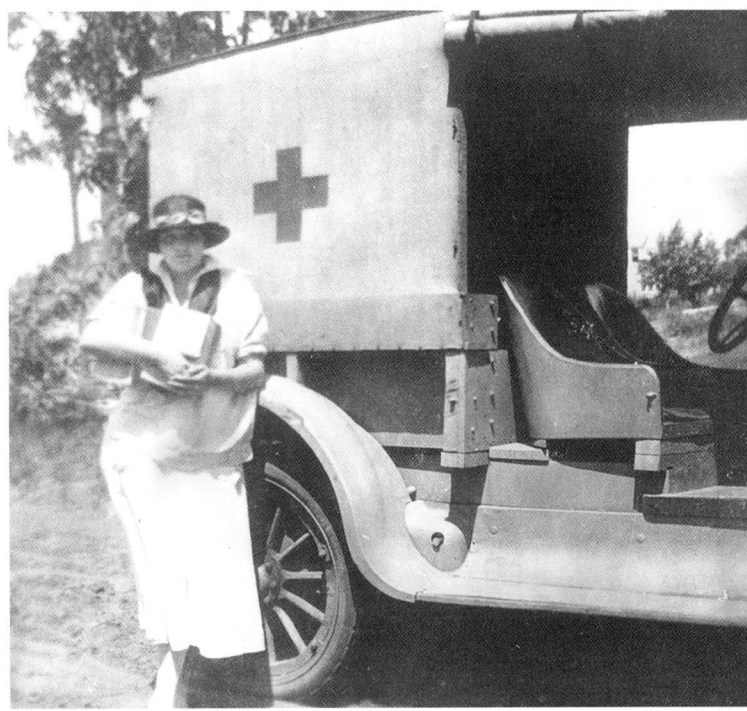

Red Cross aid worker, 1918: Red Cross recruited a total of 15,000 nurses to combat the Great Influenza Outbreak of 1918.

On Oct. 7, 1918, an emergency meeting of the Red Cross was held to determine how best to contain the virus. The next day, Mayor Charles Hubbard ordered all public meetings closed and shuttered nearly all public establishments — schools, courts, churches, draft boards, movie theaters, soda foundations, bowling alleys and pool halls. Restaurants could remain open if the facilities were fumigated from midnight to 5 a.m. Building owners were asked to daily disinfect stairs, hallways and elevators. City streets were washed twice daily and treated with formaldehyde.

Funeral homes were ordered to make ambulances available for city use, and nurses were to be transported by vehicles from car dealerships, taxi companies and private citizens.

A Red Cross emergency hospital for flu patients was converted from a detention center for women at First Street and Elgin Avenue. The facility was fumigated for 18 hours with formaldehyde, which was a popular disinfectant of the time. Jail officials burned old bedding, whitewashed walls and put in 60 sanitized cots. Mrs. Dolly Brown served as the nursing supervisor. After the epidemic subsided, money was raised to expand the hospital, which was established at 512 N. Boulder Ave. by Brown and called Morningside Hospital. Mrs. Brown later married M.J. McNulty and built a larger hospital in the mid-20s that eventually became Hillcrest Medical Center.

Dr. Clinton was named the medical director of the emergency operation. The position charged him with obtaining better medical equipment and recruiting physicians, nurses and "all patriotic people of any aptitude for caring for the sick or performing relief work, menial or otherwise, that would release a trained person for technical service to the sick," he wrote.

Strict enforcement of municipal laws on individual behavior was observed, such as an existing law banning spitting on sidewalks. A "move on" ordinance was passed to ban people from stopping on the public thoroughfares in crowds. Sneezing and coughing without using a handkerchief were forbidden, with violators subject to heavy fines and imprisonment.

By mid-October, the city was running out of caskets. A *Tulsa World* story described how 16-year-old Henry Ash built a casket for his 3-year-old sister who died of the flu.

"No county don't have to bury my sister," he said.

Another sad story featured an 18-month-old infant who was orphaned after its mother died of influenza not long after the father was killed while fighting in France. Neighbors did not know of any other family members. An October 1918 *Tulsa World* story reported hospital workers trying to locate the toddler's relatives.

First negro hospital: Frissell Memorial Hospital was burned down during the Race Riots.

Teacher Myrta E. Maxwell, then an educator at Sequoyah Elementary, wrote a letter in January 1944 to Dr. Clinton recalling the role school officials played. The city was divided into districts, and healthy teachers would check homes daily to report any new cases, status of sick people and needed supplies. One morning stood out in her memory:

"On that particular morning, there were seven deaths in my district, and after sending in this report, I found a nurse... alone in her room in a critical condition with no one to do a thing for her. I did what little I could but was unable to get her any real help until late that evening when I saw Dr. Roy Wiley about to turn in at the driveway of his home. I called him and stated the situation to him. Immediately, he went to her bedside and saw to it that she was properly cared for until the last. Death claimed her before dawn." — Myrta E. Maxwell, January 1944.

IN THE GREENWOOD DISTRICT

In 1918, Mayor Hubbard organized the Frissell Memorial Hospital at 314 E. Brady St., devoted to caring for black residents. The superintendent was nurse Elizabeth Smith, and the physicians and staff were African American. It was located near a bustling business district of black owners in the Greenwood neighborhood, known as "Black Wall Street." The move to create the hospital earned political points with one of the city's two newspapers operated by an African-American publisher.

The *Tulsa Star*, owned by A.J. Smitherman, ran an editorial predicting the re-election of Hubbard and the incumbent city commissioners. The piece praised the mayor for his gift.

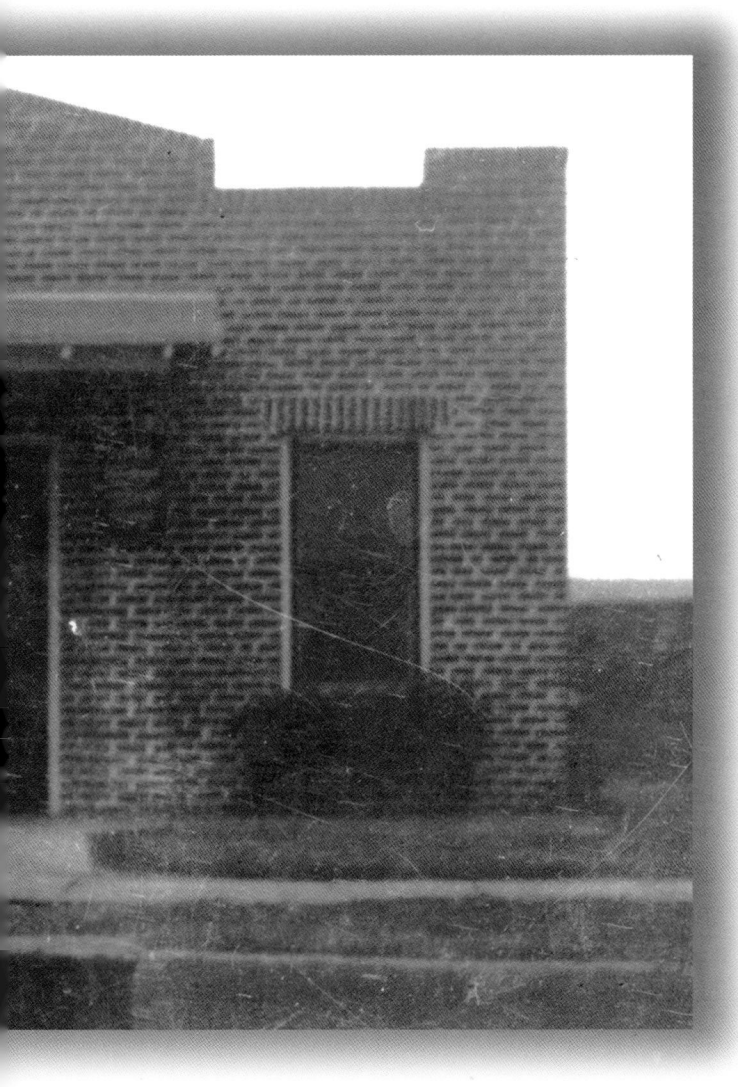

"Thrice blessed are Tulsans, to have such a place as the Frissell Hospital and its efficient and sympathetic corps of nurses... It is a gift that few areas in our country have bestowed upon our People, and it is one that everyone, male and female, should not fail to appreciate."
— *Tulsa Star*, April 1920.

OTHER HOSPITALS

In 1910, four physicians — Drs. G.H. Butler, S.D. Hawley, W.Q. Conway and R.S. Wagner — organized the Physicians and Surgeons Hospital on Carson Avenue and 13th Street in a two-story building. Dr. Butler served as chief surgeon until 1917. Then, he retired from practice to his "Peace Valley Farm" in LeFlore County. The hospital grew from 10 to 30 beds before it was sold to Mayor Hubbard, A.M. Welch, Cyrus S. Avery and J.T. Forster. It was then renamed the Municipal Hospital. In 1929, it was sold to Mrs. F.H. Atwood, who changed the name back to the original.

Sunny Side Hospital opened in 1914 on Duluth Street by graduate nurse Florence Rouleau. Her sisters later joined in the incorporation — Victoria Rouleau as a nurse and Rose Rouleau as the business manager. It was moved to a location at 512 N. Boulder Ave. in a brick building. It operated from 1916 to 1917 until it was sold to Mrs. Dolly Brown when she founded Morningside Hospital after the influenza epidemic passed.

The Grosshart Sanitorium was operating in 1909 after being established by Dr. Ross Grosshart. It merged with the Physicians and Surgeons Hospital by 1921. Located at the corner of Cheyenne and Golden Streets on a high point, the 12-bed facility was described as "commanding a most beautiful surrounding country, an ideal place in which to gain health and enjoy convalescence." ∎

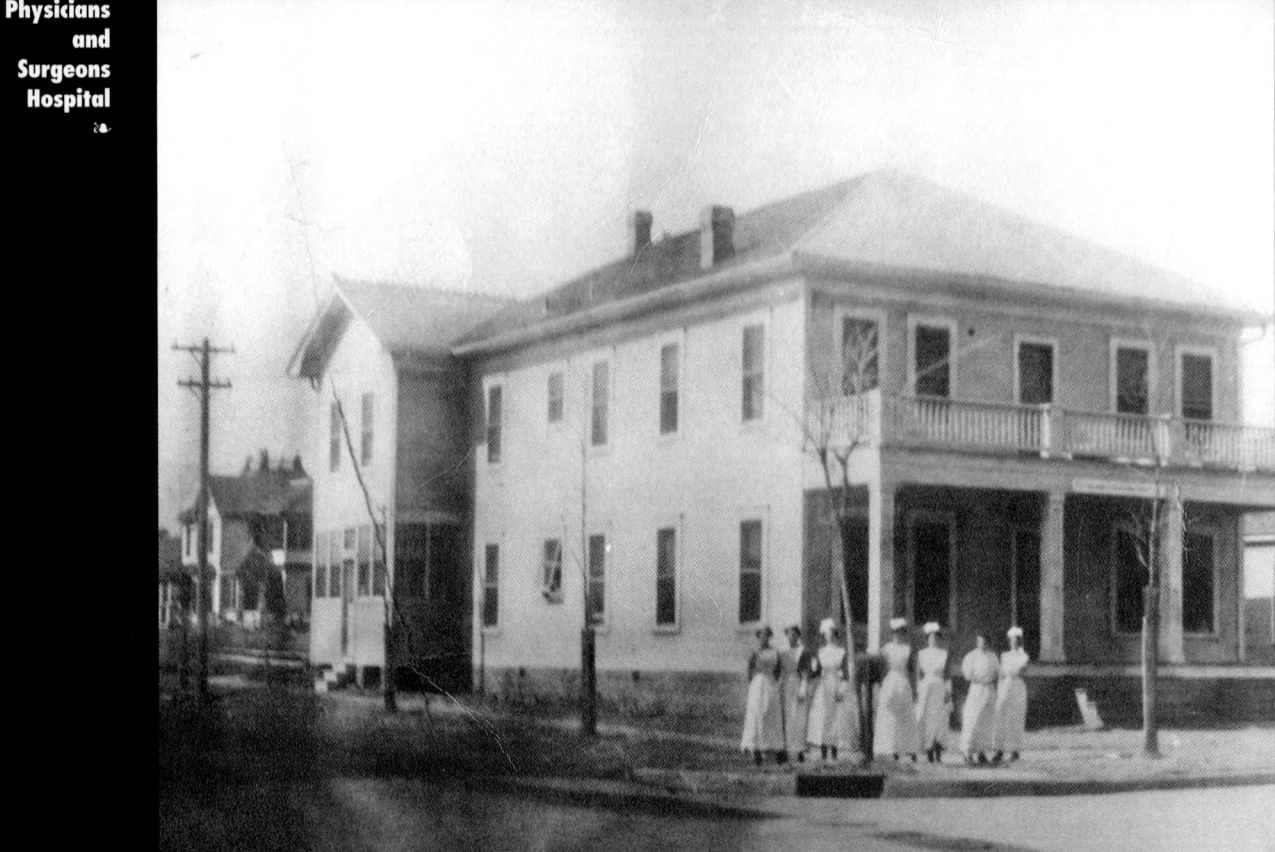

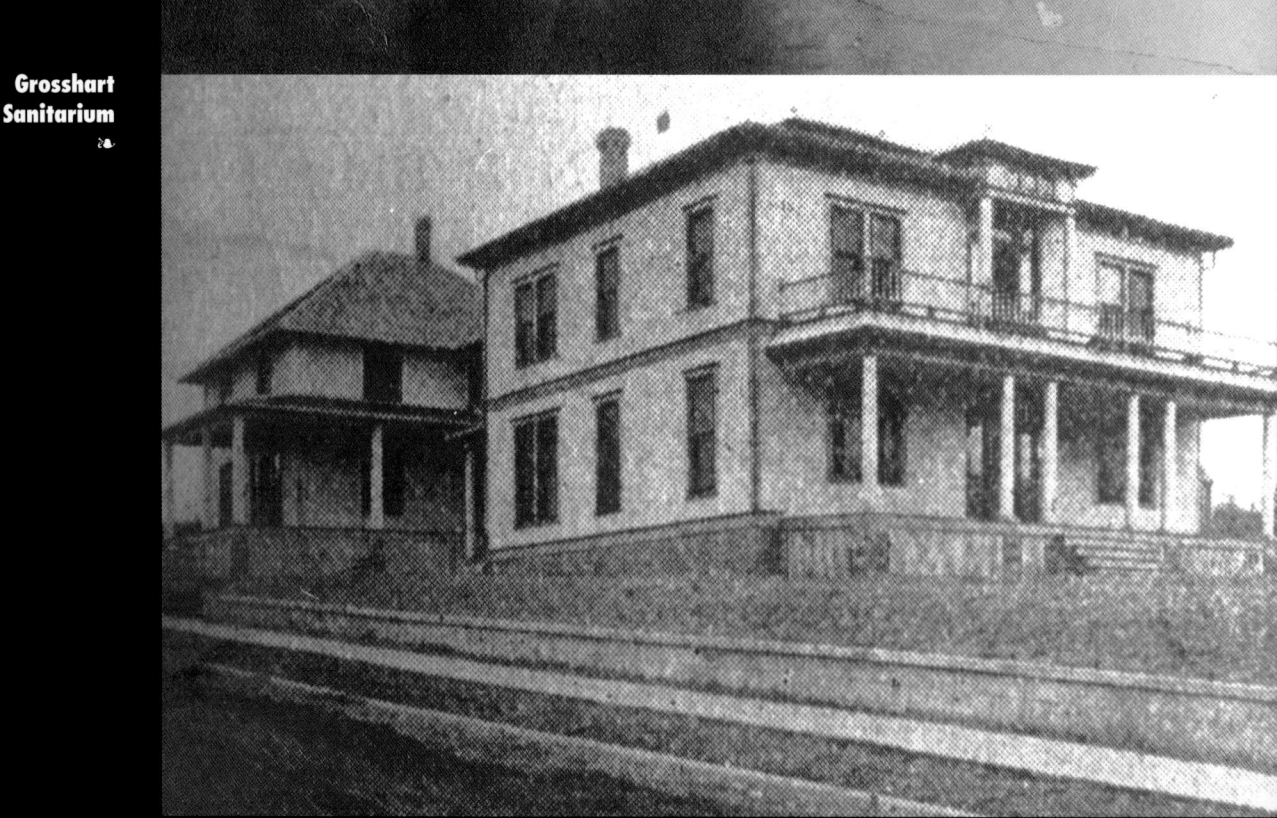

Physicians
and
Surgeons
Hospital

Grosshart
Sanitarium

CHAPTER 3
(1920 - 1929)

Bustling City

Osteopathic Hospital Nurses:
Standing on the steps of the hospital.

The 20s were a bustling time for Tulsa, which had earned the "Oil Capital of the World" title. With the Mid-Continent oilfields surrounding the city, it had evolved into the financial, manufacturing and transportation hub for petroleum. Industries were changing from coal-based energy into oil powered machinery. The population swelled to about 72,000 residents in the city and 110,000 people living in the county. It was the most densely populated and fastest-growing county in the state.

BEGINNINGS OF ST. JOHN MEDICAL CENTER

Starting in 1914, the Sisters of the Sorrowful Mother, a Catholic order from Wichita, Kansas, were invited by Tulsa's civic and medical leaders to investigate the possibility of constructing a modern hospital. Upon the first arrival, there was not a paved road into Tulsa. Yet, the sisters made repeated visits before formally requesting funds from the diocese for a hospital. The bishop in Oklahoma City approved funding on condition the Tulsa community share in the expense. By 1919, the sisters had put a $25 down payment on an 8-acre strawberry patch near 21st Street and

St. John's Hospital Ground-breaking Ceremony

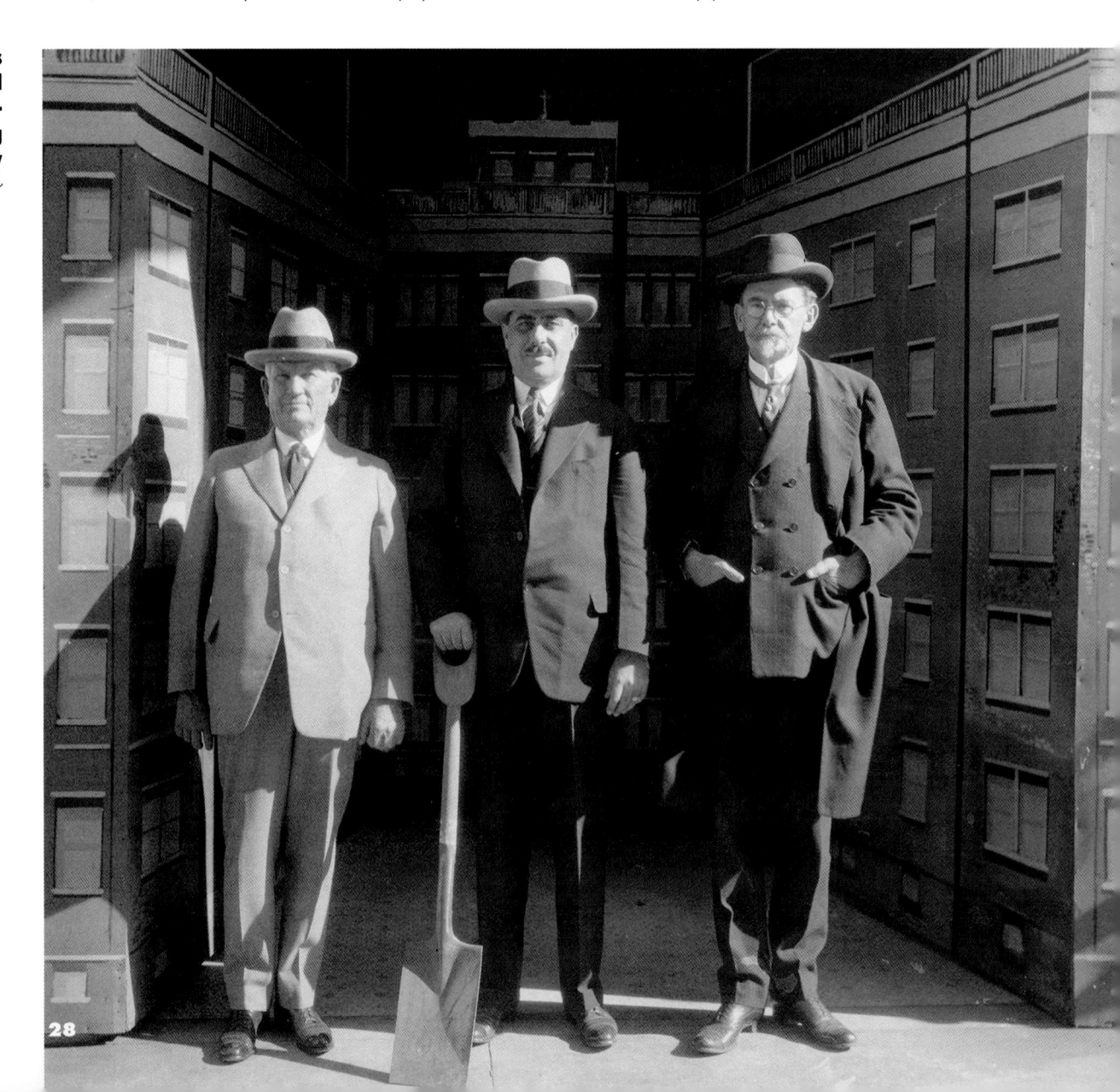

General John J. Pershing

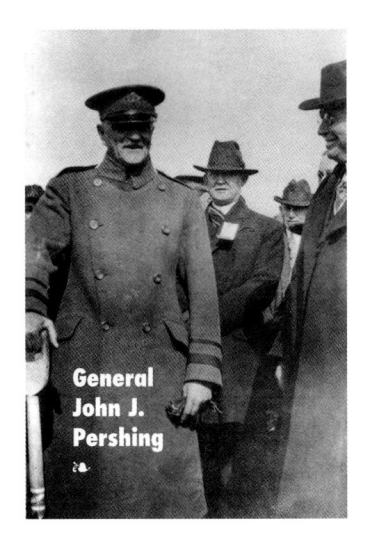

Utica Avenue. The land cost $16,000, and it took several more years of fundraising before construction could begin.

On Feb. 12, 1920, World War I hero Gen. John J. Pershing turned the first spade of dirt at the groundbreaking. He told the gathered crowd, "Let's finish it!"

Yet, construction progressed slowly as funding ran out. The five-story building sat vacant for years as an unfinished skeleton, earning the nickname "the Ghost." The Tulsa County Medical Society stepped in to finance public campaigns through newspapers and appealing to civic organizations and individuals. The construction would stop and start. The first patients were received in 1924 even though only two floors were available.

Sister Mary Alfreda was among the nurses working at the facility during this time and gave an interview in 1980 to the Junior League of Tulsa detailing the experience. Beds were placed in hallways, stairwell landings and any open space. Machines ground the terrazzo floors into place. Privacy was created by hanging sheets by strings between the beds.

"People would accept almost anything. Naturally, the sisters worked happily, cheerfully, faithfully as much as we could. And, we learned as we went, as time went on." — Sister Mary Alfreda, 1980.

A final $600,000 successful public campaign pushed the hospital to its goal for opening a significantly scaled-down 80-bed version in February 1926.

Part of the hospital's model was to emphasize training for nurses. Local newspapers had reported a shortage of nurses during this decade. The second floor of the hospital was dedicated to educating professional nurses in the St. John's Hospital School of Nursing. Until the first nurses graduated, dozens of Catholic nuns from other hospitals and schools across the nation operated the facility. Their quarters were located on a separate floor with about 50 beds available.

St. John's Hospital, School of Nursing

Without air conditioning, hospitals had to find ways to cool patients. St. John's Hospital was built with its own ice plant. Still, temperatures would reach 104 degrees in the operating rooms during summer months. The walls would not cool, trapping heat.

"So, in the operating room, we always had a basin with a hunk of ice in it and put a bath towel over it. We would ring it out and put it across the doctor's shoulders to keep them cool while they were operating. That was the cooling system we had. We had to use electric fans, which is certainly against technique. But, it was necessary for living." — Sister Mary Alfreda, 1980.

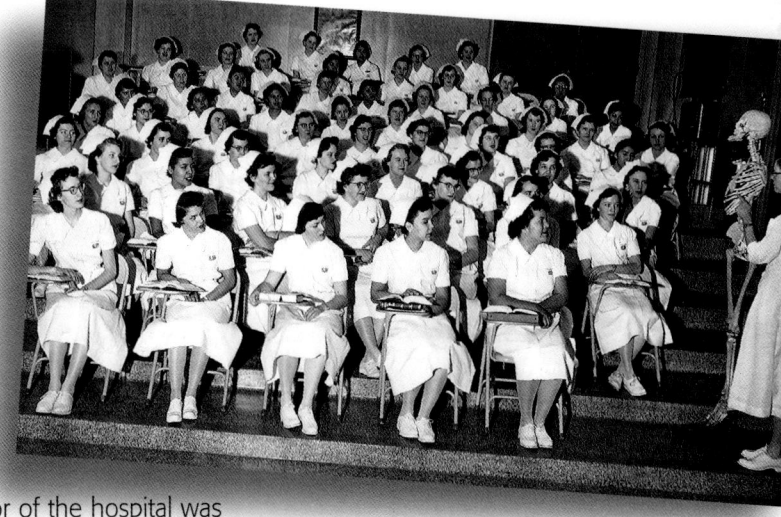

Mount Zion Baptist Church: set ablaze.

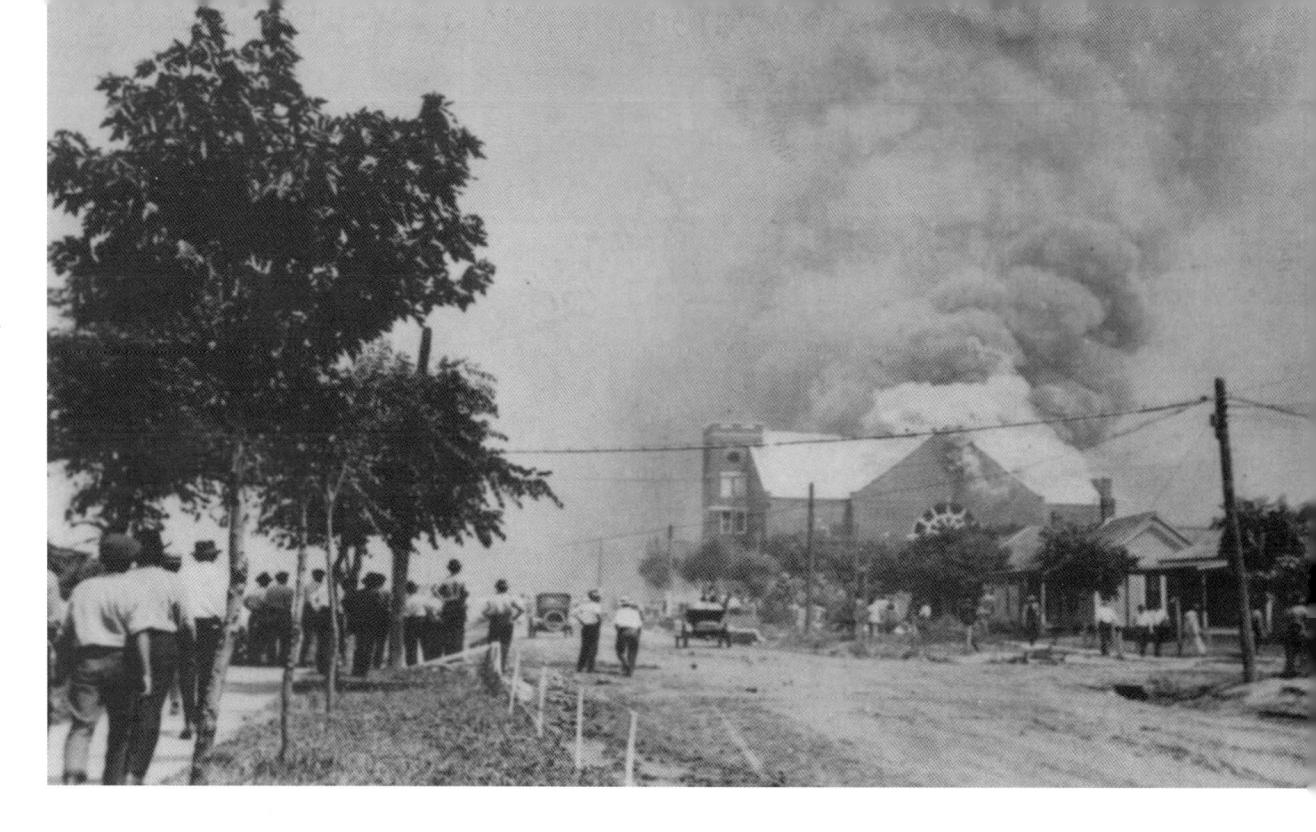

RACE RIOT

In one of Tulsa's darkest and most ugly times, a riot destroyed the Greenwood District, dubbed "Black Wall Street of America" by Booker T. Washington for its successful hub of black-owned businesses. It also had its own post office, police station, library and schools to cater to the black population during this segregated era. The challenges, recovery and moral lessons from that event have reverberated for more than a century. While some details and allegations are in dispute, some facts have been established.

It started with an incident on May 30, 1921, in a department store elevator between a black man (Dick Rowland) and a white woman (Sarah Page), who claimed she was attacked. A sensationally written story the next day in the *Tulsa Tribune* under the headline "Nab Negro for Attacking Girl In an Elevator," insinuated a sexual assault. Rumors of a possible lynching of the man spread, attracting a large crowd of white and black men to the street in front of the courthouse. After hours of a standoff between the groups, a white man and black man got into a scuffle with a gun, which fired. The white crowd looted a nearby sporting goods store of its guns and ammunition. Shooting, arson and looting moved from downtown north into the Greenwood business district. The riot lasted until early the next morning. In the chaos and haste of restoring order, about 1,500 additional police, citizens and National Guard moved into the area to take protective custody of unarmed black residents, but to many it appeared like an invading force. Residents fled north, were hidden by friends or fought in resistance. Witnesses reported seeing white residents loot black homes of clothes, jewelry and furniture.

More than 1,256 homes were burned down and 215 were looted. Only two churches, one school and a handful of homes survived. The death toll is still unknown, but 37 death certificates were issued. Of those, at least 25 victims were black men. Property damage was estimated at $1.5 million to $2 million.

The original arrest complaint against Rowland was dropped by the end of September. In a *Tulsa World* story written by Tom Latta the day after the riot: "Nothing that the mind is capable of conceiving permits a word of defense or excuse for the murderous vandalism inflicted on Greenwood."

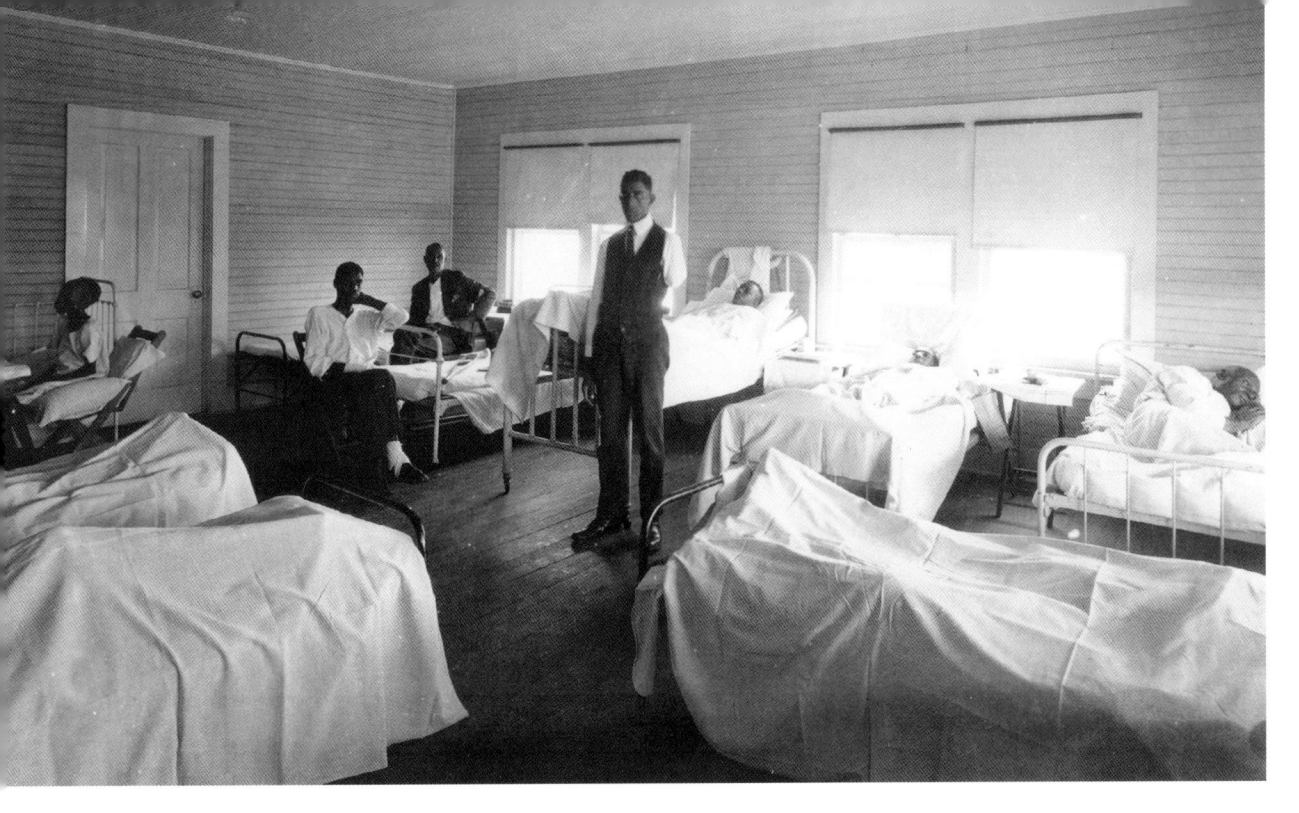

The American Red Cross: Set up a temporary ward following the Riot.

In the riot, Frissell Memorial Hospital was burned to ash. A makeshift clinic for injured black residents was set up at the National Guard Armory, which is now the Veterans of Foreign Wars Post No. 1. Maj. Paul Brown, a Tulsa physician and commanding officer of the sanitary detachment, secured beds in white hospitals for the most serious injuries among black residents.

Tulsa Race Riot: National Guard arrives in Greenwood during the Race Riot.

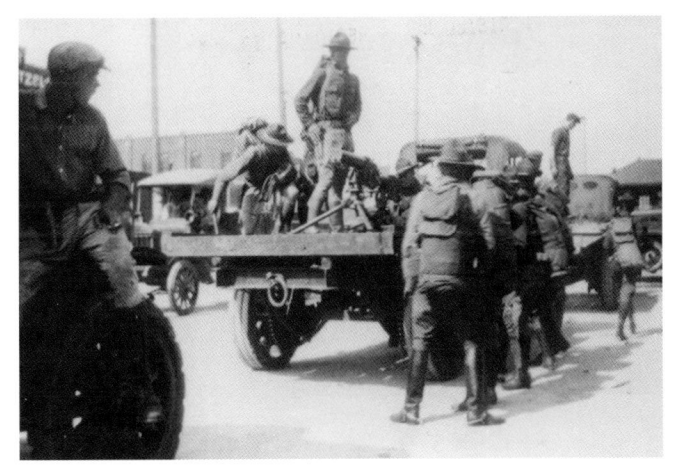

The Tulsa County Medical Society called a special session to discuss the overcrowded hospitals. Many of the city's physicians had been working shifts of 36 hours. The society helped arrange for a schedule of doctors to work more reasonable hours. The medical society reported that the 13 black physicians in Tulsa lost all their professional equipment and household possessions and were unable to care for their patients. The society raised a fund to provide $25 to each black physician and contributed medical tools to help them remain in practice. The medical association refused to help one of the black doctors, Dr. R.T. Bridgewater. It was claimed Dr. Bridgewater refused to help care for injured blacks, an allegation he strenuously denied. Dr. Bridgewater claimed he had taken time away from the relief work because his wife was ill.

The American Red Cross arrived on June 1 led by Maurice Willows, an administrator of the organization in St. Louis, to lead the relief effort. Willows had planned to retire, but the Red Cross requested he postpone his plans. In 1919, more than three dozen cities had racially based riots during the summer and early autumn months, dubbing it the "Red Summer." The Red Cross established a policy that year stating care would be extended to victims no matter the race or political party of the person.

Continued on page 33

Dr. Andrew C. Jackson

Among the tragedy and devastation left by the 1921 Tulsa Race Riot was the death of Dr. Andrew C. Jackson, a renowned 40-year-old surgeon respected by white and black Tulsans. He was perhaps the most noted victim in the deadly episode.

Born in Memphis but raised in Guthrie, Jackson was the son of an attorney. He graduated from Meharry Medical College in Nashville, Tennessee, and returned to Oklahoma for practices in Tulsa and Claremore. After developing an interest in surgery, Dr. Jackson received training in Memphis for the specialty. In 1919, he decided to make Tulsa his home with a focus on chronic diseases and surgery for women.

His work attracted the attention of Cass and John Mayo, prominent Tulsa businessmen, who described Dr. Jackson as "the most able Negro surgeon in America." His home at 523 N. Detroit Ave. was in an unusual location. It was an exclusive neighborhood with upscale homes for wealthier black residents not far from the large homes built by affluent white Tulsans. Among Dr. Jackson's neighbors were Booker T. Washington High School Principal E.W. Woods, physician Dr. R.T. Bridgewater and Tulsa Star Publisher A.J. Smitherman.

During the riot, gangs of white men went door-to-door in the black neighborhoods setting fire to the homes and occasionally attacking those inside. According to testimony by John Oliphant — a white former Tulsa police commissioner, retired judge and friend of Dr. Jackson — seven, armed white men approached and set fire to the home. Dr. Jackson was told by his white colleagues the best way to survive was to surrender and be taken into custody peacefully. However, this was not to be. Oliphant testified that Dr. Jackson was walking up to the group with "his hands in the air saying, 'Here am I. I want to go with you.'" After being grabbed into the group, two men shot him. After Dr. Jackson fell to the ground, one of the men fired again.

Some accounts say he died "in great pain" at the Convention Center but others report he died instantly or at the Armory. Oliphant called it "cold-blooded murder." One theory to motive is that the group had mistaken him for Smitherman, who had been editorializing in his African American newspaper for civil rights and writing about the slums plaguing black Tulsans.

The killers were never identified.

In the aftermath, Dr. Jackson was mourned locally and nationally. He had been serving as the vice president of the Oklahoma chapter of the National Medical Association, which is an organization advocating for African American physicians and their patients. In the June-September 1921 newsletter of the national association, Dr. Jackson was called a "valuable worker" for the black medical establishment and a "progressive and useful physician and citizen" for Tulsa.

"Let us hope that Dr. Jackson's death has not been in vain. May his untimely end be the means of creating such a sentiment against mob rule that law makers and law enforcers everywhere will see to it that the rights of citizens are so safeguarded that such conditions as obtained in Tulsa will in the future be impossible. If his death should contribute even in a small degree to that end, as it should, then we say that his death was not in vain." – National Medication Association journal. ∎

Almost immediately in Tulsa, Willows established a case management system for victims. Previously, people would be waiting in lines for hours to access relief. Under the management of Willows, a family-based structure allowed for set appointments with a social worker to determine needs. His biggest obstacle was in maneuvering local politics of the day. The business leaders at the chamber of commerce were at odds with elected leaders at City Hall over funding the relief and recovery effort. Willows managed to stay in the good graces of both camps and remained in Tulsa through the end of December. He earned the respect and admiration of black Tulsans for his leadership. In a memoir, Willows called the event a "disaster" rather than "riot" because the latter term was inadequate to describe what occurred.

An East End Welfare Board, which consisted of African-American residents, wrote a resolution to the American Red Cross, commending them for its recovery work.

"On the 31st night in May, 1921, the fiercest race war known to American history broke out, lasting until the next morning, June 1st, 1921. As a result of this regrettable occurrence, many human lives were lost and millions of dollars worth of property were stolen and burned. Hundreds of innocent Negroes suffered as a result of this calamity — suffered in loss of lives, injury from gun-shot wounds and loss of property. Many of us were left helpless and almost hopeless. We sat amid the wreck and ruin of our former homes and peered listlessly into space. It was at this time and under such conditions that the American Red Cross — that Angel of Love and Mercy came to our assistance. This great organization found us bruised and bleeding and, like the good Samaritan, she washed out wounds, and administered unto us. Constantly, in season and out, since the regrettable occurrence, this great organization, headed by that high class Christian gentleman, Mr. Maurice Willows, has heard our every cry in this our dark hour and has ever extended to us practical sympathy. As best she could, with food and raiment and shelter, she has furnished us. And to this great Christian organization, our heartfelt gratitude is extended," "Angels of Mercy," 1993 publication.

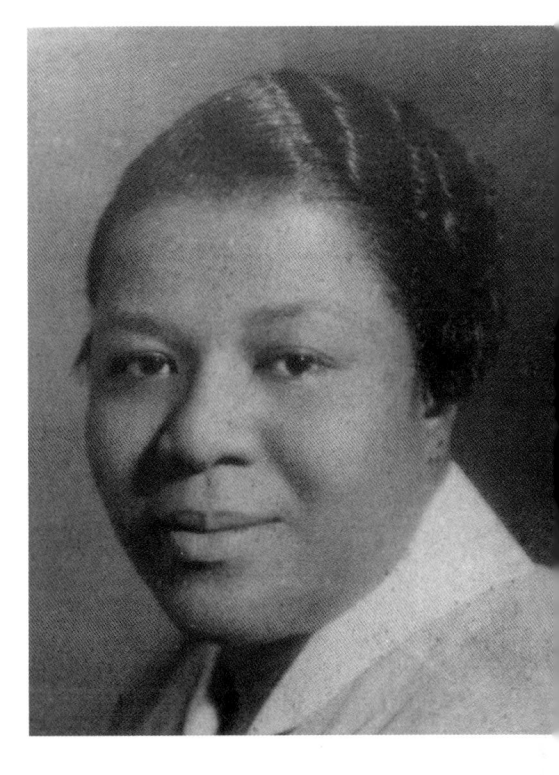

Janice Jones: Tulsa's first African American nurse specializing in public health.

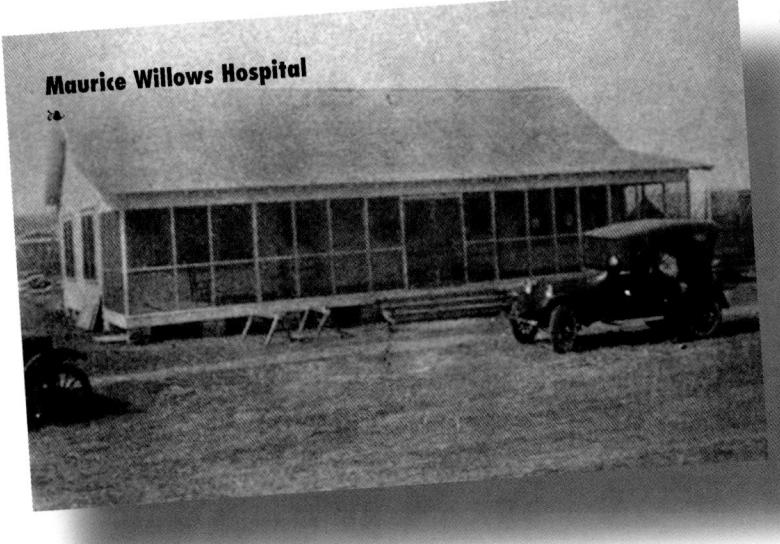

In a disaster report written by Willows, 233 people received medical care by Red Cross staff; 5 hospitals were provided emergency dressings and supplies; 1,800 people were vaccinated and 2,056 people and 8,200 families were given tents, clothing, cooking utensils and bedding. The report stated 11 black physicians and 11 white physicians were used to provide care. It also employed 38 nurses in the hospital and 8 nurses for service in the field.

Later that year, the American Red Cross opened Maurice Willows Hospital at 324 North Hartford Ave. The county commis-

Maurice Willows Hospital

sioners and board of education provided the property, the East End Welfare Board handled the labor and the Red Cross bought the materials. Black laborers built the 30-bed hospital for a total cost of about $68,000. The hospital contained male and female surgical wings, a maternity ward, women's general medical ward, fully equipped operating room and a convalescent porch. The city and county spent about $200,000 in tax money for relief and rehabilitation. By end of December, 22 patients from the race riot remained in care at the hospital. The facility was remodeled in 1932 and transferred to a community board administration. It was renamed Morton Memorial Hospital in 1941 and closed in 1967.

It would be a decades-long process to rebuild the Greenwood area and nearly all the original landmarks are gone. In the heart of that site is the John Hope Franklin Reconciliation Center. A park with a memorial was opened in December 2009.

Osteopaths Strike Out on Their Own

After Oklahoma's statehood, only allopathic doctors (M.D.) were allowed to admit patients into hospitals. At that time, medical standards for osteopathic practitioners (D.O) were not as stringent as the allopathic regulations. For example, a person could go from high school directly to medical school to become an osteopath. During this decade, a committee within the Tulsa County Medical Society started an effort to eliminate osteopaths from participating in the public school systems health departments. The differences created a contentious relationship for decades between the two types of physicians until the standards were equalized.

Without hospital privileges, it meant osteopathic doctors had to practice in a home or office or build their own hospital. In 1924, Dr. C.D. "Pop" Heasley opened the 10-bed Tulsa Clinic Hospital at 1321 S. Peoria Ave. The two-story house was the only facility available to the city's 10 practicing osteopathic physicians. With the population continuing to soar, it expanded to 25 beds by 1927. By 1930, 25 osteopathic doctors were practicing at Heasley's hospital and operated under the regulations set forth by the Bureau of Hospitals of the American Osteopathic Association.

"The history of the hospital is a story of a small but determined group of professional men and women who early on developed the habit of self-sacrifice in constructing and operating hospitals and who were never satisfied with the present except as a step to larger and ever larger institutions."— Dr. A.G. Reed.

It would eventually become Tulsa Regional Medical Center in 1989 and then the Oklahoma State University Medical Center in 2009, working in partnership with the OSU College of Osteopathic Medicine.

Junior League Steps In

In 1923, the Junior League of Tulsa formed with just 13 women who wanted to address the needs of low-income families in the city. Three years after its establishment, it started a project that would lead to the Children's Medical Center. The group established a convalescent home for crippled children in a downtown building near 5th Street and Cincinnati Avenue. In 1928, it moved to a larger cottage at 1448 S. Lewis Ave. and became known as the Junior League Convalescent Hospital. Emphasis was on the care and treatment of disabled children, mostly polio victims. This facility remained under this

Dr. C.D. "Pop" Heasley

Dr. C.D. "Pop" Heasley was the first licensed osteopathic physician-surgeon in Oklahoma when he started in practice in 1921. He had the green-colored document with the "No. 1" on display in his office at 807 S. Denver Ave.

"This was new country then – oil country. I was from oil land (in Pennsylvania) and this seemed the logical place to settle. There were big stories coming out of Bartlesville, and Tulsa only had about 40,000 people then." – Dr. C.D. Heasley, *Tulsa World*, 1968.

It also offered a land of opportunity. He founded the first osteopathic hospital in the city, starting with a two-story house at 14th Street and Peoria Avenue. It was moved to a four-story facility at Ninth Street and Jackson Avenue.

"There were very few hospitals then and a great need for a hospital to care for our patients." – Dr. Heasley, 1968.

Dr. Heasley received his bachelor's degree from Grove City College in Pennsylvania, and a doctorate degree from the College of Osteopathic Medicine and Surgery in Des Moines, Iowa. He served 15 years as the chairman of the department of surgery at the Oklahoma Osteopathic Hospital and was a former chief of staff and past president of its board of trustees.

Dr. Heasley helped establish the American College of Osteopathic Surgeons in 1928, named a fellow of the organization in 1935 and was its president from 1941-42. He was one of the group's first recipients of its highest honor, the Oral F. Martin Award.

About a year before his retirement in 1969, he reflected on changes in the profession.

"There's hardly any such thing as a general surgeon anymore. Everyone calls in specialists these days. When I first began practicing, we often had only the surgical nurse to assist in operations. Now, there's a specialist standing by for everything from giving the anesthesia to sewing them together. We didn't have all the specialized equipment and techniques then either. Medicine then was more of a personal thing. We made our own diagnosis and treatment, without all the consulting physicians and countless tests." – Dr. Heasley, 1969.

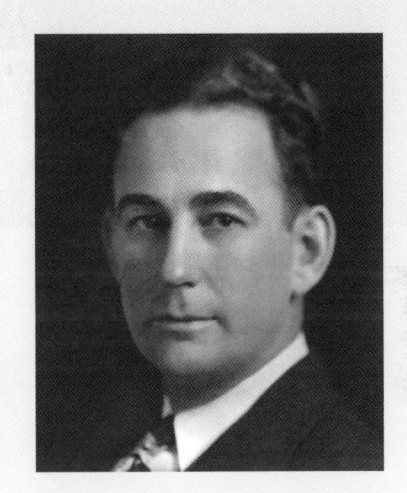

Dr. Heasley recalled that people used to only visit a doctor if seriously ill, but preventive medicine increased the needs and demands on physicians.

"Physicians are in a position to give the greatest service to humanity. Every doctor should write a book, but if I wrote one, they probably wouldn't publish it if I told the truth. It's interesting because you learn so much about humanity."
– Dr. Heasley, 1969.

Dr. Heasley died at age 86 in August 1979.

administration until after World War II, when the Junior League turned operations over to a community board. After expansions and consolidations, it became the Children's Medical Center.

From Sunnyside to Morningside

Dolly Irene (Brown) McNulty ended up in Tulsa when she responded to a newspaper story about a meeting in the city about the 1918 flu epidemic. She had been going west on a World War I troop train from New York when plans changed.

Nurse Dolly Brown McNulty

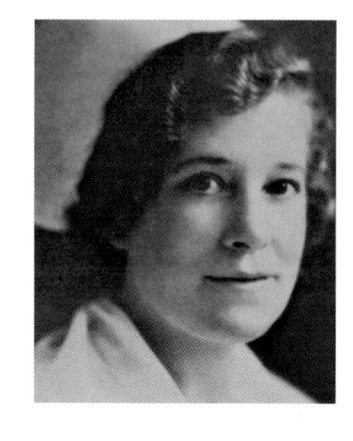

"I was on the front row of that meeting and when the doctor called for volunteers. I suppose both my hands went up at once,"
— Dolly McNulty, *Tulsa World*, 1970.

This wasn't her first experience with Tulsa medicine.

McNulty was born in Stonewall, Texas, on Christmas Eve 1889. She studied nursing at Austin Sanitarium in Austin, Texas. She became the superintendent of All Saints' Hospital in San Antonio and was called to Tulsa on medical business.

"I was staying at the Tulsa Hotel when I was taken ill. I called the desk and asked for a doctor. While we were visiting, I told him I was a hospital administrator, and he told me that he had the only hospital in town and that he didn't want me around. That was challenge enough," — Dolly McNulty, *Tulsa World*, 1970.

However, she took a detour when patriotism called her to serve in the war effort. After going to New York to enlist, McNulty answered the call to Tulsa instead.

While the Texas nurse visited schools to check students for flu symptoms, she saw how Tulsa lacked enough hospital space. She bought the Sunnyside Hospital at 521 N. Boulder Ave. from the Rouleau sisters in 1918 and added a training school for nurses. McNulty furnished the hospital with equipment purchased from Pawnee Bill, a Wild West showman. The name came after a beautiful ride from Pawnee.

She married M.J McNulty Jr. in 1923, and the couple purchased lots at 12th Street and Utica Avenue from her new father-in-law. In 1927, the first building was erected as part of a new 72-bed capacity hospital, formed in the shape of a T.

In October 1940, Morningside was acquired by a group of Tulsa businessman and re-named Hillcrest Memorial Hospital and Training School for Nurses. In 1952, it became Hillcrest Medical Center.

McNulty died on Feb. 23, 1972.

First Morningside Hospital

Morningside Hospital Groundbreaking Ceremony:
Founder Dolly Brown McNulty holding the shovel.

Dr. Charles H. Ball

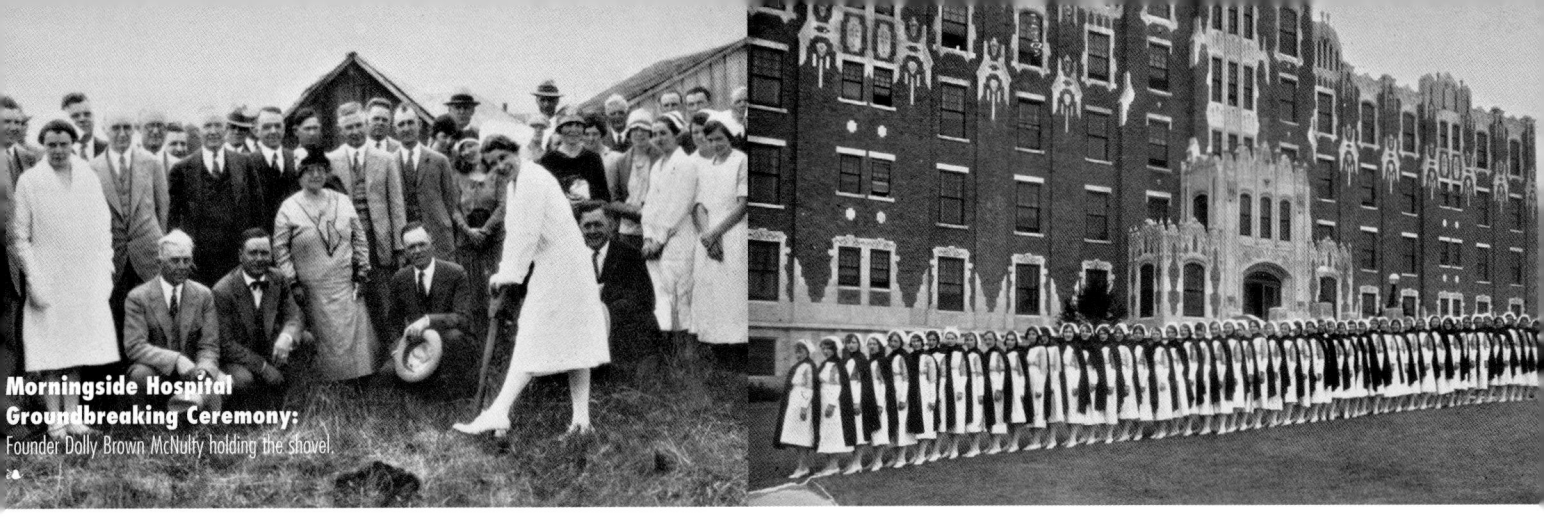

Dr. Charles H. Ball became a physician, specializing in dermatology, later in life. He was born in 1867 in Ohio and left home as a teenager to become a reporter at a newspaper in Gainesville, Texas. In 1888, he moved to Muskogee and published a newspaper and legal journal for the Choctaw, Creek, Iowa, Seminole and Chickasaw tribes. Because these were printed in the native languages, Dr. Ball became a proficient linguist. He later established the first newspaper in El Reno, and sponsored the first state fair. In 1895, he left Oklahoma to take an assistant editor job at the *St. Louis Globe-Democrat*, where he worked for 10 years. This was when he became interested in medicine.

In 1902, Dr. Ball entered the St. Louis Medical College. He studied by day and supported himself by working as a newspaper printer at night. After graduating in 1906, he practiced in St. Louis and served as an instructor in dermatology at the medical college. He also was on staff at the Free Skin and Cancer Hospital, Baptist Hospital and the Christian Orphans Home. In March 1917, he moved to Tulsa and immediately became active in the medical community. Dr. Ball became president of the Tulsa County Medical Society in 1922. His publishing roots were never too far, as he served as the associate editor of the Oklahoma Medical Association.

He and wife, Mary Elizabeth, had four children. He was a civic leader, serving as treasurer of the A.B.C. Oil and Gas Company and holding memberships in the Kiwanis, Lions and Automobile clubs.

"He holds to high professional standards and his developed skill has brought him prominently to the front as an eminent dermatologist and X-ray physician," said author Clarence Douglass. ∎

OFFICE SPACE

Doctors had a hard time finding a place to hang a shingle, particularly as veterans returned from the Great War. Doctors worked in office buildings ill-equipped for medicine with drafty rooms and poor lighting. In 1923, the Atlas Life Building (415 S. Boston Ave.) and Day Building (512 S. Boston Ave.) opened, causing a lot of physicians to move. In 1926, the Medical and Dental Arts Building started construction at 108 W. Sixth St. and was financed privately. More than 90 percent of space was sold before it opened two years later. It is considered an Art Deco style structure designed by renowned architect Bruce Goff. The effort was led by dentist Dr. Charles W. Day. The Tulsa County Medical Society heralded its opening, as related in a written history:

"It provided a concentration of reputable practitioners in a building especially designed for their needs. The need of such a specialized structure had long been felt by Tulsa doctors and dentists. Medical and dental professional men had not been particularly welcome in other buildings.

Large numbers of sick persons tended to slow elevator service, electrical

The Morningside Hospital & Training School for Nurses:
Was located at 1653 E. 12th St.

Operatory:
Medical Arts Building.

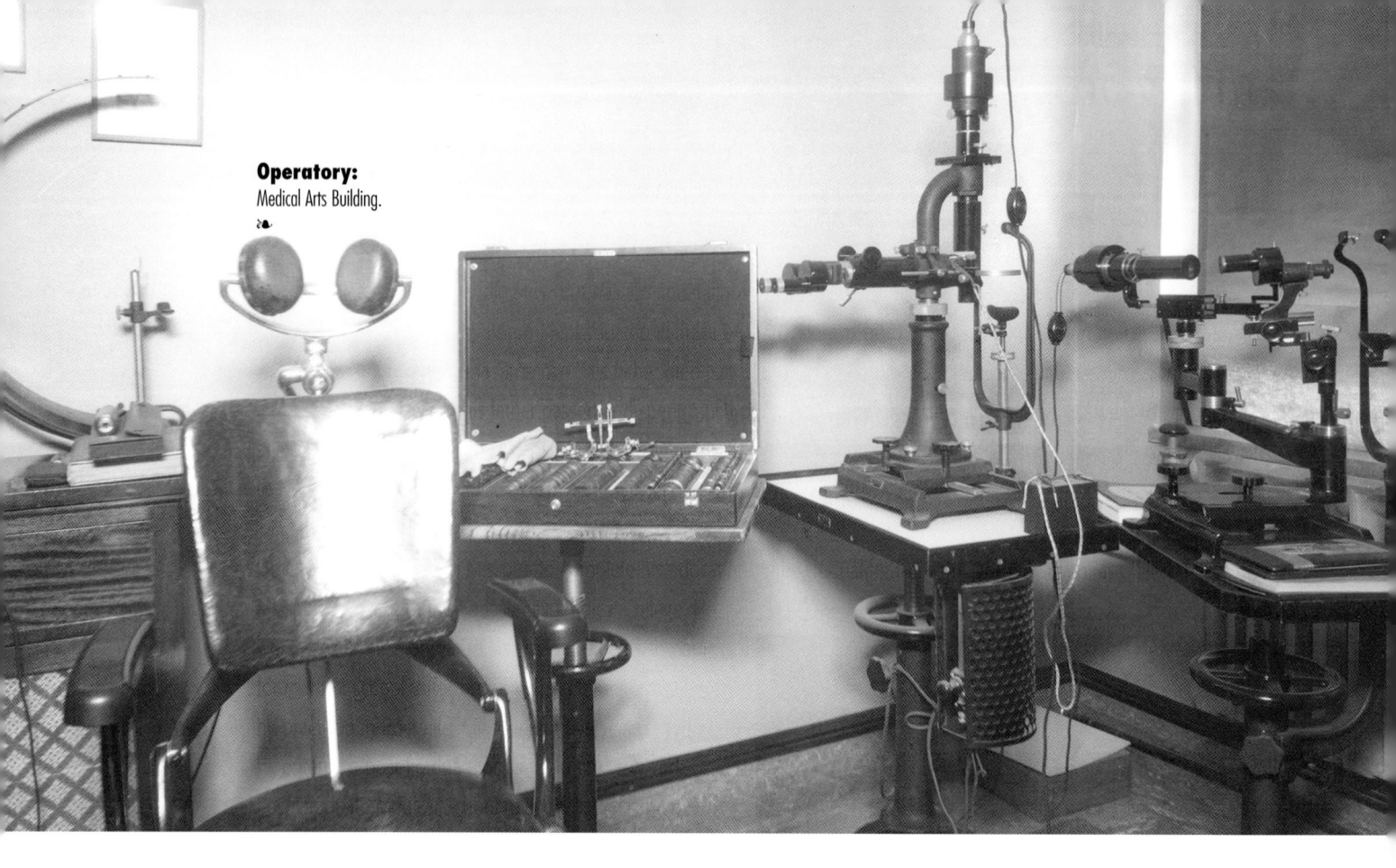

Medical Arts Building: finished in 1929.

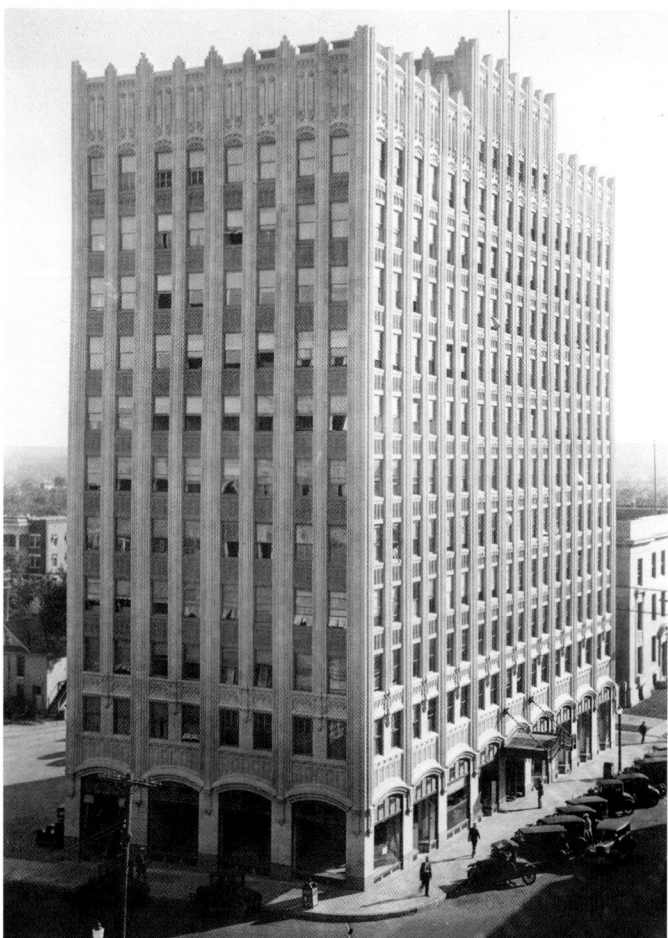

facilities were often inadequate, and in many buildings other technical requirements were substandard," — Tulsa County Medical Society.

Medical Advocacy

Throughout the decade, the Tulsa County Medical Society campaigned against illegitimate and unethical practitioners. Many applicants for membership were rejected during this time, some referred to the Board of Medical Examiners for further action.

"Frauds and quackery continued to be a major problem, not only for Tulsa but for doctors all over the state. A steady stream of victimized patients gave ample evidence of the abundant quackery," — Tulsa County Medical Society.

Continued on page 40

Dr. Hugh C. Graham

Dr. Hugh C. Graham, Sr., was among the first Tulsa physicians specializing in pediatrics. He arrived in Tulsa in May 1916 to attend Henry Kendall College (now the University of Tulsa) in the mornings and worked as a bookkeeper at the YMCA Downtown in the afternoons. In April 1917, he enlisted in the U.S. Army and worked his way to a rank of First Lieutenant. He returned to Tulsa to finish his degree then entered the medical school at the University of Oklahoma. He transferred to the University of Chicago, where he received his medical degree in 1925 and specialized in pediatrics.

After returning to Tulsa in 1928, Dr. Graham went into a pediatric practice with another physician. In 1933, he opened his own office on the first floor of his family's three-story home at 15th Street and Baltimore Avenue. Eventually, he moved to an office at 1307 S. Main St. then to the city's first suburban shopping center – Utica Square – in 1952.

Dr. Graham was a diplomat of the American Board of Pediatrics, member of the American Academy of Pediatrics, adjunct professor of biology at TU and chief of staff at St. John Medical Center and Hillcrest Medical Center.

As a civic leader, Dr. Graham served two terms on the Tulsa Board of Education, 23 years on the Tulsa Board of Health and had perfect attendance for 40 years as a member of the Tulsa Rotary Club.

Dr. Graham married Helen Marion Waggoner in 1928. She was a graduate of the University of Tulsa with post-graduate studies at the University of Chicago. She was the first president of the Tulsa County Medical Auxiliary. The couple had two children.

After their children started competitive ice skating, the couple was active in the Tulsa Figure Skating Club and as High Test judges for U.S. Figure Skating for more than 50 years.

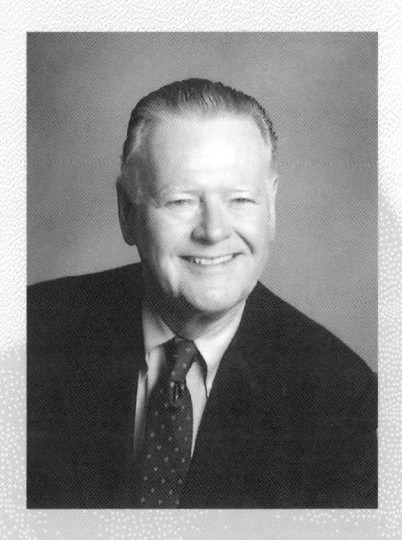

His son, Dr. Hugh Graham Jr., followed his father in becoming a pediatrician, and the two joined the Glass Nelson Clinic in 1966. The senior Dr. Graham retired in 1972 at age 77. He was named Doctor of the Year by the Tulsa County Medical Society.

In a written history of the city's pediatricians, a letter was printed from a woman, Betty Berger, to the younger Dr. Graham about his father's generosity. Ms. Berger said her daughter was born during a snowstorm in February 1944 while her husband was in England waiting to go to France for D-Day. Four months later, her husband died, leaving her a 19-year-old widow with an infant. When she took her baby to Dr. Graham for the next well-baby visit, he refused payment.

"He said if her Daddy could give his life for his country, the least he could do was to care for his daughter . . . 50 years later, I still remember and deeply appreciate what he did for my daughter and me," – Betty Berger.

Dr. Graham died on Nov. 11, 1982, at age 86.

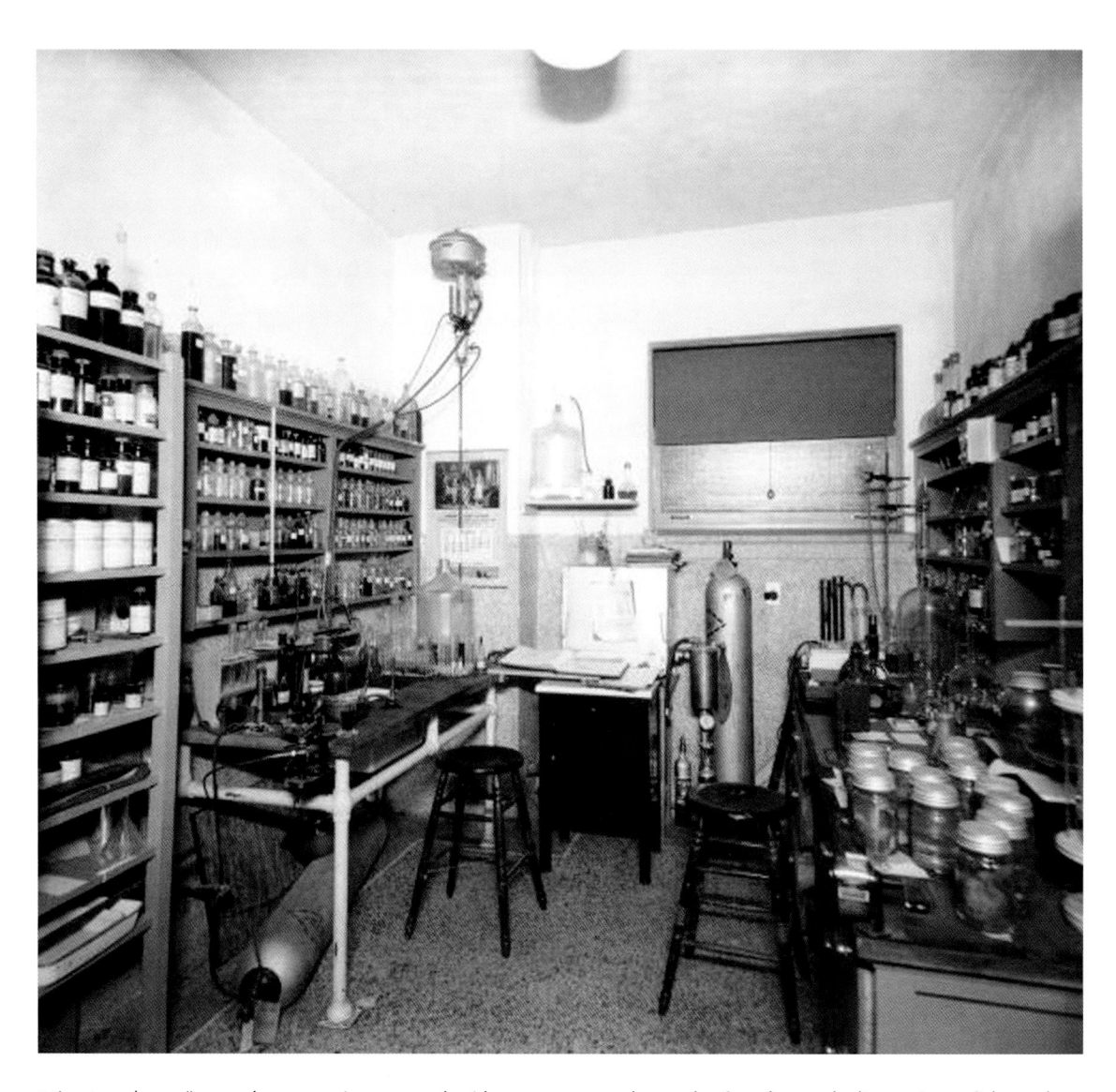

St. John's Hospital Laboratory.

Minutes show "scarcely a meeting passed without some prolonged, often heated, discussion of the subject." Part of this was whether to embrace chiropractors and osteopaths. The Oklahoma State Medical Association wanted to keep those practitioners at bay, but the Tulsa and other local societies disagreed. Instead, the local societies argued that the focus should be the promotion of scientific study.

In the early 20s, the Tulsa County Medical Society was critical of the sanitary conditions in public businesses such as hotels, restaurants and drug stores. It blamed the Oklahoma State Health Department for interfering with local enforcement. Public pressure from newspaper reports forced better conditions. The society backed the efforts of Dr. Ross Grosshart to establish the Milk Ordinance, which set the standards for grading milk and dairy products. The group also became involved in the public discussion about water quality of the Spavinaw Water System.

No matter the public issue of the moment, physicians kept focus on scientific studies. Briefly, the Tulsa Academy of Medicine was formed to present papers on living cases and medical advancements. The Tulsa County Medical Society also hosted out-of-town speakers to address the membership about scientific progresses. ■

CHAPTER 4
(1930 - 1939)

Digging Out from the Depression

Crowd outside the New York Stock Exchange.

The decade was dominated by the Great Depression and greatly humbled Tulsa, which had been enjoying the riches from growth and prosperity from the past couple of decades. In the 30s, the city laid off one-fourth of its police force and eliminated many municipal departments. Bank deposits took a nose dive, and residential construction shrank by 95 percent, from $13.6 million in 1928 to $517,000 in 1932.

The population trend turned, with the 1930 census showing 145,000 residents, compared to 170,000 just two years earlier. This set off an identity crisis, leading to a city-wide call to make sure everyone was counted.

"If you know of any person or families who have not been enumerated, call phone 3-2161, ask for the city editor, and give names and addresses of those who have been missed... Get on the job for your home city. Let's go, with the real Tulsa enthusiasm," *Tulsa World*, April 26, 1930.

The Chamber of Commerce alleged a misunderstanding between how federal and city officials considered city boundaries. Still, there was no more claim of being the state's "metropolis."

In 1931, the city's Community Fund set an ambitious $250,000 goal to help the city's poor and predicted it would not fulfill all the needs. It didn't. The fund more than doubled its goal two years later, which also did not meet all the needs.

In the early 30s, the city derided public welfare as unnecessary. At first, officials answered the growing unemployment by distributing free seeds for community gardens and sending volunteers door-to-door looking for odd jobs. By the end of the decade, the city embraced the New Deal public works programs.

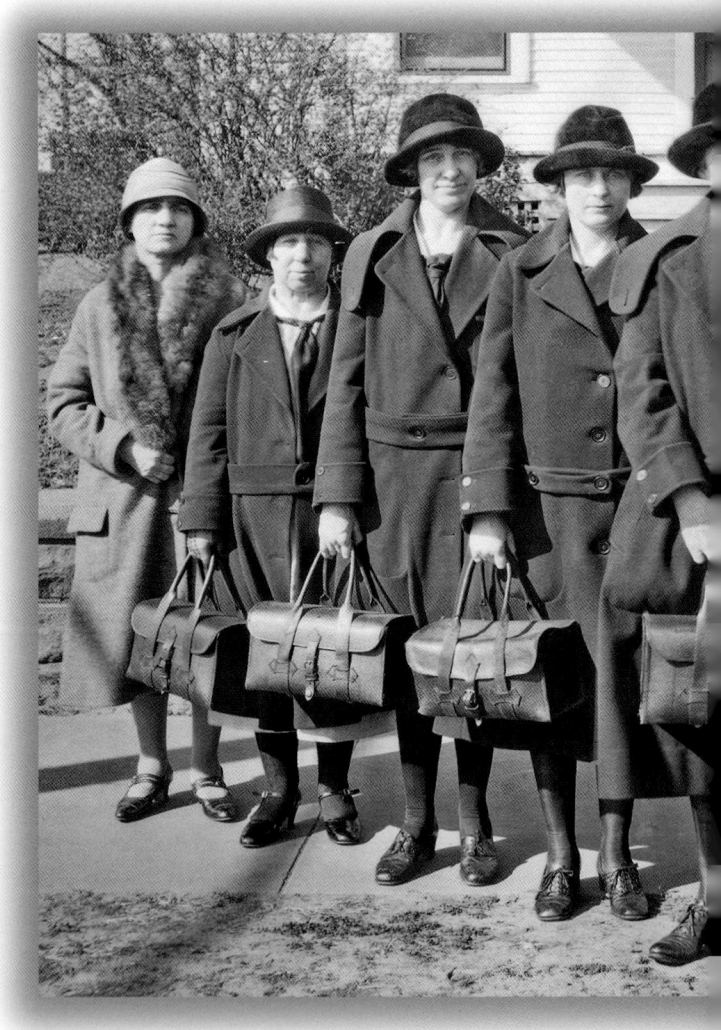

Among the programs was laying a road bed and digging a reservoir in Mohawk Park, which was described by *Tulsa World* reporter J. Nelson Taylor, who wrote first-person pieces about the experience.

In the last six months of 1933, nearly 30,000 men and women were registered with the unemployment office in Tulsa — the highest in the state. Among the New Deal workers was a man who walked seven miles in the cold to work at the Mohawk Park site for $2.40 a day. One man was fired from his 50-cents-a-shift night watch job because his boss refused to meet the new federal minimum wage of $14 a week.

"It was not a dinner bucket brigade I joined. These men don't even own dinner buckets." — Reporter J. Nelson Taylor, *Tulsa World*, 1933.

The rural communities surrounding Tulsa suffered more due to a drought that wiped out crops and whipped up infamous dust clouds. Tulsans seeking relief from the heat slept in city parks and backyards during summer months. The Tulsa airport closed for several months in the spring 1935 because of the dense dust.

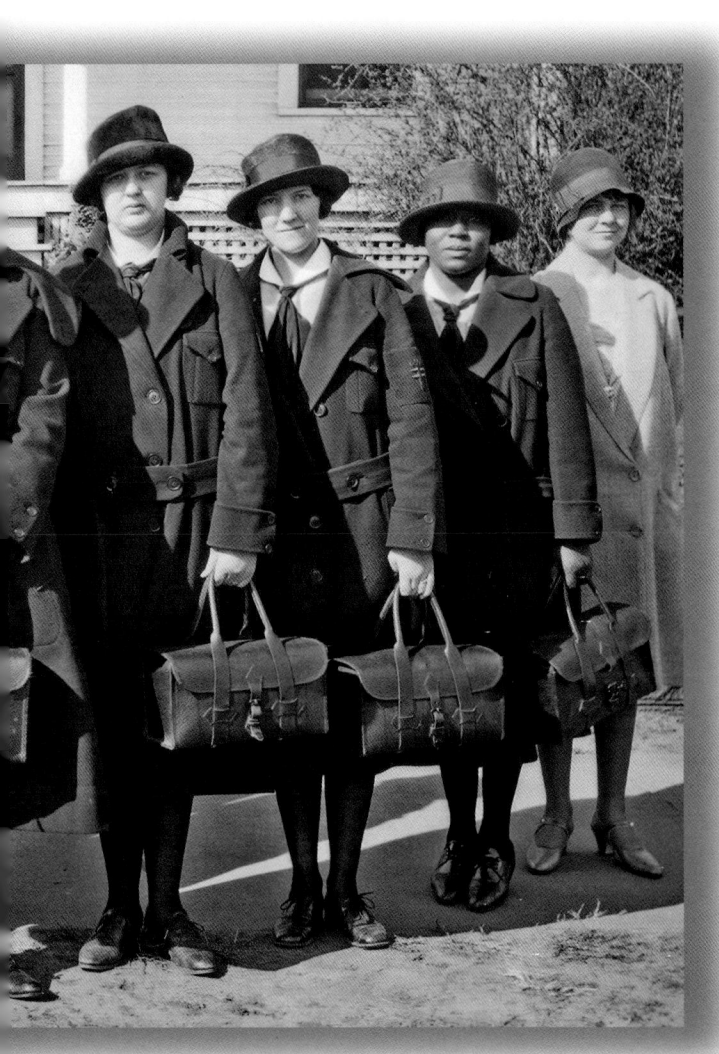

The Depression led the state to enact its first state income tax, first state sales tax and first "sin" taxes. It also instituted a large increase in oil and gas production taxes and shifted away from property and corporate taxes.

Tulsa wasn't as bad off as other communities. The state treasurer reported Tulsa County residents paid more than twice as much sales tax per capita as the state average, 16 percent more than Oklahoma County residents and five times more than some rural counties. It's unclear whether this is a reflection of the general population or skewed by a wealthy upper class.

Tulsa County medicine progressed with expansions in service and programs focused on scientific advancements. The Tulsa County Medical Society took on debates of health insurance, access and quality of care.

"Despite the gloom occasioned by increasingly bad economic conditions, the members of the Tulsa County Medical Society entered 1931 under the most favorable circumstances for the successful practice of medicine," according to the book, *A History of The Tulsa County Medical Society*.

Public Health Association Ladies Aides: During the Depression these ladies helped Tulsa children by ensuring they had proper nutrition.

INSURANCE PLANS

Against the backdrop of economic collapse and recovery, Americans worried about how to pay for medical care. Nationally, up to 40 percent of Americans were on relief. People could not pay medical bills, which decreased doctor visits and hospital demands. Before the Depression, doctors charged on a fee-for-service or on a sliding scale. The average hospital stay was two weeks

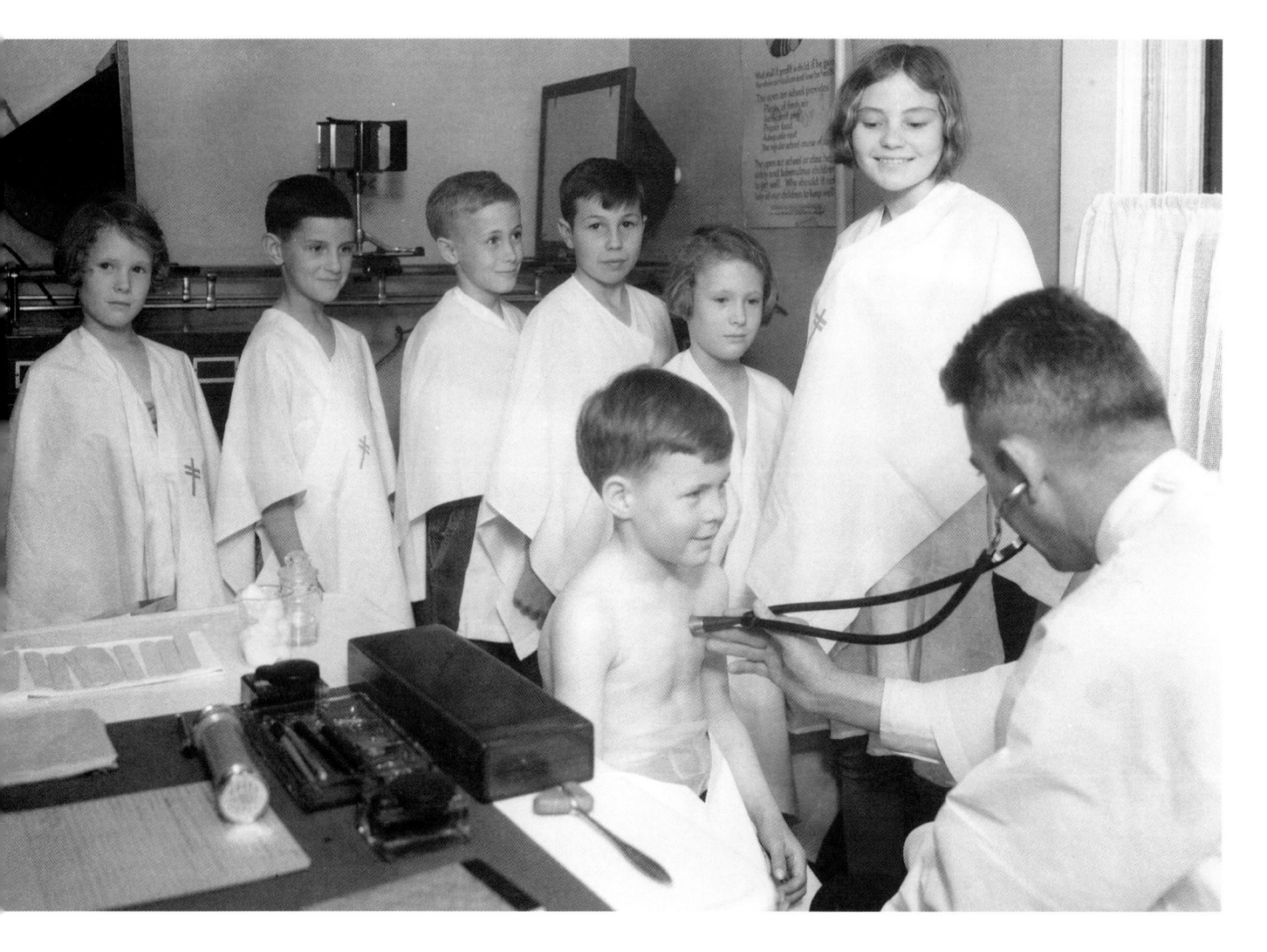

Tulsa Public Health Association: Health Screening.

in 1933. While hospital beds went unfilled, charitable donations also fell.

Congress debated whether to have a national health insurance system but did not act on it. A national health conference, held in July 1938, included a recommendation for a national health program. A Congressional bill was introduced in 1939 outlining a national public health system. It passed the Senate but died in the House.

In a poll taken in the late 30s, about three out of four Americans said they approved the government helping pay for medical care. These debates occurred on the state and local levels as well. The American Medical Association opposed the program, arguing it would eliminate doctor autonomy, and responded with a publicity campaign. State and local medical groups joined the chorus, including Tulsa County Medical Society.

"The Society conducted an investigation into the growing trends towards group practice of medicine, and into insurance plans which reimbursed physicians for services rendered on a flat pay basis. At early meetings during the year, attempts were made to outlaw these practices as far as Society members were concerned, but the well-intentioned efforts failed rather miserably. The distinctions were difficult to draw, and perhaps represented only the result of a medical trend rather than any violation of established ethics." — From the book, *A History of The Tulsa County Medical Society*.

Out of this came the Blue Cross and Blue Shield insurance plans. The American Hospital Association created the Blue Cross plan in 1933 for hospital costs. In 1939, the Blue Shield plans were added for medical and surgical costs. The AMA was dubious but ended up backing the insurance plans out of concerns of what a national government-based health plan could bring.

In 1939, the Tulsa County Medical Society developed a "master policy of surgeon's and physician's liability insurance." The malpractice policies offered by private insurers at the time did not meet the needs of doctors and were expensive. The new plan provided benefit not previously offered and saved physicians 50 percent to 60 percent in costs. Despite opposition from private insurers, it went into effect in April 1939. It was successful and eventually taken over by the Oklahoma State Medical Association as a statewide program.

ADVANCEMENTS FOR PAIN

For nearly 100 years, the most significant jump in anesthesiology was in the use of ether, which began in the 1840s after Boston physician William T. Morton successfully demonstrated its ability. Its administration was through the nose and mouth by a mask or cloth. Chloroform quickly followed for use in childbirth and later adapted for surgery and dental procedures. After the turn of the century, other strides were made, textbooks published and boards established. In 1929, the intravenous anesthetic thiopental (Pentothal) was popularized and led to other agents such as ketamine, propofol and etomidate.

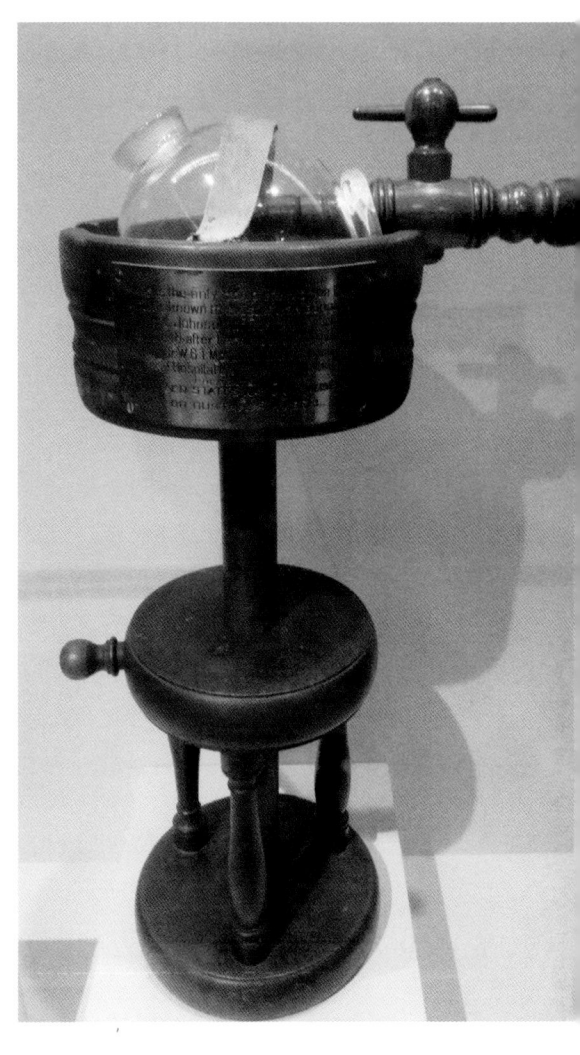

Ether inhaler: Circa 1846 by William T.G. Morton.

Harold Boyd Stewart, M.D.

The first physician to arrive in Tulsa with formal anesthesia training was Dr. Harry Boyd Stewart, who started employment at St. John's Hospital in January 1927 and continued to practice until 1963. He received his training at Ohio University. He was the only anesthesiologist in Tulsa until he hired Dr. Eugene G. Wolff in 1939 and formed the group, Anesthesia Services. Dr. Wolff was a native of Waukomis, Oklahoma, and educated at the University of Oklahoma.

RISE OF THE OSTEOPATHS

The Tulsa Osteopathic Hospital received patients from the 25 osteopathic doctors practicing in the city. The facility at 1321 S. Peoria Ave. was founded by Dr. C.D. "Pop" Heasley and operated under regulations set by the Bureau of Hospitals of the American Osteopathic Association.

Dr. Mary S. McPike

When arthritis forced Dr. Mary S. McPike to end her career spanning nearly four decades, she sobbed. She was the first osteopathic doctor to practice at the Oklahoma Osteopathic Hospital and one of the first female physicians.

In 1959, the 91-year-old Dr. McPike reflected on her life and profession. She had worked to bridge the differences between osteopathic and homeopathic approaches and standards.

"I cried when I decided to quit. I had a wonderful practice during those 37 years. I wouldn't exchange my practice with anyone — but with a surgeon perhaps. I think I would have been a good surgeon, but I felt I was probably too old when I started," said Dr. McPike, *Tulsa World*, 1959.

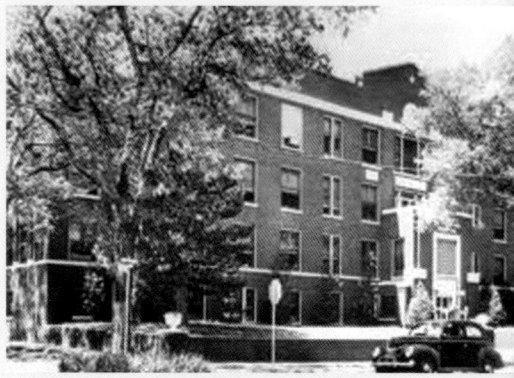

Born near Palmyra, Missouri, Dr. McPike was a married mother of four children when she entered the Still School of Osteopathy at Kirksville, Missouri, in 1902. Her husband, Dr. James K. McPike, was an osteopathic doctor. One day, she overheard a prospective patient say she would accept treatment only from a woman physician. The school she attended was founded by Dr. Andrew Taylor Still, the founder of osteopathy and osteopathic medicine.

Oklahoma Osteopathic Hospital in 1944.

"One of my sisters said to me, 'You are the one who should take that training.' I had looked at (my husband's) books when he was in school, and they looked awfully hard. But, I believed if the structure was kept in good shape, a person could keep his health... When I first entered the American School of Osteopathy, I felt I wouldn't have to treat men. By the time I got out, I was ready to treat anyone and I did," said Dr. McPike, *Tulsa World*, 1959.

Dr. McPike worked in Wichita, Kansas, after her graduation. She would travel to surrounding communities to see patients, sometimes staying as long as a week to provide medical care.

Two weeks before Oklahoma's statehood, the couple moved to Norman, Oklahoma, then to Tulsa two years later. She arrived when a horse and buggy provided transportation, the tallest building was five stories and paved roads stopped at 11th Street.

Heasley sold his interest in the hospital during this decade to the Byrne family. The hospital then became known as the Byrne Memorial Hospital by 1940.

A code book from 1939 specifies hospital amenities including one toilet in a separate, well-ventilated apartment per 12 patients. It must have hot and cold water, be free from dampness, have dry cellars and basements and be whitewashed or painted. Fly screens had to be fitted to all doors and windows from April 1 to November 1, and the building needed to be fly-free. Separate beds, pillows and beddings were provided to each patient, and babies had to be placed in individual bassinets or cribs.

By the end of the decade, it cost $5 for a private room and $3 for semi-private. New moms were

"When I came to Tulsa in 1909, I thought it was a great town. I had the best patients in town. There weren't any scoundrels. The city didn't attract that class of people," said. Dr. McPike, *Tulsa World*, 1959.

For a while, Dr. McPike was the only woman osteopathic doctor in Tulsa, but she later recruited a classmate, Dr. Ella Hicks, to join the practice.

During the flu epidemic of 1918, she worked long hours and proudly stated, "I didn't lose a patient."

She had her office at the Bliss Building, Third and Main street, for about 20 years. She then moved to the Palace Building at Fourth and Main street. Some of her clients were among the most prominent members of society including Harry Sinclair, A.L. Murphy and Charles Page.

"Mr. Page tried to get me to move my practice to Sand Springs, but I couldn't leave Tulsa. I've seen a good deal, but I have never been sorry I studied. It helps a person with his own life," said Dr. McPike, *Tulsa World*, 1959.

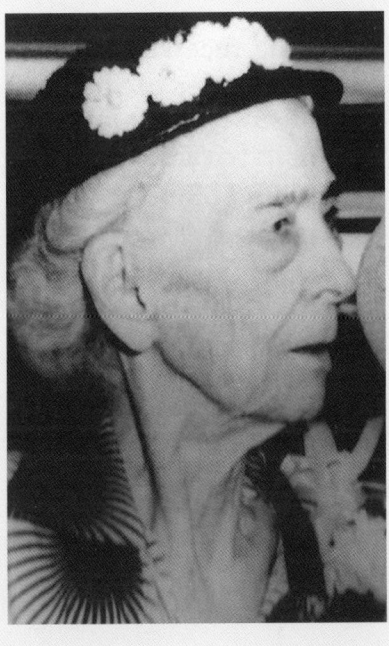

Dr. Mary McPike.

Dr. McPike would travel on outpatient calls to the countryside, "clear to 51st Street," riding on a horse named Dan. "When Dan halted and refused to go, I just got out and started walking after I tied him to something," she said.

After her first gasoline-powered car, the Hupmobile, was purchased in 1918, she didn't like the feel of it. "Being an osteopath and being used to working with my hands it wouldn't work the way I wanted it to." She switched to an automobile with a rechargeable battery and hand controls for the rest of her house calls.

Dr. McPike's husband died in 1933 and she retired in 1941. She also had a sister, Dr. Eva L. Young, who was an osteopathic physician in Tulsa, and a brother, Dr. J.R. Young, who had a practice in Beloit, Wisconsin.

At the time of her death in 1960, she had four children, 10 grandchildren and 10 great-grandchildren. ■

charged $7.50 for the delivery room, $5 for anesthesia, 50 cents a day for drugs and dressings and $1 a day for the nursery. A tonsillectomy cost $10, a red and white blood cell count was billed at $2, and its pharmacy charged 25 cents for a narcotic injection.

Medical students were on strict rotations, according to a letter from Dr. Paul F. Benien, chairman of the hospital committee, on plans for an incoming intern. The intern spent one year living at the hospital on call at all times with the exception of a half-night per week. The student provided his own uniform and received a salary of $10 a month. He collected fees for his services but had to turn it over to the hospital. Duties included scrubbing in on surgical and obstetrical cases, taking patient histories, keeping progress reports and carrying out orders left by the attending physician.

Beginnings of Family Planning

With the onset of the Depression, focus moved to the burgeoning issue of contraception for families to control births. New York's Margaret Sanger started the national conversation after opening the nation's first birth control center with a sister and friend in 1916 in Brooklyn, New York. This was before women could vote, sign contracts, hold bank accounts or divorce abusive husbands. In the 1870s, the Comstock laws made it illegal to distribute birth control and declared literature with contraception information "obscene." In 1923, Sanger opened the Birth Control Clinical Research Bureau in New York City to provide contraception and collect data on the safety and long-term effectiveness of those devices. She also founded the American Birth Control League to address global concerns of population growths. Eventually, those merged to become Planned Parenthood Federation of America.

In 1936, Sanger won a judicial victory when the U.S. 2nd Circuit Court of Appeals ruled that information and data about the impact of unplanned pregnancy and effectiveness of birth control was not obscene. It only affected three states, and it took another 30 years for married couples in all states to get access to medically accurate contraception information. It also ruled that birth control was legal under medical direction.

That same year, the American Medical Association recognized birth control as an integral part of medical practice and education. North Carolina became the first state to recognize birth control as a public health issue and provided contraception services to indigent mothers.

Margaret Sanger: Seated behind desk.

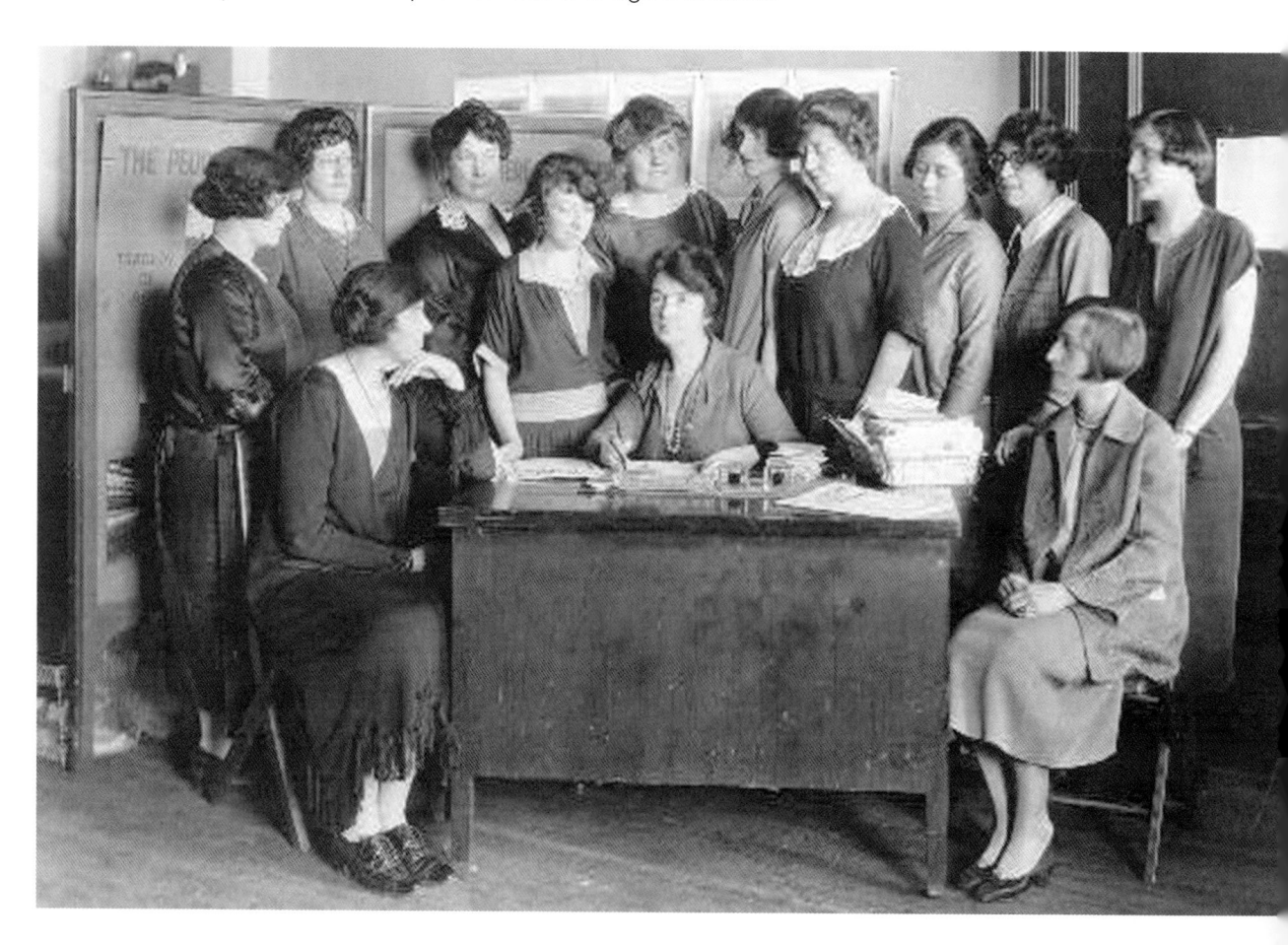

On March 17, 1937, Tulsa opened its first birth control clinic at the Tulsa General Hospital, 755 W. 9th Street. The Tulsa Birth Control League was the founding organization of the clinic, but quickly changed the name to the Tulsa Maternal Health League to sound less controversial.

Georgia Lloyd Jones, wife of *Tulsa Tribune* publisher Richard Lloyd Jones, was the first board president. The clinic was staffed by volunteers with a yearly budget of about $600. It held clinic hours twice a week. Women accepted for services must have been referred by a charitable organization and already had one child. The typical client was married, had about five children and lived in poverty. The founders said opposition was widespread with harassing phone calls and condemnations from churches.

The first day brought in six mothers with varying medical needs. One woman with tuberculosis had two children, ages 2 and 4, with a husband working day labor. She was seeking contraception. Another woman with tuberculosis and five children worried that having more children would risk her health. A 19-year-old with tuberculosis, two venereal diseases and an infant sought birth control, concerned another child would be fatal to her. Two other women had at least two children each and husbands with "irregular" work and did not want to have more children. A 35-year-old woman with six children said her husband was on relief for four years and that if they had any more children "she did not know how they would care for them," stated a *Tulsa Tribune* story.

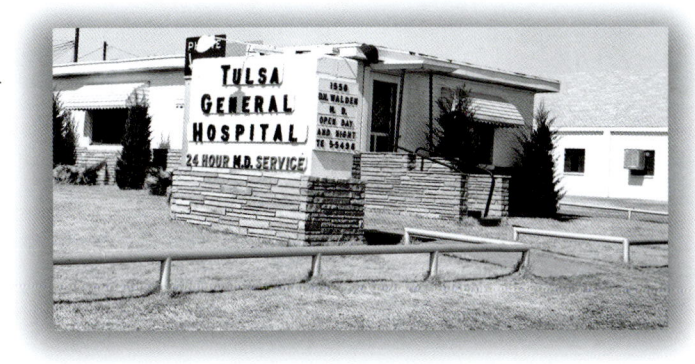

Tulsa General Hospital

"Frightened, uncertain but desperately in need of help, five mothers went to the first birth control clinic of the Tulsa Maternal Health league this morning to receive information to save either their lives or the lives of their children... Competent and busy physicians donated their time to examinations. They were fitted with birth control appliances and told to report next week for further examination." — *Tulsa Tribune*, March 17, 1937.

By 1951, the clinic changed its named to Planned Parenthood and joined the national organization.

SPECIALIZED TCMS CLINICS

As a reflection of the times, the Tulsa County Medical Society faced how to best treat indigent patients. Under the leadership of Dr. Walter Larrabee, the society relied upon studies for the most effective course of care. Discussions about a possible free clinic began in 1936.

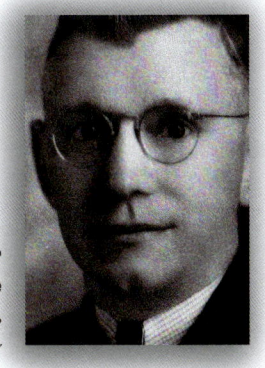

Walter Larrabee M.D.

"The question of treatment of charity patients had long puzzled Tulsa County physicians... Tulsa doctors had long been displeased with the method of administering curative medicine for county indigent patients, the relatively high costs of the old system, and the lack of proper regulation by a medical agency," — From the book, *A History of the Tulsa County Medical Society*.

In 1939, the Tulsa County Medical Clinic for indigent patients opened with public financing in partnership with the county health department. The main

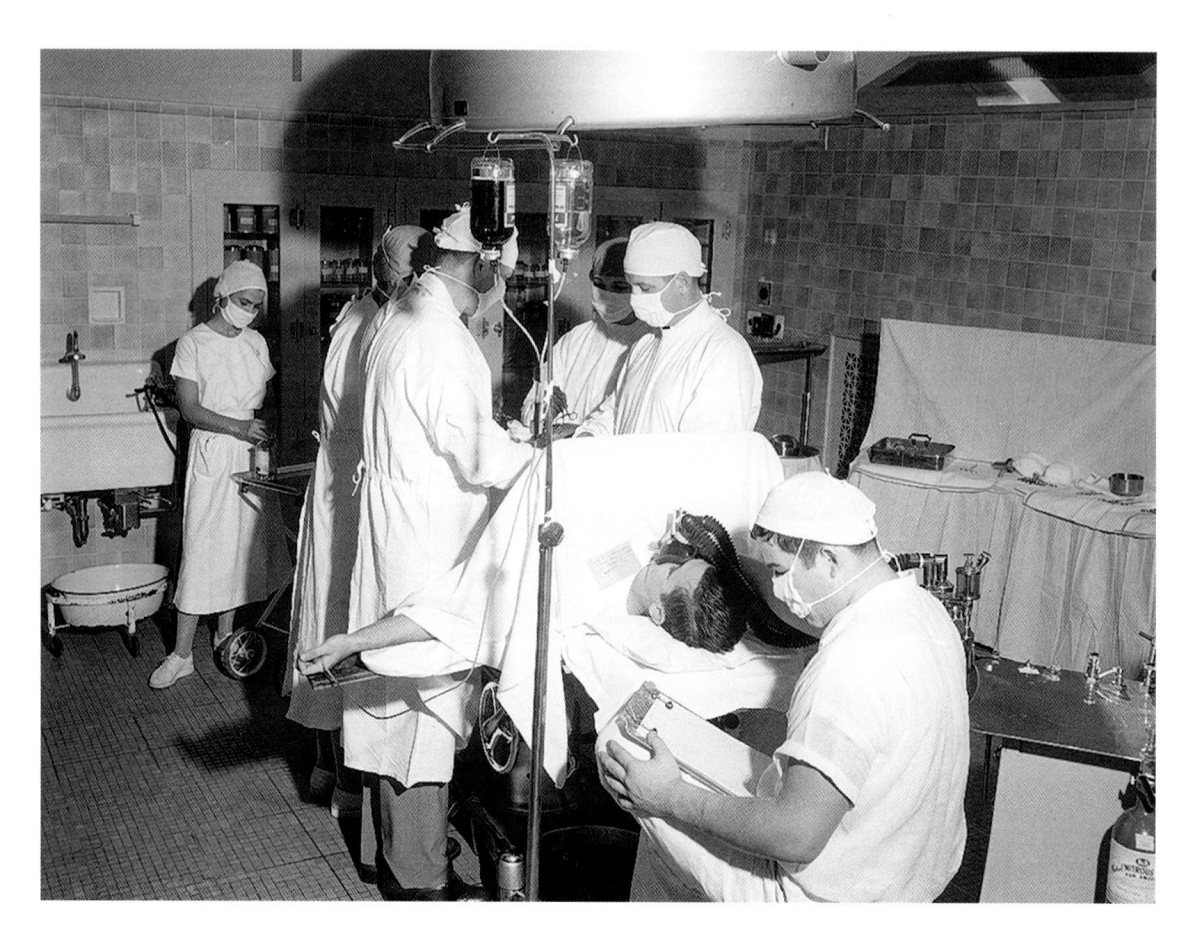

Surgical team at work.

obstacle for implementing the clinic had been consistent denials of support from the county commissioners. After Tulsa County Medical Society established an executive office and secured the 12th floor of the Medical Arts Building, a public campaign won support of the local newspapers and a majority of residents. The contract with the county included medical society members donating time to the clinic, the medical society organization maintaining supervision of the clinic and clinic expenses being paid by the county.

During the first month, about 1,500 patients were examined, and charity medical expenses at the hospital dropped sharply. It is estimated taxpayers saved between $30,000 to $50,000 a year with the clinic's opening.

"Tulsa County indigent patients received the finest medical care available in the county without cost. Facilities were available to them, which the average moderately situated family would not be able to afford from a private doctor. The benefit was mutual, however, as physicians were enabled to conduct clinical studies." — From the book, *A History of The Tulsa County Medical Society.*

In 1937, plans were underway for the creation of a venereal disease clinic under the operation of the Tulsa County Medical Society and the Oklahoma State Health Department. It would later grow into the Tulsa Cooperative Clinic, which treated syphilis and gonorrhea. That year also brought the society's assistance in the organization of the Women's Field Army for Control of Cancer and support for a study of the decentralization of the University of Oklahoma Medical School. ■

CHAPTER 5
(1940 - 1949)

Advancing Medicine in War-Time

2,403 Americans died in the Pearl Harbor attack.

The era ushered in a world war, polio epidemics, rise of osteopathy, antibiotics and a G.I. Bill that encouraged more Americans to study, advance and practice medicine.

For years, Tulsa newspapers — along with other national publications — had been filled with stories of possible war. The country was divided on its role in the growing European war. The front pages of the *Tulsa World* gave a glimpse of what was to come: Local National Guardsmen going through extended training, draft boards appointed in secret and a National Guard aviation outfit added at the Tulsa airport. The federal government nationalized the Pensacola Dam on the Grand River, claiming national defense needs. The regional economy got a boost of tens of millions from the Douglas bomber plant in Tulsa and the government ordnance facility under construction in Baxter Springs, Kansas. In the week before the attack on Pearl Harbor in Hawaii, national wire stories covered President Roosevelt's latest hard-line negotiations with the Japanese Emperor Hirohito over his war with China and alignment with Nazi Germany.

Still, the Japanese bombing was a shock. An editorial in the *Tulsa World* on Dec. 9, 1941, stated, "It was hard for Americans, inured to peace, to realize their security, their liberties, their lives were

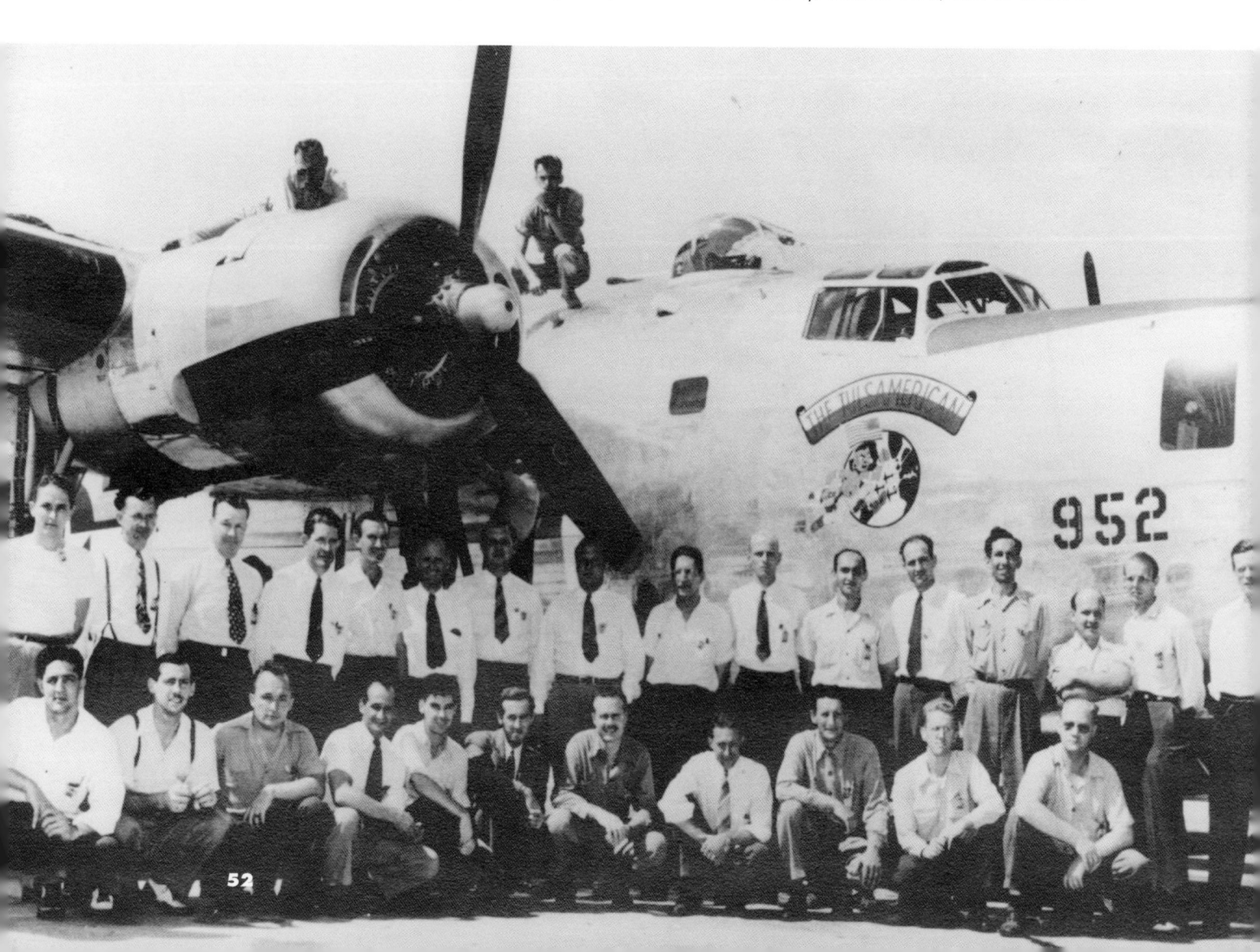

The Tulsamerican:
B-24 Liberator

involved in the insane and infinitely cruel Axis war upon democracy. There had been hopes that, somehow, we would escape."

Daily accounts were published about local men going to and returning from war. Some stories reported on families who received telegrams with news of their loved ones who died in action. On the homefront, the Douglas plant produced the B-24 Liberator, which was the highest produced American aircraft. It then switched to the A-24 Dauntless dive bombers and the A-26 Invader. Men and women flocked to Tulsa to fill the jobs. It's estimated at least 20,000 pilots earned their wings at the Spartan School of Aeronautics and another 5,000 students were trained as mechanics.

Prior to the war, Tulsa had been ranked 33rd nationally in manufacturing. The city jumped to 18th in the U.S. due to war supply and facility contracts. Manufacturing jobs increased from 11,000 in 1930 to 42,000 during the war. Tulsa grew by almost one-third, to 185,000 people.

After years of economic depression, this infusion of cash led to a financial boon. Local department stores reported a 41 percent jump in sales. In the two years ending in December 1945, Tulsa bank deposits rose by nearly $100 million, which was a 40 percent increase. Prosperity showed in other ways — one downtown movie theater added a "swing shift" showing at 1:30 a.m. and the Cain's Ballroom continued to swing with live music.

Hillcrest's Nurses and Staff serving in WWII.

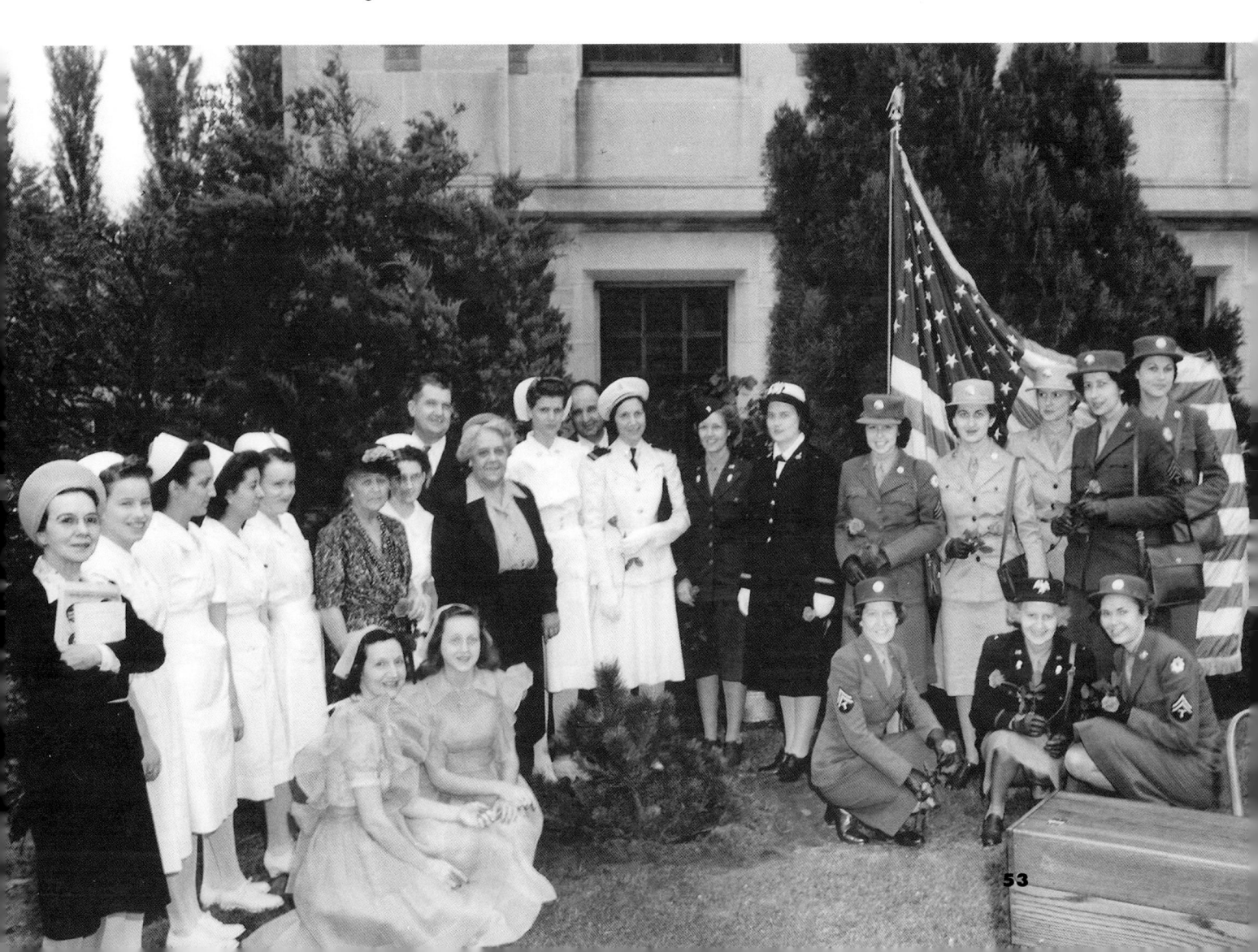

Doctors Go To War

During this era, the Tulsa County Medical Society remained active, hosting health conventions and advocating in the area of payor options and physician training.

In 1940, the Tulsa County Medical Society assisted in the organization of the Group Hospital Service of Oklahoma, a unit of the Blue Cross hospital insurance plan. The plan launched in April 1940. It had been opposed by some doubting physicians and a sizable group in Oklahoma City. The Tulsa physicians pushed the plan through, convinced of its success based on the model of using a physician-dominated board of directors. The plan quickly grew and was almost in every county by 1945.

Consolidated B-24 Liberator Taking Off.

That same year, the Medical Society hosted a "Hall of Health" at the Tulsa Coliseum on the fairgrounds, featuring displays explaining medical progress. More than 26,000 people attended, but it had a significant drawback:

"It was perhaps one of the most unique expositions ever conducted in Tulsa. It represented weeks of hard work on the part of the Tulsa County Medical Society members and employees. While tremendously successful as an educational feature, it's unforeseen expense plunged the Society into a bankrupt condition from which it did not readily recover." — From the book, *A History of the Tulsa County Medical Society.*

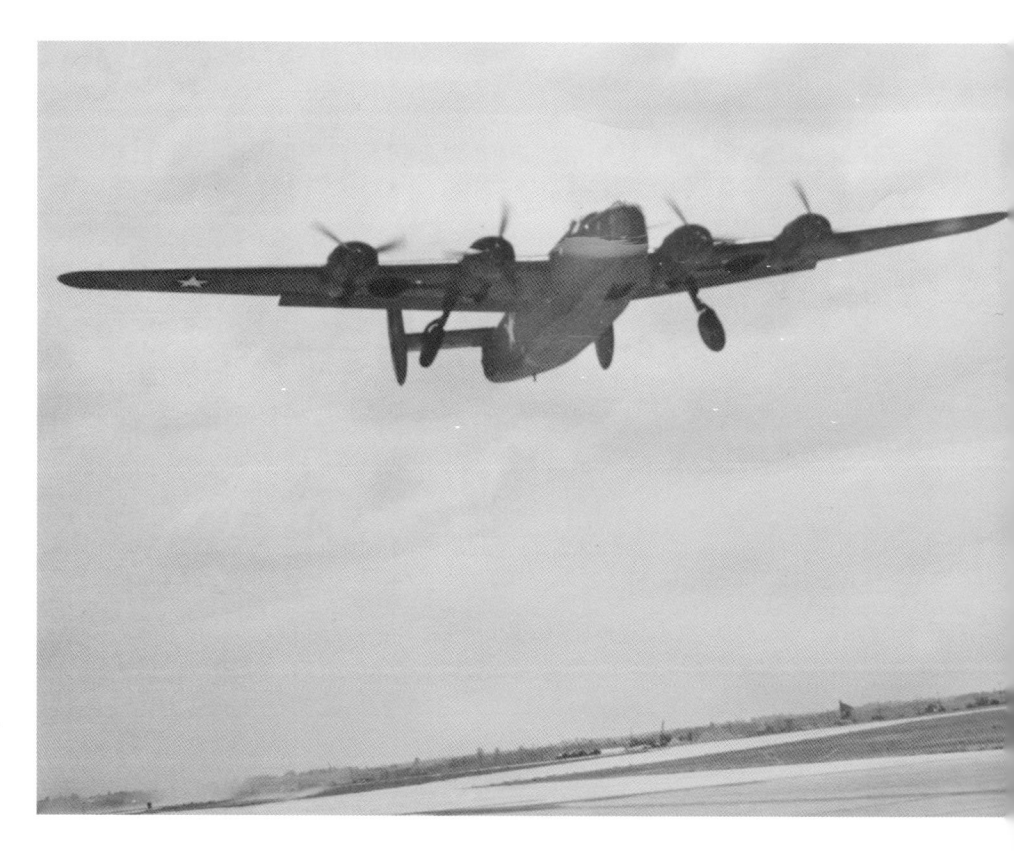

When World War II began, Tulsa County physicians began to leave their practices to serve. It meant changes in the society's activities. Dr. H.B. Stewart, a nationally known anesthesiologist, served as the group's president through the first year of the war.

"He faced a multitude of problems, most of which arose from the unsettled and complex economic and social conditions occasioned by the conflict. With his characteristic energy and directness, however, he prosecuted a valuable program of activity throughout the year," *A History of The Tulsa County Medical Society*.

Tulsa doctors entering service at the start of the war usually went into the Army medical corps. As the Pacific fighting increased and expanded the American Naval fleet, local physicians joining after January 1944 usually entered the Navy.

In Tulsa, about 35 percent of its physicians went to war — 55 doctors. All but two were members of the Tulsa County Medical Society. This does not include interns or medical students. Most were assigned overseas.

At least two Tulsa doctors were injured in combat. Dr. Jack O. Atkins lost his right leg due to machine-gun fire at the Salerno landings. Dr. Logan A. Spann, an eventual co-founder of Doctors' Hospital, was slightly wounded in a landing at Guam as a Navy flight surgeon assigned to the 3rd Marine Division in the South Pacific.

One of the few women practicing medicine in Tulsa also served in the war. Dr. Anna "Luverne" Hays, was a medical officer in the U.S. Navy. She was a lieutenant commander when she retired from the military in 1945. She was a graduate of the University of Michigan School of Medicine in 1926 and specialized in pediatrics. Dr. Hays was an instructor of pediatric medicine at the University of Illinois and spent a year in fellowship training at the University of Vienna in Austria. She came to Tulsa in 1933 and practiced until 1944, when she enlisted in the Navy. Dr. Hays retired from medicine in 1958 and died in December 1965. The Tulsa County Medical Society has a scholarship in her name.

"The loss of a good percentage of civilian practitioners placed a heavy burden on the remaining doctors. The population was rapidly swollen by the local Douglas Aircraft Corporation and by other military defense installations in Tulsa employing large numbers of workers. Increased availability of funds for medical purposes also prompted a greater degree of medical care. The result was long hours for the Tulsa doctors. The penalty proved severe in physical strain and the loss of a number of physicians... was keenly felt." From the book, *A History of The Tulsa County Medical Society*.

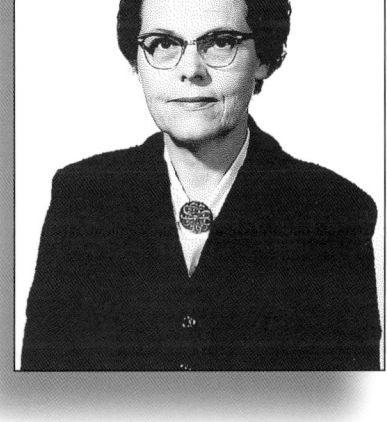

Dr. Anna "Luverne" Hays

The Tulsa County Medical Society set up committees to deal with war-time measures such as rationing of materials. Some projects included prepaid surgical and obstetrical services. It continued to host regular meetings and annual conventions and fight fraudulent practitioners. It had restored its budget by 1943 with a surplus.

By 1945, the society had occupied the entire 12th floor of the Medical Arts Building, had a mailing list reaching 1,000 physicians, operated the Tulsa County Clinic and oversaw the Medical Credit Bureau.

More Doctors
The military recognized the need for more doctors and created specialized training programs in 1942. These would allow a soldier to finish his college education and get started in medical school.

A person enrolled in these programs would be on an accelerated schedule to return to service. The Servicemen's Readjustment Act of 1944, known as the G.I. Bill, encouraged troops to attend higher education. Before the war, most physicians practiced in general medicine, with some specializing in surgery or obstetrics. The change in more veterans completing medical school training coincided with the rise in subspecialties such as neonatologists, pulmonologists, cardiologists, hematologists, enchronologists and ophthalmologists.

Economist Milton Greenberg stated the G.I. Bill added 67,000 more doctors and 22,000 dentists to the workforce. In addition, it brought 450,000 engineers, 240,000 accountants, 238,000 teachers and 91,000 scientists. For every $1 invested by the bill, the return to the American economy by the graduates was $7.

As an example of how the military education programs influenced the number of doctors in Tulsa, Dr. Robert Kendall Endres listed a few in a local history of pediatrics.

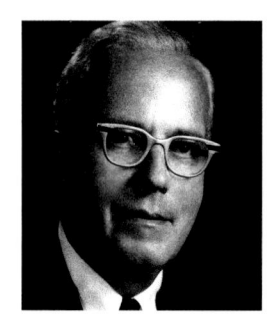

- Dr. Walter F. Sethney (1912-1980): Received a medical degree from Columbia University College and residency in pediatrics at Children's Hospital in Detroit before entering the Army in 1942. Served in Africa and came to Tulsa upon his discharge. He arrived in the middle of a polio epidemic, handling about 126 cases. He established the first poison control center in Tulsa and received a community service award from the Tulsa Chamber of Commerce for his work.

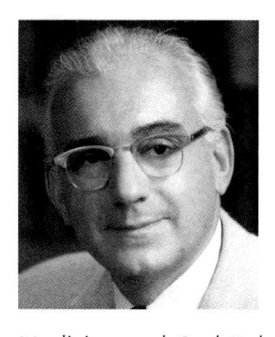

- Dr. Herschel J. Rubin (1912-1996): Earned a medical degree from Hahnemann Medical College in Philadelphia and completed residencies at Willard Parker Hospital in New York and Boston's Massachusetts General Hospital. He entered the Army in 1940 and discharged in 1945. He returned to the Boston hospital for additional training then arrived in Tulsa in 1947. He may be the first to streamline office practices, such as hiring assistants to take notes on patients. Dr. Rubin was a clinical professor for the pediatric departments at the University of Oklahoma-Tulsa College of Medicine and Oral Roberts University.

- Dr. Leon Horowitz (1925-2011): Served as a combat infantryman from 1943 to 1945 and was a prisoner of war. After discharge, he went to medical school at New York University College of Medicine and specialized in pediatrics. Later, he subspecialized as a pediatric allergist, becoming one of the first to become board certified in that area.

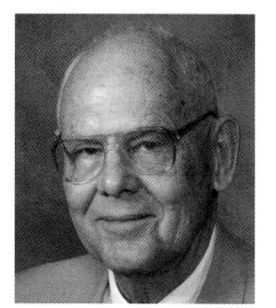

- Dr. John C. Kramer (1926-2010): A graduate of Harvard Medical School, he finished residencies in internal medicine and pediatrics when he was drafted by the Army in 1953. After arriving in Tulsa in the late 50s, he was immediately busy with a polio ward at Hillcrest Hospital. He is best known for his work with cystic fibrosis, becoming one of the first board-certified pediatric pulmonologists in the country. He also became an

Continued on page 58

Dr. Charles Bate

A native of Tennessee and graduate of the Meharry Medical School in Nashville, Dr. Charles Bate came to Tulsa in 1940 and became the first black member of the Tulsa County Medical Society.

When Dr. Bate attended medical school in the mid- to late-30s, few schools accepted black students and internships and residencies were also hard to find. In a 1980 interview with the Junior League of Tulsa oral history project, he said his cost per quarter for his undergraduate at Tennessee State University was $69 and tuition per semester at Meharry was $250.

After finishing his residency, Dr. Bate considered joining the Army, but the military did not accept or promote black soldiers in the same way as white troops. He opted to follow the suggestion of some schoolmates, who said "Tulsa had a strong African American community."

"Tulsa was a city within a city. There were about 20,000 blacks in an area about less than four square miles. I had never seen living conditions in a city like they were in Tulsa. I'd never seen it. I saw 25-foot lots with three houses on one lot. And you'd have to go through the first two houses to get into the last house. There were outdoor privies everywhere. And none of the streets were paved in the Negro area of Tulsa. They didn't get paved up until the late 40s or 50s. Just mud streets everywhere. And very narrow. It was interesting enough to see a church on almost every corner — just all over the place. And another thing that was interesting was the railroad train went right up to Greenwood, which was the main thoroughfare." — Dr. Charles Bate, 1980 Junior League of Tulsa interview.

Yet, Dr. Bate was drawn to the city: "The spirit of the people in Tulsa was tremendous. They had very little, but I mean the people were spiritual."

Dr. Bate explained the expectations of African American doctors from their communities: "The role of the Negro doctor has been a rather interesting thing because he's had to wear many hats. In every community, you found the Negro doctor or the family doctor a strong pillar in the church. Participated in church activities and school activities, the Chamber of Commerce, everything that was trying to upgrade the people you'd find the black doctor committed to it."

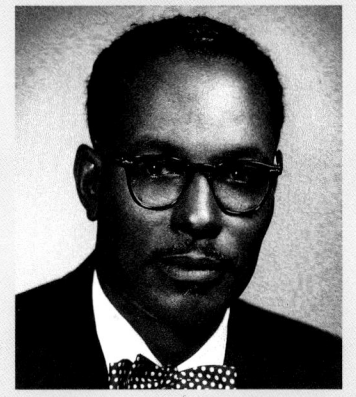

While Dr. Bate worked with many white doctors, his privileges were restricted to Moton Health Center, which served north Tulsa's black community. He said several white physicians argued to include his work in clinical conferences held in Tulsa, especially when some featured topics centered on his cases.

In 1952, Dr. Bate gained membership to the Tulsa County Medical Society. The society held a two-hour special session to amend its bylaws to create a "scientific membership" category. That allowed him to use all of the society's medical facilities and attend all of its medical-related activities and forums. But, it did not carry with it admission to the society's social events. Dr. Bate eventually received full membership.

He was a longtime board member of Moton Health Center, where he was a physician from its opening in 1941 until it was phased out in 1967. He began a personal war on poverty in 1966 with "Operation Hope," a program designed to train high school girls and dropouts for work in medical offices. In 1978, he was named Doctor of the Year by the National Medical Association, an organization of black physicians. The auxiliary to the Tulsa County Medical Society named him and three others as Doctor of the Year in 1982.

Dr. Bate wrote and published a history of black doctors and nurses in Oklahoma, *It's Been a Long Time (And We've Come a Long Way)*, in 1986.

He retired in 1990 and died at age 90 in 2004. He and his wife, Ercelle, had five daughters and 10 grandchildren.

When asked of his proudest accomplishment: "One of the best things would be when we did all this surgery on poor people who needed it. I didn't hardly get enough money out of it to buy a car... but I had a lot of fun doing it and did a lot of good."

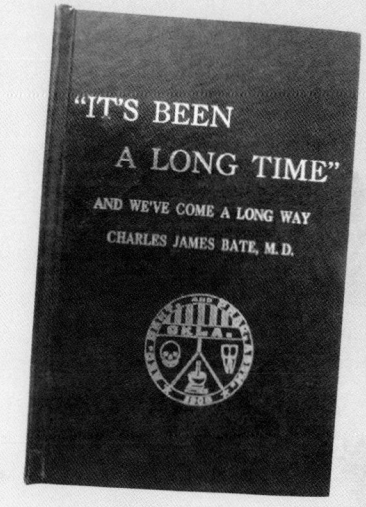

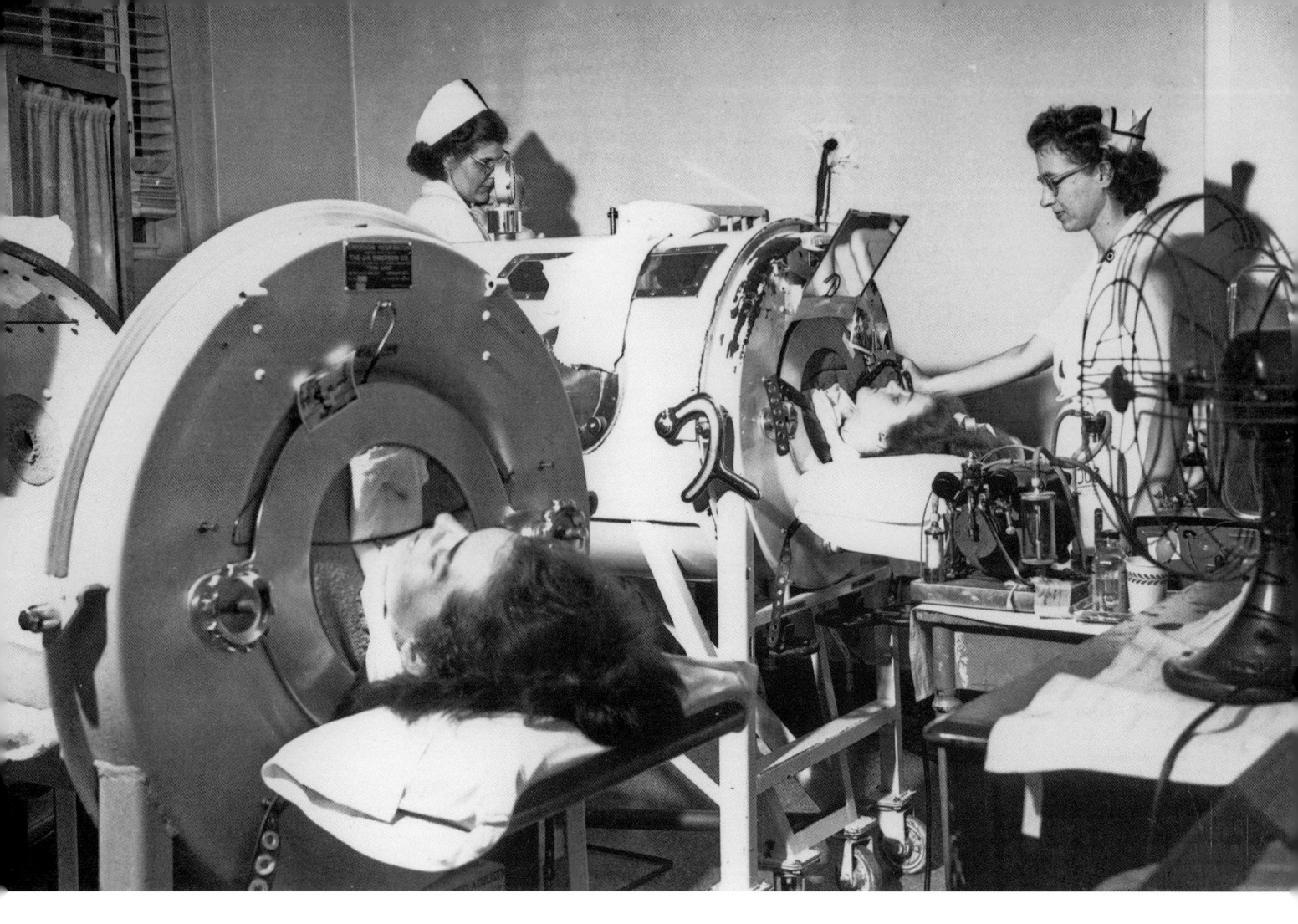

Hillcrest Medical Center's Iron Lungs.

infectious disease specialist, helping to speed up data collection between drug companies and the U.S. Food and Drug Administration.

POLIO EPIDEMICS

Families were often paralyzed in fear during this era as polio outbreaks hit the Tulsa area in the summers of 1916, 1931, 1943, 1949 and 1952. Children were kept from swimming pools, movie theaters and other places with crowds. It is a disease known as infantile paralysis and affects nerves that cause muscle control.

In recalling his experience contracting the disease in 1949 at age 18, Tulsan Doyal Knowles said doctors at Hillcrest Hospital originally thought his back pain and fever were symptoms of appendicitis. The usual diagnostic test was a spinal tap using a large needle to remove fluid.

"I remember one time that in this acute ward not only were all the rooms filled, but they had to put beds in the hall, and they strung electrical wires down the corridor to plug in iron lungs. It seemed like between most every door and room there was either a bed patient or an iron lung," Doyal Knowles, *Tulsa World*, 1997.

Many polio patients were placed in coffin-sized "iron lungs" to help them breathe. They would be on their backs with only their heads poking out while the machine moved oxygen into their bodies. Some might be there for months or years. In Oklahoma, 1949 was the worst year, with 1,323 cases and 66 deaths. The country that year reported 42,033 cases with 2,720 deaths. The worst year for the nation was in 1952 with 57,879 cases and 3,1879 deaths.

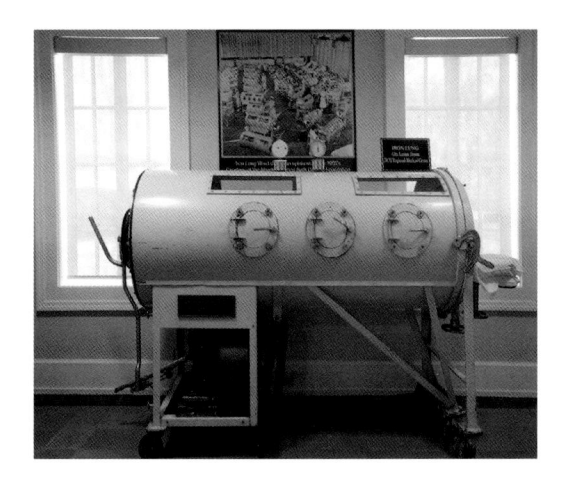

Knowles did not need an iron lung but was wrapped in layers of boiling hot, wool Army blankets with a plastic sheet to trap the heat. The blankets were layered with dry blankets.

"I can remember in July with it being 100 degrees outside, the windows would fog because of the hot packs," — Doyal Knowles, *Tulsa World*, 1997.

The hospital, like most facilities, did not have air conditioning.

Tulsa newspapers wrote about the daily polio total just like sports scores, often printing the names and addresses of local victims. Because much was not understood about the disease transmission, false information took root, such as claims it was related to diet or the color of a person's eyes.

Sand Springs resident Carol Hammans became a March of Dimes poster girl to help raise money for the nonprofit to benefit polio research and treatment: she sat on top of a pile of pennies for a photo to promote the penny drive fundraiser. Hammans was 3 when polio struck her in 1943. The hospitals were full, so she and her family were quarantined before she could be admitted. She spent nearly six years away from home, at St. John Medical Center, Hillcrest Hospital and the Junior League's convalescent home.

Hammans remembers a nurse sending her postcards from vacations and Dr. Ian MacKenzie, who reportedly saw more polio patients than any other Oklahoma Doctor.

"He was wonderful. I thought he was great. I thought he was the best doctor in the world. He just seemed to really care about all the kids and took time for us." — Carol Hammans, *Tulsa World*, 1997.

MacKenzie, a leading orthopedic surgeon, was founder and head of the polio center at Hillcrest until he resigned in 1952. He died at age 50 from injuries sustained in an October 1953 car collision.

Albert Sabin and Jonas Salk developed vaccines that turned the tide in the polio epidemic. In 1963, the Tulsa County Medical Society undertook a massive

Continued on page 62

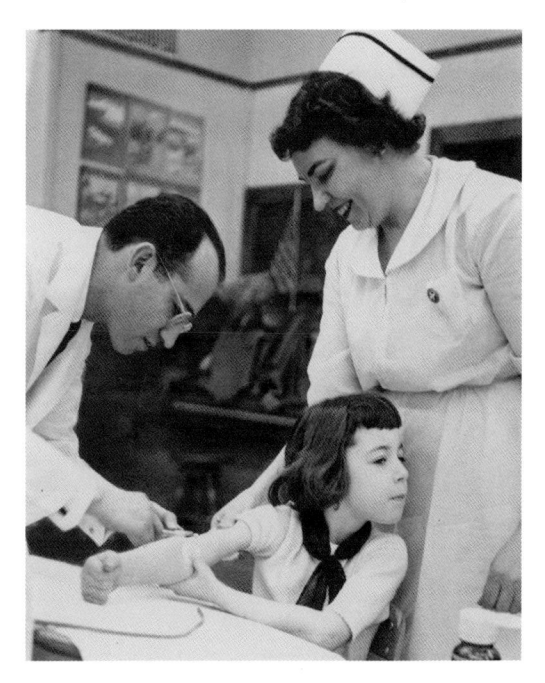

Dr. Ian MacKenzie.

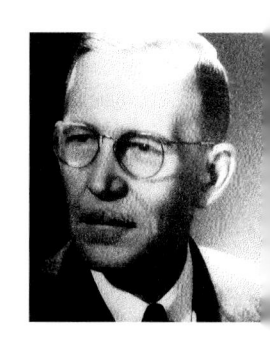

Dr. Jonas Salk: Inoculating a child with the Polio Vaccine, ca. 1954.

The Unspoken Disease Unveiled

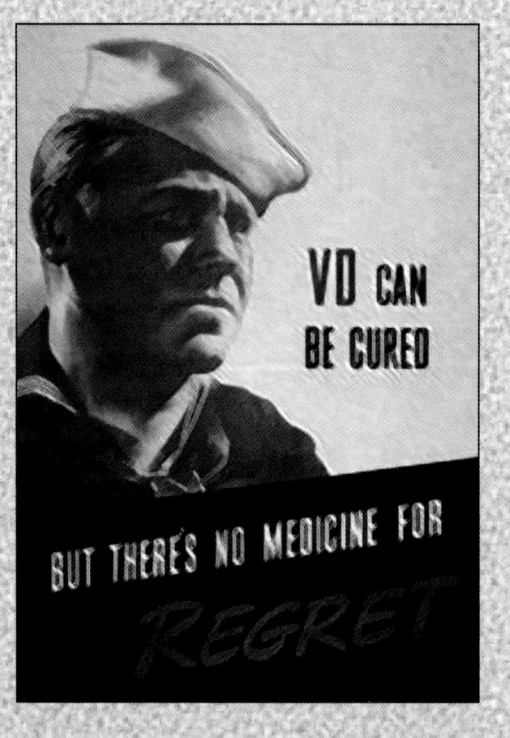

The biggest newspaper investigation of the late 1930s centered on a disease considered too scandalous to speak aloud. Syphilis.

Tulsa World reporter Walter Biscup wrote a six-part exposé in December 1936 on the sexually transmitted disease, which afflicted 200,000 Oklahomans and 9,000 in Tulsa County at that time. It was the most prevalent communicable disease behind measles.

The stories were roundly praised, from ministers to physicians. The U.S. Surgeon General and dozens of residents wrote letters of support in January 1937.

"It was the state's biggest health problem, and something had to be done," Biscup said years later.

This taboo health crisis was described by Dr. W.A. Showman, a Tulsa physician who arrived in the city in August 1927 specializing in dermatology and syphilology. During his residency and speciality training, the clinic in St. Louis, Missouri, would see between 3,000 and 5,000 syphilis cases a week.

"It wasn't nearly spoken about in those early days and that made it more difficult to handle." – Dr. W.A. Showman, 1980 interview.

The *Tulsa World* stories were reprinted in newspapers across the country. Booklets were made with all the stories and given at no cost to civic groups and individuals. Only the New York Times had written about the disease, according to a history written by Gene Curtis of the *Tulsa World* in 2007.

Dr. George Osborn, president of the Oklahoma Medical Society, hailed the work for "removing the mask of secrecy from the hideous features of syphilis." He added, "While medical science has determined the cause of syphilis and evolved methods of diagnosis and treatment, society must recognize its responsibility and cooperate."

Not everything in the series has been found to be accurate. Officials blamed prostitution for more than half the cases and stated 40 percent of victims caught it through casual contact with toilet seats, door knobs, swimming pools or sharing eating utensils or clothes. It was also believed to be transmitted by receiving services from barbers or hair stylists.

Still, it prompted a reform of the state's laws.

In 1943, the state Legislature cracked down on prostitution and empowered health officials to require blood test from people suspected to have syphilis. In 1945, lawmakers passed a bill requiring premarital blood tests for the disease. That mandate remained until 2004.

When that law was removed, Oklahoma health officials said only five new cases of syphilis had been confirmed in the 60,000 tests a year for the previous five years. The decline was credited to better tracking of cases through health agencies and better treatment.

Dr. W.A. Showman

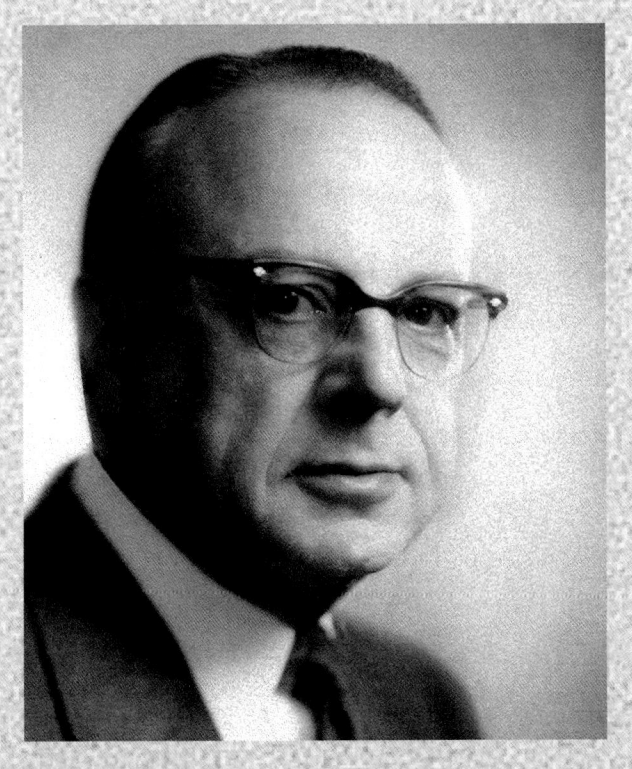

Before penicillin, the most common treatment was with arsphenamine, known as Salvarsan or compound 606, and took about 18 months. The drug is an organoarsenic compound and first modern chemotherapeutic agent. Today, a single dose of penicillin can cure a case.

During World War II, the two worst venereal diseases affecting the troops were gonorrhea and syphilis. Though treatment had improved with sulfa drugs and penicillin, it was still a loss of time, cost and redirection of needed medical resources.

The military started a campaign with slogans such as "Venereal Diseases Aid the Axis" on equipment and food ration containers. Brochures about sexual health were distributed emphasizing safe sex, stating "most prostitutes" have a disease and "manhood comes from healthy sex organs." The military also provided free condoms — six per man, per month. Chemical prophylactic kits were issued to men in case they feared coming into contact with the disease. It contained a tube of 5 grams of ointment (30 percent calomel and 15 percent sulfathiazole) direction sheet, soap cloth and cleansing tissue.

It was World War II that discovered effective treatment for patients in the early stages of syphilis. In 1943, doctors at a U.S. Marine Hospital on Staten Island in New York applied an antibiotic to cure four patients, and experiments started. In 1944, an academic paper was published stating penicillin injections should be administered every few hours for eight days.

Two American studies of syphilis treatment during the 1930s and 1940s resulted in scandals and apologies decades later. U.S. scientists conducted medical experiments on impoverished patients through the Tuskegee Institute and in Guatemala without informing those in the study.

Reporting of syphilis cases to the U.S. Centers for Disease Control and Prevention began in 1941 and totaled 485,560, for a rate of 368.2 people per 100,000 with the disease. The height of the epidemic was in 1943 with 575,593 new cases in the U.S., for a rate of 447. In 2014, the CDC states 63,450 syphilis cases reported for a rate of 20.1, which is the highest total since 1995.

Dr. Showman recalled how advances in pharmacology revolutionized this sexually transmitted disease. He said the treatment evolved to encourage a patient to "run down the contacts" of others who may be infected as a way to control the spread.

"When penicillin came along, it almost immediately got rid of infectious syphilis. Our speciality — dermatology and syphilology — dropped the syphilology because there was no syphilis to speak of." — Dr. W.A. Showman, 1980.

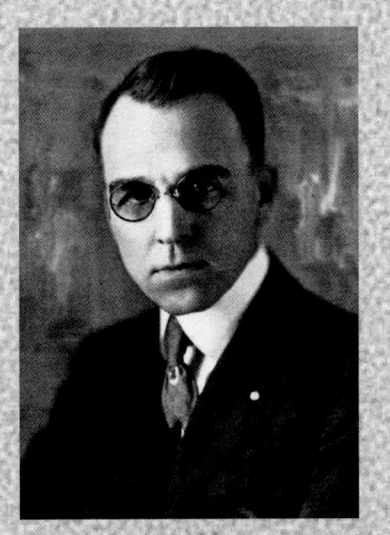

■

Dr. George Osborn

immunization campaign, enlisting more than 1,000 volunteers and staffing nearly 50 clinics to distribute the oral polio vaccine. By the end of the campaign, area residents had taken 780,224 doses of all types of the vaccine. Public health authorities said that more than 70 percent of the total population had been immunized.

Today, the disease is eradicated throughout most of the industrialized world. Internationally, polio cases have fallen by 99 percent between 1988 and 2014, from 350,000 to 359 reported cases, according to the World Health Organization. Only two countries — Pakistan and Afghanistan — have never stopped transmission of polio. There remains no cure for polio, only prevention. The WHO points out as along as the poliovirus remains, it can be imported into a polio-free country and spread rapidly among unimmunized populations. Polio vaccine, given multiple times, can protect a child for life.

Hospitals Evolve

In 1941, changes started on the former Maurice Willows Hospital, which was founded to serve north Tulsa in the aftermath of the devastation of the 1921 Race Riot. In 1932, the hospital was incorporated into a larger facility at 603 E. Pine St. and was known as the Tulsa Municipal Hospital No. 2.

Robert Russo Moton.

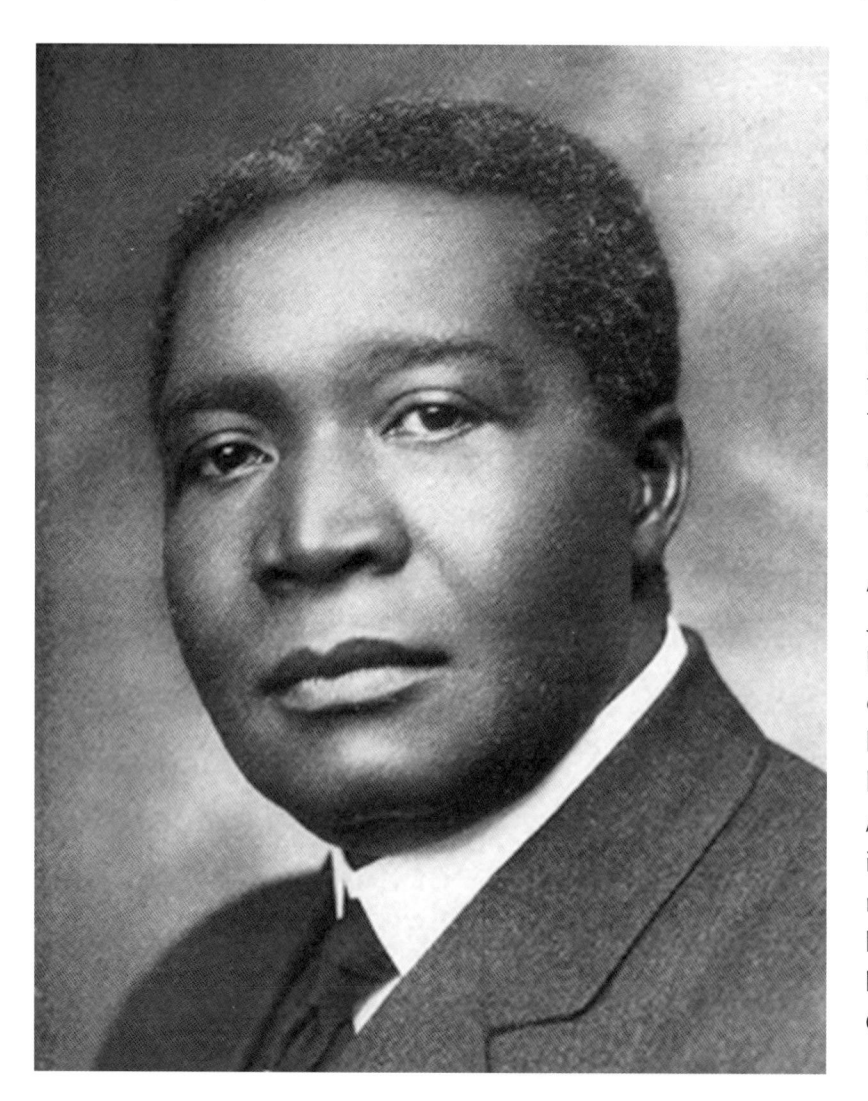

In 1941, the City of Tulsa transferred management of the municipal hospital to a board of community representatives. It was renamed Moton Memorial Hospital after Robert Russa Moton, a former principal of the Tuskegee Institute who died in 1940. It was a 27-bed private hospital.

After World War II, the Junior League of Tulsa began to change and expand its convalescent home for crippled children located at 1448 S. Lewis Ave. It started to withdraw its administrators and move to a community board. By the early 50s, it had become the Children's Medical Center.

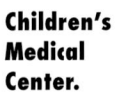

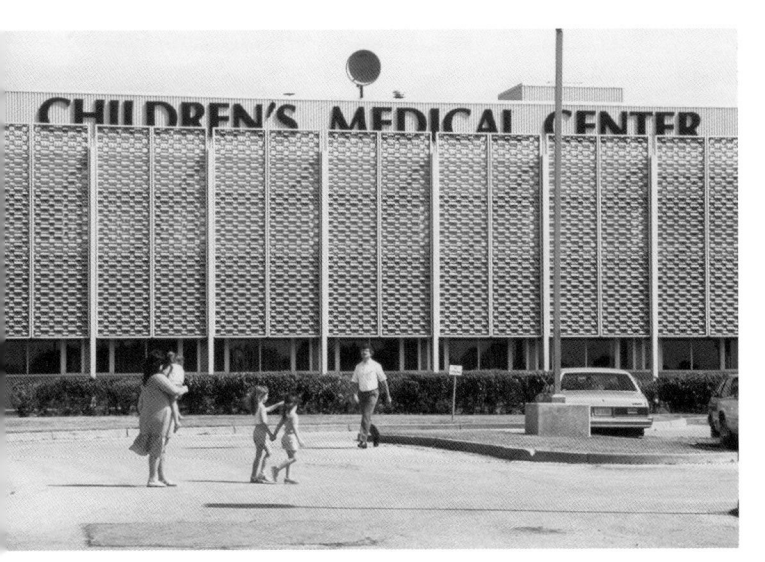

Founding of Oklahoma Osteopathic Hospital

Osteopaths were denied volunteer service in the Medical Reserves Corps for World War I and World War II. It is estimated that 45,000 medical doctors were enlisted to serve and care for the 7.5 million American military force. This left osteopaths on the home front and reforms began that transformed the profession. Before the war, the American Medical Association branded osteopaths as "cultists," called it dishonorable to consult with a D.O., and banned professional relationships between the two.

Children's Medical Center.

"This repudiation of service would lead to legislative and educational advances that allowed osteopathic medicine to reform, grow, and professionalize into the early framework of what it is today," *The Journal for the American Osteopathic Association*, June 2012.

The osteopathic profession increased standards for student admission into schools and added higher quality faculty to increase the percentage of students passing state-required medical licensing requirements. As veterans returned, they were recruited into the programs. These changes led to the federal government supporting the osteopathic schools and institutions.

In Tulsa, the demands on osteopathic doctors were growing, and physicians needed a larger hospital facility. The Byrne Memorial building was inadequate. During this time, the facility known as the Tulsa Hospital at Ninth Street and Jackson Avenue had morphed into the Westside Hospital. By 1943, the building was seized by mortgage foreclosure and placed up for auction.

Dr. John W. Orman quickly moved into action to buy the hospital. On Jan. 12, 1943, he called a meeting at an office at the Palace Building to finalize the articles of incorporation for the Osteopathic Hospital Founders Association. Names on the document include Dr. Roman, Dr. C.P. Harth and Dr. C.D. "Pop" Heasley. The founding trustees, all osteopathic doctors, listed are: H.C. Baldwin, Paul F. Benign, John E. Halliday, C.P. Harsh, C.D. Heasley, G.H. Meyers, John W. Roman, L.A. Reiter, A.G. Reed and Louis M. Shea. The following September, Dr. Meyers resigned from the board and was replaced by Dr. Robert D. McCullough, who is considered a founder.

The articles were filed with the Secretary of State for Oklahoma at a fee of $4.60. Among the statements in the articles:

"That the purpose for which the corporation is formed is charitable and nonprofit, and to establish and maintain a hospital for the care of the sick, to prevent and treat disease, to treat personal injuries, crippled or deformed bodies, and render similar service as may be proper to the care or relief of human ailments, injuries or physical suffering."

When the articles were drafted, minutes show that 49 osteopathic doctors were invited to become members. Each founder contributed $1,000 and sought other private donations to buy the building. On Nov. 1, 1943, Dr. McCullough took the bid of $35,000 to the Tulsa County Courthouse on the day of the auction. It was the only bid for the building, which was once appraised for $350,000. By the end of the month, the founders decided to call the building the Oklahoma Osteopathic Hospital and contacted Tulsa architect Joseph Koberling to lead renovations. He stayed with the hospital through expansions and remodeling through 1975.

Oklahoma Osteopathic Hospital Building Committee.

It is believed to be the first hospital completely made of solid brick. Dr. James F. Routsong, who interned at the hospital in 1948, explained its solid construction to the authors of *Dreams, Challenge and Change*, a history written for the hospital's 50th anniversary:

"When it was demolished (in 1981), the contractor thought one throw of the wrecking ball would take out a whole corner. I have a series of slides showing that it took 18 blows with the ball to loosen the first brick. Before the addition (in 1953), there was a discussion as to whether to build on to the original building or move to a new location to build a totally new hospital. In his report, the state hospital engineer said, 'This is the best constructed building in the state; continue to add to it.'"

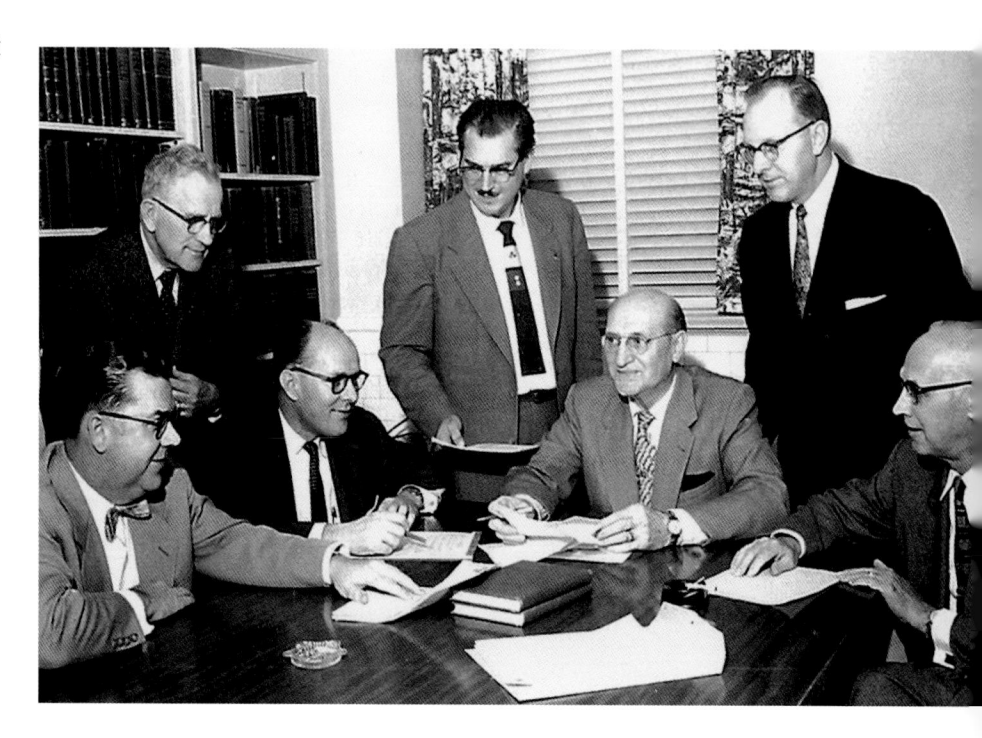

Renovations were estimated to cost $125,000. Local osteopathic physicians donated about $45,000 total. This was at a time when a house call or an hour's work in the office was charged at between $3 and $5. A fundraising company based in Kansas City, Missouri, led a public capital campaign that raised $45,000 and other loans and large donations were secured.

The modernized hospital opened in 1944, and shortly after, the federal government granted approval to treat emergency maternal and infant patients and for the administration of premarital and other examinations. The hospital shared proportionally with other Tulsa hospitals in the receipt of blood plasma distributed by the Oklahoma Health Department.

Leading up to the official opening on Dec. 17, 1944, public festivities were planned. More than 100 inches of newspaper space was purchased for promotion, 2,500 opening invitations were mailed and 2,500 brochures printed. Hundreds of residents arrived the first day for tours. The building had 60 beds and 14 bassinets, including a $4,600 nursery, new labor and delivery rooms and an enclosed porch for use as a solarium.

Charges for use were $4 daily on a general ward, $5 for a semi-private room, $6 for a private room without a bathroom, $7 for a private room with a bath and $8.50 for a private room with a bath and telephone. Operating room costs for a major procedure was $15 and $10 for a minor procedure. A tonsillectomy and/or adenoidectomy was $6. In the first five months of operation, 215 babies were born there. The first patient was a 26-year-old defense worker needing an appendectomy.

Oklahoma Osteopathic Hospital

The rift between osteopaths and the allopaths remained, including the difficulty in getting the American Red Cross to approve allowing its nurses to work at the hospital. Many young doctors wrote the hospital seeking positions because they could not serve as a medical officer in the military. In a letter written by a soldier stationed with a construction battalion in Gulfport, Mississippi in 1944:

"In the letter, he explained that after receiving a D.O. degree and advanced training in radiology, he had supervised the X-ray department at the Naval Air Station in New York for 16 months. In spite of his education and experience, he was ranked only as a pharmacist's mate at his new base, and there was no room for him in radiology. He hoped (Oklahoma Osteopathic Hospital) would request him, thus releasing him from service."— *Dreams, Challenge and Change.*

It is unknown what happened to this man's request.

In 1947, the board expanded to include non-physicians to gain experience to complement the existing medical expertise. They were allowed to vote on all non-medical matters. The first lay members of the board were Paul Estill, of Sand Springs Home Interests; William Gates, owner of a hardware business; Paul Hedrick, oil editor of the *Tulsa World*; Dan P. Holmes, insurance salesman; Jack McCarter, of the First National Bank; and Paul I. Johnston and J.W. Satterwhite, who were involved in the oil business.

A women's auxiliary formed in 1948 to focus on patient needs. In December 1948, a celebration of the first four years of operation attracted about 800 Tulsans. That year, the hospital treated 1,030 patients, handled 1,657 surgical cases and recorded 670 births.

Medical Breakthroughs

The war brought a pressing demand for better treatments of injuries, disease and infection. The advancements in penicillin is heralded as one of the most important discoveries in this decade. Before this, the sulfa drugs were the most common pharmaceuticals in use. Howard Florey and Ernst Chain developed a usable form of penicillin in 1940, and a year later the clinical trials showed abilities to cure life-threatening conditions. Several strains were developed. The 1945 version of penicillin was 20 times more potent than what was available in 1939. The drug was used en masse on D-Day in wound dressing to prevent gangrene while the injured waited for surgeons.

In 1944, Selman Waksman discovered streptomycin, an effective antibiotic to fight tuberculosis. It led to further types of antibiotics including chloromycetin in 1947. Also, the war launched better treatment into malaria, due to mosquito bites in the Pacific Theater, and in research on blood transfusions.

Statewide Medical Expansions

The issue of a national health care program had not gone away. President Harry Truman had made suggestions of a socialized-type system. The American Medical Association assessed each member $50 to campaign against that idea.

In November 1945, President Truman outlined a five-part program for improving the health and health care of Americans. The Hospital Survey and Construction Act was passed in response to the first part of the proposal, which called for the construction of hospitals and related health care facilities. It was designed to provide federal grants and guaranteed loans to improve hospital facilities and provide 4.5 beds per 1,000 people. It required a certain amount of free or reduced-charge care, have emergency room doctors on staff and allowed for anyone to seek help in emergency rooms. The bill made it illegal to racially discriminate in hospitals but did allow for segregation. That provision was struck down by the courts in 1963. The AMA gave its approval.

Oklahoma had about 56 percent of the beds to meet the minimum standard of the law with rural areas most in need. Some patients in southeast parts of the state travelled more than 75 miles for a health facility. By August 1956, the state had built more health centers to attract doctors into underserved areas, cutting down the distance for patients to less than 25 miles. When the law was passed, several state health agencies examined gaps in the health care system.

Between 1947 and 1956, more than 2,000 hospitals or additions to medical or surgical facilities were built or in the planning stages of construction. The total cost was about $26 million, with $16 million paid by the state and the rest by the federal government. The University of Oklahoma Medical School set up a program where doctors in small towns took on senior medical students for training. Research stepped up from 17 projects in 1945 using $2,257 in outside funding to 86 projects in 1955 with assistance from $262,577 in grants. The expansions benefited the outpatient capacity of the Convalescent Children's Home operated by the Tulsa Junior League. ■

CHAPTER 6
(1950 - 1959)

Modernizing Medicine

Patient Receiving Cobalt-60 Therapy.

The 1950s ushered in a more modern era for Tulsa in terms of culture, business, communications, education and medicine.

Bell's Amusement Park opened in 1951 and remained a staple of Tulsa entertainment into the next century. The Golden Driller statue went up as a display at the International Petroleum Exposition and became a lasting Tulsa symbol. The Tulsa Ballet was founded in the decade along with the gift of the Gilcrease Museum to the city. As part of the celebration of Oklahoma's 50th anniversary, Tulsa buried a 1957 Plymouth (named the Belvedere) in the Tulsarama time capsule at Sixth Street and Denver Avenue, and it was opened a half century later.

Utica Square opened in a stylish neighborhood in 1952 as the city's first shopping center. By 1959, the city boasted 21 shopping centers, five others under construction and applications for 20 more. Just two months before the dawn of the decade, KOTV-Channel 6 launched the city's first television broadcast. Three more would be added by 1959: KVOO-Channel 2, KOED-Channel 11 and KTUL-Channel 8. The Oklahoma Educational Television Authority (OETA) was established, and network cable hookups started appearing.

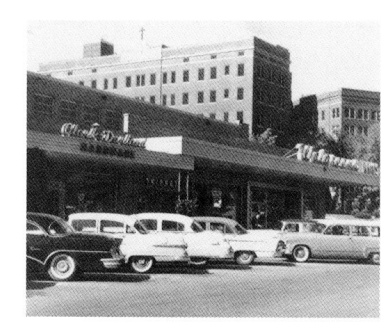

Utica Square Shopping Center: Circa 1954.

Tulsa's infrastructure grew as the population took leaps, beginning with 182,740 residents in 1950 and growing by 43 percent in the next 10 years to 261,684 people. Lake Eucha and a second pipeline from Lake Spavinaw added to the city's water supply. The Tulsa Metropolitan Area Planning Commission was established, which continues to oversee zoning and the comprehensive development plan for the city. Tulsa's land mass more than doubled, annexing nearly 26 miles into the city with the greatest expansion in the south and east. It increased the city's size from about 24 square miles to about 50 square miles. The only de-annexation during this time was the city ceding control of the fairgrounds to the county.

Tulsa Water Needs Meeting.

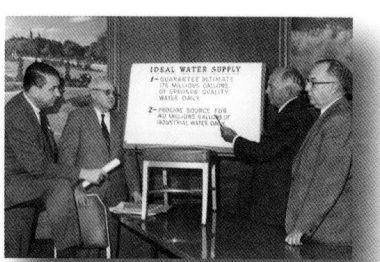

All this change attracted physicians, medical professionals, specialists and a boon in hospital expansions. At each facility, the administrators reported not being able to keep up with the demands of such a burgeoning city.

CREATION OF THE
TULSA CITY-COUNTY HEALTH DEPARTMENT

Efforts to consolidate city, county and school health departments into one agency began in the late 1940s and became reality in 1950. The move was to provide more money and resources to meet public health needs. It was a consolidation endorsed by the Tulsa County Medical Society.

Street Commission Discussing Tulsa's Expanding City Limits.

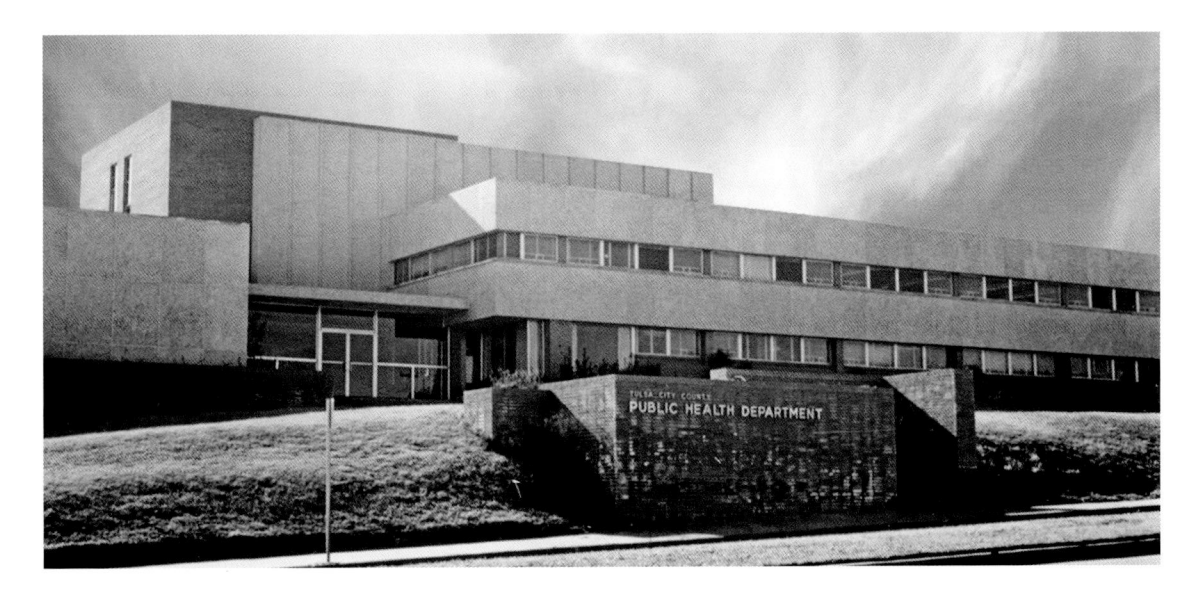

Tulsa City-County Health Department: located at 4616 E. 15th Street.

Before this time, public health care was provided by a variety of sources, including city, county and a voluntary group called the Tulsa Public Health Association, which focused on nursing care and controlling tuberculosis. School officials had opposed the merger. In a December 1948 school board meeting, Tulsa school board president Ben O. Kirkpatrick said no district official has been authorized to move forward with consolidation.

"The health program of the Tulsa school system is recognized by school authorities throughout the country as one of the best in the nation, and we are constantly answering inquiries from other school systems which desire to pattern their health activities along Tulsa lines. We intend to continue to maintain an excellent health program," — TPS School Board president Ben O. Kirkpatrick, *Tulsa Tribune*, Dec. 3, 1948.

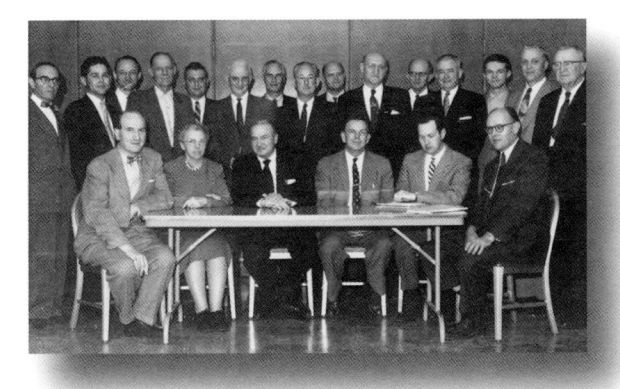

A response from Charles Follansbee, chairman of the chamber of commerce health committee, warned against making decisions too early. He said the merger was in the study phase, but that the school health budget was $22,000 annually. A consolidated agency would be about $300,000 a year budget, using local and federal funds.

"For the school board to attempt to block the program before it is even informed on it, considering the small part they would be asked to contribute, is unfortunate," said Charles Follansbee, *Tulsa Tribune*, Dec. 3, 1948.

The school was successful in staying out of the merger. On Feb. 6, 1950, the Tulsa City Commission and county commissioners signed an agreement for a cooperative health department to be overseen by a superintendent of health. The state law had not kept up with the structure, leaving no legislative authority for such an integrated city-county health organization. In 1955, the Legislature passed a law to establish the agreements for Tulsa and Oklahoma counties. Tulsa officials then amended its agreement to reflect state law, calling the agency the Tulsa City-County Health Department and changing the top administrator's title from superintendent to medical director.

Above: Tulsa's Public Health Committee.

The nursing personnel of the Public Health Association were housed with the health department. Nurses from the Public Health Association provided home-based, direct patient care while the health department nurses provided traditional public health services. The Public Health Association had its own board and was mostly funded by the United Way. Eventually, the association separated from the health department and became the Visiting Nurses Association of Tulsa.

Dr. T. Paul Haney, M.D., led the agency from its inception, hired from St. Petersburg, Florida, at a salary of $12,500 annually. The city paid $10,000 and the county paid $2,500. The other 1950 medical personnel at the department included Dr. James H. Neal, M.D., as assistant superintendent of health, Dr. Margaret G. Hudson, M.D., as director of maternal and child health division, Dr. David V. Hudson, M.D., as director of division of communicable disease and Dr. Richard Apffel, M.D., as director of child guidance. The first annual budget was $254,660.

Speaking in support of consolidation in 1950 were the League of Women Voters, physicians, health-care

Hillcrest Medical Center: After 1950s expansion.

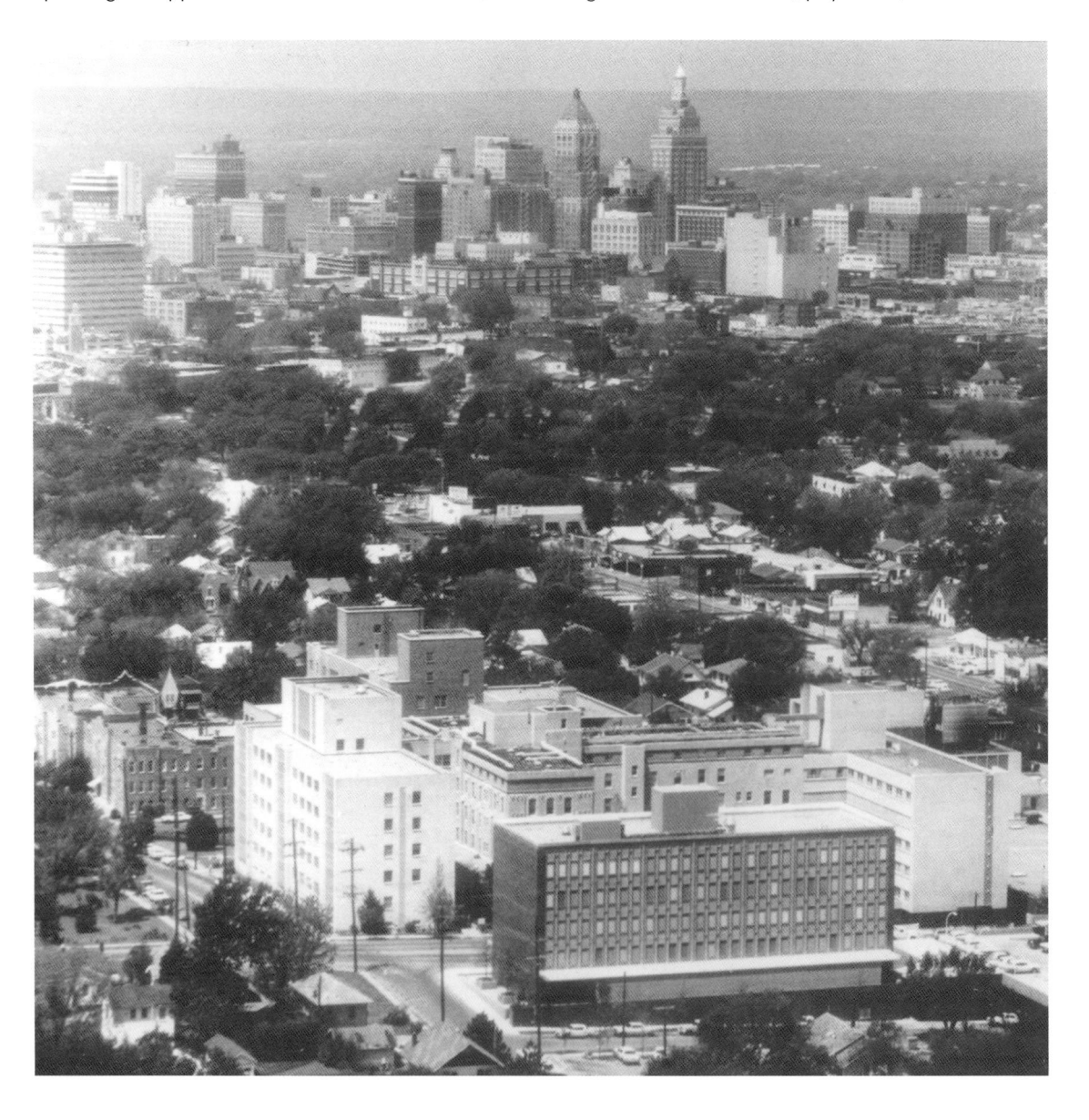

workers and several elected officials. James Slater, sanitary engineer, told the county commissioners at a meeting that the merger would mean city and county residents would get the same health services.

"Disease doesn't stop at the city boundaries. It means a healthy county increases the economic value of the city and means efficiency in government," — said James Slater, *Tulsa Tribune*, Jan. 2, 1950.

Locations of the health department were at 521 N. Boulder Ave. and 536 E. Oklahoma St. In 1954, new health centers were constructed at Bixby, Broken Arrow, Skiatook, Collinsville and Sand Springs. In 1957, the building that served as the main center for decades was built — at 4616 E. 15th Street, near the fairgrounds.

One of its first actions the city-county health department launched was in June 1950 against "doctored" hamburgers. The agency sought an ordinance to regulate what could be added to hamburger meat. It was reported that meat being sold contained chemical preservatives, powdered milk, potato flour, cereals and other substances to give body and weight. The agency sought labeling of hamburger to show whether it was pure ground beef or veal. The department's board also swiftly passed an ordinance that same month requiring all meat sold in Tulsa be inspected. Veterinarians from Oklahoma A&M (now Oklahoma State University) and state health officials found only one-third of meat sold to Tulsans had been government inspected. The move created a division of meat and poultry inspection within the health department. Health department sanitation workers also started handing out tickets for refuse violations, $2 for a first offense and $4 for each fine after that.

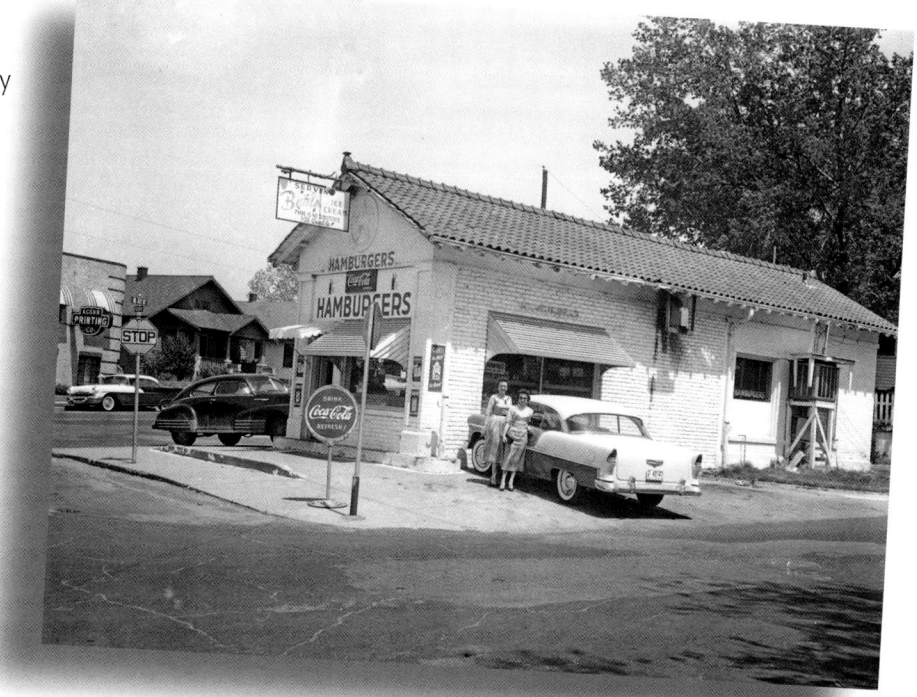

A Typical Hamburger Joint.

Other initial projects included working with municipalities for improved water supplies and sewer systems, helping schools with health education, adding more maternal and child care clinic programs and getting more effective results from the venereal disease clinics. It also worked with a group called the Pilot Club to provide dental care to low-income children.

TULSA GETS FLUORIDE

Community fluoridation of water became the policy of the U.S. Public Health Service in 1951, and Tulsa joined municipalities in adding fluorides to drinking water. Also like other cities, it was not without opposition.

The policy came from more than two decades of study into fluorosis, which causes brown stains and mottling of the teeth. It was found that low concentrations of the mineral fluoride, which exists in nearly all water supplies, serve as a prevention of cavities by building enamel of teeth and healthy bones. This is particularly notable in young children.

In minutes from a Jan. 6, 1953, public meeting about the fluoridation of Tulsa water, those against fluoridation questioned the purported benefits while those in support cited scientific research. The debate was in a presentation to the Tulsa city commissioners. Water Commissioner Glenver McConnell told the commissioners that the Oklahoma Department of Health gave approval for fluoridation of Tulsa water with details of how the process would be completed and regulated.

"The State Department of Health has no doubt that Tulsa's Water Personnel is quite competent to add the fluorides to the city water supply," the minutes state.

A crowd of about 125 people attended the meeting, and each side chose a spokesperson. Dr. Fred E. Simms, president of the Tulsa Dental Society, spoke in favor of fluoridation, reading a short statement about the merits. He cited a need to "respect beliefs and teachings" of other groups including the American Medical Association, American Water Works Association, American Dental Association and other technical and professional organizations. He stressed the groups support a controlled fluoridation to be beneficial.

> **I am wondering why New York City, a hot-bed for communism has not even proposed fluoridation.**
>
> Walter J. Madson, President of the Tulsa Organic Farm and Garden Club

Walter J. Madson, president of the Tulsa Organic Farm and Garden Club, took his allotted time to speak directly to Dr. Simms about his reasons for opposing the move. Among his statements:
- "I am wondering why New York City, a hot-bed for communism has not even proposed fluoridation."
- "If fluoridation will do what dentists say, will it not put 90 percent of the dentists out of business?"
- "If an excessive amount of fluoride is put into the water, is there an antidote?"

In response the last question, Dr. Simms replied, "We are speaking of controlled fluoridation. There are any number of communities that have a natural fluoride content in their water far above the 1 ppm (parts per million) we are recommending for Tulsa." Another physician added that lime water or alum prevents poisoning by fluoride.

"How do you explain the increase in heart disease, polio, nephritis, and numerous other dread diseases after Detroit began fluoridating their water supply?" asked Mr. Madson.

"Detroit is not fluoridating their water supply," answered Dr. T. Paul Haney.

After a burst of laughter from the room, Madson said he meant Grand Rapids, Michigan. Then, a statement was made that Tulsa would be adding less than .05 parts per million in fluoride. The minutes reflect that Madson "took up a great deal of the morning session with his questioning" and cited a University of Texas study pointing to fluorides causing cancer.

Dr. Max Armstrong countered this statement with a published paper from the Texas Department of Health titled "Facts Relative to Rumors That Fluoridation is Harmful." It outlined problems with that university study and added other more professionally and scientifically accepted research. It was discussed that young people would benefit the most, fluoride could not be eliminated by boiling and fluorides taken from the air and earth is more complicated than those from a laboratory.

William L. Wall spoke for the Christian Scientist group stating they felt it was an infringement on the constitutional rights of American people to worship as they pleased and to select the type of medication which they desired. Others in opposition spoke about waiting for more facts or about the legal liability if fluoride hurts the residents. The city attorney cited three court cases allowing cities the right to treat its water. All those in favor of fluoridation were physicians or members of the health department.

Tulsa moved forward with fluoridation. By 1960, the national fluoridation movement reached about 50 million people. By 2006, nearly 70 percent of the U.S. population was on public water systems treated with fluorides. In 2011, federal officials renewed its support for fluoridation, stating the optimum level is .7 parts per million.

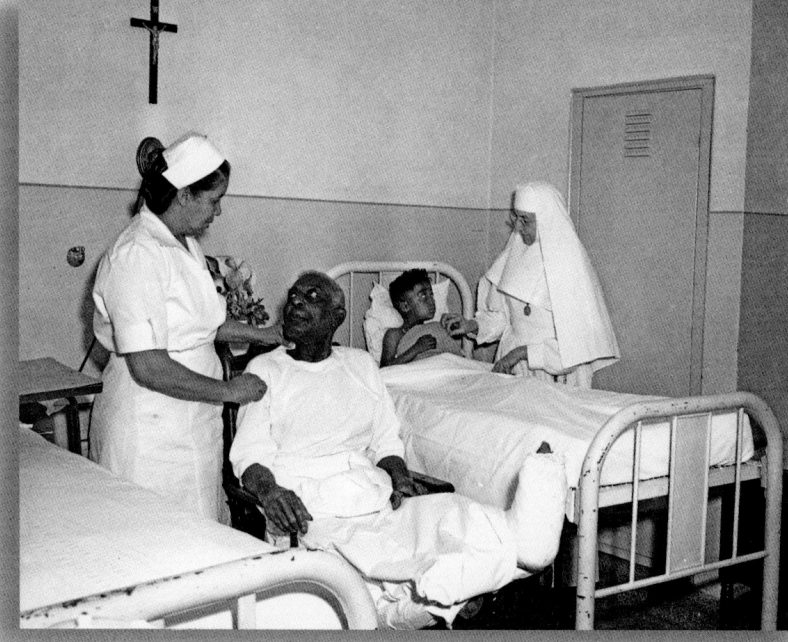

CHARITY CARE

An increase in population meant more growth in lower-income and struggling families. In April 1952, Tulsa county commissioners were asked to study the need to increase payments for charity patients cared for at local hospitals. Soaring costs were forcing Hillcrest and St. John's hospitals to seek a reimbursement higher than the $6 daily rate, according to news reports. Between July 1951 and April 1952, the county spent $44,872 on charity patients, leaving only about $149 in that account. At a meeting on June 9, 1952, hospital officials told the county commissioners it was upping the charity daily rate to $9.80. When County Commissioner Claude Bailey said he wanted to put the nonprofit hospitals on the tax rolls for raising rates, he was told the Oklahoma Constitution would need to be changed.

Nurses Caring for Patients at St. John's Hospital.

"That's a hell of a constitution!" Bailey responded.

St. John's Hospital business manager Kenneth Wallace stated a survey of 124 Oklahoma hospitals found the average daily cost per patient was $13.75. The daily charity rate was to cover all services including surgery.

Continued on page 76

Dr. Margaret E. Hudson

Starting in the 1930s, Dr. Margaret E. Hudson quietly led a forceful charge to prevent disease in children through education, knowledge and a practice of good health.

In a 1949 *Tulsa World* story about Child Health Day, Dr. Hudson was described as a "quiet-spoken, mild-mannered woman whose work is never done." At that time, she was the chief of the city health department's division for maternal and child hygiene, which had been created in 1946. Within two years, at least 400 pre-school children were visiting the clinics monthly.

"When she says, 'There is nothing more important in the world than our children's health,' you get the idea the declaration is a worn phrase. It is. She repeats it many times a day as she directs child health conferences at points in the city and the county."
– *Tulsa World*, May 1949.

Known as "Dr. Margaret," she oversaw 14 nurses and staff in the department. They fanned out across the city in home visits, schools and clinics to reach each child. If parents were not able to afford medications, the staff directed them to a free county program.

"I'm just one person in an organization that is charged with a great responsibility. All of us realize the importance of the work we're trying to do successfully. None of us will feel our program is successful until everybody is aware of its vital necessity."
– Dr. Margaret Hudson, May 1949.

Hudson often shied from the spotlight, letting the work speak for itself and giving credit to her staff, but she would speak up when it came to explaining what families and children in need require to flourish. She pointed out health is not limited to the physical but also envelopes the emotional and social.

"Health is a state of complete physical, mental and social well-being, not merely the absence of disease or infirmity. The requirements for health now go beyond the old definitions."
– Dr. Margaret Hudson, May 1949.

Born in rural Pennsylvania to Dr. Leon and Frances Grove in 1898, Dr. Hudson taught in a one-room schoolhouse before entering Pennsylvania State University. In 1920, she entered Johns Hopkins Medical School in Baltimore, Maryland. Among her 80-member graduating class, 12 students were women. The 20s era brought out opportunities for women, including the right to vote, wear short skirts and go on a date unescorted.

Hudson met her husband, Dr. David V. Hudson, while the two were attending medical school. She was a year behind him, and the couple married during her senior year. David took a surgical residency at Peking Union Medical College in China, where he was born to missionaries.

Upon Margaret's completion of her internship in preventative medicine and hygiene, she joined her husband and completed a residency in a Presbyterian Hospital. In 1927, the couple became medical instructors at the Iowa State University. They arrived in Tulsa in 1930. David set up a private practice specializing in urology and became involved in the Tulsa County Medical Society, serving as its executive secretary for many years and establishing a medical library. Margaret worked in the Medical Arts Laboratories from 1933 to 1941. Both became interested in public health.

"Margaret and David were concerned for the people who could not afford medical attention, health care or even food for their families. Margaret spent a lot of her time at health conferences examining babies and giving new mothers valuable tips on how to care for them." – Janet Hudson Colton, granddaughter, in a 2015 video biography of the couple.

After World War II, the couple joined the Tulsa City-County Health Department, where they became best known. Margaret led the maternal and child division, and David served as chief of the communicable diseases area. They had an outlook based in missionary work, seeking to help the most vulnerable, poor and disenfranchised.

"I just wish some people could go with me at times and see the misery we find. There's a lot more than the average person suspects." – Dr. Margaret Hudson, *Tulsa Tribune*, May 21, 1960.

Dr. David Hudson began his work in venereal disease clinics, working with young people on preventing sexually transmitted diseases. In 1946, the police took an approach of giving women seen loitering around beer taverns a ticket to appear in his clinic for a checkup. The girls would receive health information. The clinics branched out to include all communicable and social disease prevention.

Dr. Margaret Hudson handled all aspects of maternal and child health and eventually took a special interest in prenatal care for teenage mothers. Her mission started out working with disabled children, but expanded to include well-child visits, prenatal care and family health. In 1951, she started a program of school health in the country schools.

As the economy rebounded in the 1950s and a baby boom was underway, the couple kept a focus on the under-served populations.

"Even in this time of economic strength, there were people in Tulsa who were struggling. David and Margaret Hudson, through their work at the Tulsa City-County Health Department, did the best they could. Margaret was very creative – too many people needing medical treatment were being turned away. According to Margaret: 'I would just call a private physician and say I had someone in need of care. I haven't had a doctor say no.'"
– Janet Hudson Colton.

During their careers, the couple also raised two sons – David Hudson Jr. and John Hudson. They had one grandchild, Janet Hudson Colton.

"Dr. Margaret herself is largely responsible, having devoted her career to doing everything possible to help parents raise healthy children." – *Tulsa World*, Feb. 21, 1963.

In 1964, the Hudsons were selected by the Tulsa County Medical Society as Tulsa's "Doctors of the Year." Margaret retired in 1962 due to poor health, and David retired in 1967. At her retirement, she had been handling all the child conferences for the public health department. To replace her, 35 private physicians volunteered to take on her caseload.

"I've thoroughly enjoyed public health work, and I have very mixed feelings about leaving. I hope the private doctors enjoy it such as I have. Heaven knows where they will find the time, but they are certainly enthusiastic." – Dr. Margaret Hudson, *Tulsa Tribune*, June 14, 1962.

In 1968, health department officials named a new program in her honor. The program provided an education and health care to teenagers who became mothers. It was originally financed through Model Cities; Oklahoma Crime Commission; Health, Education and Welfare and private donors.

"She did so much in her field, the trustees named the unit the Margaret Hudson Program for School-Age Parents as a living memorial to her."
– Mary Hughes, program coordinator, *Tulsa World*, Jan. 29, 1973.

Dr. Margaret Hudson died in January 1973 at age 75. Dr. David Hudson died in January 1976 at age 79.

The Margaret Hudson program has grown into an influential Tulsa-area nonprofit with a school in midtown and another in Broken Arrow. The program has served more than 9,000 teenage mothers and their children with comprehensive services including education to finish high school or vocational training, child-care, health screenings, case management for benefits and social services for mentoring, counseling and parenting skills. It is a United Way-supported agency operating through private and government grants on a budget of about $2.3 million annually. Between 130 and 170 girls and their children are enrolled in the program each year. ■

"I hope you do build your own hospital," Wallace told the commissioners. "You'll find your costs, when you begin paying for the professional services you'll need, will run $25 a patient a day."

The commissioners voted to raise the rate to $7 daily and stated it would likely need to increase the following year. But, Hillcrest and St. John's refused to take patients while the osteopathic hospital agreed to the rate. Eventually, the parties came to an agreement for low-income patients to continue treatment.

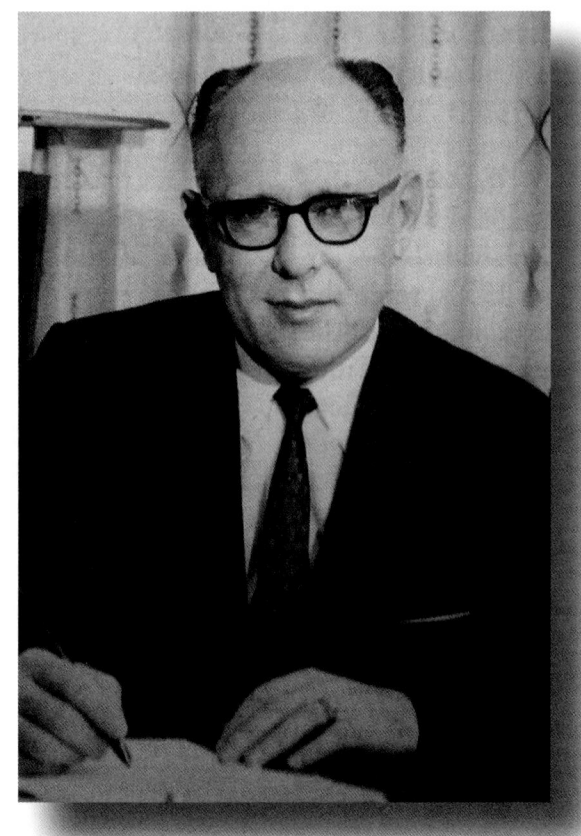

Administrator leads the way

Taking the Oklahoma Osteopathic Hospital into the next part of the century with grand plans was administrator L.C. Baxter, who joined the facility in September 1953. Under his leadership, he led three expansions of the hospital and updated practices and policies. He was a native of Texas who became a licensed embalmer and funeral director before serving as business manager of the Fort Worth Osteopathic Hospital. In a history book of the hospital published during his retirement, Baxter remembers his impression of the facility when reconsidering a job offer.

"When I came to Tulsa, there was just the first old building. I was impressed because OOH had no debt; it even had about $60,000 in the bank. The little hospital I left in Fort Worth had several mortgages on it. My beginning salary at OOH was $600 a month; I thought I was rich since I'd been making $450. The hospital didn't volunteer moving expenses so I didn't ask, but I did insist on being called administrator."

One of Baxter's first moves was to re-evaluate the board of trustees. He helped shift the board membership to a majority of physicians because he viewed the group as setting policy for the medical staff. He also had the hospital join the American Osteopathic Association and host national speakers.

Administrator L.C. Baxter.

"Another necessary step was to establish control over buying. At that time, if a doctor went to a convention and saw something he wanted for the hospital, he just bought it and had it shipped. I stopped this by refusing shipment on one order, just sent it back. It was a little embarrassing for the doctor involved but it got purchasing squared away."

Acquiring land was the most significant legacy of Baxter. Through his vision, he bought surrounding land as it became available, allowing for expansions in 1953, 1959 and 1966 and initiated construction for a 1975 addition.

"The only way I could see this hospital growing was with more space. So I set out to convince the board that with every opportunity and every few dollars we had, we ought to buy a piece of property. First, we bought seven or eight houses where the ambulance entry is now; bought them one at a

Nursery, Tulsa Osteopathic Hospital, Tulsa, Okla.

Oklahoma Osteopathic Hospital Nursery.

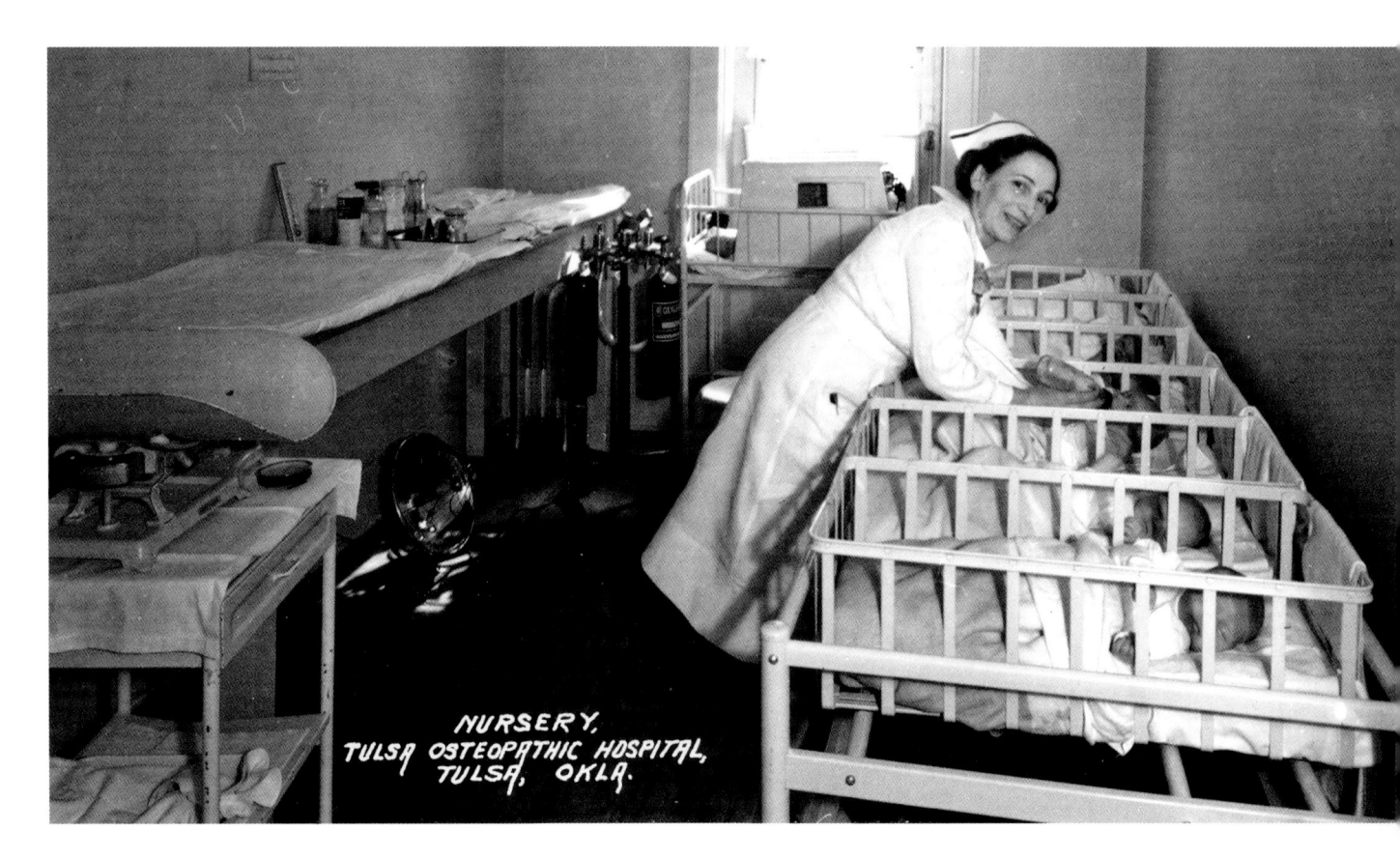

time, petitioned the city to close the alley, and did the second expansion along Eleventh Street."

Baxter then focused his buying efforts on the block to the north, which included the city's bus repair plant and several houses. He recalled one man who refused to sell.

"He led us on a merry chase until he finally said he'd sell if we'd let him live there the rest of his life. He wanted $12,000 for the house and yard, plus the hospital was to take care of the property. When the papers were drawn up and it came time to pay, he wouldn't take a check, wanted cash. So, I went down to the bank and got that old gentleman $12,000 in thousand-dollar bills. After that, he called us every two or three days because the yard needed mowing or a faucet dripped. He really outsmarted the hospital."

The land acquisition then went house-to-house across the street then an urban renewal project allowed for the purchase of nearly every structure on Houston Street. The hospital worked its design around the highway plans.

The project in 1953 cost about $900,000 for an addition, two elevators and air conditioning the old hospital. The new construction added a pharmacy, orthopedic unit and 40 beds, bringing capacity to 105 patients. In the capital campaign, osteopathic physicians contributed $100,000 and an auxiliary helped with landscaping, grounds clean-up and smaller fundraisers. The women of the auxiliary raised $25,000 selling sloppy joes and cakes at the Tulsa State Fair. The federal government also made $270,000 available to the hospital through funds from the Hill-Burton Act, which provided money for the care of lower-income people. These changes made the hospital the first completely air conditioned hospital in Tulsa.

When the new structure opened on Jan. 1, 1956, it was immediately full. The overflow resulted in beds being placed in waiting rooms and corridors to handle the osteopathic referrals from surrounding areas. It led to plans for a second addition. After two years of study, ground was broken in February 1958 for a $1.25 million project to add 45,000 square feet and 108 beds. Half the funds came from the federal government and the rest was from a bank loan.

This second project placed the Tulsa facility as the third largest osteopathic hospital in the United States. The design resulted in an E-shaped hospital, with the new wing lining Jackson Street. The kitchen and surgery were located in the middle, and parking space was created to the west. The modern facility boasted of seven operating rooms, a meal-pack system in a stainless steel kitchen, motorized beds, public cafeteria, long-term patient areas, two recovery rooms and piped-in oxygen to all areas. It created a larger radiology department and added a pathology department. The facility had 102 physicians, five residents and 14 interns on staff with about 200 hospital employees. For its dedication ceremonies, President Eisenhower wired a message:

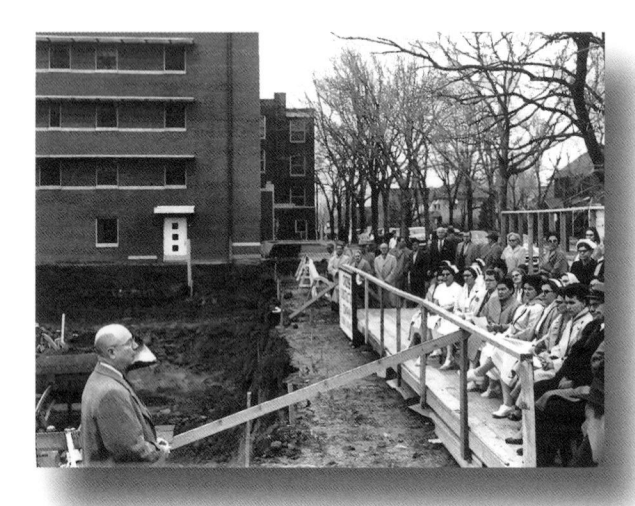

Oklahoma Osteopathic Hospital's 1950s Expansion Project.

"This fine new addition will strengthen your service to the people of Tulsa and surrounding areas."

Another credit to Baxter was his routine that kept him in touch with staff. He would go by the switchboard in the morning, have coffee with the doctors, swing by the business manager's office then do rounds to check with nursing staff and other employees.

"For years I could call everyone in the hospital by name; I could talk with everyone. This way I really knew what was going on in the hospital. I thought it was important."

During his time with the Tulsa hospital, Baxter also served as a trustee, president, executive committee member and chairman of the building committee of the American Osteopathic Hospital Association. He was a charter member of the American College of Osteopathic Hospital Administrators, board member of the Oklahoma Blue Cross Blue Shield, president of the Tulsa Hospital Council and member of the Tulsa Area Health and Hospital Planning Council. He turned over operations of the hospital in 1973 but followed a construction project on a part-time basis through 1974.

Baxter died on Dec. 30, 1999, at age 82. The Tulsa Regional Medical Center dedicated a room named the L.C. Baxter Memorial Library.

BABY BOOM CONTINUES

The birth of the Baby Boom started right after World War II ended, with more babies born in the U.S. in 1946 than any year before (3.4 million, or 20 percent higher than in the previous year). The babies kept coming — 3.8 million in 1947, 3.9 million in 1952 and more than 4 million every year between 1954 and 1964. By the time the trend begin to fade in the mid-60s, 76.4 million Baby Boomers made up 40 percent of America's population.

Tulsa hospitals experienced this baby invasion. A 1954 *Tulsa World* story provided details about the St. John's Hospital nursery at capacity. The room was designed to accommodate 60 babies, but 90 infants have been housed in the nursery. Beds for expecting and recovering mothers was at 67, but "a common sight on the OB floor is a new mother on a cart, waiting for someone else to go home." The hospital reported 571 babies born in 1935. It jumped to 1,685 babies in 1945 and to 3,579 in 1953.

"The waiting room for fathers and relatives shows the wear and tear in the worn terrazzo floors from miles of pacing — in the tons of half-smoked cigarets carted out and in the well-thumbed magazines which are sometimes read upside down." — *Tulsa World*, April 26, 1954.

Help for the obstetrics ward was coming with the planned $3.5 million wing. The addition was to turn the fourth floor over for obstetrics patients.

"Although the conditions on the OB floor are critically crowded, it doesn't seem to keep the mothers away. One woman has returned for the delivery of each of her seven children." — *Tulsa World*, April 26, 1954.

Continued on page 83

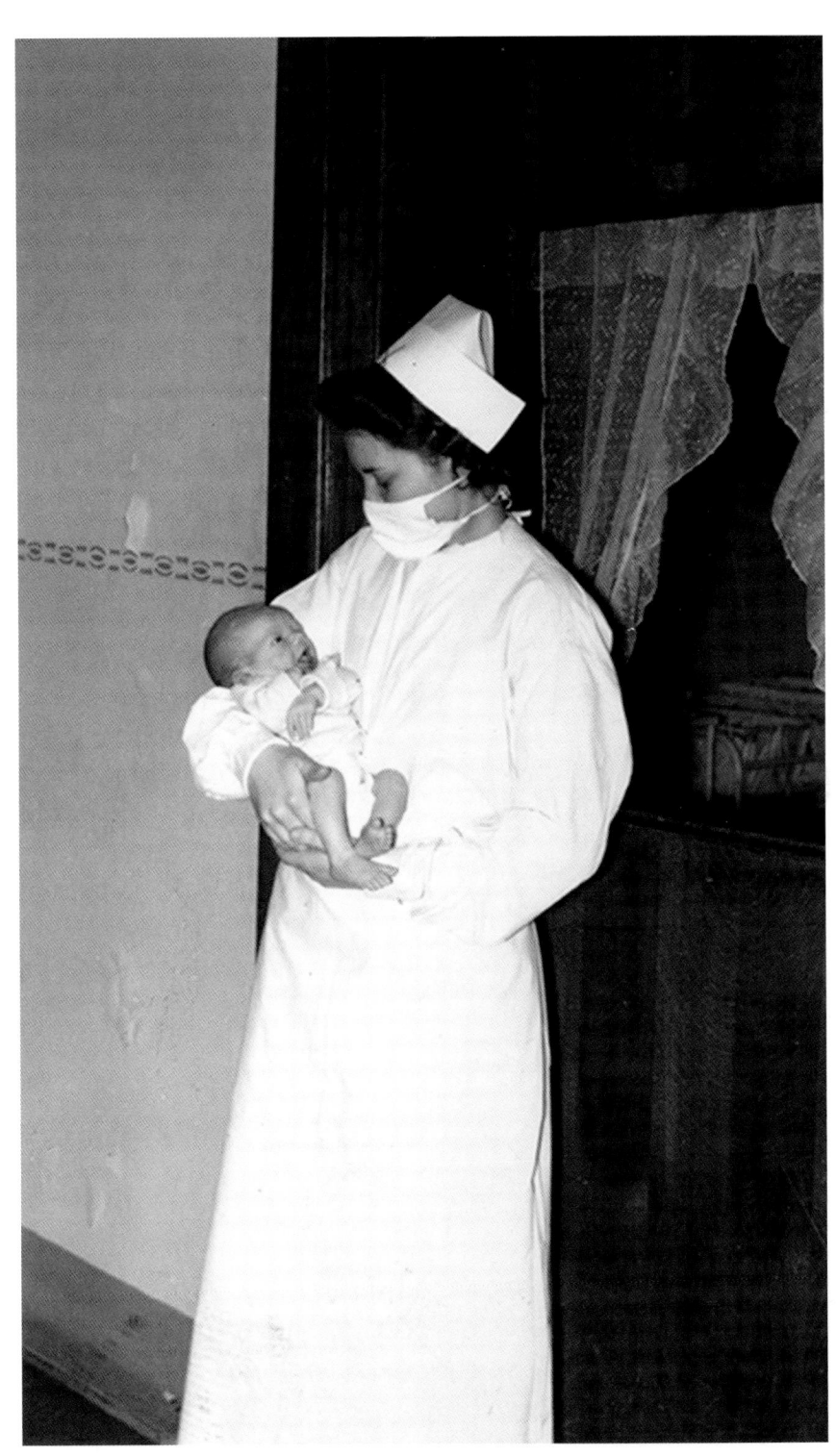

A Baby Receiving Care at Hillcrest During the Baby Boom Era.

Junior League of Tulsa
and
Care for Children

Spanning decades, a medical home for children was founded and administered by a group of Tulsa women who formed a nonprofit to fill needs in the community. While the children's facility remained a major project from the 20s through the 50s, the later part of the 20th century saw significant changes.

In 1923, Mrs. W. Albert Cook gathered several women to form the Junior League of Tulsa to serve the community and to give women a chance to develop their leadership potential. One of its first actions was funding a public health nurse and raising money for a facility for disabled children. A donation to use a home at 1101 E. Fifth Place by Sand Springs philanthropist Charles Page allowed the Convalescent Home for Crippled Children to open on Oct. 1, 1926.

In 1927, an effort launched to raise money for a new home. Donations were made by leading Tulsans including $25,000 from Mr. and Mrs. R.M. McFarland, $10,000 from oilman Waite Phillips and $5,000 from W.G. Skelly. Total cost was expected to be about $80,000.

A 1927 "*Tulsa Tribune*" story detailed some of the ailments children faced:
- A 2-year-old girl from Checotah arrived in January that year with clubbed feet and described as "sickly, and life seemingly held no happiness in store for her." She was released six months later in leg braces but no clubbed feet: "She was a normal, happy child — a living testimony to the value of the Junior League work for crippled children."
- A 12-year-old Claremore boy arrived in June 1927 struck with infantile paralysis since age 1. His only method of movement for a decade was to drag his body with his arms. He received therapy and leg braces to help him improve walking. "He has equal chances with other boys of his age to succeed in life, a privilege which would have been denied him had he continued to be without the use of his legs."
- A Tulsa 12-year-old boy entered the home after receiving treatment at St. John's Hospital. The child had been severely burned while feeding wood into a fire. His arm was burned to the point of no longer being able to move and nearly required amputation. His recovery was at the convalescent home, "In no way could his parents have provided for treatment at a hospital and paid for it." He regained use of his arm within three months.

The newly constructed Convalescent Home for Crippled Children was built in 1928 at 4900 S. Lewis Ave., which was five miles from the city at that time. It was the only such facility for children in Tulsa. Within two years, the debt was cut in half, and the organization hosted a series of lectures on occupational therapy. The home was surrounded by a large acreage and trees, according to Junior League's "The Gusher" magazine in February 1963.

After children underwent surgery, they were brought to the home for recovery. Doctors volunteered their time, and it was provided at no charge to the families of the patients. Children received an education while at the home through public school teachers provided by the Tulsa School Board. Funding for the building was raised through private donations and its tea room, which sold 15-cent cinnamon rolls, 5-cent coffee and average of 60 cents for lunch. However, it was not enough to keep up with rising health care costs and needs during the Depression. Fundraisers were added including the addition of luncheon fashion shows, group dinners, lectures and theatrical shows. Newspaper stories showed the recreation children were offered, including turning the surrounding acreage into a camp.

"President Roosevelt's interest in polio and handicapped children gave an added interest to our own main project, the Convalescent Home. Fortunately, we had many talented and hard-working members with original ideas for Ways and Means. Each month the bills maintaining the Home were somehow paid." – Bernice Tibbens McKay, Junior League of Tulsa president in 1933-1934 in the group's 40th anniversary magazine.

By 1938, the mortgage on the children's medical home was paid off. World War II created difficulties for the organization as women took on other community projects to support the war effort and moved to accommodate the entrance of their husbands into the military. At the war's end, the economy boomed and the convalescent home underwent improvements. In 1948, the home was expanded to a capacity of 38 children, from the previous 21 beds. A psychotherapy room was enlarged, a new pool was added for exercise treatment and a floor was resurfaced with non-skid material. Two years before, a donation led to the purchase off new Super de Lux Ford station wagon to transport children. In 1948, the home had 14 children with a 38-bed capacity, leading to concerns about its usefulness.

In 1949, a polio outbreak led to the home providing convalescent care for 106 children, who stayed an average of 64 days. That year, the children's home was in debt, and a report from the Children's Bureau, Federal Security Agency based in Dallas, Texas, suggested changes in organization, medical staff, housekeeping and updated equipment. The members voted on June 24, 1949, to keep the home open for 18 months and cover the $15,000 in costs, and place administration under a community board. The board was made up of 13 men and women including a judge, businessman, physician and Junior League members. By that time, more than 1,000 children had been cared for at the home since its formation. Eight months later, improvements met the recommendations of the federal report while holding down costs.

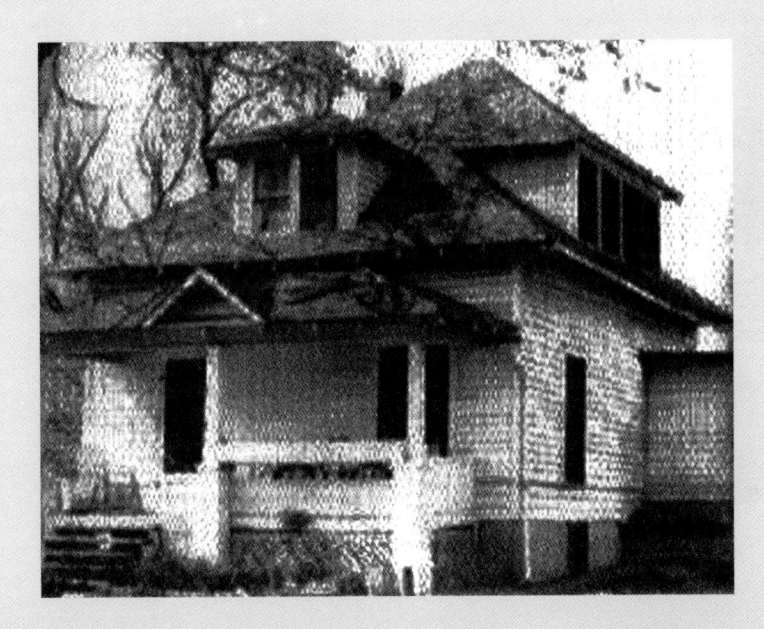

On May 19, 1950, the community board voted the changes permanent and reported 40 children in care with a capacity of 50 beds. One-third of the children were polio patients, but needs were showing in orthopedics and occupational therapy. The financial structure changed with some children qualifying for aide from a fund and others paying, at a rate of about $6.54 a day. On Oct. 10, 1951, the transfer became official and the name changed to the Junior League Children's Hospital for Convalescents. Within the year, the hospital was at capacity, with a waiting list and plans for the addition of two wings made, creating an L-shaped building. On Sept. 19, 1953, more than 150 physicians and surgeons were among the spectators at the opening of the first wing. It cost $200,000 and housed the dental, orthopedic, cerebral palsy, speech, hearing, X-ray, laboratory and child guidance clinics.

Convalescent Home for Crippled Children.

During the 50s, polio treatments dominated news reports about the convalescent home focused on different therapies and programs, such as the creation of an outdoor gym by a nurse and the installation of a "gadget board" donated by an occupational therapist. All children participated in activities such as gardening programs, model airplane classes and a hospital newspaper published by children. Beauty product and equipment companies donated everything for a children's salon. Appeals for volunteers were made to staff all the programs.

In June 1961, the Junior League voted on a series of motions that changed the name, turned control to a community board of trustees and expanded services and facility. Since 1949, which had been the last reorganization, the home had served about 300 children in convalescent care and operated at about 92 percent capacity.

"By the league's vote today, the hospital will be incorporated under its own name with a membership charter, giving the board of trustees a legal entity to operate as a community institution. The hospital was originally planned as an orthopedic hospital only, but increasing needs have widened the variety accepted in the last two years." *Tulsa World*, June 13, 1961.

It was named the Children's Medical Center and officially moved to the control of a 22-member community board in 1962. The vote also approved the construction of a $150,000 wing and the addition of outpatient services. This consolidated the physical and administrative functions of several agencies in the Tulsa – the Tulsa Child Guidance Clinic, Sunnyside School, Child Study Clinic and Vocational Training Center. It brought together clinical facilities for the emotionally disturbed and physically handicapped children and provided evaluation and treatment in child psychiatry, psychological counseling, physical rehabilitation, occupational therapy, mental retardation, vocational training, and education problems.

Though the Junior League was no longer the primary administrator or majority on an oversight board, it continued to monetarily support the facility with fundraising, including raising $8,000 the following year after hosting a pro-am golf tournament. By this time, the Junior League of Tulsa had grown in membership to about 245 members and branched out into many fields of philanthropy, providing financial and/or volunteer support to 53 agencies. A *Tulsa World* editorial praised the league for giving $1 million to the community and 1 million hours of volunteer service within its first 38 years of existence.

"Perhaps the League's outstanding contribution to Tulsa is the Children's Medical Center," the editorial stated.

In 1975, the Children's Medical Center moved into the former Sinclair Research Laboratory at 5300 E. Skelly Drive. In 1994, the center became part of Hillcrest HealthCare System and specialized in behavioral and rehabilitative care for children and adolescents. It had grown into a 185,000-square-foot facility on about 28 acres. It was licensed for 108 beds and served more than 14,000 children annually.

In 2000, Children's Medical Center closed its facility and moved patient care into Hillcrest Medical Center and Tulsa Regional Medical Center. Economics was the driving factor in the decision, citing a $4 million loss in the center that fiscal year, according to a Jan. 7, 2000, *Tulsa World* story.

Even though the Junior League of Tulsa handed control of the children's hospital to a board decades ago, it has remained one of its more powerful legacies. Since then, the organization has continued to keep children's issues as its touchstone. It has given support for foster children, disabled children, schools, arts programs for youth, maternal leagues and projects to benefit underprivileged children. Some Junior League members were also listed in news reports as being on other boards supporting women, children and families. As stated in Naomi Harrington's closing remarks as Junior League of Tulsa president in the 1942 annual report:

"If the Junior League of Tulsa is to continue to maintain its position of leadership in the community, every member must pledge herself to do a little more than her share, both as an individual and as a member of the League. We are going to be called on for many sacrifices in the times to come, but if each of us as individuals realize that our sacrifices are small compared to those some others are making, it should make ours less burdensome. The heritage of our children is in our hands," she said. ∎

St. John's Hospital Grows Wings

In 1952, St. John's Hospital announced a fundraising effort to build a wing on the north side of the facility. The hospital had opened a $3 million, six-story wing on its south side in 1948, but the patients continued to arrive in record numbers. This was also a time more doctors entered into more specialties.

"Considering the crowded conditions and the need for expansion of special departments, such as surgery and the outpatient department, we have decided our pressing obligation to the people of the Tulsa community is to alleviate the crowded conditions and to expand our facilities both for beds and for these special departments." — Sister Mary Agatha, *Tulsa World*, Dec. 29, 1952.

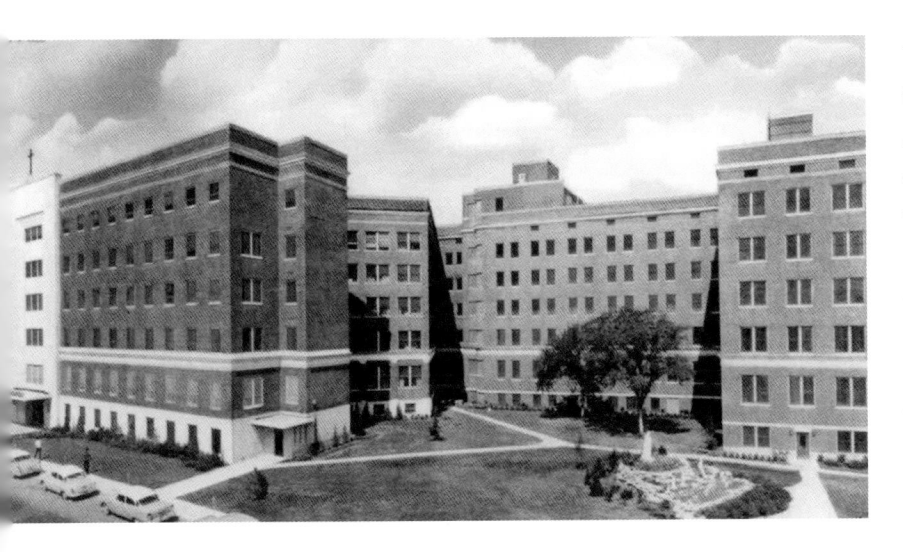

The wing established the hospital's first psychiatric department and expansions in the surgery, emergency, pharmacy, physical therapy and outpatient department. It added beds and enlarged the records department.

A 1957 photo of St. John's Hospital's West Side Expansion, now called the Heyman Building.

Ken Wallace, business manager at the hospital, told an advisory board in February 1953 that the city's population has outpaced medical infrastructure. Elective medical and surgical cases were waiting at least three weeks for a bed. He cited figures from the state health department stating Tulsa needed at least 200 more beds.

"At present, there are very few standby beds that would be available in the event of any catastrophe. During the recent flu epidemic, a number of cases were necessarily refused admittance to the hospital." — *Tulsa Tribune*, Feb. 12, 1953.

The project added the construction of a two-level parking garage, across from Utica Square on the southeast part of the site. The 225-automobile structure was designed for later expansion to at least four stories. Hospital officials attempted to purchase nearby land for the parking facility but were not successful. The parking garage was put into a location previously used as a garden and recreation area.

"The garden was not utilized this year because of the severe drought. But in previous years, it was worked extensively by the sisters. And, during the Depression, supplied a large portion of the vegetables used in the hospital." — *Tulsa World*, Oct. 10, 1954.

The project grew to a cost of about $3.5 million and also added improvements to the laundry and kitchen. The dedication of the wing was held in May 1957 conducted by the Rev. Eugene J. McGuinness, bishop of Oklahoma's Catholic Church.

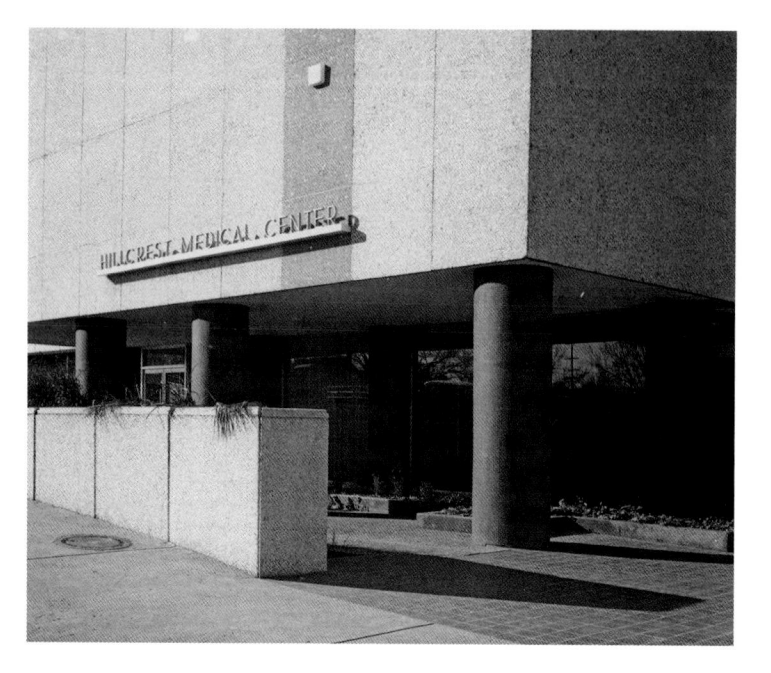

HILLCREST TRANSFORMS

In 1952, the Hillcrest Memorial Hospital & Training School for Nurses became Hillcrest Medical Center. It followed the same upward trends in construction, patient growth and additional services and specialties.

Former administrator James Harvey described the decade as having "explosive growth," which was often measured by the number of beds a hospital could boast. The crowded facilities often had patients recovering in hallways and vacant offices. Also, hospitals didn't have medical groups. Doctors were self-employed.

Hillcrest Medical Center.

"They all came from different directions. There wasn't a common platform so what you had was a very heterogeneous medical staff. Not that that was bad because they were doing a good job. However, there would be as much controversy and acrimony between doctors as there was between doctors and administration and doctors and nurses. They ran things, no question about it." — James Harvey, *Tulsa World*, Sept. 16, 1997.

At Hillcrest, the 50s established a ward for mentally ill patients, added wings and opened one of the largest outpatient clinics in the state. The 25-bed "neuropsychiatric unit" opened with the aid of a donation from W. Wilson Dye, president of Western Supply Co. after he was informed it was the most pressing need in Tulsa. A newspaper report stated it was the first such hospital unit in Oklahoma and one of the few in the nation.

"For the first time, Oklahoma's mentally ill will receive treatment in the same manner as that provided to patients with ordinary illnesses," — *Tulsa World*, Nov. 6, 1949.

The unit was not used for patients requiring custodial care or showing symptoms of degenerative brain disorders such as dementia. Among the equipment used was an electroencephalograph, which attached wires with clay to a patient's head to carry currents of electricity from the patient to a recording machine. Hospital administrator Bryce Twitty said treating patients with mental health needs in large hospitals was showing success nationally.

"They have found it represents a saving in time, money and minds. It allows the mental patient to receive treatment without the stigma of being confined to an institution." — Bryce Twitty, *Tulsa World*, Nov. 6, 1949.

In 1952, Hillcrest opened an outpatient clinic with 15 specialty clinics. When it launched, it was not exclusively for charity cases but was intended to be an option for people who could not afford a private physician. Fees were based on a patient's ability to pay. The clinic operated in cooperation with health and social work agencies.

"It can be built into one of the biggest medical centers of its kind in the country," Dr. A. Ray Wiley, director of the hospital's outpatient department, *Tulsa World*, July 27, 1952.

At the 1952 dedication of a wing adjoining the hospital with a west structure, Dr. Louis H. Bauer, president of the American Medical Association gave the featured remarks. The wing was to be a foundation for a future multi-story building.

"This triad of physicians, hospitals and community, all cooperating in volunteer efforts in the spirit of free enterprise is an unbeatable combination. If we fail, there will be no more free enterprise, but government supervision, government control and government red tape." — Dr. Louis H. Bauer, *Tulsa World*, Sept. 22, 1952.

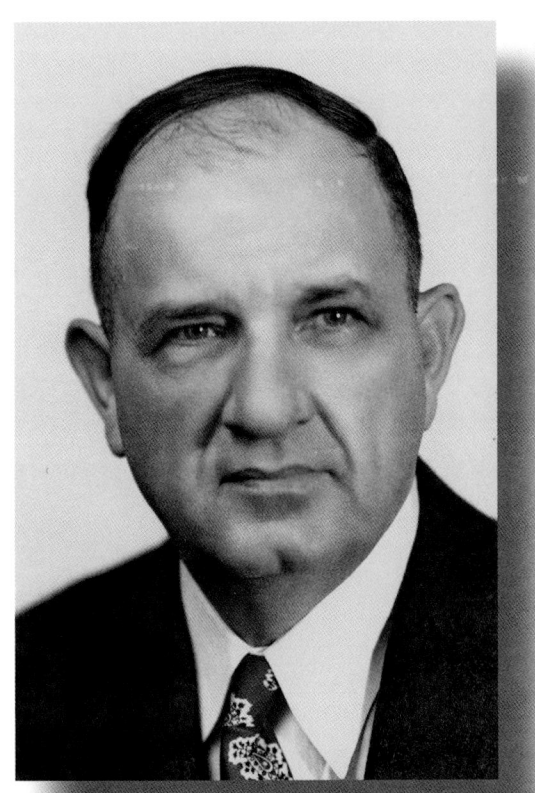

Bryce Twitty: Hillcrest Medical Center Administrator.

In 1954, plans were announced to construct a physician's building facing west on Utica Avenue and three-story parking garage In 1955, construction plans were announced for an eight-story, 294-bed addition. The new wing went at the end of the main building's north-south extension, parallel to the east-west wing, which fronts on 12th Street between Utica and Troost avenues.

The following year, administrator Bryce Twitty, who had led the hospital since it was incorporated in 1940, gave public speeches about his vision for the next 15 years. He predicted gains in mental health treatment that would require more space, a need for a cancer hospital for research and treatment and the moral obligation to care for children. In a foreshadowing of the future design of the medical profession, he backed the pending plans for a physician's building to adjoin the hospital.

"To a person thinking only of a small hospital sitting on a hill doing mediocre medicine, a medical arts building is not necessary. But to one who takes a long and constructive look at a great and beautiful medical center of influence and service, it will be impossible to do without the physicians nearby." — Bryce Twitty, *Tulsa World*, Nov. 12, 1955.

THE STRANGE CASE OF NANNIE DOSS

Tulsa's most notorious serial killer was a 49-year-old, plump grandmother who confessed to killing four husbands with poison in 1954. The case dominated headlines locally and nationally and shined a light on the work of pathologists.

Nannie met two of her husbands, including Tulsa's Samuel Doss, through a "lonely hearts club" magazine. Doss was taken ill after she laced his prunes with rat poison. After he was released from the hospital, Nannie served him coffee with a large dose of arsenic. He died the next day. The doctors became suspicious.

"Had she done it in any of a hundred smaller communities in the state, it is likely she would have been free to marry again. Big cities have pathologists at their major hospitals, and these physicians are Oklahoma's first line of offense in the detection of death by poison." — *Tulsa World*, Dec. 11, 1954.

Nannie agreed to an autopsy, and tests showed Doss "had enough arsenic in him to kill a horse." She said Doss was killed "because he got on my nerves" by not letting her read true detective magazines, have a radio or visit neighbors to watch television.

She admitted to the poisoning deaths of Doss, Frank Harrelson of Jacksonville, Alabama, Arlie J. Lanning of Lexington, North Carolina, and Richard L. Morton of Emporia, Kansas. Only her first husband, Charley Braggs of Alabama, got out of the marriage alive. When Doss died, Nannie was lining up her sixth husband, a North Carolina dairy farmer to whom she had sent a cake. Two of her daughters, ages 1 and 2, died mysteriously in 1924 when their bodies turned black after their deaths. Her mother, Sue Hazle of North Carolina, died while in Nannie's care, and a later autopsy revealed arsenic poisoning.

Police believed she committed the murders for convenience and money. Family members testified she seemed to enjoy planning the funerals, including hiring photographers to document the events. Psychiatrists stated they believed Nannie to be "mentally defective" after observing her for 90 days at Eastern State Hospital in Vinita, but a jury ruled her sane. Doss sold her story to *Life* magazine to pay for her defense.

She pleaded guilty to the Tulsa murder and on June 2, 1955, was sentenced to life in prison. The case resulted in the Oklahoma Legislature passing a law requiring an examination by a medical examiner of all individuals who die without being attended by a physician.

Nannie was described as a model prisoner, and told a *Tulsa World* reporter who visited her in prison: "When they get shorthanded in the kitchen here, I always offer to help out, but they never let me." She died of leukemia on June 2, 1965, exactly 10 years after going to prison.

SEGREGATION OF MEDICAL SCHOOLS END

George W. McLaurin, 61, challenged the 1896 Plessy v. Ferguson Supreme Court "separate but equal" ruling by applying for admission to the University of Oklahoma Medical School in 1948. He held a master's degree from the University of Kansas and taught at Langston University, an all-black school. NAACP attorney Thurgood Marshall, Tulsa attorney Amos T. Hall and Black Dispatch newspaper editor

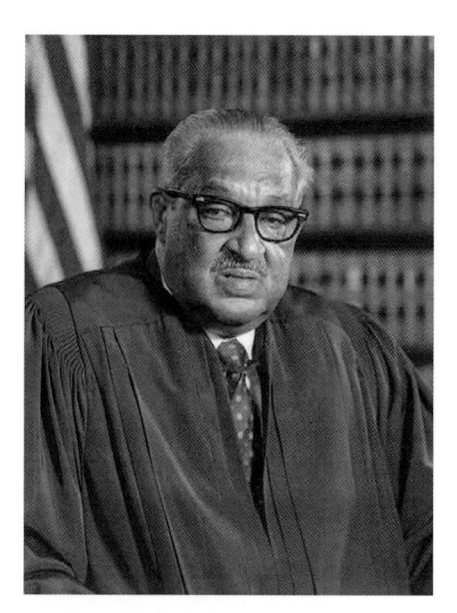

Former Supreme Court Justice Thurgood Marshall.

Roscoe Dunjee backed McLaurin's effort, along with those of five other African Americans who were applying for other professional, graduate degrees at OU. One of those students was Ada Lois Sipuel Fisher at the OU Law School.

The federal court ordered OU to admit McLaurin. But, like Fisher, he was segregated into his own classrooms, library, cafeteria and restroom areas. Marshall successfully argued in McLaurin v. Oklahoma State Regents for Higher Education that this treatment violated the Fourth Amendment. In 1950, the U.S. Supreme Court ruled that universities must provide the same services and treatment to black students as to those of other races.

Leap in Technologies

This decade brought forth revolutionary research leading to more effective medications, tools, medical practice and public health safety.

Within the specialty of ear, nose and throat, antibiotics developed in the 40s and 50s were the first transformative technology. Then, along came high-powered microscopes. Before the first sulfonamide and penicillin, the only treatment for infections was incision and drainage. The medications were successful in nearly eliminating bacterial infections such as scarlet fever and diphtheria. The next jump came with the development of the Zeiss binocular operating microscope in Germany. It allowed for the hearing mechanism and delicate structures of the middle ear and eardrum to be magnified, providing for a greater reliability of diagnosis and treatment. The scope was meant to remove disease and restore hearing.

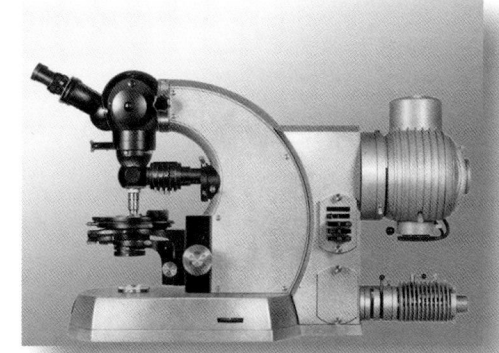

Zeiss Microscope.

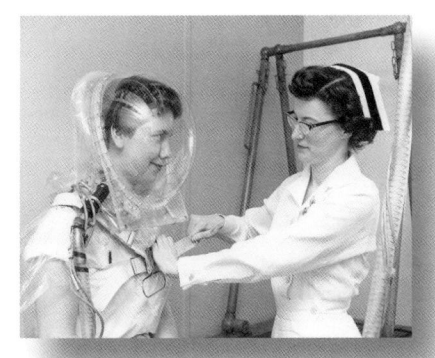

The first Ziess operating microscopes arrived in Tulsa in 1958, appearing almost simultaneously in three places — St. John's Hospital at the request of Dr. Donald Mishler and in the offices of both Dr. Royal Stuart and Dr. Roger E. Wehrs. The microscopes were developed primarily for surgery of the chronic ear. A backlog of patients developed almost immediately after having no previous treatment for eardrum perforations, draining ears, cholesteatoma and chronic mastoiditis.

"In addition to the otologic surgery, there were marked strides made in nose, sinus and throat surgery. As infection could now be controlled with antibiotics, there emerged new and extensive surgery that could be carried out on these structures. Magnification, utilizing the Zeiss operating microscope and lens of long focal length, the armamentarium of instruments to treat diseases and surgery of the larynx and even the nose and sinus were developed. It was this atmosphere that enabled the residents at that time to experience extensive and valuable training in the changing field of ENT surgery." — "The History of Otolaryngology in Tulsa, Oklahoma, 1950-1970."

Part of the expansion at St. John's Hospital included the addition of a radioisotope laboratory in its radiology department. The tool was used to treat certain types of cancer, brain tumors and blood disorders.

Above: Metabolic Research.

"Atomic medicine is already a big field and it is going to be bigger. What atomic energy can do to help man live is of far greater importance in the long run than what the bomb itself can do to make people die. St. John's is entering this field of medicine as early as possible because the hospital recognizes how important this field will be in the near future." — Dr. Lucien Pascucci, head of the St. John's Hospital radiology section, *Tulsa World*, Jan. 7, 1953.

When the "cobalt bomb" tool was installed in 1957, Dr. Pascucci explained the significance.

"This is a most valuable tool in treating cancer and other malignancies. It penetrates deeper than X-ray, yet produces less skin reaction. It will allow us to place more radioactive units deep into the source of the tumor. We feel this machine will eliminate much of the radiation sickness, which is experienced with deep and prolonged X-ray treatments. You might say this radioactive cobalt has a soft touch for surface and normal tissue but packs a might wallop for cancerous tissue. The machine can provide multiple port penetrations, that is, the patient is moved by the machine slightly each time the element is used. This method allows a minimum amount of radioactive force to pass through surface tissues yet the core or seat of the trouble gets repeated doses from the cobalt element." — Dr. Lucien Pascucci, *Tulsa World*, Aug. 28, 1957.

Cobalt Therapy Penetrates Deeper than X-rays.

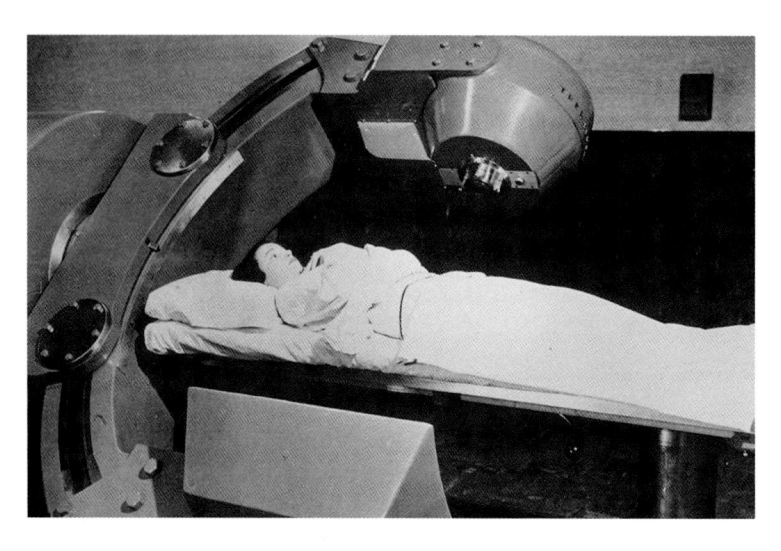

Tulsa's Health Status

A headline on Christmas Day in 1957 proclaimed "Tulsa's Health Is Better Than Other Cities in State," with details on the mortality and disease of residents. Heart disease stood as the No. 1 killer with 591 deaths, but stated the number was likely higher because hundreds more deaths were categorized as vascular disorders. The Tulsa City-County Health Department had given about 50,000 polio shots that year. Only one polio death was reported, and the story stated the victims had not received the vaccine, developed by Jonas Salk in 1953.

Other notable facts from the report:
- Two large hospitals with a slated combined capacity of 1,500 beds;
- Largest osteopathic hospital in the southwest;
- The 42-bed Moton Memorial Hospital serving black residents;
- A unique health department with a city-county model supported by local, state and municipal funds;
- Tulsa County Medical Society reports 345 members; and
- The city had 10 African-American physicians. They were voted "scientific memberships" in the medical society. No black doctors had been elected to the staff at either of the city's major hospitals.

CHAPTER 7
(1960 – 1969)

Constructing New Heights in Care

President Lyndon Johnson Signing Medicare Bill.

Tulsa expanded rapidly. The Medical Arts Building on 6th Street downtown was demolished to make way for the new Petroleum Club. The movie theaters – The Ritz, Orpheum, Rialto, and Majestic – disappeared. New shopping centers sprang up citywide, such as Whittier Square, Utica Square, Southland and Southroads Mall, Woodland Hills Mall, and a variety of shopping "communities" such as Brookside and Cherry Street. Baby Boomers entered adulthood as the Vietnam War raged, space exploration expanded science and "sex, drugs and rock-n-roll" became a mantra.

Medical advancements sprang forward eradicating polio, allowing reproductive freedom with a pill, repairing heart conditions through surgery and improving diagnosis through progressive scans. The federal government instituted an expanded health care coverage for the elderly and disabled that shaped the way medicine is practiced. Tulsa hospitals grew, a new one was founded and specialists began to flock into private practices.

A Pink Hospital on the Hill

While hospitals traditionally started small with investments from doctors, one Tulsa oilman decided to go grand — opening a multi-million dollar pink hospital loaded with the latest medical technologies and research-based programs.

In 1955, oilman William K. Warren announced his foundation would build a hospital called Saint Francis. The original thought was to place it near Woodward Park at 21st Street and Peoria Avenue. Then, the foundation chose a 38-acre spot near 21st Street and Darlington Avenue for the hospital. However, plans were scuttled after coal mine shafts were found beneath the property. Warren was scouting other possible location by helicopter when he spotted tracts of farmland flanking Yale Avenue at 61st Street.

The foundation spent $8 million to construct, equip and staff the facility. The other hospitals were at capacity and fully staffed. This addition to the city was meant to attract new physicians, offer a research facility and offer patients more options. It also shaped development of south Tulsa from farmland into the city's more expensive expansions. Warren's son, W.K. Warren Jr. said his father had an empathy for people with illness and believed

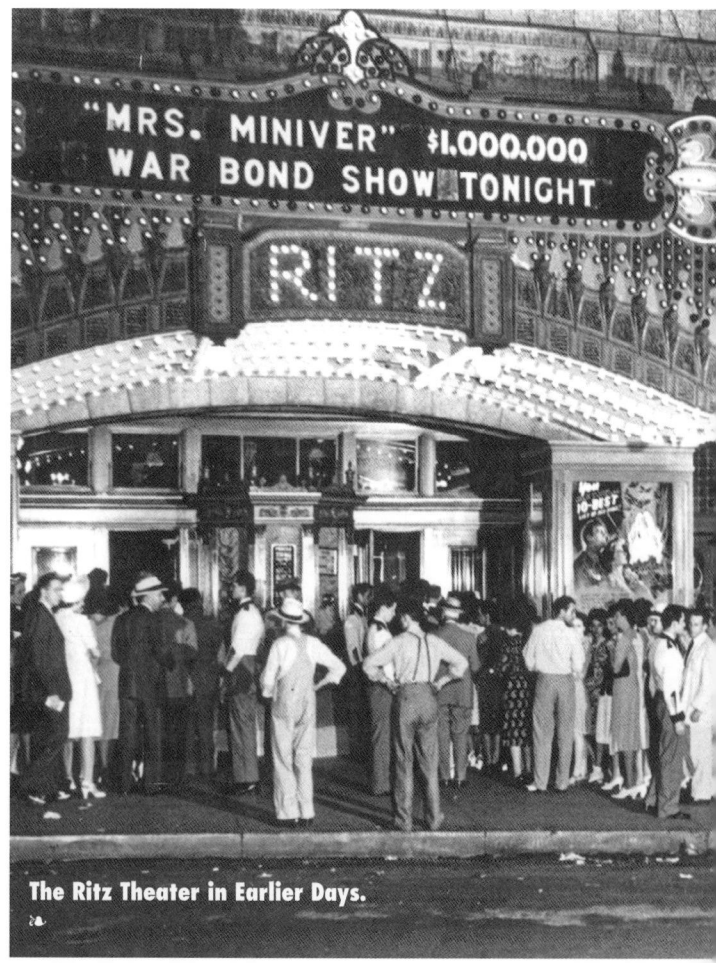

The Ritz Theater in Earlier Days.

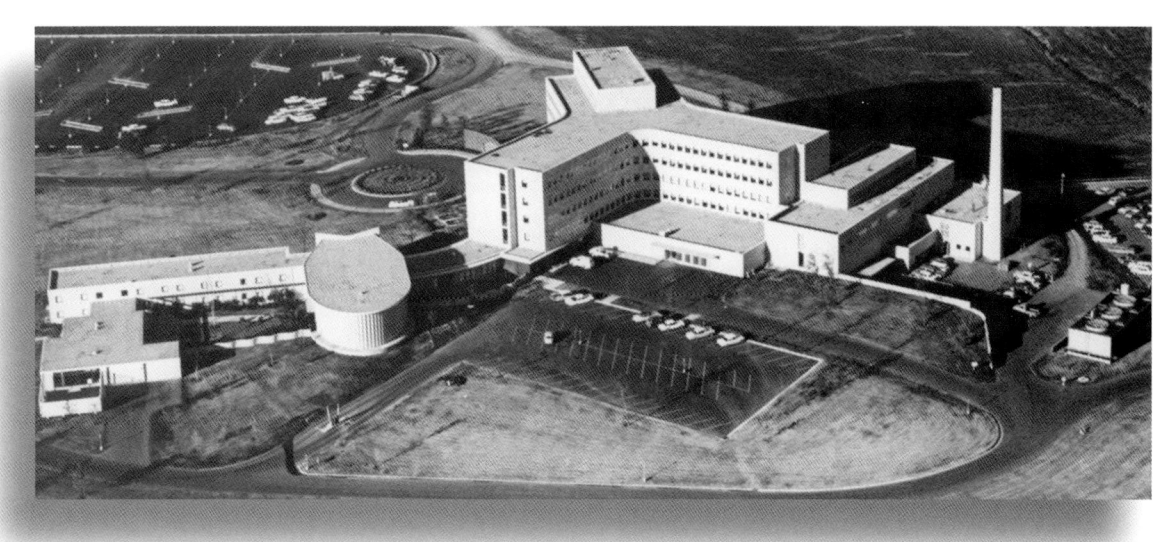

Aerial View of Saint Francis Hospital in 1960.

a faith-based institution was critical. That's why he included a chapel, a chaplain's quarters and a convent in the plans.

"I feel he felt a great empathy for people who are told they have cancer or diseases so traumatic to that person's heart. He felt if they would follow their faith, the Lord would hear their prayers," said W.K. Warren Jr., *Tulsa World*, Oct. 1, 2010.

The foundation spent two years planning the facility and another two years in construction. Pink became the hospital's trademark look. Natalie Warren, his wife, chose the hospital's exterior to be made of Italian pink modur. Each piece is about 40-inches square and three inches thick. It is a chalky composite with an aggregate of white and gray silver stone. The selling point is that it is impervious to light, holding its color indefinitely. The Warren matriarch choose pink — her favorite color. She provided no other alternatives.

For two days in September 1960, an open house was held to introduce the hospital. Aerial photos show a traffic jam on the two-lane Yale Avenue, stretching for miles and a line extending along with the hospital's exterior. Women wore dresses, and men wore suits as they toured the state-of-the-art hospital. The *Tulsa World* called it "a polished jewel set in an emerald green field" in a October 1960 special section. The *Tulsa Tribune* seven months earlier placed the headline, "You Name It... New Hospital Has It" and quoted doctors saying it was "nothing like they've ever seen before."

"As you drive to the hospital entrance, you will see its arms spread wide in greeting. Spare, clean and modern, the hospital is decorated in a way to combine pleasant surroundings with quiet, restful results." *Tulsa World*, Sept. 18, 1960.

Each visitor received a 16-page, pocket-sized booklet explaining different aspects and technologies in the building. Aspects noted were the patient-controlled radio panels, televisions, electronically operated beds, intercoms from rooms to nursing stations and private rooms. Closed-circuit televisions allowed for broadcasts from the hospital's chapel, and for a family to see a newborn from the nursery. The medical rooms included the emergency room, nursery, surgery and radiology, which touted the city's "largest X-ray equipment." The machine could produce a photo in 6 1/2 minutes, considered seven

Continued on page 94

Dr. Leon Horowitz

Tulsa's first certified pediatric allergist set a standard for medical care, which is evident in the thriving Allergy Clinic of Tulsa. He was also the husband of Betsy, a well-known community activist who ran for mayor three times and led efforts to preserve the historic Maple Ridge neighborhood.

The Horowitz's were a popular couple involved with Jewish causes and other philanthropies.

Dr. Horowitz spent his youth in Brighton Beach, New York, graduating from Lincoln High School in Brooklyn. He entered the U.S. Army as a combat infantryman, serving from 1943 to 1945 in the European Theater. He was taken as a prisoner of war by the Germans and was awarded four campaign ribbons.

As a 19-year-old, he was captured by the Germans in late 1944 and fell ill just before the Nazis shipped all the Jewish prisoners in his stalag to the Berga slave labor camp.

"I was so sick, I collapsed unconscious on the barracks floor. Everybody thought I was dead. They even sent the burial detail for me. They really thought I was a goner." – Dr. Leon Horowitz recalled in the book *Given Up for Dead*, by Flint Whitlock.

The Germans had a coffin ready with his name on it. He missed out on the transfer to Berga but got better. A few months later his camp was liberated, and he weighed 85 pounds. He was sent home for recovery.

After his service, he graduated cum laude and Phi Beta Kappa from New York University College. He then used the G.I. Bill to pay for his education at the New York University College of Medicine, graduating in 1952.

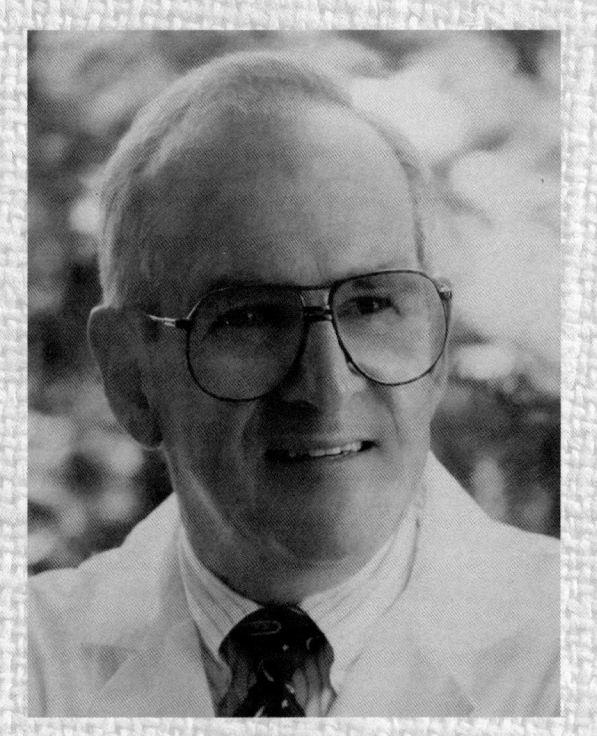

That same year, he married Betsy. She studied retail at New York University and had been working as a production assistant for television shows, including *I Love Lucy*. Years later, she attended law school at the University of Tulsa.

Dr. Horowitz completed an internship at Lennox Hill Hospital then took his pediatric residencies at Bellevue Hospital, New York, and at Lenox Hill Hospital. He moved to Tulsa to join Dr. Herschel Rubin in practice from 1955 to 1958. Then, he left for an allergy fellowship at the Kaiser Foundation Hospital in San Francisco and one at the University of Oklahoma Allergy Clinic.

The family returned to Tulsa in 1961. Dr. Horowitz was the city's first board certified pediatric allergist and the 37th physician to be certified by the board. He was integral in starting the Tulsa Pediatric Society and was a member of several other societies. He was a diplomat of the American Board of Pediatrics, American College of Allergists and had been elected to the Cardiopulmonary Council of the American Heart Association.

Under his guidance, the Allergy Clinic of Tulsa flourished as he strove to implement the latest in scientific research and technology. In 1975, the clinic started a program to provide daily pollen counts as a public service. It would issue pollen alerts when conditions could be difficult for patients with asthma and other allergy conditions.

Through the decades, Dr. Horowitz was a main source for stories related to allergy care. In a Nov. 7, 1987 *Tulsa Tribune* story about ways to treat allergies, he summed up the life-long struggle some people face.

"Allergy is not outgrown, it just expresses itself in different ways at different ages," Dr. Horowitz stated.

Dr. Horowitz was also a regular author of guest editorials in the city's newspapers. In a 1989 piece, he wrote about the failures of the Soviet Union after he went on a medical trip to the country. Two years before, he weighed in on a controversy after a racially insensitive logo appeared on the Tulsa State Fair's marketing campaign. The fair's theme was "The Orient Expressed." In an opinion piece, Dr. Horowitz wrote, "The time has come for all of us to develop greater sensitivity. We must be more aware of the other fellow's feelings; it's too late to say, 'No offense meant.'" He was also a leading voice in the anti-smoking campaigns. In one editorial, Dr. Horowitz argued the city needs to ban smoking like it did leaf burning.

"It took a long time for us to accept the fact that tobacco smoke polluted the body of the smoker. Now, no one doubts the fact that tobacco smoke causes emphysema, lung cancer, heart trouble, bladder cancer, bronchitis, etc. Persons exposed to second-hand smoke — side-stream smoke from burning cigarettes, cigars and pipes and exhaled smoke — are at risk of developing these diseases, just as are the smokers themselves." – Dr. Horowitz, *Tulsa Tribune*, Jan. 9, 1987.

The couple, particularly Betsy, was known for community activism and contribution. Three years after returning to Tulsa, the family was featured in the *Tulsa World* newspaper for their restoration of a mansion at 305 E. 19th St. It would be a precursor to their dedication to the neighborhood. It was in this house they raised five children.

"To give their children an appreciation of charming homes of the past which were designed for gracious living and to provide them with comforts of the present, Dr. and Mrs. Leon Horowitz decided to buy and restore a three-story Georgian Colonial house in Maple Ridge Addition. Their decision was made after a long search for a house and was based on their findings that they could get more space in the older house at a price they could not match by building a new house of the same size." – *Tulsa World*, Sept. 30, 1964.

When a zoning issue arose just blocks from their home in 1961, Betsy and several neighbors organized the Maple Ridge Association, which became the model for Tulsa neighborhood associations.

In 1968, the city made plans to build a "Riverside Expressway" to connect downtown Inner Dispersal Loop through the west wide of the Maple Ridge neighborhood. It would have run next to the playground at Lee Elementary, near 19th Street and Cincinnati Avenue. Betsy became the face of the organized protest to save the school and neighborhood, becoming a common figure at City Hall.

Betsy earned such nicknames as "the Maple Ridge Gadfly" and "LaFortune's Misfortune," referring to Robert J. LaFortune, a future Tulsa mayor, who was street commissioner at the time. The campaign included protests at city commission meetings, petitioning state lawmakers and meeting with congressmen in Washington, D.C.

"It was a great political battle. What was at work was government agencies saying this is what is best for you. I was shocked at their arrogance," she said in a 1992 *Tulsa Tribune* story.

In 1972, the state highway department abandoned plans for the Riverside Expressway after Horowitz and other opponents filed a federal lawsuit, making it impossible to get the funds in time to complete the loop. Betsy observed in later newspaper interviews that the River Parks developed because of the effort to end the expressway plans. Betsy ran unsuccessfully for mayor three times and once for the city's finance commissioner.

The couple took many mission trips and was active in the Jewish community. Dr. Horowitz was a member of the American Ex-Prisoners of War organization and was a recipient of Temple Israel's Isaiah Award for service to the temple and for representing Jewish values in the community. Betsy died in May 2009 and Dr. Horowitz died in September 2011. ■

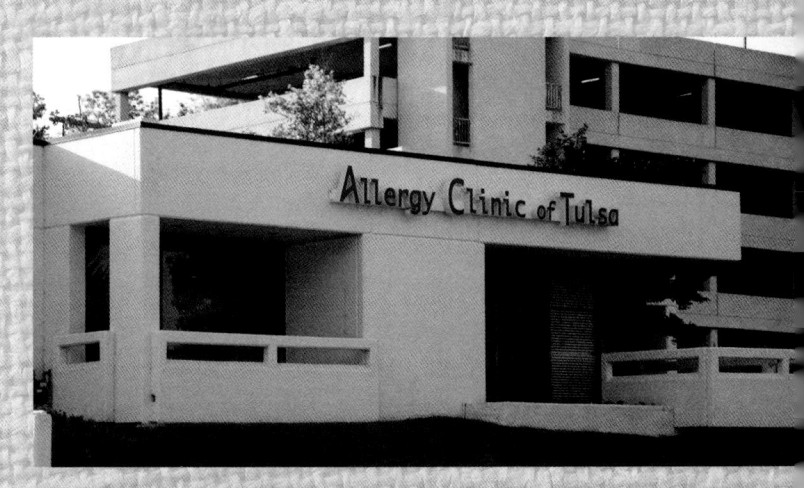

Allergy Clinic of Tulsa's Utica Office.

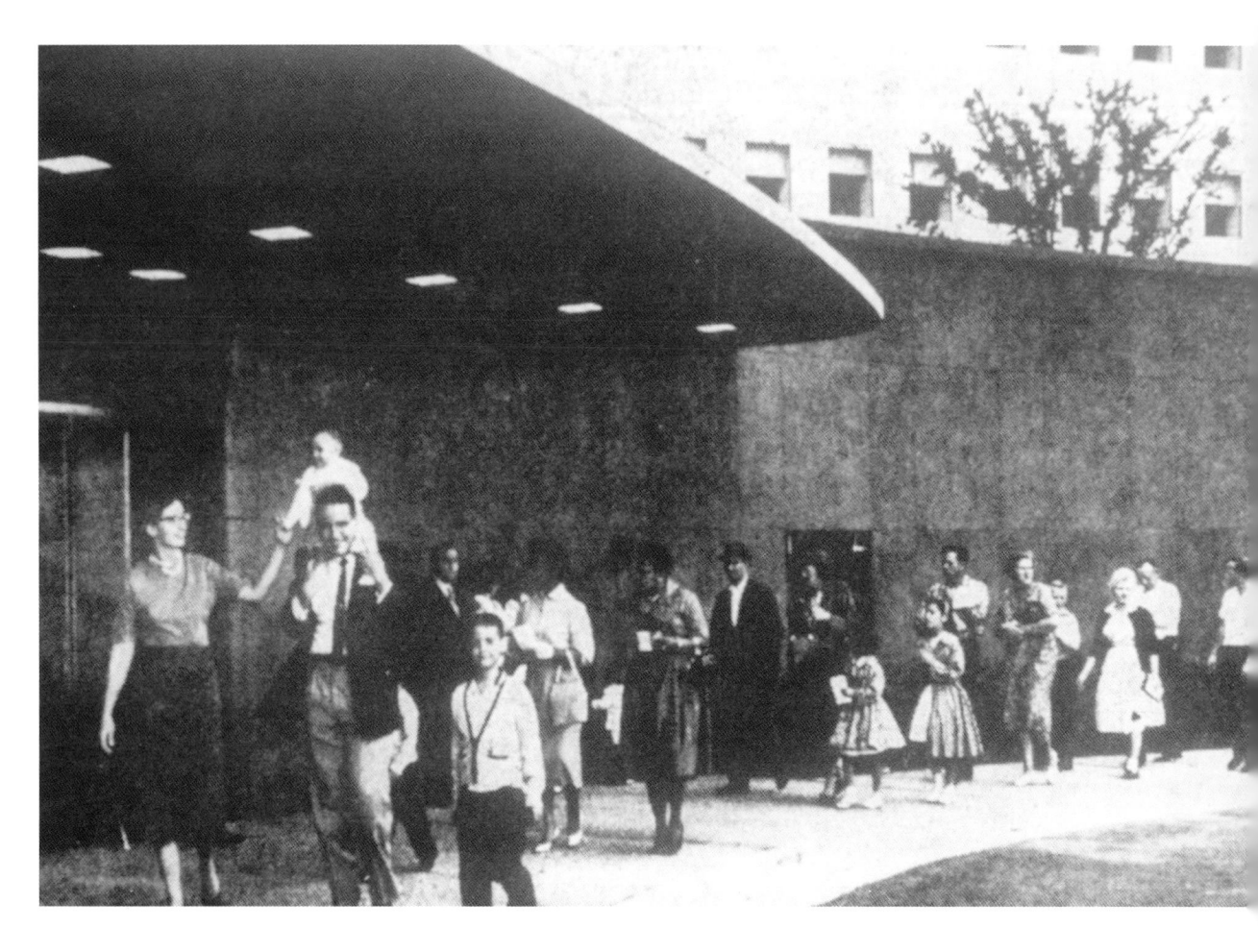

Saint Francis Grand Opening in 1960.

times faster than the old method. More than 20,000 people passed through the corridors in the two-day period, attracting thousands more than anticipated.

"On behalf of the nuns, the staff, Mr. Warren and myself, I want to express our thanks to the visitors for their consideration and orderliness. We feel it was most remarkable that there was no damage to the building, equipment or the ground," said Natalie Warren, *Tulsa Tribune*, Sept. 26, 1960.

The towering six-story hospital, built in the shape of a "Y," had 275 beds when it opened. The hospital was officially dedicated by His Eminence Francis Cardinal Spellman on Dec. 3, 1960, on the feast day of St. Francis Xavier for whom the hospital was named. Semi-private rooms cost $17.50 a day and private rooms $22.50 a day. The prices were about the same as other hospitals. St. John's charged $13 to $21 for semi-private rooms and $15 to $27 for private rooms, and Hillcrest rates were $15.50 for semi-private rooms and $20 to $25 for private rooms.

In the nursery, new mothers were offered a photo of their baby the day after giving birth. It was a new service with a "modern automatic camera" in the nursery. In the few months the hospital was open in 1960, there were 786 babies born at the hospital. The first baby was born the day it opened — Oct. 1, 1960 — to Mr. and Mrs. Leroy Holley. They named their son Warren Otis Ricky Holley in honor of the hospital's founder. The first person to check into the hospital was Georgia H. Lloyd Jones, wife of Richard Lloyd Jones, publisher of the *Tulsa Tribune*. She was admitted for a medical checkup.

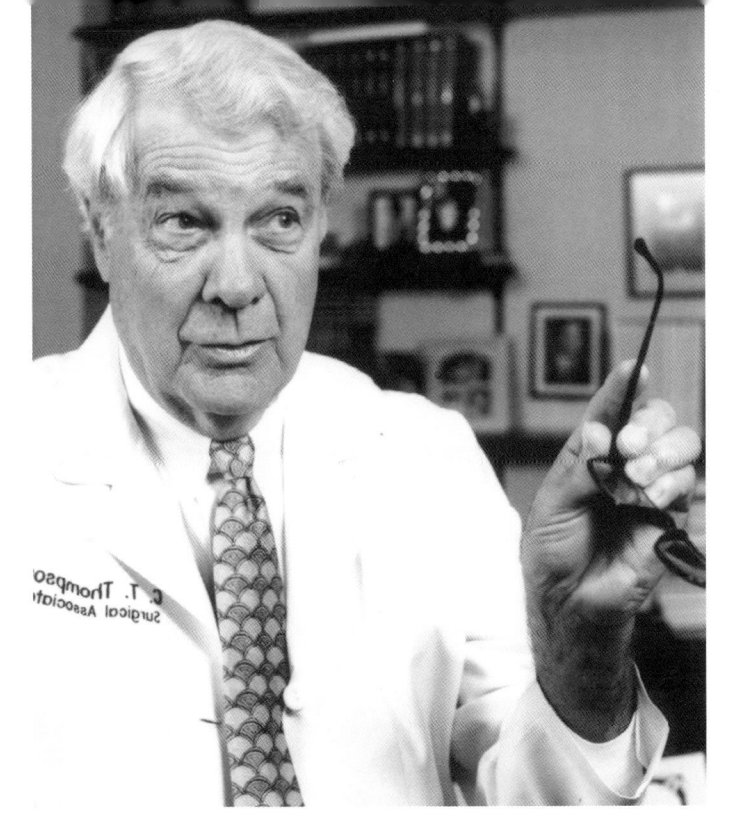

Dr. C.T. Thompson.

It was a slow go with patient admissions, with the first month of operations averaging 28 patients a day. By May 1961, it was losing about $90,000 a month for at least seven months and had about 110 patients. The deficit was covered by the foundation. Reasons cited by city doctors were the distance. Dr. C.T. Thompson, former executive vice president and chief operating officer, said that doctors spent a good portion of time driving from hospital to hospital caring for patients: "When St. Francis came on the scene, it began to polarize practice."

Eventually, physicians and medical groups located near the hospital as the William, Kelly and Warren Medical Buildings, the Warren Clinic and the Warren Place office complex were built. Physician groups were being formed at record rates and many aligned themselves with specific hospitals. Surgical Associates was among the first to work with Saint Francis and helped it grow. Dr. C.T. Thompson, a founder of the group, who is credited for recruiting numerous doctors to the hospital in its first decade, practiced at Saint Francis until 1996 and served as an interim chief executive officer. Dr. Gerald Gustafson of that surgical group was instrumental in developing trauma treatment, which led to the development of the Hospital Emergency Ambulance Radio system by Motorola.

"At that time, the funeral homes were running ambulance services. It was crazy, I didn't understand why we couldn't connect ambulance to hospital and hospital to ambulance. But the problem was, there were two handfuls of radio frequencies for emergency services, and we wanted the same access the Tulsa sheriffs had. So we politicked." — Dr. Gerald Gustafson, "Saint Francis 50."

Dr. Gerald Gustafson.

Saint Francis Hospital admissions steadily increased, and August 1961 marked the first month the hospital made a profit. By 1964, the hospital hit its first full capacity and reported an 87 percent average occupancy rate.

"Our patients are our best boosters. When a person has been a patient here, he or she tells family members and friends. For this reason, I know we will succeed." — Sister Hildalita, a member of the order of Sisters Adorers of the Most Precious Blood, *Tulsa Tribune*, May 16, 1961.

In the hospital's expansion in 1968, another Y-shaped wing would be added, in which the two bases of the Ys joined to resemble a cross or X design. It expanded the facility to about 650 beds and cost about $15 million.

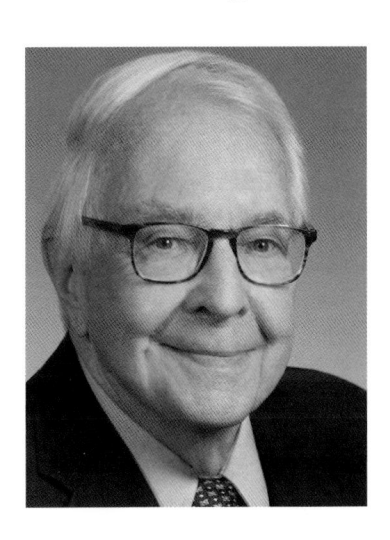

One of the attractions for doctors and patients were the technologies available. During the decade, several of these were featured in media, such as a gastric hypothermia machine to treat ulcers without surgical removal, an X-ray machine that rotates patients and a sonar machine. Also, a piece covered the "ultrasonic sound wave" machine that cleaned surgical instruments in three minutes, compared to 15 minutes by hand washing. In 1962, one of the first document copiers (a Xerox 914) was installed, prompting a newspaper feature story on the "duplicating machine."

"The principle of mechanically duplicating records is an old and trusted one in business. Hospitals, however, have been leery of tampering with their lab procedures. At stake is a patient's health, and a mistake can be costly if a life hangs in the balance. St. Francis official happily cited three major boons from the machine. (1) It turns out plenty of copies without the threat of error. (2) It cuts time and energy spent on manually making copies. (3) It gives the patient's doctor a handy complete lab record on one sheet." — *Tulsa World*, Jan. 24, 1962.

In 1962, Saint Francis opened the city's first intensive care unit followed by a radio-frequency paging system in 1963.

As the decade ended, the hospital changed management to the Sisters of Charity of the Incarnate Word from Houston, who took over from the order of the Sisters Adorers of the Most Precious Blood. The next leaders ushered in a new era of medicine with advanced technology. The core of the administrative team was Lloyd Verret and Sister Mary Blandine Fleming with Dr. Thompson serving as a liaison between medical staff and administration.

"A perfect storm was brewing. The growth of the city, an explosion of doctors and the introduction of Medicare. It led to enormous need for hospitals. That's what contributed to the growth of Saint Francis. That and the exodus of doctors from other institutions, particularly in the surgical ward. They came in groups." — Dr. C.T. Thompson, "Saint Francis 50."

Doctors' Hospital

On Aug. 29, 1966, a 100-bed hospital operated by a group of 18 general practitioners opened at 2323 S. Harvard Ave. It was formed as a nonprofit after the doctors were concerned about admitting privileges and amount of control doctors would have at the other hospitals. The $1.2 million facility was built on a 10-acre campus centered around a wagon-wheel building design with wings extending out. It was a public hospital with an open staff, meaning any legally qualified medical doctor could apply for staff membership. Also, it was the first hospital west of the Mississippi River built completely with private funds.

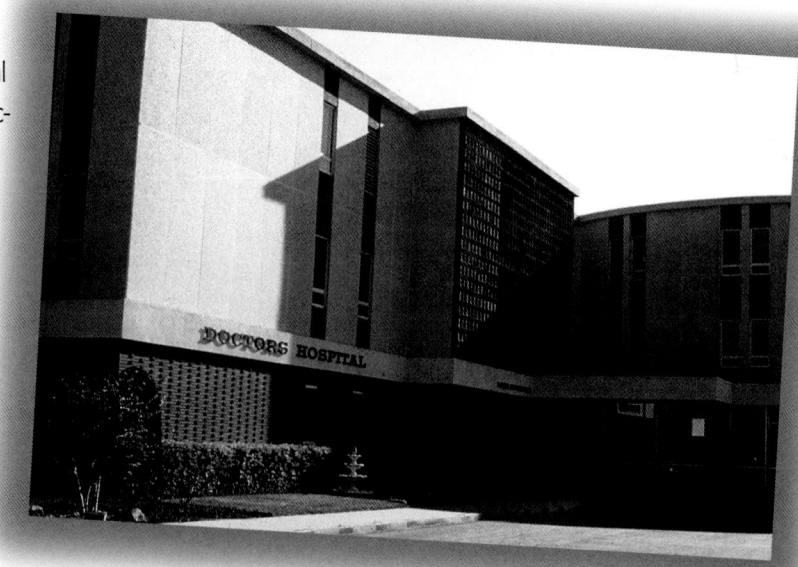

"We are building the hospital because we feel it will attract many general practitioners to Tulsa. Tulsa is badly in need of more GPs," said Dr. Harlan Thomas, president of Doctors' Hospital, *Tulsa Tribune*, June 1, 1964.

The rooms and halls were decorated in warm colors to provide a home-like atmosphere and in a French provincial style, news reports stated.

"Every detail has been looked into, even down to the selection of specially planned color coordinated wallpaper. After consulting with a color therapist, we choose in-depth wallpaper. The patient will not be staring at a blank wall, but one that makes the room seem larger," said Roy Finley, Doctors' Hospital administrator, *Tulsa Tribune*, June 15, 1966.

The hospital was the first facility in the country to carry the emblem of the American Academy of Family Physicians — an image of two overlapping rings, one framing a family and the other a doctor. It designated the hospital as specializing in family care.

The trustees and original incorporators were: Harlan Thomas, president; Herbert Oor, vice president; Charles Wilbanks, secretary; Logan Spann, treasurer; Curtis Clifton; William Ewell; Warren Gwartney; Charles Lilly; Joseph Salamy; Theodore Williams; Fred Woodson; R.Q. Atchley; John Capehart; Earl Lusk; Hugh Nicholas; Martin Leibovitz and John Brasfield. Two doctors — M.O. Hart and Buel Humphreys — were original incorporators but died before the hospital opened.

> **Doctors' Hospital was the first hospital west of the Mississippi River built completely with private funds.**

In 1975, a $2 million expansion was added and included a 40-bed extended care facility, a 100-bed nursing-convalescent center, and a multi-story professional office building. A $1.5 million administrative building was added.

In September 1983, the hospital was sold. The sale proceeds were used to establish the Founders of Doctors' Hospital, which is a nonprofit supporting the charitable activities backed by the retired family doctors. It has given at least $50 million in grants to medical, educational, civic and social projects in the Tulsa area. Hillcrest Healthcare Systems bought the facility in 1999, but financial problems led to its closure in December 2000.

The last living founder of the hospital, Dr. Joseph Salamy, died in August 2010.

"We all felt sad. It's just like losing a part of the family. But things change. Gotta accept it," Dr. Joseph Salamy, *Tulsa World*, Dec. 20, 2000.

Promises in Hissom

In what was considered an advancement for the lives of children with developmental and intellectual disabilities, the Hissom Memorial Center for the Mentally Retarded opened in 1961 to serve 19 counties. It was named after Wiley B. Hissom, who donated his $220,000, 227-acre farm in Sand Springs for the school. The Oklahoma State Board of Mental Health approved the programs and hired the Tulsa architectural firm of Murray-Jones-Murray to design the $6.5 million campus, which was located on 85 acres. The facility was considered modern with programs including trained teachers, art therapist, physical therapists, psychologists, physicians and caretakers.

"Wiley Hissom and his wife had no children of their own, and they wished to help the children of others," said Carl K. Bates, head of the State Board of Public Affairs, *Tulsa World*, July 2, 1961.

It wasn't until the 50s medical schools started to change its approaches on developmentally disabled children, including using the classifications from psychologist H.H. Goddard of Idiot (less than 25 IQ), Imbecile (25 to 50 IQ) and Moron (50 to 70 IQ). Children with these disabilities were usually warehoused in institutions in Vinita, Enid and Paul's Valley at the suggestions of physicians. Few families cared for children with intellectual disabilities in their homes, and no job or housing programs were in existence for developmentally disabled adults. Hospitals would separate babies with Down's Syndrome and prevent the mother from bonding with their newborn.

In the planning of Hissom, officials were unsure whether to call it a school or hospital, reflecting the shift in mindset and culture. Settling on "center," much was debated and written about the possibilities. It was designed and built while under the supervision of the Oklahoma Mental Health Department. But within two years, it was transferred to the state's Welfare Department.

"This is a long, tough job with no assurance of success. But if it isn't done, there will be no chance to reclaim the lost asset of these Oklahoma citizens. At Hissom, Oklahoma will give it a good try. Hissom's nearness to a city the size of Tulsa makes it a prime spot for another facet of the fight against mental ailments. It is here that the state will inaugurate a full-scale training program in a variety of technical fields — all aimed at the problem of wasted minds." — *Tulsa World*, May 3, 1962.

The center was intended to be a new model of education for people with intellectual disabilities.

"The center will care for all types of retardation, with emphasis on education, research and psychiatric and medical treatment. The goal will be to return the patient to a normal home life. The research and education programs will attract students from universities of the state, and the two student quarters will provide accommodations." — *Tulsa Tribune*, April 11, 1961.

After about two years, some concerns were made about aspects of the original design of the building. The center had 300 cage-like beds for some bedridden and severely disabled children. These bleak-looking beds were surrounded by bars and screens with metal-door latches. A group of dignitaries touring the center in 1963 reported being disturbed by the sight, calling them "animal-like cages." The outcry about this poor treatment reached a Legislative Council in November 1963. By the end of that month, lawmakers forced the transfer of those cribs to the McAlester State Penitentiary, where they were torn apart and repurposed for furniture. The amount of glass used in the architecture was also troubling to a newly appointed director of the center. Dr. Joseph C. Denniston said about one-fourth of the children were considered "hyperactive" with the possibility of breaking glass. In 1965, the school windows were replaced with tempered glass to prevent breakage.

"You can't build a perfect institution for every type of child," said Dr. Joseph C. Denniston, director of Hissom, *Tulsa Tribune*, Nov. 8, 1963.

Through the decade, programs and buildings were added to the campus. In June 1968, it opened a $650,000 activities center with Gov. Dewey Bartlett delivering comments. The event featured a bell-ringing choir performed by children at the school. It was intended for recreational therapy and contained a gymnasium, auditorium and swimming pool with smaller areas for music therapy and locker rooms.

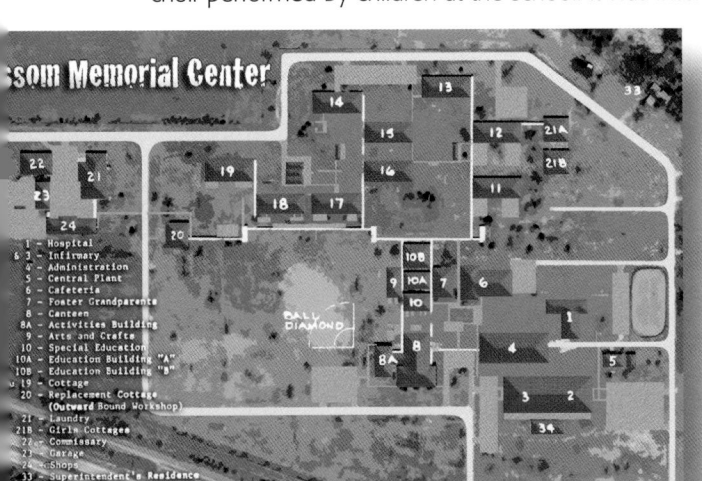

Hissom Memorial Center Map.

"The real dedication of a building is to take advantage of the physical aspect to the fullest — to see programs put into effect (which will) develop our children. Progress has been made, but more progress must be made to see that our state stands at the forefront in the area of mental retardation." — Gov. Dewey Bartlett, *Tulsa World*, June 11, 1968.

As part of the growing popularity of the Special Olympics started in 1968 by Eunice Kennedy Shriver, astronaut James Lovell served as head coach for a team of Hissom children at the Southeast Special Olympics. The Southeast Tulsa Jaycees sponsored the two-day event in 1969 to attract about 1,000 developmentally disabled children from six states. Lovell spoke to the Jaycees in March 1969 as a guest of the Joseph P. Kennedy Foundation to back research and activities for people with intellectual disabilities.

Within 20 years, the facility did not live up to expectations and some say became dangerous. In May 1985, Homeward Bound Inc. filed a lawsuit against the Hissom center and associated state agencies. Plaintiffs were parents of children who were living at the center. The allegations included negligence and abuse, injury, unnecessary physical and chemical restraint, and lack of adequate medical care, clothing, food and rehabilitative services. The six children in the original complaint suffered multiple bites, scratches and cuts among their injuries. Other signs of neglect included broken teeth, rashes and fungal infections. The living conditions were described as patients spending most their days sitting idly in chairs or benches resembling those at a bus station while being provided little to no services to how to function in daily life. Sleeping areas were described as being large areas partitioned into small areas with multiple beds and little privacy. Personal toys were kept locked in a closet and rarely provided to the residents.

In July 1987, a federal judge ordered the institution closed and children moved into community-based settings. The U.S. Court of Appeals affirmed the decision in May 1992. Two years later, it officially closed.

MOTON — FROM HOSPITAL TO CENTER

After decades of serving the largely black and low-income neighborhoods in Tulsa, Moton Memorial Hospital closed in June 1967 after being plagued by financial trouble and a dilapidated facility. The hospital, 603 E. Pine St., could no longer meet Medicare standards. When it closed, it was a 27-bed hospital with nine black doctors on staff.

The local agency spent $900,000 for renovation and modernization of programs in 1968, and later that year was awarded a $1.15 million grant from the U.S. Office of Economic Opportunity to continue the effort. The project was to serve the 25,000 low-income people living within eight square miles of the facility. Of those, about 4,000 were Medicaid eligible and able to use the facility, though no one would be turned away. It was one of 48 such health centers in the country.

After six months, the hospital emerged in February 1969 with a new name — Moton Health Center — and a mission of outpatient services. The City-County Health Department ran the clinic, which was funded largely by the federal government. Services included physical therapy and rehabilitation, pharmacy, X-ray, laboratory, dental and exam rooms. Transportation was provided and a nursery available while parents were receiving treatment.

"I think the most important facet of the center is its philosophy. We are using the family approach. ... Nearly every family is multi-problem. We are giving them a one-door facility to solve all their health needs, not just medical," said Dr. Walter Atkins, health department assistant director and project coordinator, *Tulsa World*, Feb. 6, 1969.

Moton Municipal Hospital.

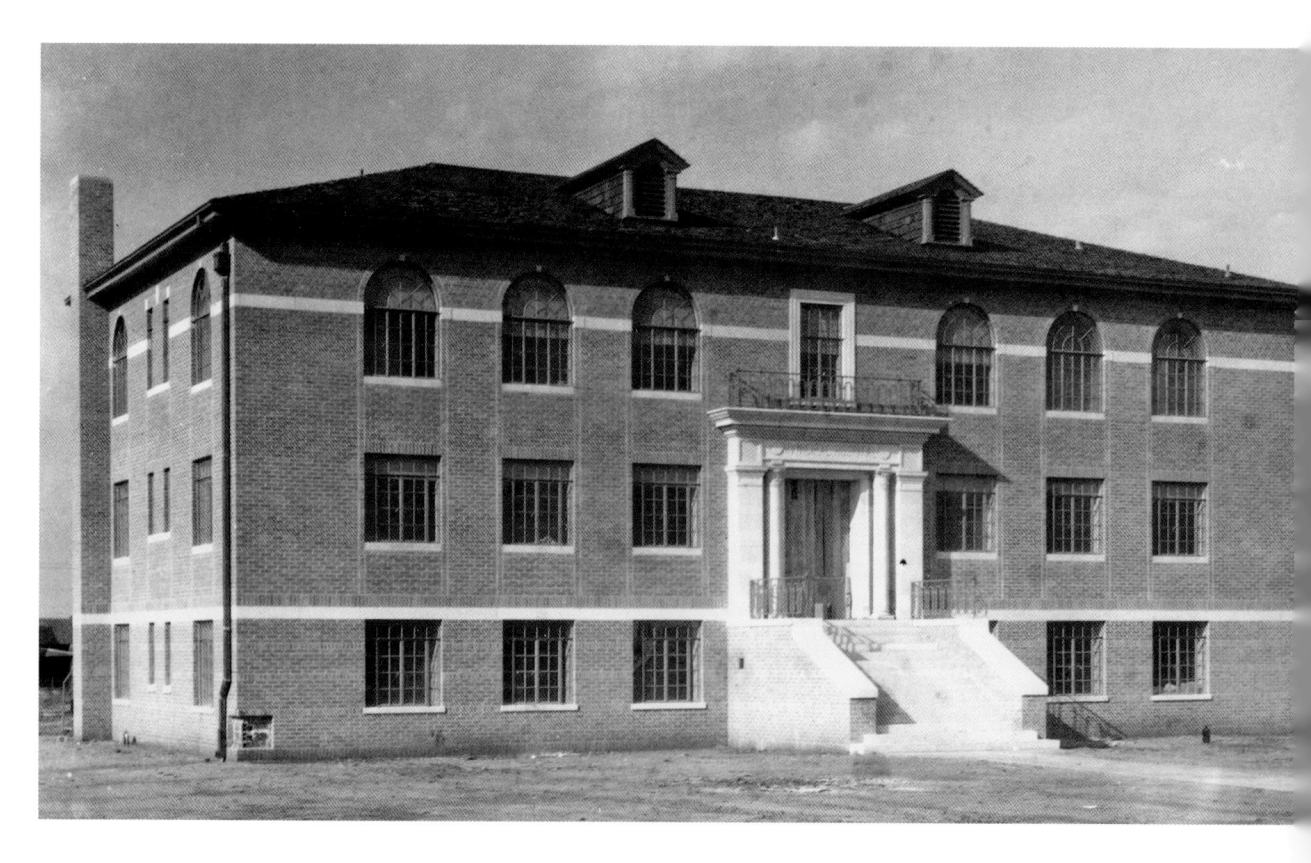

At the center's opening in April 1969, race was a central theme in the remarks made by Charlotte Moton Hubbard, daughter of the facility's namesake and deputy assistant secretary of state for the U.S. Department of Public Affairs.

"Of course I am aware of the color of my skin, but I feel human. I feel human first. If I've learned anything, it is to look at the individual. A building like this has meaning only if it benefits those it is supposed to serve. A hungry child or a person needing medical care do not need food or attention because of color but because they need those things," said Charlotte Moton Hubbard, *Tulsa World*, April 28, 1969.

A year later, the Moton dental clinic was the only one in the city serving indigent patients and scheduled 30 to 50 appointments daily. For people who did not show up for any medical service, staff went to the homes to check on them. A writer describes some of the patients on a typical day: A man with legs gnarled from childhood polio leaning on crutches patched with tape, a woman waiting to have nine teeth pulled, a mother of four children with varying illnesses, a woman experiencing her first doctor's visit and a diabetic man with a swollen foot with no toes seeking dietary and pharmaceutical assistance.

Moton Municipal Hospital Exam Room.

"These are the poor, the dirty, the hungry. These are the ones whose main thought is how to scratch out today's existence in a time when it is harder than ever for them to survive. Poverty is everywhere, in every town and city, gasping for air in rickety shacks huddled together in sidestreets and alleys where no one dares to go. And poverty, with a face that is mostly black, is here in Tulsa," *Tulsa Tribune*, July 29, 1969.

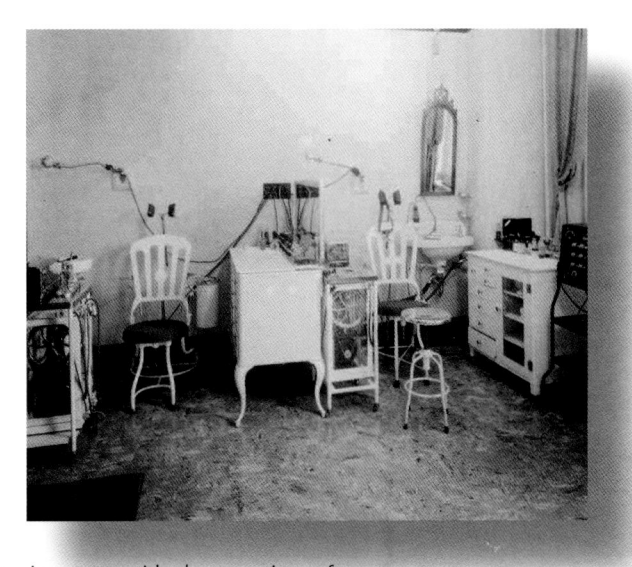

Medicare

One of the most transformational laws regarding health care came in 1965 with the creation of Medicare. President Lyndon Johnson signed into law the Social Security Amendments to provide health coverage for about 19 million people aged 65 and older and elevate other benefits. It consisted of hospital insurance (Part A) and supplementary medical insurance (Part B) and went into effect July 1, 1966. It came with controversy. Tulsa hospital officials stated the city was already facing overcrowding and that the federal program would cause a further shortage of beds and a crisis in nursing recruitment. Many said the federal funding would not keep up with actual costs, creating debt on hospitals and leading to less quality care. The American Medical Association opposed the legislation.

"Medicare is going to cause changes in Tulsa hospitals that we never dreamed of, and that is putting it mildly," said Kenneth Wallace, assistant administrator at St. John's Hospital, *Tulsa Tribune*, Aug. 2, 1965.

The flip side of the argument stated Oklahomans would receive $76 million in extra benefits from the amendments in the first year of operation. It would provide more financial stability for hospitals facing large indigent populations by expanding health care to a vulnerable population.

The Democrat Oklahoma senators split on the vote, with A.S. Mike Monroney supporting its passage and Fred Harris against it. On the House side, Oklahoma congressman voting for the legislation were Democrats Carl Albert, Ed Edmondson and Jed Johnson Jr. The congressmen voting against the measure were Democrats John Jarman and Tom Steed along with Republican Page Belcher.

A long-time projectionist became Tulsa's first resident to participate in Medicare. Carney A. Burton — who worked 31 years at the Ritz Theater and little more than 5 years at the Rialto — turned 65 the year it became available and signed up at the Social Security Board office. He paid $3 a month with the federal government matching the cost. His coverage included "liberal hospitalization," 80 percent of diagnostic costs and financial aid for physician services. Five months before the program launched, about 12 million Americans had signed up for the voluntary program, which was on par to exceed the 80 percent participation figure cited by officials.

"I can think of no other time in history when 12 million people have agreed in the space of five months to pay $3 a month on a continuing basis for anything," said Robert M. Ball, commissioner of Social Security, *Tulsa Tribune*, Feb. 4, 1966.

Hospitals then had to pass inspections to participate in the program. These standards were wide-ranging and included nurse ratios, types of equipment, governing bodies, medical records maintenance, fire safety and civil rights compliance. By April 1966, only about 60 of Oklahoma's 167 hospitals had been accredited by the Joint Commission on Accreditation of Hospitals. But, those represented 73 percent of hospital beds.

By June 1966, Hillcrest Medical Center and the Oklahoma Osteopathic Hospital were the only Tulsa hospitals approved to participate in the program. Mercy Hospital in Oklahoma City was the other approved facility in the state. In the era of desegregation, the approval for Saint Francis had been held up by federal officials pending an investigation for compliance with the Civil Rights Act, which passed the previous year. Concerns cited by government officials were no black physicians with hospital privileges and a low rate of black patients — 2.4 percent of black patients compared to the city's 9.2 percent of the total population. Hospital officials stated the location was furthest from the largely black neighborhoods in north Tulsa and that all physicians are considered equally, without preference to race. By mid-June, Saint Francis was given clearance under the Civil Rights Act to participate about two weeks before the July 1, 1966, deadline.

Administration of federal health care program in Oklahoma was divided between Blue Cross and the Aetna Life Insurance Co. Blue Cross handled the hospitalization portion while Aetna processed medical claims. The installation of computers was part of the program and began the modernization of medical billing. At Blue Cross, 13 employees were tasked with operating the computer. The company would compute and certify costs before sending them through digital codes to its headquarters in Maryland. To handle this type of accounting, Blue Cross bought the two-story Remington Rand Building at 1203 S. Boulder Ave. A *Tulsa Tribune* reporter described the information as being coded to numbers "which the computers gobble up like strawberry shortcake." The coded patient information was sent on a high speed tape, routed through a computer in Chicago for storage. It ended up in the computer system at the Social Security Center in Baltimore.

Continued on page 104

Dr. Myra Peters

An Alabama native became a woman of many firsts in medicine. Dr. Myra Peters, one of nine children and daughter of a locomotive engineer, was inspired by the women working in the medical field.

"Across the street from our house lived a nurse by the name of Mrs. Knight and my mother had a first cousin who was also a nurse. Between the two of them I developed my interest in medicine and started thinking about making a career in medicine. The first time I mentioned it to Mrs. Knight, I told her, 'When I grow up I'm going to be a nurse like you.' She said, 'No you're not – you're going to be a doctor.' And from then on I would say, 'I'm going to be a doctor.' And everyone would laugh at me. So, when I was in high school that was my thing. I took all the high school courses that I needed to — chemistry, physics and biology. By the time I finished and went down to the University of Alabama, I enrolled in premed courses," Dr. Peters, July 21, 2002, interview.

Dr. Peters graduated from the University of Alabama at age 20 with a 3.8 grade point average. She enrolled at the Medical College of Alabama in Birmingham with eight other women. Seven of them graduated from the program in 1949. She then became the first woman accepted into the orthopedic surgery program at the Mayo Clinic.

While at the Mayo Clinic, she befriended Mr. and Mrs. John Dunkin, prominent Tulsans, after completing a spinal fusion on their ranch foreman. The couple recruited her to move to the city. There were few female physicians in Tulsa. Of the nine orthopedic surgeons in Tulsa, none were women. She received privileges at St. John and Hillcrest hospitals.

"I think there was only one orthopedist that didn't like me because I was a woman. However, later we became good friends," said Dr. Peters, July 21, 2002, interview.

Dr. Peters was a charter member of the Tulsa Orthopedic Society and always held a membership to the Tulsa County Medical Society. She served on the board and then was elected president in 1968, becoming the first woman to lead the board of the Tulsa County Medical Society. When she took office, only about 2 percent of the membership was women.

"I was always interested in the politics of the association. I served on committees and was a delegate to the Oklahoma State Medical Association from Tulsa. … (Becoming president) was really a very proud moment for me – to think that my fellow doctors would vote for me because they felt that I was an asset to the association and the community. The county medical society serves a local brotherhood. It is important for physicians to become involved – they need to be taught the importance of working together for the good of medicine. The county society must provide an interface between physicians and the community," Dr. Peters, July 21, 2002, interview.

The next time a woman would lead the Tulsa County Medical Society board would be in 2000 with the installation of Dr. Barbara Hastings, a neurologist. When she took office, about 15 percent of the membership was women.

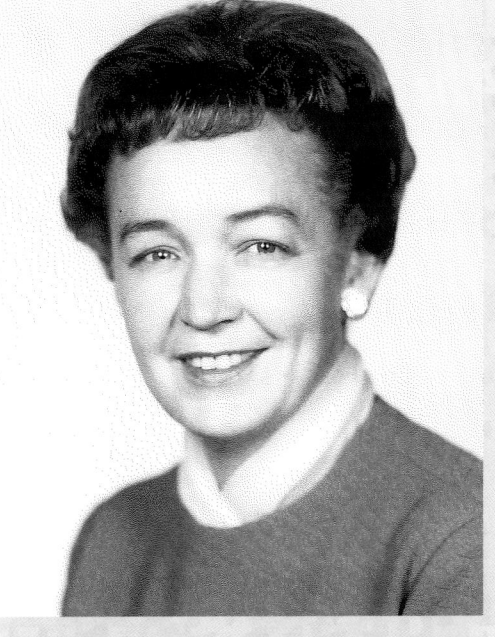

"We couldn't administer the Medicare program if it weren't for our computer, and the big one at the Social Security Center in Baltimore. The computers do most of the job," said W. Ralph Bethel, vice president of the Oklahoma Blue Cross Blue Shield, *Tulsa Tribune*, July 1, 1966.

The year leading up to the Medicare launch detailed the preparations and expectations, from dire to optimistic. The American Medical Association had passed a resolution encouraging doctors to shun the government forms for payment and require patients to submit the forms themselves. By doing this, patients would pay upfront then seek reimbursement. Tulsa physicians largely ignored the AMA resolution and most said a clerical worker in their offices would be handling the paperwork.

"It's sorta like lining up for a race with an opponent you've never met. Officials of three of Tulsa's major hospitals are braced for the starting gun of a profound financing program on July 1. Although optimistic that there will be no problems which can't be met, they freely admit that predictions about the precise nature of Medicare's impact remain a matter of conjecture. There seems to be no doubt that prospective Medicare clients are 'saving their ailments' until after July 1," *Tulsa Tribune*, June 17, 1966.

On the day Medicare started, nearly all the submissions from Tulsa hospitals were for existing patients who qualified for the federal program. New patients under the Medicare program included six from Hillcrest Medical Center, 16 from St. John's Hospital and 10 from the Oklahoma Osteopathic Hospital. No one kept track at Saint Francis Hospital, but officials estimated between 30 and 40 patients were on Medicaid.

"The fear that Medicare would gobble Tulsa's medical facilities like a lion among sheep proved false Friday. Medicare marched in like a lamb. Friday's first day of government-financed medical care for the aged proved to be a quiet one. There was not a flood of patients now that Medicare will help pay the bill; there didn't even seem to be a wavelet," *Tulsa World*, July 2, 1966.

At the one year anniversary, there were mixed reactions to the program, with conflicting statistics and opinions.

"At one extreme of the reaction spectrum is the federal government, and at the other the medical profession and hospital. In the middle are the insurance companies," *Tulsa World*, Aug. 10, 1967.

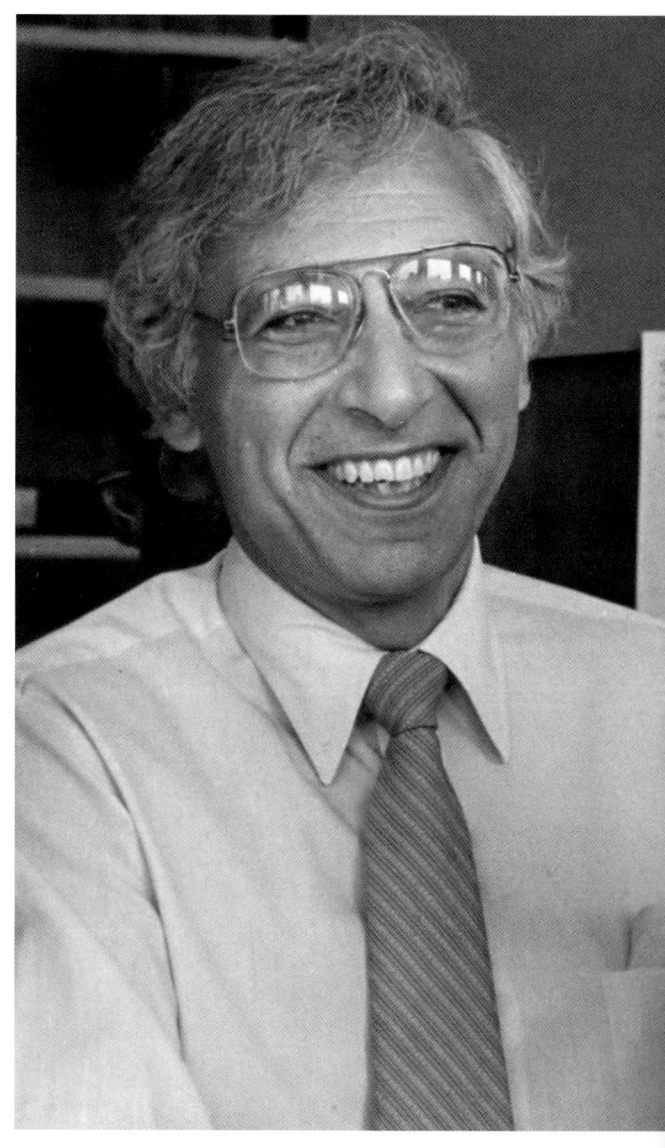

Dr. Robert C. Gallo, former biomedical researcher best known for work with HIV, and Dr. Albert B. Sabin, who developed an oral polio-virus vaccine.

At the second anniversary of the program, Medicare enrollment in Tulsa County had risen 3.2 percent over the previous year, with $8.94 million in 18,000 claims paid to the city's hospitals. Statewide, $46.5 million flowed from the federal program into hospitals, surpassing the first year's $33.2 million, for a 40 percent increase.

"Oklahoma's over 65 population has apparently become accustomed to Medicare. When the gigantic federal program of medical care for the elderly checked in to the state two years ago Sunday, it was not received with the immediate impact predicted. But as Medicare winds up its second fiscal year of operation Sunday, hospital administrators and paying agents directly involved with the program are only mildly surprised that year 2 of Medicare has witnessed significant increases over year 1," *Tulsa World*, June 30, 1968.

At its third year, Oklahoma had 145 hospitals and 41 extended-care facilities approved for Medicare. More than 297,000 hospital stays had been covered by Medicare and helped in more than 10,900 admissions for post-hospital care. Payments under the state hospital program totaled more than $134 million, and about $59 million had been paid under the medical insurance program.

A Sugar Cube and Polio Vaccine

It was in this decade a disease that disabled and killed its victims was finally eradicated. Polio was conquered with the help of a sugar cube. Dr. Albert Sabin, a scientist at the University of Cincinnati, developed an oral vaccine for polio. For the previous decade, an injected vaccine developed by Dr. Jonas Salk had been used to reduce the number of people affected. It was successful, considering 651 cases were reported in Tulsa within five years during the 50s compared to 10 cases in 1962. The oral vaccine was touted to be 100 percent effective while the injected version was 85 to 90 percent effective.

Problem was the taste, especially for children. So, the liquid vaccine was put onto sugar cubes to help the medicine go down.

The Tulsa County Medical Society distributed 780,000 doses of the Sabin vaccine to 70 percent of the county's population. The first doses (265,710), called type I, was received in January

Continued on page 108

William K. Warren

It was an oilman who changed the landscape of Tulsa medicine starting in the 1960s by building a pink hospital.

William K. Warren Sr. arrived in Oklahoma at age 18 after hearing about the potential for riches in the oilfields from the wife of a former mayor of Sapulpa. Warren grew up in Tennessee and was delivering newspapers at a Nashville hospital when he chanced on meeting Myrtle McDougal. She told young Warren exciting tales of the Sooner State and the opportunities for prosperity. In spring 1916, he arrived in Sapulpa by train, and McDougal helped set him up with a job. Within a week, Warren left for a position in Tulsa with Gypsy Oil, a subsidiary of Gulf, which was one of the big firms coming out of the Spindletop discovery in Texas. Gypsy was one of 80 companies operating in Tulsa.

Warren worked as an accountant for the company and did contract work at night for other oil companies. In 1919, he left to gain field experience as a tool pusher for Gilliland Oil Co. in Texas, and was later put in charge of payrolls, tank farms and other operations. He resigned in March 1922 to start his firm in Tulsa based in the Atco Building. He made his fortune by creating a market for a liquid by-product of oil — natural gasoline. Sometimes called white water or casinghead, it is the gasoline that came from the ground ahead of crude oil. Up until that time, fortunes were made in refining oil. Warren hit on the idea of natural gasoline. His company — Warren Petroleum Co. — started with two employees, Warren and his wife, Natalie.

The couple courted long distance while Warren made his way through the Oklahoma oilfields. Natalie Overall was born in Murfreesboro, Tennessee, and graduated in 1920 from Vanderbilt University. She studied chemistry, was one of the founders of the Nu Omicron chapter of Alpha Omicron Pi. The couple married in the fall 1921 and had seven children — six girls (Dorothy King, Natalie Bryant, Elizabeth Blankenship, Patricia Swindle, Marilyn Vandever and Jean Marie Warren) and a son (William K. Warren Jr.).

The couple had an unusual arrangement of faith with W.K. being a devout Catholic and Natalie a Methodist. The daughters were raised Methodist and son raised Catholic.

The company quickly grew. By May 1926, it controlled 31 gas processing plants in five states. In 1930, Warren bought the entire natural gasoline production of Amerada Petroleum Corp. and set a shipping record the following year. By the early 40s, Warren held the largest fleet of liquefied petroleum gas tank cars in the Southwest. By 1956, Warren Petroleum had become the world's largest marketer of natural gas and merged later that year with Gulf Oil Co. When it merged, Warren Petroleum had 2,000 employees and produced about 17,000 barrels of oil a day. The company was later purchased by Chevron USA Inc.

Rather than retire after the merger, Warren sat on the boards for Warren Petroleum International and Gulf Oil. It was during this time, he led the project to raise a hospital in the country, changing the landscape of Tulsa and trajectory of city expansion. The city's hospitals were filled, and doctors needed room to practice.

In December 1955, the William K. Warren Foundation announced it would build a hospital named Saint Francis to be operated by the Sisters of The Precious Blood, who operated a hospital in Wichita, Kansas. The location was not known, but it was planned as a state-of-the-art facility. The foundation had been established in 1945.

"Mrs. Warren and I are most anxious to build and maintain this hospital in Tulsa. Tulsa has done a lot for us, and we like it here. There will not be any solicitation for funds for the construction, equipping or maintenance of the hospital. The foundation will take care of all costs and whatever is necessary for maintenance. Under such conditions we feel confident we will be able to acquire a proper site." said W.K. Warren, *Tulsa Tribune*, Dec. 3, 1955.

It took a little more than two years of planning and another more than two years of building before Saint Francis Hospital opened in 1960 after the foundation spent $8 million in costs. The hospital had 275 beds, parking for 450 cars, dining for 200 and two 494-ton air conditioners. During construction, Natalie Warren drove to the construction site nearly everyday to watch the building rise.

While Saint Francis Hospital is the most visible and significant of Warren's philanthropy, it was just part of his ongoing charitable giving. The foundation led the construction of the William, Kelly and Warren Medical Buildings, the Warren Clinic and the Warren Place office complex. The Warrens were also supporters of other community causes.

William and Natalie Warren.

In 1984 when a flood devastated much of Tulsa, many of Saint Francis employees were affected. They were able to take loans of between $3,000 and $5,000 interest-free from the hospital. The payback was taken out of their checks. They could buy food from the dining supply at cost for six months.

"I knew him when he was running Warren Petroleum. He owned a bank, and he put me on the board there. He used to give me a cashier's check to take to the widow of a fallen fireman or policeman. They would want to know who sent it. I told them I was just the delivery boy. He sent many, many cashier's checks. Since he owned the bank, he didn't have to put his name on them. That was how he wanted it." – Henry Zarrow, fellow oilman, philanthropist, Saint Francis Hospital trustee and member of the hospital board for nearly 40 years.

For Warren's contributions, he was given the "Outstanding Layman" award in 1978 from the Oklahoma State Medical Association's House of Delegates. He was cited for "distinguished service" to the medical profession and citizens of Tulsa in 1979 by the American Medical Association. He received the Award of Merit of the Oklahoma Hospital Association.

In 1960, he received the Humanitarian Award from the National Jewish Hospital and National Asthma Center. He was a member of the Oklahoma Hall of Fame and inducted into the Tulsa Hall of Fame. He was a trustee of the University of Tulsa and contributed funds to endow lectureships at Vanderbilt University.

Warren held honorary degrees from The University of Tulsa, the University of Notre Dame, Catholic University and Villanova University. In 1964, he received the distinguished service citation from the University of Oklahoma as the state's "outstanding citizen."

Before his death, Warren's last major contribution through his foundation was the Laureate Psychiatric Clinic and Hospital, 6655 S. Yale Ave. The $20 million, eight-building facility licensed for 135 beds was opened in March 1990.

He died June 11, 1990, at age 92 and was given a funeral service at Christ the King Church. Natalie died in 1996 with a funeral held at Boston Avenue Methodist Church. At the time of her death, they had 25 grandchildren and 31 great-grandchildren.

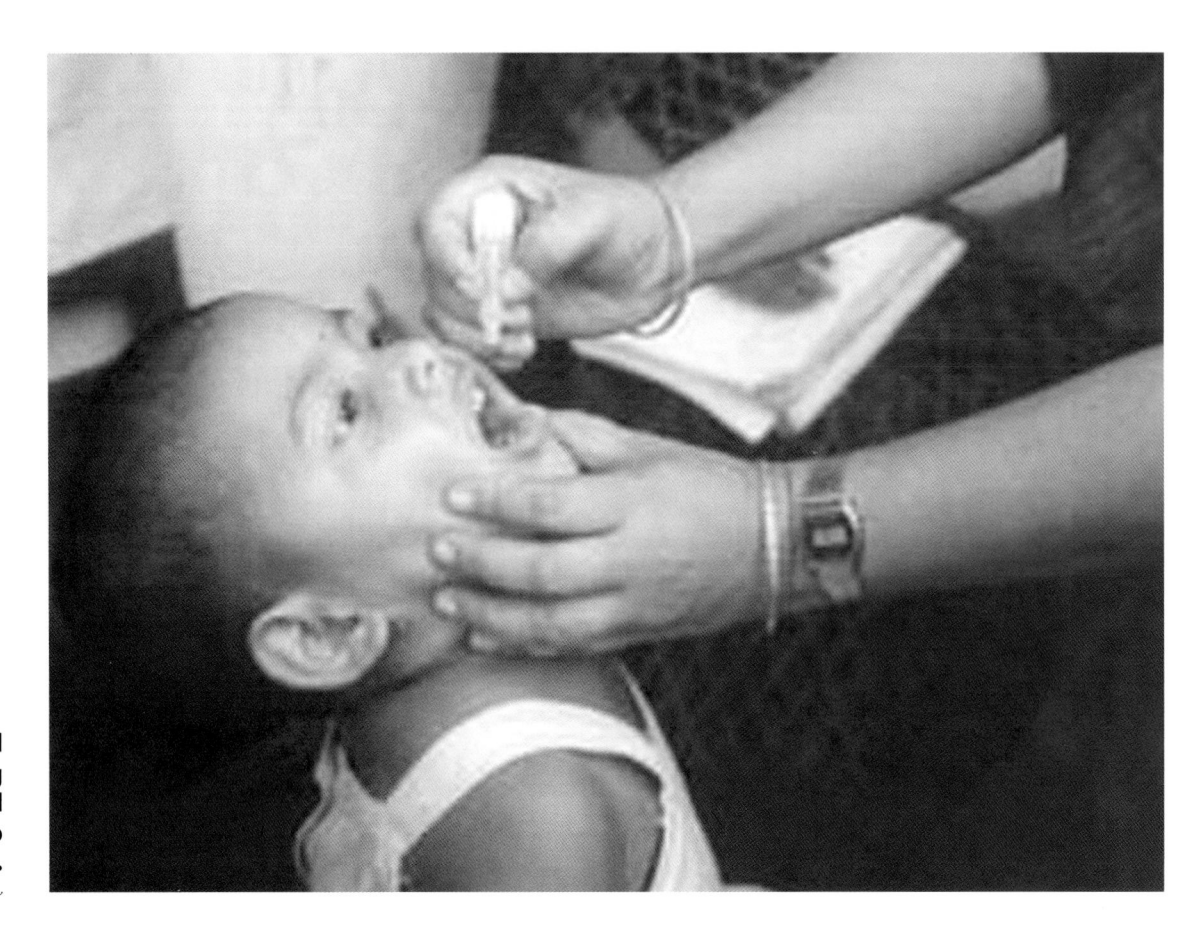

A Child Being Administered Oral Polio Vaccine.

1964, followed by type II (257,000 doses) in March 1963 and the third round (253,064 doses) in late April and May 1963. Each dose was to be taken six to eight weeks apart and was believed to give a lifetime immunity.

More than 2,000 volunteers in Tulsa including doctors, nurses, pharmacists, Boy Scouts, school principals, Civil Defense patrolmen and others staffed 40 clinics, schools and the Armory to dispense the vaccine-loaded sugar cubes. In a March 10, 1963, front-page *Tulsa World* story, an illustration of a syringe dripping liquid on a sugar cube featured "Get Your Type II oral polio vaccine TODAY?" across the top. An accompanying story stated the vaccine was being given at 43 locations that day and each recipient was asked to contribute 25 cents. If someone could not pay, no one would be turned away. Only 162,615 people arrived at the clinics for that second dose. The low turnout was blamed on rain and a wave of illnesses in the city, with many children absent from school with flu and chicken pox. A makeup clinic the following weekend resulted in 95,339 people showing up.

Oklahoma's last polio case was reported in 1969. The last case of polio in the U.S. was in 1979.

OTHER MEDICAL LEAPS

As technology helped Americans reach the the moon, it also allowed them to live longer. Hearts became healthier as the first transistorized self-contained pacemaker was introduced in 1960. Seven years later, Dr. Michael DeBakey developed the coronary bypass, and Dr. Christiaan Barnard performed

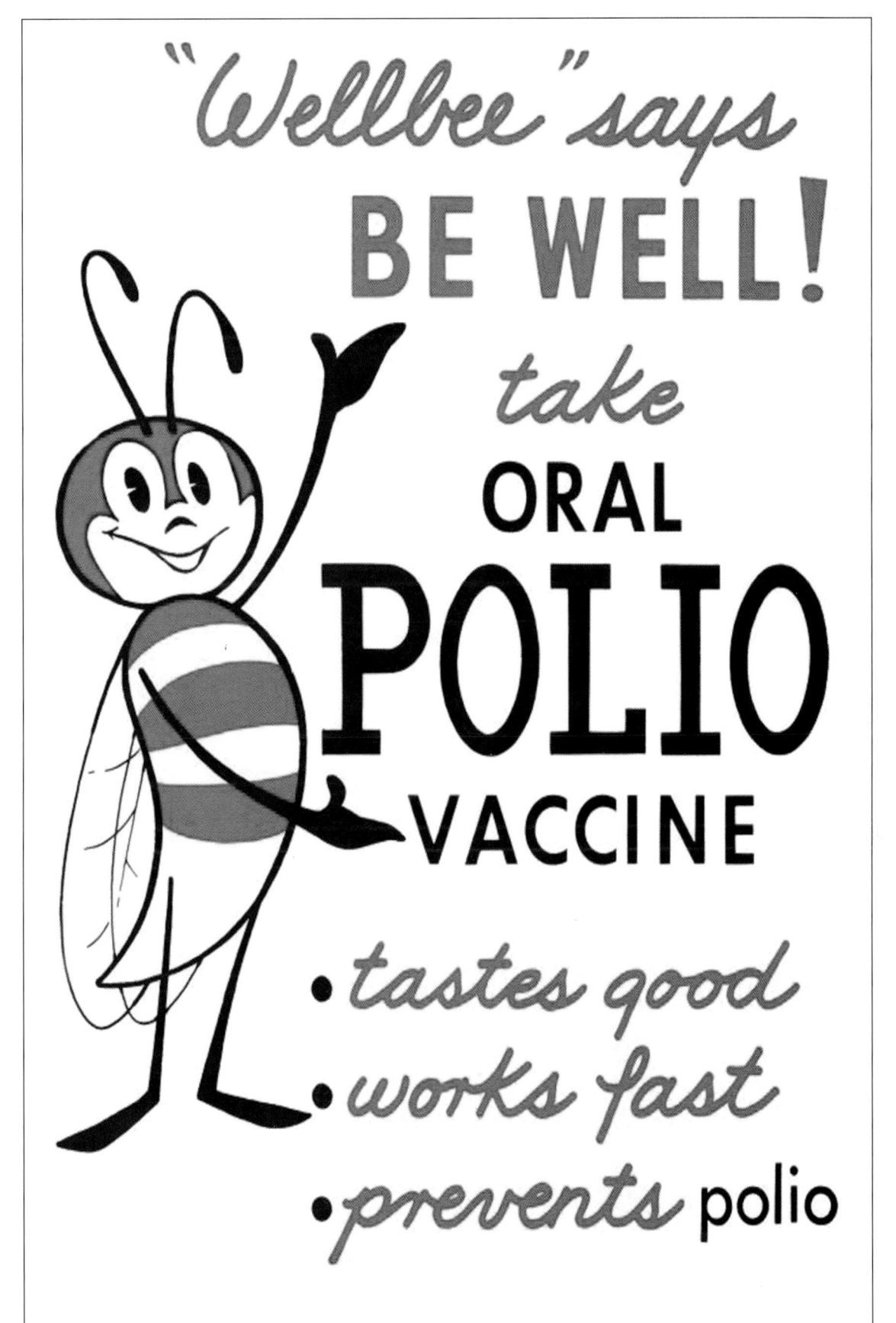

Notices such as this one were used to encourage use of the oral polio vaccine.

the first heart transplant. The following year, angioplasty was being used for arterial treatment and diagnosis. On the prevention end, guanethidine — a noradrenaline release inhibitor — was developed in 1960 to treat high blood pressure. Then, a beta-adrenergic blocker appeared in Britain and alpha-methyldopa was used clinically by the early 60s to control blood pressure. Heart attack deaths were reduced by 40 percent in the decade. Aspirin and streptokinase taken within hours of an attack was found to improve mortality.

In a history of Tulsa cardiac medicine written by Dr. R. Wayne Neal, M.D., in 2002, he wrote about the state of heart care in the year he became the director of cardiovascular services at St. John's Hospital in 1968. He had become board certified in cardiovascular disease and a fellow in the American College of Physicians the previous year.

"There was a cardiac catheterization laboratory in the Radiology Department. Heart catheterizations had been performed by Dr. C.S. Lewis and Dr. William Moore. The pressures were recorded by a Sanborn direct writer machine. The same machine was taken to the operating room where pressures were recorded during the heart operations. I made my catheters which were used for percutaneous insertion. This was done by placing a flexible wire through the catheter material, heating it over an alcohol burner until the material was soft, and pulling it out to a taper. The tapered end was then cut to fit snugly over the guide wire. The catheter was then inserted into the patient's artery or vein to measure pressures, take blood samples or inject contrast for purposes of taking an angiogram," Dr. R. Wayne Neal, 2002 history.

In 1969, Dr. Neal observed a coronary bypass operation by Dr. George Morris at the Methodist Hospital in Houston. He reported his observations to Tulsa cardiovascular surgeon Dr. Albert Shirkey.

"With his abilities and understanding as a surgeon, he began to successfully perform this operation. These, along with many other cardiovascular surgical procedures, have been successfully performed at St. John Medical Center in subsequent years by Dr. Bill P. Loughridge, Dr. Robert Blankenship, Dr. Frank Fore, Dr. Robert Garrett and Dr. George Cohlmia," Dr. R. Wayne Neal, 2002.

As physicians came to Tulsa, they formed into groups serving the various hospitals.

Anesthesiologists Howard Bennett and Ted Wenger moved from the St. John's group and formed a new practice in 1960 to provide anesthesia coverage at Saint Francis Hospital. The practice, Associated Anesthesiologists, hired Dr. Victor Neal, who had just completed his residency at the University of Oklahoma. Dr. Neal administered the first anesthetic on a patient at Saint Francis Hospital on October 1, 1960. It was an uncomplicated Caesarian section. At the Doctors' Hospital, Dr. Fred Woodson divided his time between the new hospital and Hillcrest Medical Center providing anesthesia services. In 1967, Dr. Thomas L. Ashcroft resigned from a clinical staff teaching position in Chicago to develop the department of anesthesia at Doctors' Hospital.

As the decade drew to a close, public health issues such as smoking, automobile safety and packaging information foreshadowed some of the medical problems lying ahead. Tulsa would continue to attract physicians, specialists and an education program in the next decade. ■

CHAPTER 8
(1970 - 1979)

Emerging Schools and Treatments

Classroom at ORU Medical School.

Tulsa going into the 70s was still riding an economic wave that continued development to the south and a hip arts scene gaining international attention. The Mabee Center on the Oral Roberts University campus opened in 1972 to host performers including Elvis Presley, Johnny Cash, Tom Jones, Neil Diamond, the Bee Gees and Natalie Cole. In August 1976, the state's largest mall — Woodland Hills Mall — brought together 169 stores and restaurants on 71st Street near Memorial Drive. The city's nightlife exploded with the Tulsa Sound, an evolution of blues, rock, and country created by musicians including Leon Russell, J.J. Cale, Elvin Bishop, Dwight Twilley and the Gap Band. It brought to the city visiting musicians such as Eric Clapton and George Harrison for recording sessions.

Local television launched the careers of actors Gary Busey and Gailard Sartain, who was Dr. Mazeppa Pompazoidi on the late-night weekend show *The Uncanny Film Festival and Camp Meeting*. Beginning in April 1970, Sartain and colleague Jim Millaway (playing Sherman Oaks) created the inventive, off-beat sketch comedy show that wrapped around old horror movies and Busby Berkeley musicals. Busey joined in 1971 as Teddy Jack Eddy. It ran until 1973.

ORU Mabee Center Opened in 1972.

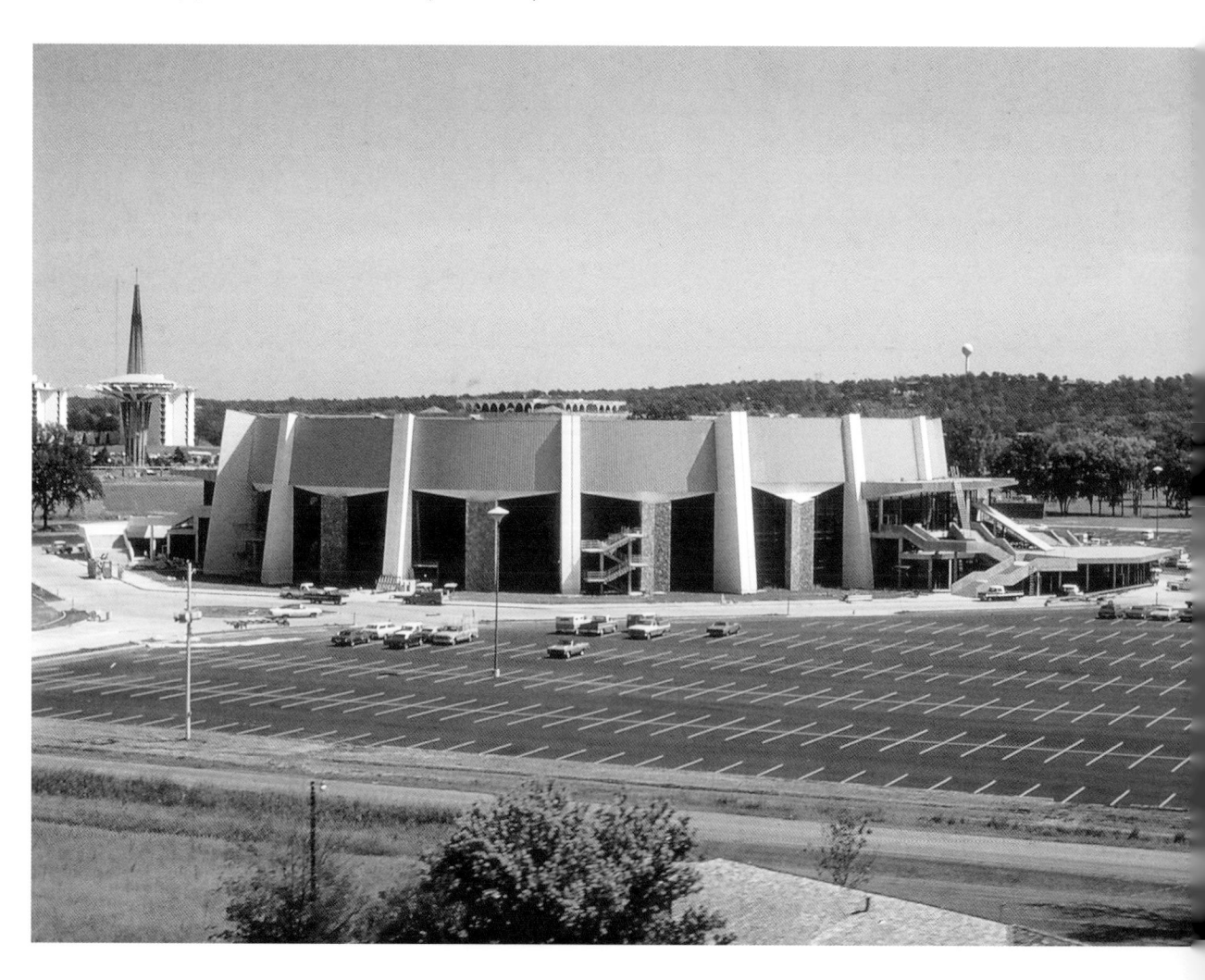

The Brookside neighborhood along Peoria from about 31st to 41st streets was known as the Restless Ribbon for its cruising teenagers. The Williams Center tried to bring people downtown in 1978 with the Forum, featuring an ice skating rink, movie theater and three levels of shopping and dining.

On the economic front, in 1970, the Port of Catoosa officially connected the Tulsa region to international trade through a series of river navigation systems to the Mississippi River and Gulf of Mexico. The decade was the waning days of Tulsa's boast of "Oil Capital of the World," with the last International Petroleum Exposition — a symbol of Tulsa's leadership in the industry — held in 1979.

An energy crisis that gripped the nation in the mid 70s wasn't felt as much in Oklahoma because of its rich natural gas supply. Other parts of the country depending on home heating oil were hit worse. The country was already dealing with gasoline shortages when Arab nations imposed an oil embargo in 1973 in retaliation for supporting Israel. However, Oklahoma experienced a revenue bonanza in 1974 in gross production tax on crude oil and higher gasoline taxes. Gasoline rose from 35 cents a gallon to 48 cents in 1974 at a time when cars averaged 13.5 miles per gallon. While Tulsa motorists didn't have long lines at the gas tanks like other cities, it did impose other energy saving tactics. Tulsa gas stations closed on Sundays, and the Oklahoma Highway Patrol lowered the speed limits to 55 mph, though it was raised to 65 mph in 1987 and 75 mph in 1996. Tulsa Mayor Robert LaFortune

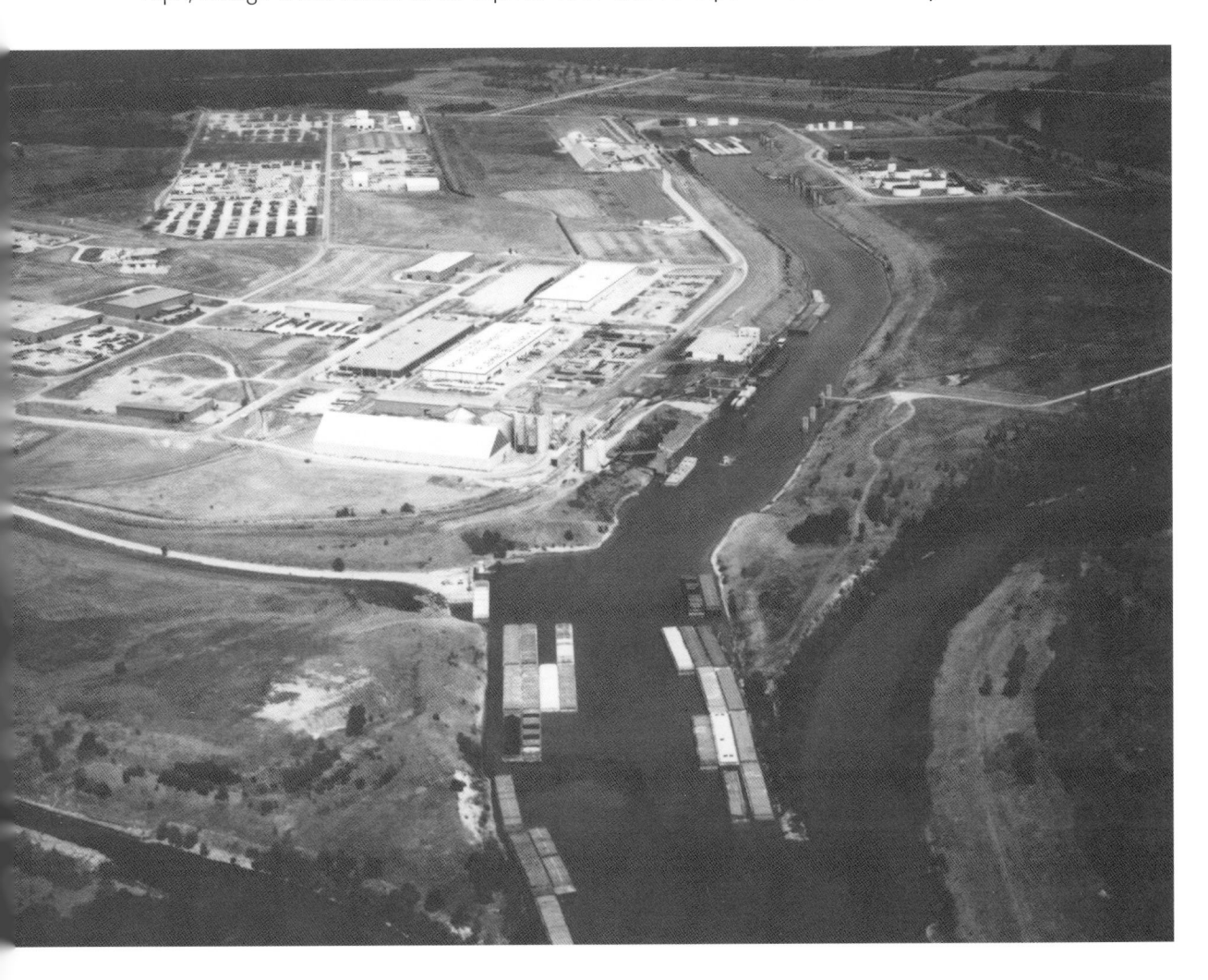

Port of Catoosa.

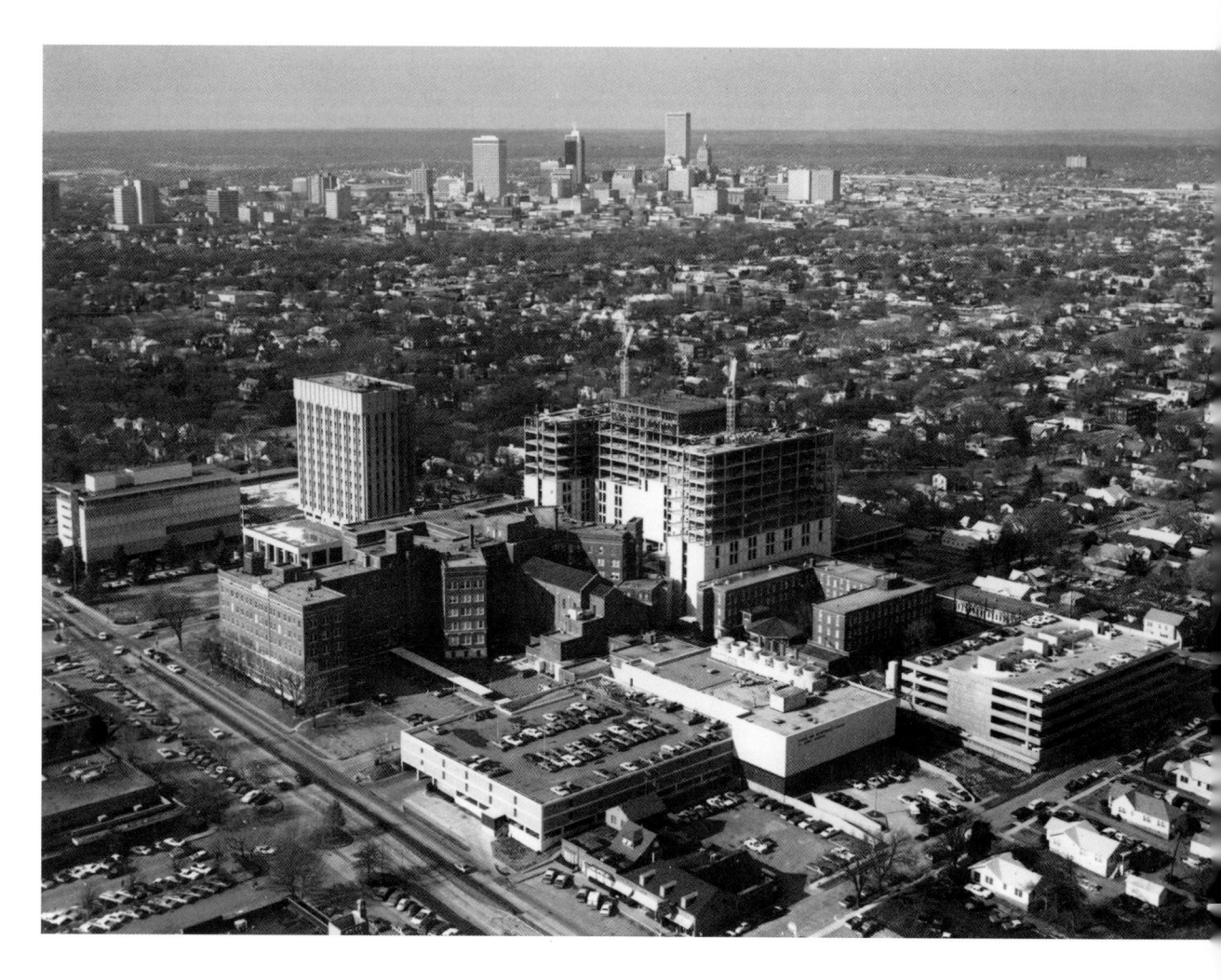

Construction on St. John Hospital's North Tower in 1975.

ordered every other lightbulb removed from City Hall corridors and downtown Christmas lights were turned off at 10 p.m.

In Tulsa County medicine, medical schools went from none to plentiful, hospitals morphed into businesses, specialists formed their own practices, vaccines proved effective and a Supreme Court decision came down that continues to cause controversy.

ANOTHER TOWER RISES

St. John's Hospital received a major, $44 million facelift that included a 14-level medical-surgical tower on the northwest corner of its two-block property, an energy plant and renovation of 400 rooms. Under new standards of the U.S. Health, Education, and Welfare department, the rooms needed to be upgraded, and the hospital increased capacity to 723 beds.

The construction included a connection between the tower and the west wing, remodeling the old wing and building an underground parking facility for doctors. It razed the original building and changed the front door entrance. The tower was designed for further expansion to 800 beds. The dedication of the tower was held on the 50th anniversary of the hospital in February 1976. Among the floors in the tower as it opened:

- **Underground** — A cancer treatment center; consultation rooms for specialty physicians.
- **Ground floor** — Offices, pharmacy, general stores, central processing and connection to the power plant.
- **First floor** — Module arrangement for diagnostic radiology.
- **Emergency department** — An 18-room trauma center, which remained at the entrance.
- **Second floor** — Rehabilitation for in- and out-patient needs and respiratory therapy.
- **Third floor** — The surgical floor with 23 suites designed for specific procedures such as open heart surgery, brain procedures and other specialty operations. A 16-bed intensive care to minimize movement for critical patients.
- **Fourth floor** — Houses all mechanics for the "H" shape of the tower.
- **Fifth floor** — Consolidation of all laboratories once scattered throughout the hospital.
- **Sixth floor** — Obstetrics floor with 14 private rooms, 32 semi-private rooms, five delivery suites and a nursery.
- **Seventh floor** — A 65-bed children's area divided into age categories and a pediatric intensive care unit.
- **Eighth floor** — Heart and medical intensive care beds with 42 intermediate care beds.
- **The rest of the floors** — no 13th floor — are specialty and general care facilities.

During the construction, workers came across a copper box welded shut that contained religious medals and mementos placed at the cornerstone when the original structure was built. Sister M. Therese Gottschalk, the hospital's board president, explained some of the items, including medallions of their nuns' order, Seven Sorrows rosary, a regular rosary and rosaries named for Saints Anne and Philomena. The Sisters of the Sorrowful Mother owned and operated the hospital.

"There were some tiny little statues of the Blessed Mother, St. Therese (the Little Flower) and the Infant of Prague. Each was in its own little metal box, not more than an inch-and-a-half long and about a half-inch wide. People must have carried them in their purses or pockets. But the one which amused us most was a medal of St. Christopher (patron saint of travelers). On the back was a model of a touring car," said Sister Therese Gottschalk, *Tulsa World*, Aug. 31, 1978.

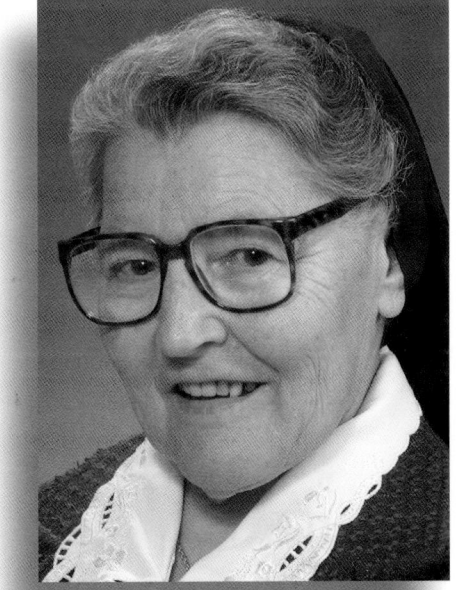

The items were given a "gentle scrubbing" to bring them back to their original condition. They were placed into another copper box for preservation in a cornerstone marking the connecting unit between the St. John's north tower and the portion of the medical center built in 1967. The new cornerstone also contained papers related to the north tower and other hospital history, medallions honoring the 1975 Holy Year and Elizabeth Seton — the first American woman canonized — and a relic blessed by Sister Mary Frances Streitel, the mother foundress of the Sisters of the Sorrowful Mother. Sister Therese had no predictions for when the items would be opened again.

St. John's Hospital Administrator, Sister Therese Gottschalk.

"I hope it will be at least another 50 years," said Sister Therese Gottschalk, *Tulsa World*, Aug. 31, 1978.

When the traditional "topping out" ceremonies were held during construction of the connecting link, the Bavarian pine placed at the top was later planted on the grounds. The custom originated in Bavaria, which was where the Sisters of the Sorrowful Mother came from.

In October 1979, Dr. David Edwards donated seven porcelain pieces by renowned artist Edward Marshall Boehm to the hospital to be on permanent display. The almost life-size Boehm birds are in a special case and feature some of his famous favorites — bob-o-link, catbird, yellow warbler, mockingbirds, crested flycatcher, tufted titmice and rufous hummingbirds. Boehm's works have been gifted from U.S. diplomats to foreign dignitaries and royalty. His "Birds of Peace" mute swans were given by former President Nixon to Pope Paul VI for placement in the Vatican Museum.

Medical Schools Emerge

In 1972, the Oklahoma Legislature passed two bills to establish medical colleges and training in Tulsa through the University of Oklahoma and Oklahoma Osteopathic Hospital. Televangelist Oral Roberts added a medical school to his private university in 1978 with the creation of the City of Faith.

Early University of Oklahoma Medical School Facility in Tulsa.

"All three schools are different in philosophy and affiliations but the end result is the same — to train doctors, particularly those of the Marcus Welby, the family practice type. Why is it happening? Most confirm it is a result of need for doctors, especially family practitioners, and that fact was recognized by the state Legislature. Money followed the recognition." — *Tulsa World*, Dec. 7, 1975.

The first to launch was the osteopathic medical college. The second was the founding of the OU-Tulsa Medical College, which was for third and fourth year students. ORU broke ground in 1976 and opened two years later.

"These state-supported medical schools are different and destined to remain separate in location and facilities. Although basic training of the M.D.s and doctors of osteopathy is similar, the curricula and emphasis in education varies significantly. There is a potential for cooperation between the OU branch and ORU here, particularly in the last two years of medical training when much of the student's time is spent in doctor's offices, clinics and hospital." — *Tulsa World*, Dec. 7, 1975.

Oklahoma Osteopathic College of Medicine Opens, Hospital Grows

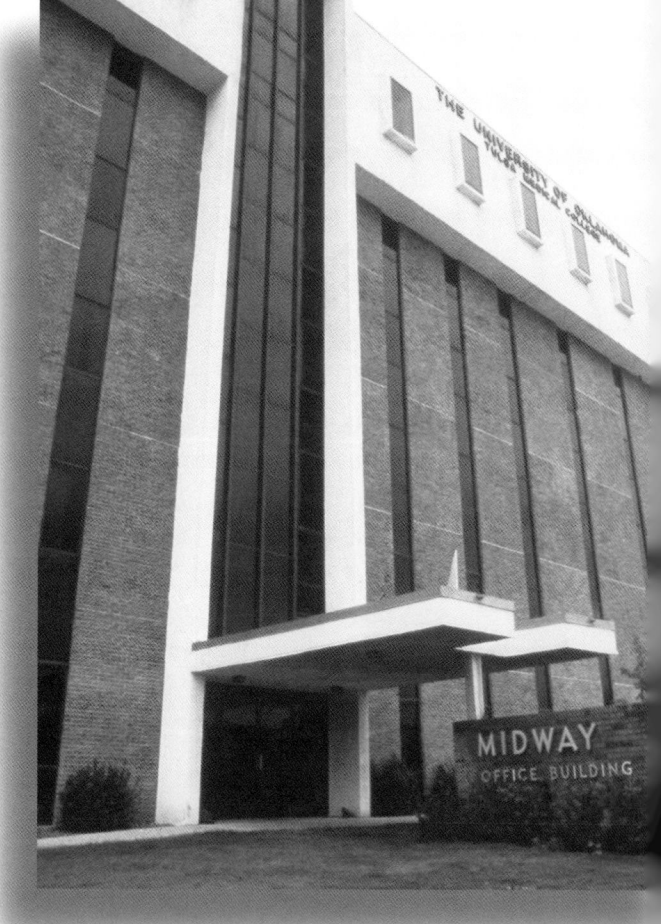

With the passage of Senate Bill 461, the Oklahoma College of Osteopathic Medicine and Surgery opened and kept Tulsa's hospital as a central component to the curriculum. The staff and students came to the hospital in the morning for training. The emphasis remained on general practice, but the school extended into specialties to meet demand. The first class of students entered in 1974.

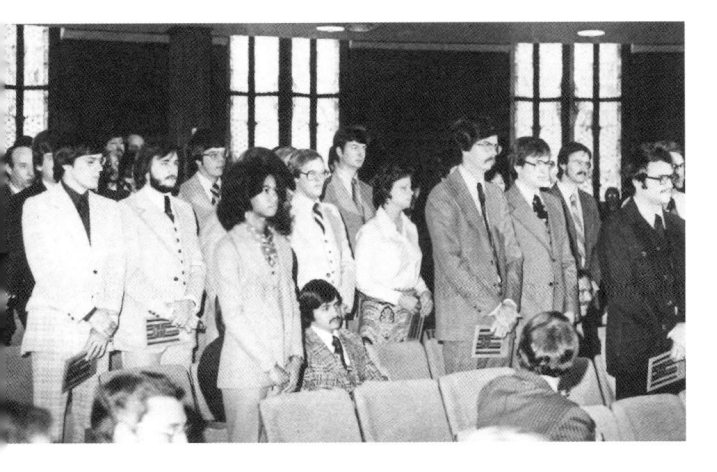

"During the 70s, the medical and surgical procedures attained new pinnacles of sophistication worldwide, particularly in the areas of eye surgery, thoracic surgery, kidney dialysis and medical imaging." — *Dreams, Challenges and Change*, 1994.

Oklahoma College of Osteopathic Medicine and Surgery's Convocation, Oct. 30, 1976.

While the medical school side grew, so did the hospital. A fourth addition was completed in July 1975, costing $12 million. The construction closed 65 obsolete beds in the original, first building and added 200 beds, resulting in a total of 443 beds. It also housed the physical therapy, dietary and expanded emergency department. Building of the west tower began in 1972, but excessive rain and a shortage of materials and skilled workers led to delays.

In 1974, the hospital started a clinic to check pacemakers, which were used to keep a steady heartbeat in cardiac patients. In 1976, the hospital was granted approval to offer open heart surgery and cardiac catheterization, becoming the first osteopathic institution in the southwest with these specialty services. The cardiac team performing open heart and revascularization procedures was composed of Drs. Larry Dullye and Paul Koro, and the lab director was Dr. Ernest Pickering. In 1983, Dr. Robert L. Archer, a thoracic and cardiovascular surgeon, joined the team.

"We started with a lot of support from many people — from the whole hospital. It was amazing when we did our first case, which was a young lady on whom we performed a valve repair. There was a staff meeting that night and after the surgery, we went down to the meeting and staff members stood up and applauded because... well, this staff was very proud of what went on in our hospital, and they were as excited about it as we were. Of course, they all knew (Dr. Dullye) because he had been here for seven years and was responsible for setting up our program. They staff believed in him and gave their support," said Dr. Paul Koro, *Dreams, Challenge and Change*, 1994.

The hospital's Renal Dialysis Center opened in 1977, but a two-year battle followed in getting Medicare reimbursement. Two state agencies — the Oklahoma Health Systems Agency and the Oklahoma Health Planning Commission — approved the dialysis unit. But, the U.S. Department of Health, Education, and Welfare twice denied federal funding, which was a major blow considering 80 percent of the cost of dialysis program is covered by Medicare. The federal agency's argument was that it was not necessary to the city. A federal lawsuit was filed by the hospital. In November 1979, U.S. administrative law judge John M. Slater ruled a "need did exist in 1977 for four additional dialysis stations in Tulsa" and approved the application for Medicare reimbursement. The hospital had been picking up the cost to offer the service, but the ruling included reimbursement for back pay to the institution.

The Tulsa hospital also became the first osteopathic institution in the nation to own and operate a computed tomography scanner, known as a CT scanner. Drs. Jon Knight and William Lavendusky shared the responsibility of operating the scanner in the hospital's radiology department.

Leading the institution during this era was Jon Pirtle, who joined the hospital in 1968 as an assistant administrator then promoted to associate administrator in 1971 and administrator in 1973. He started an annual employee recognition banquet, kept an open-door policy, established a public relations department and placed emphasis on patient care. One such program was giving new parents a candlelight dinner. He also promoted local charities. In 1979, Pirtle set a national record in pledges earned during the Walk for Mankind. The walk was a fundraiser for Project Concern International, which established primary health care centers in areas with little medical services. Pirtle organized a team from the osteopathic hospital, calling themselves the "Pirtle's Platoon."

"Pirtle took the stance that every OOH employee is a public relations person. He believed that a patient's impression of the hospital is a compilation of the individual impressions each employee gives... Pirtle strongly believed in the employees, feeling they were his most important asset... Pirtle believed that the high morale of employees made them eager to do the kind of job that would bring patients back." — *Dreams, Challenge and Change*, 1994.

UNIVERSITY OF OKLAHOMA OPENS TULSA MEDICAL COLLEGE

University of Oklahoma-Tulsa Medical College.

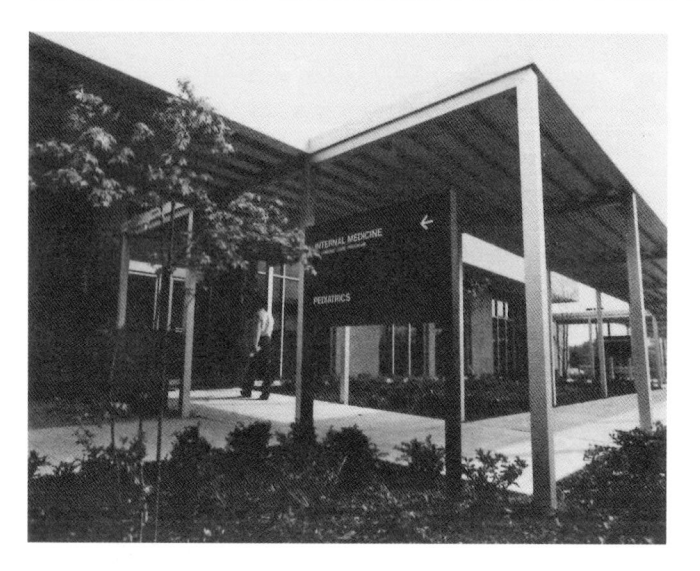

The University of Oklahoma started its presence in Tulsa with a partnership in 1957 with the Tulsa City-County to offer a Library and Information Studies graduate degrees. The program averaged 50 students each year and was among the first programs in the Tulsa Graduate Center, which became University of Central Tulsa (UCT) in 1982.

The state legislature created a clinical branch of the OU College of Medicine in Tulsa with the 1972 passage of Senate Bill 453. The state provided $435,000 and a grant from the U.S. Veterans Administration added $1.5 million over a seven-year period.

On Aug. 14, 1974, the University of Oklahoma officially opened its Tulsa Medical College with 16 third-year students. The newspapers and local officials called it a "historic event." Upon its inaugural year, there was no centralized base. Students studied under faculty and private physician supervision in four hospitals for two years, calling that time a "clerkship." The majority of the class planned to enter family medicine, then the fastest-growing specialty in medicine. Though, physicians also entered obstetrics and gynecology, pediatrics and surgery. By 1979, there would be two classes totaling 100 students.

OU President Paul Sharp addressed the class on their first day and cited the use of community hospitals for their training, saying "the whole community is a laboratory." He called the college an "unusual venture in cooperation" and encouraged students to be part of finding solutions to the problems in health-care delivery. Between 800 and 900 physicians were needed to meet national averages in providing care. Oklahoma was facing a shortage of residency opportunities, with only 85 positions available in the state. About 60 percent of each medical school graduating class had to train elsewhere.

"It is an exciting educational experience we are launching and are about to live through... I would urge all our fellow citizens that this is the kind of move this state desperately needs, a pooling of resources, creativity and imagination." — Paul Sharp, OU president, *Tulsa World*, Aug. 15, 1974.

The OU-Tulsa Medical College's first entering class students were: Ralph Dell Bernier, Robert Bruce, Charles Clayton, Donald Elgin, John England, Randall Henthorn, Sharon Manor Henthorn, Gary Hill, Robert Johnston, James King, Michael Lundy, Charles McEntee, James Kelly Mahone, Shelley Monroe, Arlis Garel Ray and Noel Eugene Stalnaker.

It grew quickly. By 1977, the OU-Tulsa Medical College had opened two family medicine centers to see patients. The first was at 1044 N. Sheridan Road and the second at 9912 E. 21st St. In August 1976, the Tulsa Pediatric Center was opened under the supervision of the college faculty and replaced long-standing clinics at St. John's and Hillcrest hospitals. It was based at the Utica Center Building, 1578 E. 21st St., and Dr. Robert Block — then an assistant professor of pediatrics at the college — served as director of the program.

"When a pediatrician goes into practice, he spends an average of 80 percent of his time in an office (rather than a hospital). We needed to find a setting in which to teach this kind of care," said Dr. Robert Block, *Tulsa World*, Aug. 8, 1976.

That same year, the Oklahoma regents approved that the medical college rent two floors in the Midway Building, 2727 E. 21st St., to serve as the school's headquarters. The college had been leasing space in the Ranch Acres Medical Building, the Harvard Center Building and the physician's building across from Hillcrest Medical Center. This space consolidated those offices.

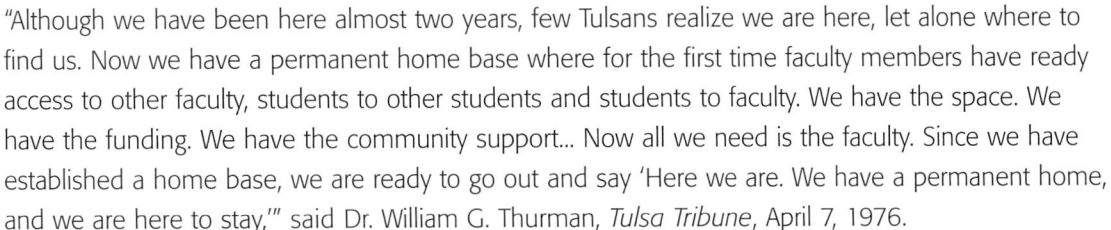

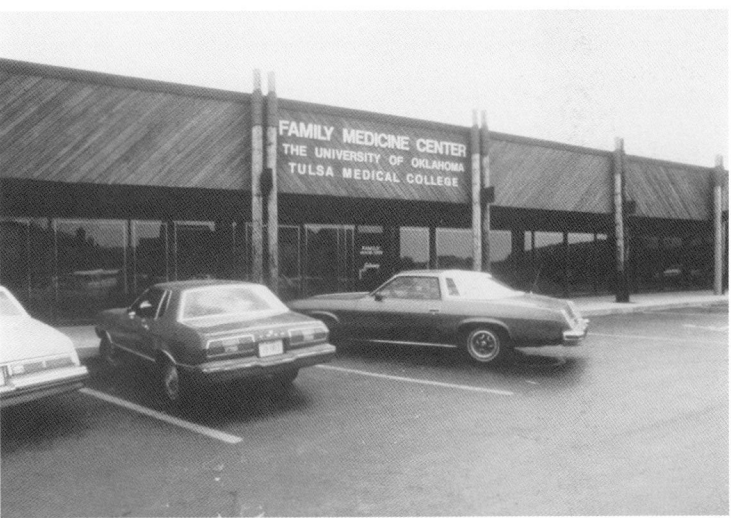

OU-Tulsa Medical College's Family Medicine Center.

"Although we have been here almost two years, few Tulsans realize we are here, let alone where to find us. Now we have a permanent home base where for the first time faculty members have ready access to other faculty, students to other students and students to faculty. We have the space. We have the funding. We have the community support... Now all we need is the faculty. Since we have established a home base, we are ready to go out and say 'Here we are. We have a permanent home, and we are here to stay,'" said Dr. William G. Thurman, *Tulsa Tribune*, April 7, 1976.

Continued on page 121

Oral Roberts

To understand the City of Faith and the medical school, a person must know about Roberts. He was born into poverty as Granville Oral Roberts Jan. 24, 1918, in Bebee, Oklahoma. He claimed his Christian ministry began with his own miracle healing of tuberculosis at age 17. Roberts preached at revivals in Oklahoma and Georgia while studying at Oklahoma Baptist University and Phillips University.

A turning point in his ministry came in 1947, at age 29, when he said he picked up a Bible and it fell to 3 John 2: "Beloved, I wish above all things that thou mayest prosper and be in Health, even as they soul prospereth." The next day, he said God appeared to him, instructing him to heal the sick. He resigned his pastoral ministry with the Pentecostal Holiness Church and founded Oral Roberts Evangelistic Association, conducting faith healing crusades around the world. In November 1947, he started *Healing Waters* which was a monthly magazine to promote his meetings. Roberts kept the ministry headquarters in Tulsa.

The crusades attracted thousands of sick people waiting in line for Oral Roberts to pray for them. He stated his dream was to teach the sick to hail "how they might obtain from God" relief from their ills. While others called him a "faith healer," he rejected the notion, often stating "God heals, I don't."

"I don't claim to have the miraculous power to heal any afflicted person. All I do is try to persuade people to join God's work and to convince them that faith in God can cure man's ills after medical science has failed. I suppose that you could call me a middle man for God and His great work," said Oral Roberts, *Tulsa World*, Sept. 8, 1948.

Roberts pioneered the seed-faith ministry, which is the teaching that everything received by faith starts with a seed. He originally called it a "blessing pact," but then it changed to "seed faith." It comes from Matthew 17:20: "If you have faith as a mustard seed, you will say to this mountain, 'Move from here to there,' and it will move; and nothing will be impossible for you."

From the start, his brand of ministry created controversy. In 1955, Roberts went to Johannesburg, South Africa, and attracted 125,000 in attendance. Newspapers criticized the fundraising aspects and attacked his claims of healing.

A headline in the *Sunday Express* stated: "Religion Is Not Found in Pounds, Shillings and Pence." Another story was headlined: "Amen, Mr. Roberts, Now Please Get Out of South Africa." Another: "20,000 Went and Prayed and Paid." Roberts stated 20,500 were converted and/or healed during that crusade.

When Roberts added television cameras to the services in 1954, it brought his ministry to the masses through the programs *The Place for Miracles* and *The Abundant Life*. Roberts was viewed on more than 100 television stations, cable and satellite networks and now his programs have a presence online.

In 1963, he founded Oral Roberts University on 500 acres near 81st Street and Lewis Avenue. It was the countryside then. He served as the university's president until 1993 and chancellor until his death in 2009. In 1977, Roberts said a vision came to him in the form of a 900-foot-tall Jesus, who told him to create the City of Faith Medical and Research Center. It was to merge "the healing power of medicine and prayer."

In a fundraising appeal in 1980, Roberts described a dream where a 900-foot Jesus Christ encouraged him to continue building the institution. A May 25, 1980, fundraising letter stated: "I told you that I would speak to your partners and, through them, I would build it!" Partners is the term Roberts used for donors. Roberts stated it was the second time he had met Jesus. In 1983, he said Jesus came to him in person, tasking him to find a cure for cancer. With the City of Faith appearance, Roberts said Jesus came to him about 7 p.m. while praying in front of the City of Faith.

"I felt an overwhelming holy presence all around me. When I opened my eyes, there He stood... some 900 feet tall, looking at me; His eyes... Oh! His eyes! He stood a full 300 feet taller

120

than the 600 foot tall City of Faith. There I was face to face with Jesus Christ, the Son of the Living God. I have only seen Jesus once before, but here I was face to face with the King of Kings. He stared at me without saying a word; Oh! I will never forget those eyes! And then he reached down, put His hands under the City of Faith, lifted it, and said to me, 'See how easy it is for me to lift it!'" – Oral Roberts fundraising letter, *Tulsa World*, Oct. 16, 1980.

In 1987, Roberts announced God would "call him home" unless he raised $8 million for scholarships for medical-school students. In a biography published later, Roberts stated God told him to keep the center afloat or be prepared to perish.

"I'm asking you to help me extend my life. We're at the point where God could call Oral Roberts home." – *Associated Press*, Jan. 10, 1987.

Roberts ended up raising $9.1 million, though the center closed in 1989. In his biography, he states the ORU medical school left "a lasting impact on the understanding by many medical professionals of the importance of treating the whole person – body, mind and spirit." ■

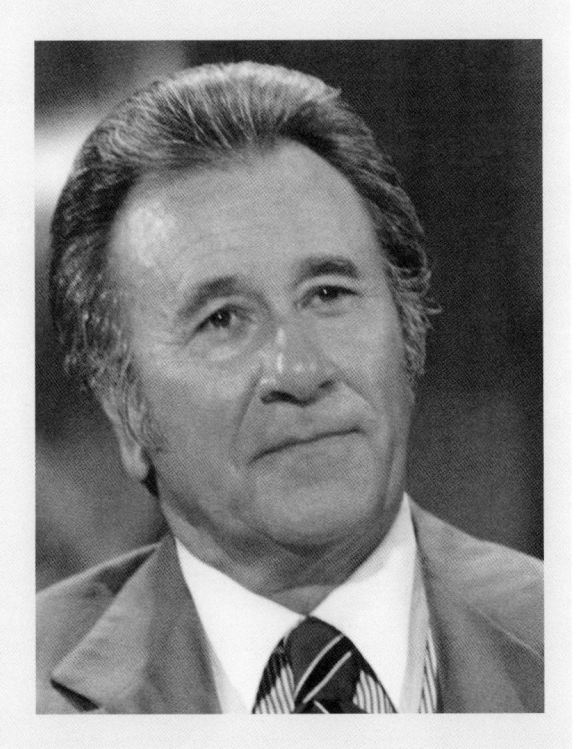

In 1978, the school added an adult ambulatory medicine facility at its headquarters. The internal medicine clinic assigned each patient to a resident, who would stay with that person through the three-year residency. The program was overseen by Dr. F. Daniel Duffy, then the chairman of the OU-Tulsa Medical College internal medicine department.

"This is important in two aspects. First, it makes for a more realistic educational experience for the resident, since he gets to follow and know a patient and his family over the course of several years rather than simply treated isolated cases. It is also better for the patient to know he always has a doctor to call," said Dr. F. Daniel Duffy, *Tulsa World*, Aug. 4, 1976.

In 1999, the college purchased the 40-acre campus near 41st Street and Yale Avenue, led by a $10 million donation from the Charles and Lynn Schusterman Family Foundation. It was the former research facility for Amoco. The facility was renamed the Schusterman Health Sciences Center and continues to house OU-Tulsa's growing medical education and research.

ORAL ROBERTS UNIVERSITY'S SCHOOL OF MEDICINE

Tulsa's most famous televangelist turned a dream into a City of Faith. The idea came to him while sleeping, he said. It was interpreted as a calling to merge faith with medicine. The plan was to build a $60 million to $100 million facility on the grounds of the university on Lewis Avenue near 81st Street to offer graduate programs in medicine, dentistry, theology, business, nursing and law.

It came with pushback from other medical institutions and accreditation agencies, which questioned the need for another medical school. Gov. David Boren stated it was causing him a "great

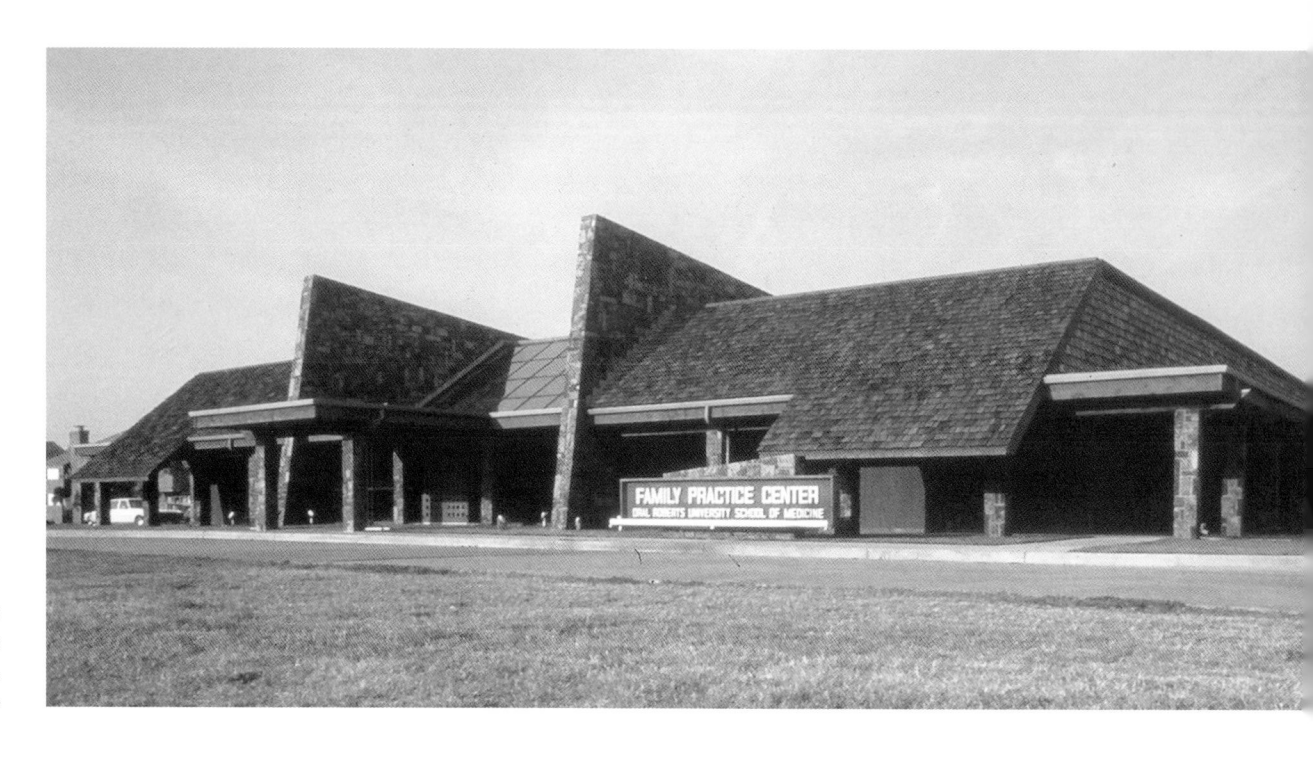

ORU's Family Practice Center.
~

deal of concern" because the school could endanger establishing the OU-Tulsa Medical College. Then, other groups expressed doubt. Hillcrest Medical Center and Saint Francis Hospital sought a district court decision to put a moratorium on hospital construction in Tulsa.

"I don't think the state is large enough to handle that many schools financial wise," said Dr. Arnold G. Nelson, president of the Oklahoma State Medical Association, *Tulsa Tribune*, April 29, 1975. He added the money should be placed in one center "rather than spreading it all around."

The ORU response was that the program's reach would be well beyond the state's borders. Officials pointed to the undergraduate enrollment attracting about 80 percent from out-of-state.

"We are proud to be in Tulsa and feel the program will help meet the medical education needs of Oklahoma... But the primary focus will not be on Oklahoma, but on a national basis, although I imagine a few graduates will stay in Oklahoma," said Dr. Carl Hamilton, ORU Executive Vice President for Academic Affairs, *Tulsa Tribune*, April 29, 1975.

At the groundbreaking on Jan. 24, 1976, Roberts was joined by 34 others with golden shovels to turn the first dirt, including comedian Jerry Lewis, who spoke on behalf of "the crippled children of the world." Lewis called the school's addition "one more tremendous cog in the wheel of victory" against muscular dystrophy.

The dental school opened in August 1978 with 20 men and five women and a plan to grow the enrollment to 50 a class. It was the 60th dental school in the nation and second in Oklahoma. OU opened a dental school in 1972.

Dr. Frank Bowyer, president of the American Dental Association, welcomed the first class, commending

Roberts for "bridging the gap" between religion and education and calling the school "like none other in the whole world." Dr. Bowyer said the "whole person" philosophy has made ORU an "integrated university" where students are: "Spiritually alive, intellectually alert and physically disciplined."

On the medical school side, a sticking point was securing a hospital affiliation for student training. Negotiations with Tulsa hospitals broke off in 1977 when Roberts announced plans for a 777-bed hospital as part of the City of Faith. The facility was to be a student training ground and to serve the followers of Roberts. Officials at Tulsa hospitals were shocked by the magnitude of the plan, stating it would create too many beds, causing a community problem. Hillcrest was the first to reject any affiliation.

"We could not divorce the hospital component from the other two components. We understand their contention that they would draw their constituency from outside the Tulsa hospital service area. However, that's a matter of opinion and conjecture. We think the project could get under way on a much smaller scale, but that is not our decision," said Hillcrest Administrator James Harvey, *Tulsa Tribune*, Dec. 22, 1977.

St. John's Hospital agreed to a limited affiliation in September 1978 by a physician vote of 79 to 66. Part of the agreement was that the hospital receive all the patients from the ORU family practice residency program, which officials said was not a deciding factor.

"The swaying point was that the majority of physicians wanted to teach... We will not be Oral Roberts' hospital. We will continue to be St. John," said Joseph L. Parker, chairman of the St. John board of directors, *Tulsa World*, Sept. 29, 1978.

Five months later, provisional accreditation was approved for the ORU School of Medicine by the Liaison Committee on Medical Education, which is made up of members of the American Association. Full accreditation could not be granted to a school until the year a first class graduates, which was to be 1982 at ORU.

Future site of COF with ORU campus in background.

"We are deliriously happy. Accrediting officials were very complimentary of our basic sciences (program) and of the plans which we have in effect for the maturing of the St. John affiliation, and for the growth of the science and clinical faculties," said Dr. Carl H. Hampton, ORU Provost and Executive Vice President for Academic Affairs, *Tulsa World*, Feb. 17, 1979.

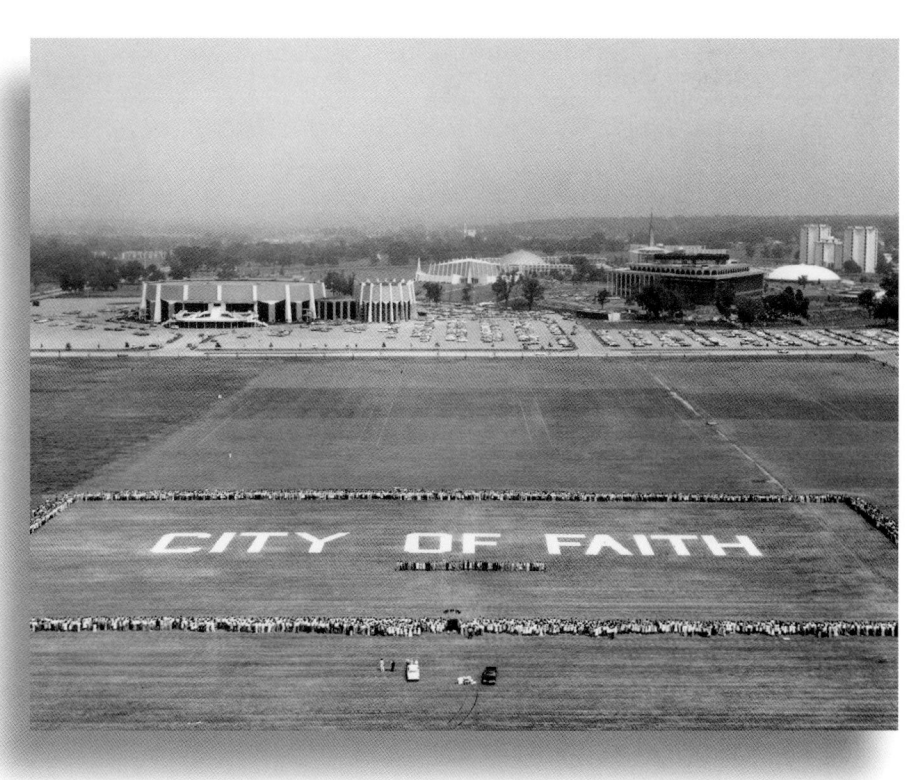

Continued on page 125

In January 1973, a 25-year-old Vinita native diagnosed with kidney failure became the first patient in a Tulsa hospital to undergo a renal transplantation. At Hillcrest Medical Center, Danny Parker received a kidney from his father, Sanford Parker, 47, after a 4-1/2 hour operation.

Kidney transplants had been performed in Oklahoma at the Veterans Administration Hospital in Oklahoma City by surgeons affiliated with University Hospitals at the University of Oklahoma Health Sciences Center.

Doctors leading the Tulsa transplant procedure were Dr. Victor L. Robards Jr., Dr. Roger V. Haglund, urologists, and Dr. Maurice Fuquay, a thoracic and cardiovascular surgeon. A nursing team led by Mimi Brunton assisted with the operation. Dr. Thomas R. Medlock, director of the cardio-renal laboratory at Hillcrest, had stated that the hospital was prepared for two months to do the transplant.

Parker had fallen ill in June 1972 while working as a draftsman in Beaumont, Texas. The diagnosis was a shock to the family, who told local reporters that he had never been seriously sick before then. He was transferred to St. John's Hospital, where he spent a month going in and out of critical condition.

From the start, Parker was considered a candidate for transplantation. After release from St. John's Hospital, he entered the Hillcrest dialysis program. He was one of about nine patients waiting for a transplant. Kidneys for transplant come from living family members or donors after death with uninjured organs. Tissue typing is conducted to determine a successful match. A first round of testing of Parker's parents and two siblings found no match. A later review of the results determined a flaw in the father's laboratory tests. An evaluation determined the father was most suited as a donor. After the transplant, the two were reported in good condition with the kidney starting the function almost immediately, according to physicians.

"All the credit goes to God, this hospital and the doctors," said Mrs. Sanford Parker, *Tulsa World*, Jan. 11, 1973.

By this time, kidney transplants were no longer experimental but had become the most common and successful type of organ transplant surgeries. Public education was a significant part of launching the Tulsa program: Patients needing to be aware of transplant availability and that organs of newly deceased people have been successful. A few initial candidates had declined a transplant with cadaver donors.

The first patient to receive an organ from a non-related, deceased person was William O. Meisenheimer, 39. He was the third person in a Tulsa hospital to receive a transplanted kidney, which came from a 19-year-old Fayetteville, Arkansas, man following an accident. The kidney was found for Meisenheimer through a national computer system search. It was shipped by airline to Tulsa that night, and the surgery was performed at Hillcrest the following morning.

Hillcrest Becomes Kidney Transplant Leader

After the first renal transplant, it was estimated between 40 and 50 patients in northeastern Oklahoma annually would be candidates for the procedure. A study released in March 1974 by the Tulsa Area Health and Hospital Planning Council estimated about 100 kidney transplants annually will be asked of the city's hospitals by 1980. Also, about 375 patients annually were expected to be in need of dialysis care. Part of this influx was credited to Medicare's expanded coverage of renal transplants and dialysis which began in the summer of 1974. As the only hospital in the Tulsa region performing kidney transplants, Hillcrest was expected to complete 30 renal operations in 1974 and 50 in 1976.

By 1977, the Oklahoma Kidney Foundation estimated that dialysis machines were costing about $2,300 a month for patients. Dialysis is a life-support treatment filtering wastes, salt and excess fluid from blood, which is the function of a kidney. The treatment gained widespread use in the 60s. In that era, about 8 percent of patients going on dialysis died within a year and about half of the dialysis patients died within 7 years. The longest anyone had lived on dialysis was 14 years.

"The dialysis machine just can't do as good a job as a natural kidney. As a result, dialysis patients are more susceptible to cardiovascular disease, bone deterioration and infections," said Bill Harwell, R.N., coordinator of the Hillcrest transplant program, *Tulsa Tribune*, Dec. 22, 1976.

Dialysis has continued to be an expensive treatment, though the federal government pays 80 percent for most patients. Private health insurance and Medicaid also help with costs. Like all medical technology, improvements have been made. Life expectancy on dialysis depends on a person's medical condition and how well the person follows a treatment plan. Average life expectancy on dialysis is 5-10 years. Some patients have lived for 20 to 30 years on dialysis.

By 1994, Hillcrest had performed a total of 416 kidney transplants since its beginning. Ten years later, it was transplanting kidneys in between 30 to 40 patients annually.

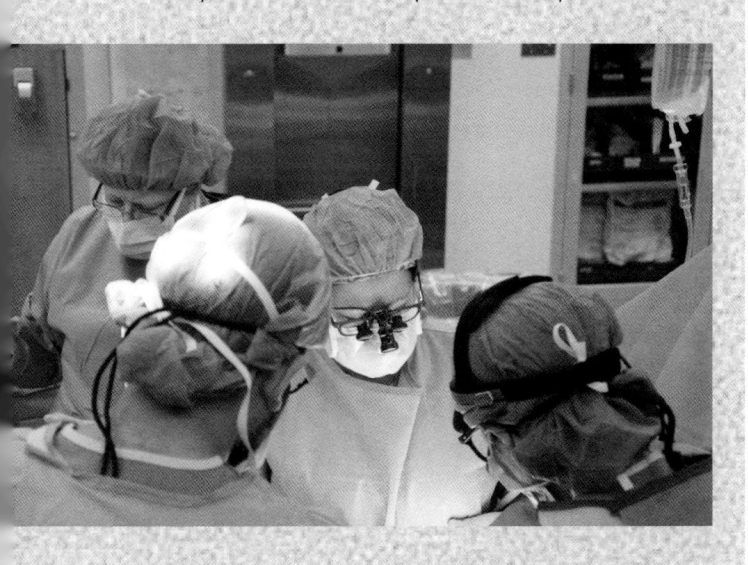

Since 1992, St. John Medical Center has provided kidney transplant services, and Saint Francis began offering renal transplants in 2005. As of January 2016, the United Network for Organ Sharing, which is the national organization registering waiting transplant patients and matching with potential donors, has about 101,000 people waiting on a transplant. Of those, more than 600 are in Oklahoma. It is estimated about 3,000 patients are added to the waiting list nationally each month, and about 13 people die monthly while waiting on a possible donor. ■

Kidney Transplant Surgery.

A Special Focus

While 1960s Tulsa built hospitals in record expansions and experienced a heavy recruitment of doctors, the next decade saw an evolution into specialty groups.

In otolaryngology, Drs. Don Mishler, David Merifield, Munson Fuller and Rollie Rhodes were in practice at the Springer Clinic by the mid-60s. In 1973, Dr. Charles Heinberg joined the physicians, who two years later established a group specialty practice at the Kelly Building and practiced at Saint Francis Hospital. The group then added Drs. Anthony Lohr and Robert Nelson. Other otolaryngologists arriving in Tulsa were Drs. Jack Preston, John Campbell, Thomas Dodson, Richard Brownson, William Zollinger and Richard Freeman.

"Thus, by the 1970's Tulsa was adequately covered by an excellent staff of ENT physicians... An early example of camaraderie between the Tulsa practitioners of ear nose and throat was the formation of The Tulsa Otolaryngology Society. This organization was formed for social, as well as medical reasons. The members would meet at each other's homes every month or two. After some drinks and hors d'oeuvres, one of the group would present a review of an interesting case or a summation of an article from a medical journal. One of the beneficial aspects of this society was that it brought together all the Tulsa otolaryngologists, who because of their different hospital affiliation rarely encountered each other's company. This organization eventually evolved into a regional and state society, The Oklahoma Academy of Otolaryngology-HNS," said Dr. Roger Wehrs, "The History of Otolaryngology in Tulsa, Oklahoma, 1950-1970."

In 1974, Dr. Harley Galusha, of the Oklahoma Osteopathic Hospital, performed the state's first intraocular lens implant. He

Dr. Harley Galusha.

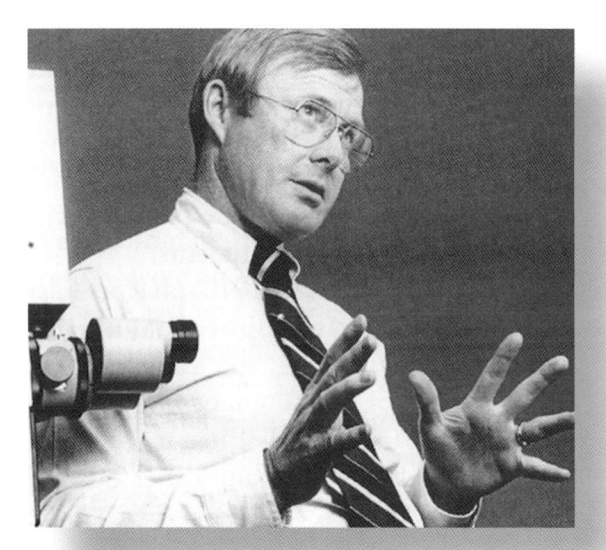

described it as "a trial of all my skill and courage," and one of the most difficult procedures he had in his career to that point. The lens implant procedure revolutionized cataract surgery, and Dr. Galusha perfected the operation after training in California and Europe. He arrived in Tulsa in 1960 and was the first in the osteopathic profession to limit his practice, from its beginning, to ophthalmology. The hospital established the department of Eye, Ear, Nose and Throat separate from the Department of Surgery in 1968, which was the year Dr. Richard Mills became its first ophthalmologic resident.

"Because the osteopathic profession has an emphasis on general practice, and even though the Eye, Ear, Nose and Throat specialty appeared in our profession in 1919, we were not as quick to divide this large field into subspecialties as the medical profession in general. Until I established this exclusively from the beginning of my practice, an ophthalmology practice had resulted from the discontinuance of ENT by a doctor who formerly did EENT," said Dr. Harley Galusha, *Dreams, Challenge and Change*.

In 1972, Cardiovascular Surgery, Inc. was founded by Dr. Albert Lauck Shirkey with Dr. Bill Loughridge joining shortly after. Both had been with Surgery, Inc. The two teamed up to perform the first heart valve replacement surgeries in eastern Oklahoma and were affiliated with St. John Medical Center and Saint Francis Hospital. Both served as professors and mentors to medical students at the OU-Tulsa Medical College and the Oral Roberts University School of Medicine. Dr. Loughridge performed more than 10,000 surgeries in his career. After Dr. Shirkey retired in 1981, he worked on electronic instruments for physical therapy as the founder and president of the Inola-based Rich-Mar Corp.

Saint Francis Hospital opened its cardiac catheterization lab in 1970 and the Natalie Warren Bryant Cancer Center in 1975. The cancer center was named after founders Mr. and Mrs. William K. Warren's second daughter, who passed away from breast cancer at age 49.

A consequence of the doctors going into specialized medicine meant a decline in general practice, which became known as family medicine. Nationally, the percentage of physicians going into general practice fell from about 50 percent in the 40s to 8 percent by the 60s. In 1969, the American Board of Family Practice was established about the same time medical schools started growing family medicine departments, including those at the OU-Tulsa Medical College, osteopathic college and Oral Roberts University. In 1972, there were 96 family practice residency programs in

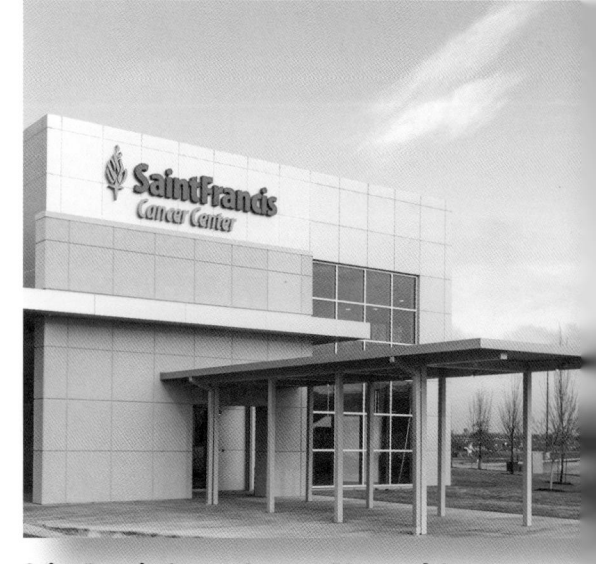

Saint Francis Cancer Center, 51st. and Garnett Ave.

the nation, and that grew to more than 300 by 1978. For doctors wanting family practice certification, they must complete a three-year residency to take the board exams. A grandfather clause was added to allow doctors with at least six years' experience to take the exams. The purpose was to demonstrate that family medicine doctors were as qualified as any specialist.

"The G.P. was dying. All the doctors were going into subspecialties. As medicine progressed, the hospitals started crowding out the G.P.s, saying that they didn't have enough experience. Also, the G.P.s didn't have any input in medical education... Legislators have picked out the family physician as the answer to a lot of health care problems. The goal of many medical schools is to get at least 50 percent of their graduates into primary care, and half of those into family practice. That will help solve a lot of patient care problems," said Dr. Lesley Walls, associate professor of family practice at the OU-Tulsa Medical College, *Tulsa World*, Sept. 4, 1977.

The reasoning behind the renewed emphasis in family medicine was to streamline care.

"It's an ideal way to practice medicine to me. There's no reason one doctor can't take care of 80 percent of someone's medical needs. And, the more you know about someone, the better you can treat them. The more I know about someone, the more comfortable I am taking care of them," said Dr. Don Roller, then a third-year resident at the OU-Tulsa Medical College, *Tulsa World*, Sept. 4, 1977.

Some residents in family medicine at the time spoke about a philosophical difference with the subspecialty practices.

"Internal medicine seems a little too academic and not as patient-oriented. Most health problems are neither physical nor emotional — they're both. And practically, you don't learn how to deal with the real common things in other specialties. Family practice represents a little more basic and practical approach to health care. It is somewhat a specialty in learning how to deal with everyday things," said Dr. Doug Wilsey, who had completed a family medicine residency in the mid-70s, *Tulsa World*, Sept. 4, 1977.

> **"I like all fields of medicine, and family practice is the only field where you get to do a little of everything. And, you develop a closer relationship with your patients."**
>
> Dr. Doug Cox

Oklahoma medical schools were reporting that about half of the graduates were expressing interest in family medicine. As a third-year student, Dr. George Caldwell told a newspaper reporter that credit goes to medical school faculty who "has talked about the attributes and the needs for it, and the students have responded to that."

Dr. Doug Cox, who later became an elected state lawmaker and an emergency room physician in

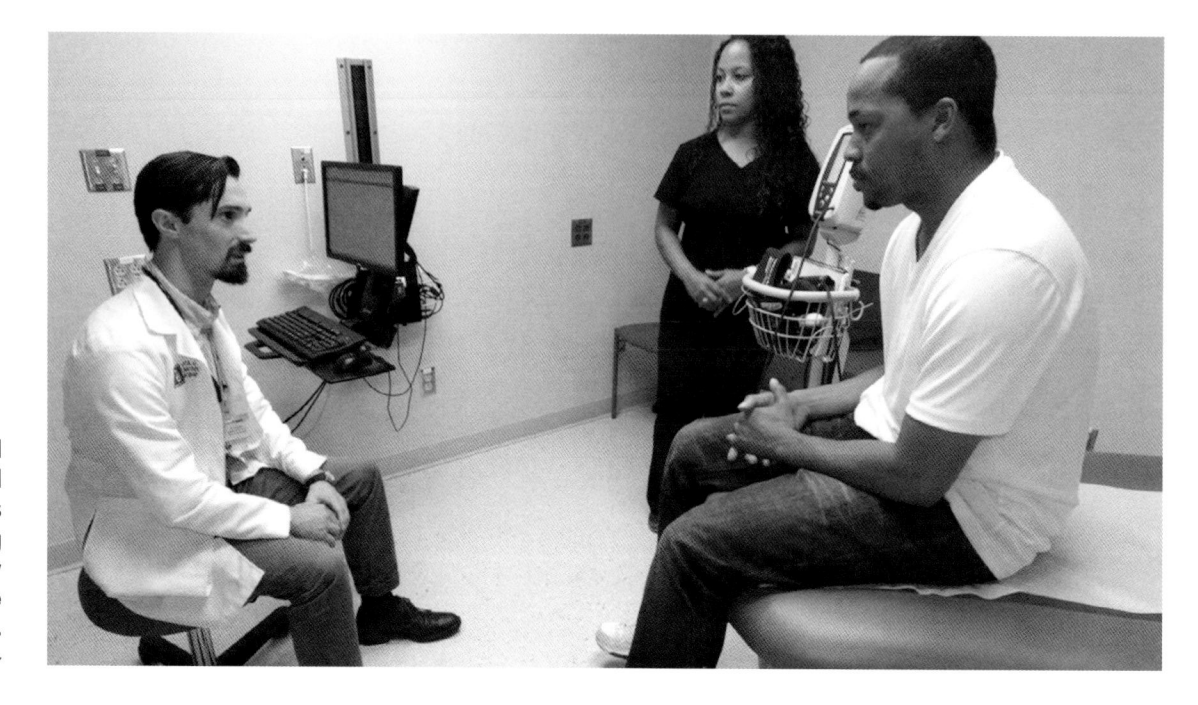

OU-Tulsa and OSU Medical Schools Focus on Training Family Medicine Physicians.

Grove, Oklahoma, was a fourth-year student when stating that because family medicine training has improved "the other physicians have begun to look more favorable toward them."

"I like all fields of medicine, and family practice is the only field where you get to do a little of everything. And, you develop a closer relationship with your patients," said Dr. Doug Cox, *Tulsa World*, Sept. 4, 1977.

THE BUSINESS OF HOSPITALS

Hospitals have always required a certain amount of economic acumen, but the modern era ushered in a more complex financial health care system. It more clearly defined the tug-of-war of health care between a system of public trust and business. As government programs came into the marketplace as a way to provide care to more Americans, it started different streams of funding — private pay, insurance pay and Medicare and Medicaid.

In a piece about growing health-care costs in 1977, the Doctors' Hospital administrator cited a growing number of government-paid patients. At that time, about 40 percent of its patients were eligible for Medicaid and Medicare, which provided about $1 million less a year than its traditional charges. The increase in government programs also brought more regulations for tracking data and processing claims. Most hospitals and physician practices had to upgrade its accounting systems into the first generation of computerized models. At Doctors', the average hospital stay was reduced between 1973 and 1977 from an average of 8.2 days to 6.5 days.

"The same basic laws of economics apply to a hospital as any other business. It must have an excess of revenue over expenses to meet obligations and create a reserve for future expansion and purchase of new equipment. The term 'nonprofit' means that there is no distribution of earnings to owners — of, in a legalistic sense, no inurement of benefits to any proprietor, partner or stockholder," said Bill

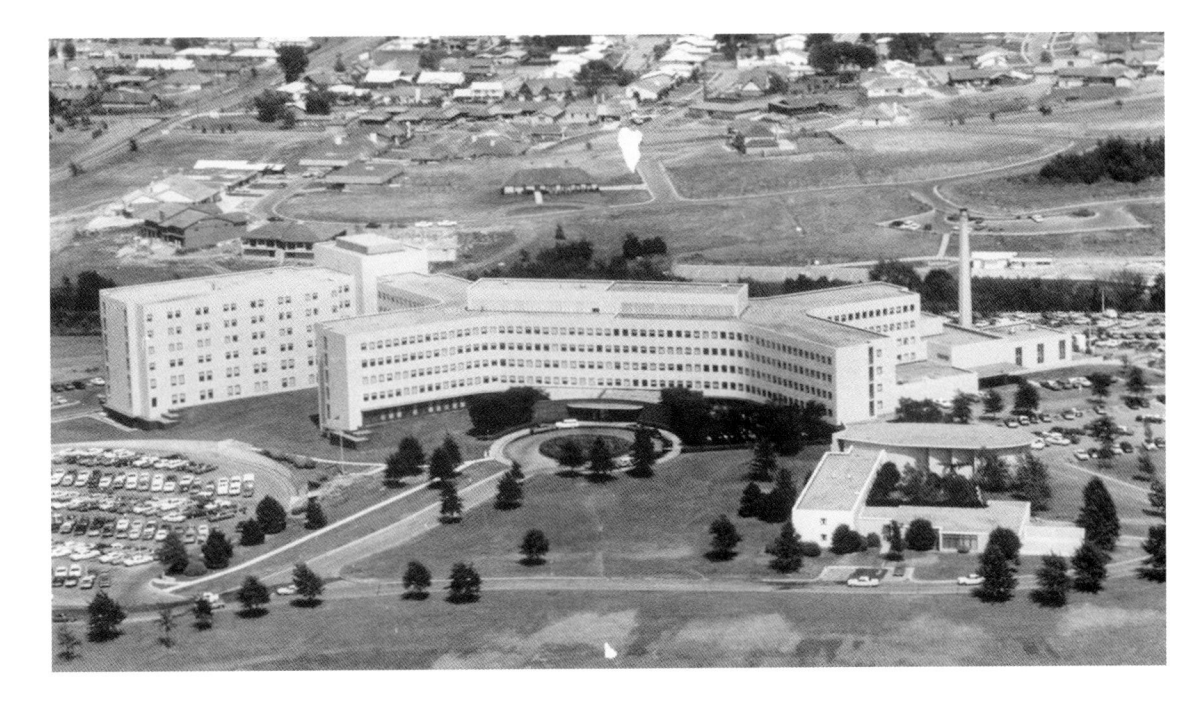

Arial View of Saint Francis Hospital in 1970.

Humphrey, administrator of Doctors' Hospital, *Tulsa World*, Aug. 28, 1977.

Hospital officials started reporting on efforts to keep beds available to acutely ill patients as a way to control costs. By the mid-70s, hospitals were announcing raises in daily room rates. In 1975, Saint Francis announced room-rate raises, citing the need for cost-of-living increases for staff. The room costs went up by a range of $4.50 daily for a semi-private room (to $59.50) to $33.50 daily for cardiac intensive care (to $160). The Hillcrest Medical Center rates were $59 daily for a semi-private room up to $151 for intensive care. Doctors' Hospital charged $50 for a semi-private room up to $125 for intensive care. Oklahoma Osteopathic Hospital quoted daily rates as $64 for a semi-private room up to $155 for intensive care. The St. John's Hospital rates were $57 for a semi-private room up to $160 for cardiac intensive care units.

The room rates stayed in headline news as rising inflation forced spikes in costs. In 1978, several hospitals made more increases, with private rooms nearing $100 a day. Hillcrest president James Harvey stated in January 1978 that patients in Tulsa should expect bills to rise about 6.8 percent by the end of the year.

"We are squeezing down our margin considerably to dampen the inflating effect," said James Harvey, *Tulsa Tribune*, Jan. 4, 1978.

Beginning in July 1973, Medicare was expanded to all people, regardless of age, who were receiving disability payments under Social Security. Hospital officials blamed Medicare and Medicaid for the soaring inflation costs at the facilities. The monthly premiums began climbing almost immediately after Medicare. It climbed to $4 a month in 1969 and reached $6.30 by 1973. In 1976, Medicare recipients were required to pay the first $104 of their hospital bills, up from $92, compared to $40 deductible in 1967. By mid-1978, the five Tulsa hospitals received between 28 percent and 47 percent of their rev-

Continued on page 131

It the dawn of the 70s, an Irish nun and a Louisiana military man took Saint Francis from an administrative crossroads to a foundation of expansion and prominence.

The Adorers of the Most Precious Blood – under the direction of Sister Superior Mary Hildalita and later Mary Marcellina – administered the Catholic hospital for nearly a decade. Then, a different philosophy and vision developed between the order and the hospital founder, William Warren, who wanted to grow the facility. The nuns preferred to maintain the status quo. In 1969, the order resigned the post.

Sister Blandine Fleming and Lloyd Verret

That's when Sister Blandine Fleming and Lloyd Verret arrived.

Sister Blandine was tapped as the administrator on behalf of her order, the Sisters of Charity of the Incarnate Word, based in Houston. She was born in County Cork, Ireland, the third youngest of eight children. At age 15, she joined the order and received a master's degree in hospital administration from Xavier University, training as a medical records librarian for 10 years. She came to Saint Francis at age 35 after working at St. Elizabeth Hospital in Beaumont, Texas.

Verret grew up in Lake Charles, Louisiana, attending Southwest Louisiana Institute in Lafayette. In 1951, he enlisted in the U.S. Air Force, assigned to the Lake Charles Air Force base and two years in Morocco. He became interested in hospital administration during his service and earned a master's degree from Northwestern University in Chicago. After an internship at Ochsner Hospital in New Orleans, he took an administrative position at Saint Patrick's Hospital at Lake Charles, which was run by the Sisters of Charity of the Incarnate Word.

"She was 36-years-old, and he was a burr-headed Cajun from Lake Charles. It was a big step up for both of them. They took it and ran. There were very few hospitals connected with Blandine's order – the Sister of Charity of the Incarnate Word – that had a foundation behind it like Saint Francis did. It was an opportunity to start in on the ground floor and build and develop," said Dr. C.T. Thompson, "Saint Francis 50," 2010.

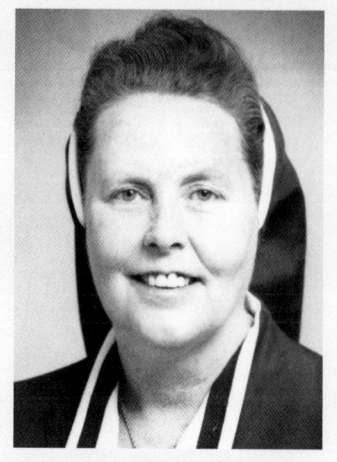

Sister Blandine Fleming.

The next era brought leaps in advancements – diagnostic machines, lasers, X-rays, nuclear medicine. The hospital-affiliated doctors and staff worked on a plan to concentrate in areas of trauma, cancer, neonatal and heart care. The administrators and Warren backed the emphasis moving forward.

On the 15th anniversary of the hospital, the doors opened to the Natalie Warren Bryant Cancer Center. It was among the first centers where radiation therapy, chemotherapy, laboratory and support services were placed in a single location for a patient.

In 1975, the $4.5 million Kelly Building was completed. It was 12 floors with 100 offices and 160,000 square feet. Two years later, the west wing of the hospital was dedicated.

In 1979, Life Flight launched out of the focus on trauma led by Dr. Gerald Gustafson, who was inspired by his Vietnam War experience. It was a helicopter service transporting critically ill or injured patients to a hospital. It was the first such service in Tulsa. That year, a fetal maternal medicine unit and skilled nursing facility were added.

Sister Blandine served as the top administrator though she and Verret often operated in tandem.

"She could be very stern. She'd send you home if

Lloyd Verret.

you were wearing too low a neckline or too short a skirt. One reason I was afraid of her were the stories I would hear. But, at the same time, I'd hear these wonderful stories. I know she could get mad, and she wanted things a certain way. If there was trash on the floor, she'd bend down and pick it up. And I would do the same thing, because I was so proud of the hospital. This was her home, and we were all her children," said Linda Crow Hughes, Saint Francis choir leader and administrative assistant, "Saint Francis 50," 2010.

Sister Blandine served until November 1993 then was posted as an administrator at CHRISTUS Schumpert Medical Center in Shreveport, Louisiana. She left that position June 2013 to return to her order.

"Reflecting on her many years in ministry, Sister Blandine said that one of her happiest experiences was when she was at St. Francis Hospital, Tulsa, Oklahoma, where the staff and physicians worked hard to develop a strong family spirit. This effort enabled them to focus on the Healing Ministry of Christ as their first priority in health care." — Sisters of Charity, website, 2010.

Verret served at Saint Francis as an assistant administrator, second to Sister Blandine, until August 1993. He then served as administrator until September 1994. He was a life fellow of the American College of Healthcare Executives. He died in December 2007.

"He had the reputation of being quick of wit, with a keen sense of humor that brightened a room. From 1969-1994 he guided the future of Saint Francis Hospital, garnering the coveted designation of one of the top 100 hospitals in the country. Even though the scope of his position demanded a great deal of his time, he never lost sight of the reason that Saint Francis was founded – to serve the people. At least once a day Lloyd Verret could be found on the floors, giving encouragement to the patients and to the staff... Even though he spent 25 years in the Midwest, he never lost his Cajun drawl or his love for Cajun food. In fact, his fried turkeys became a tradition at Saint Francis Hospital," *Tulsa World* obituary, Dec. 26, 2007.

In 1998 when Saint Francis Medical Center launched its Hall of Fame, the inductees were William K. and Natalie Warren, Sister Blandine Fleming and Lloyd Verret. ■

enue from the government programs. The primary reason was the lower rate of payments made by the federal government than what facilities charged.

"It's affecting not only hospitals in the Tulsa area, but even more drastically hospitals in rural areas where the percentage of Medicare and Medicaid patient load is higher. If your hospital has 75 percent Medicare and Medicaid occupancy reimbursed on a cost basis and when you add in bad debt, you have very few patients who actually pay hospital charges. A lot of small hospitals are getting into a financial bind because of it." — Ben White, senior vice president of the Oklahoma Hospitals Association, *Tulsa Tribune*, May 17, 1978.

CHARITY CARE

In 1973, Hillcrest Medical Center was among national hospitals reporting problems with price control tactics put into place by the federal government. The institution reported an outstanding balance of $113,000 in old Medicaid cases and was required to dip into a reserve fund to replace worn-out equipment.

"Hillcrest's problems are not uncommon to institutions which carry money-losing responsibilities for charity care and medical education and those paying back loans from earlier construction. The problem, although monumentally complicated in hospital budgeting processes, is basic: Under the price controls, officials say, hospitals have not been able to raise rates to generate enough dollars to meet zooming prices the institutions are paying for supplies and services." — *Tulsa World*, July 22, 1973.

In 1972, Hillcrest lost $600,000 and the indigent patients were increasing. By 1974, 34 percent of all indigent patients in the state were cared for at Hillcrest Medical Center and University Hospital in Oklahoma City. A study conducted by a committee for the state Health Planning Commission found that hospitals in the metropolitan areas were bearing a disproportionate amount of the cost for charity care. It was also discovered that some hospitals were requiring deposits and turning away patients who didn't pay. The committee proposed pooling funds for indigent care and to establish an open-door policy for all nonprofit, voluntary and local or state government-sponsored hospitals.

More than half of the patients treated at charity clinics in Tulsa in the early to mid-70s were at Hillcrest. Saint Francis Hospital was pulling in more patients who were paying full private pay costs. Though, officials at the time said 40 percent of patients came from outside Tulsa. Hillcrest was left with more of the indigent patients, and the institution was battling a need to modernize and increase capacity with shortfalls in the budget. Administrator James Harvey said about 20 percent of its income was written off as charity care in 1974.

"Caught in the crunch of government controls, inadequate payment for services and increasing competition for the private patient, Hillcrest officials believe they must either trim their community service burden or face eventual financial collapse." — *Tulsa Tribune*, Jan. 28, 1974.

This was the same time the hospital launched a 6-year, $31-million construction plan. It transformed the look and capacity of the hospital. The first phase was a four-level building at the northeast corner of 12th Street and Troost Avenue. Plans eventually changed to make that a 10-level building. The second stage was a seven-level bed tower with about 50 beds on each level, replacing an outdated west wing. It brought the bed capacity to 738. The third phase connected the tower and facility. Each stage included expansions of surgery, laboratory, pharmacy, special stores, ambulatory care and emergency services.

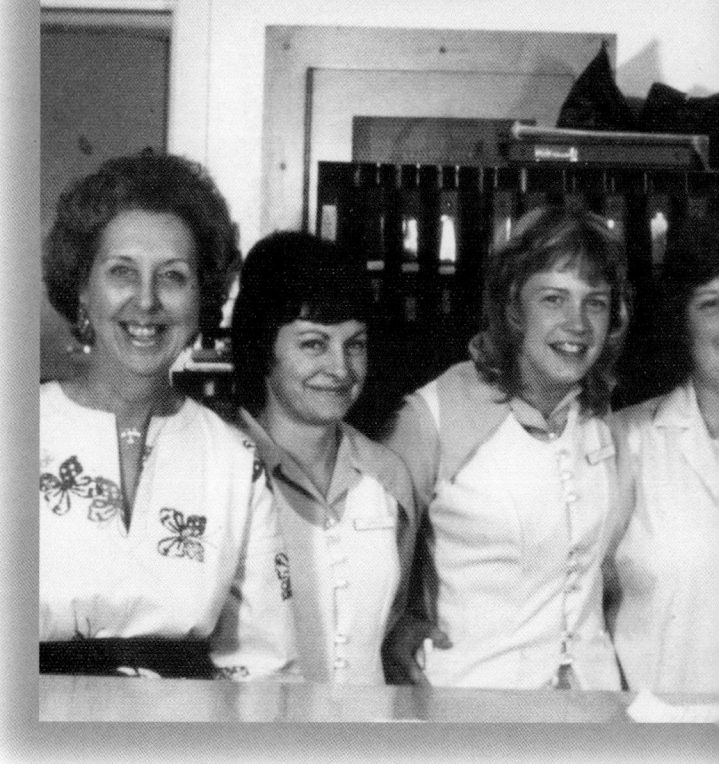

"A national trend — experienced also in Tulsa — involving growing use of emergency rooms for routine care has brought a need for more space." — *Tulsa World*, May 5, 1974.

The plans came after a year-long study in the community needs and hospital infrastructure. Though acknowledging finances were tight, especially with a commitment to charity care and medical education programs, hospital leaders felt it needed upgrades to compete and retain quality care.

"Essentially, we found we had no option but to remain a viable community institution. We think the best answer to accomplish that is what we're describing. Hillcrest, in this process of making numerous decisions, is facing up to its future. But this is a Tulsa question, not just a Hillcrest question. It's a matter of having a health care system in Tulsa which is adequately financed," said Hillcrest Administrator James Harvey, *Tulsa World*, May 5, 1974.

Hillcrest officials took advantage of other innovative financing strategies, landing often in business newspaper stories. A July 31, 1977, *Tulsa World* story about how it made money through the bond market, the headline stated, "It's Complex, but Hillcrest Trades Old Bonds for New to Save Millions in Interest." By mid-decade, finances turned from red to black. Key people on the board of trustees were credited for the financial transformation — Tulsa attorney William H. Bell, who served as chairman; Paul E. Taliaferro, chief executive officer of Sunray-DX and a former board chairman; Jack E. Roth, vice president of Getty Oil Co.; and Walter H. Helmerich Jr., chairman of Helmerich and Payne, Inc.

"Using business rather than political or emotional approaches to solving problems, they have been instrumental in not only a turn-around in profit but on several other vital fronts as well," *Tulsa Tribune*, Feb. 14, 1975.

Hillcrest Nurses.

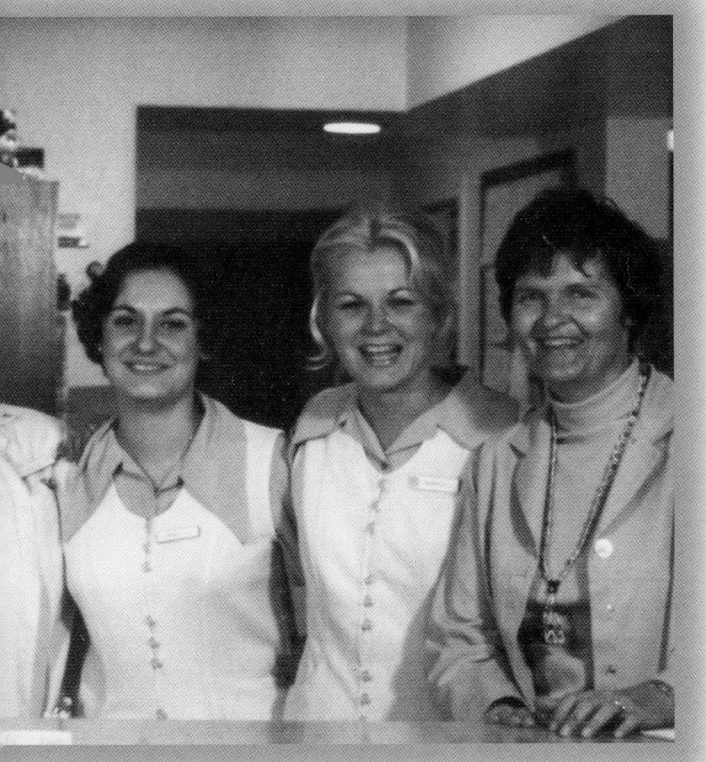

The expansion got underway by using a bond issue sold to Goldman Sachs. A physician recruitment program was put into place followed by the identification of niche programs for the hospital. Those leading trustees took notice of details while raising funds, such as adding benches to parking areas and using vinyl with tile in the bathrooms.

The hospital also received attention of its programs, such as one that promoted siblings holding siblings in a nursery. In May 1977, NBC's *Today Show* taped a segment at Hillcrest on its child abuse and neglect prevention program. Tulsa pediatrician Dr. Donald Pfeifer and pediatric mental health nurse Catherine Ayoub started the project at a clinic just west of Utica Avenue on 21st Street. Public relations officials with the hospital — Maggie Jewell and Missy Kruse — contacted the network after it broadcast a piece on violence in families. The Tulsa program had been showing success in treating at-risk parents by bringing in social workers with the medical staff. They had home visits, safety plans and regular communication with the parents.

VACCINES AND IMMUNIZATIONS

Smallpox was largely considered eradicated in the U.S., leading to national debate about the need for continued mass vaccinations. In 1969, two researchers from the National Communicable Disease Center, the precursor to the U.S. Centers for Disease Control and Prevention, recommended discontinuing the routine vaccinations. They argued the benefits of small vaccinations for children no longer outweigh the risks. Physicians, including those in Tulsa, disputed this claim, saying the disease is contagious and, though rare, it spreads quickly before it can be contained and cured. Just three years earlier, smallpox accounted for between 500,000 to 1 million deaths a year worldwide.

"This kind of talk has been going on for many years. But the great majority of professionals think that the few serious reactions are much less of a risk than letting smallpox become an epidemic again. We haven't had smallpox in this country for a good many years, and this is reason to keep vaccinating. With worldwide travel as it is, smallpox could be brought into this country. Smallpox was once a serious epidemic in this country and still is in other parts of the world," said Dr. George W. Prothro, director of the Tulsa City-County Health Department, *Tulsa World*, Nov. 16, 1969.

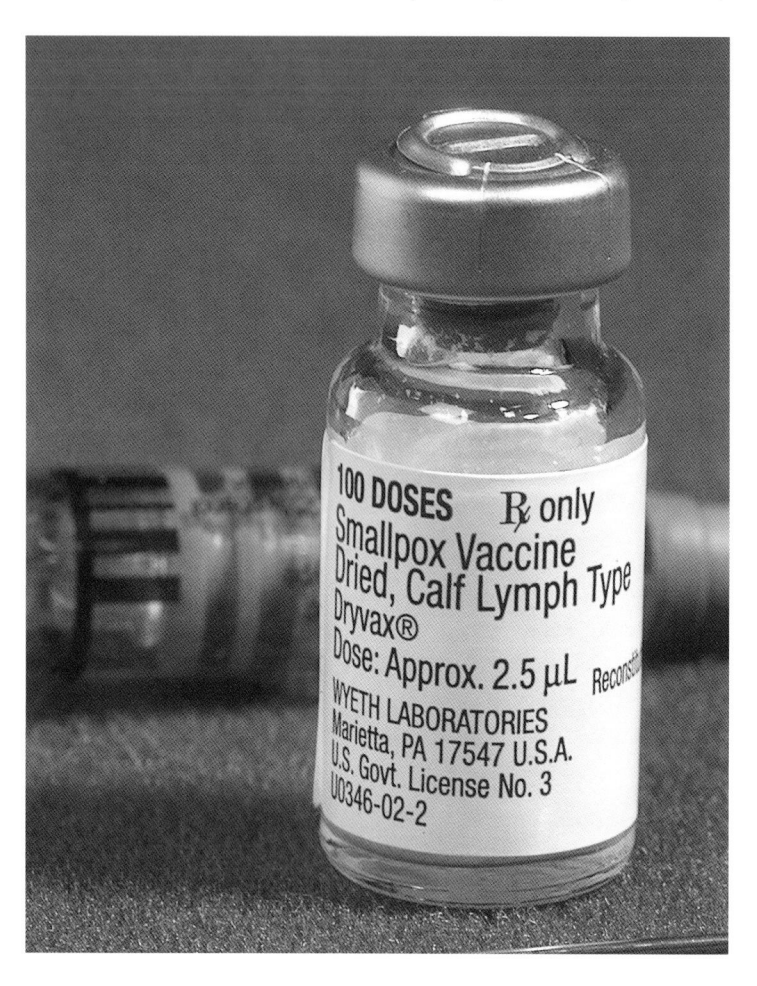

In 1972, smallpox reappeared in Yugoslavia, with 149 cases reported within four months including 22 deaths. In 1973, England experienced a smallpox outbreak and prompted measures requiring travelers to that country prove they have received the vaccine. The following year, one of the largest international health stories was the smallpox epidemic in India, killing at least 20,000 in 1974 and afflicting more than 125,000.

"I have been concerned with the problems that if we let up on vaccination requirements, we will start seeing more of the disease. That's what's happening," said Dr. George W. Prothro, director of the Tulsa City-County Health Department, *Tulsa World*, April 11, 1973.

In June 1974, a 3-year-old girl in Tulsa became ill with what was believed to be exposure to a person who had been given a smallpox vaccine. The girl, Jenny Ann Joyce, had a immune deficiency and was treated with serums from the U.S. Centers for Disease Control and Prevention and blood transfers from people with the smallpox immunity. She was hospitalized at St. John's Hospital then transferred to Children's Memorial Center in Oklahoma City. She developed lesions on her legs and mouth, making it difficult to swallow and causing some disfigurement. Months later, it was found that her blood did not contain smallpox antibodies. Physicians were considering the case as possibly an "id reaction," a type of allergic reaction not involving actual infection. Jenny recovered but required plastic surgery.

Items from a smallpox vaccination kit.

By 1980, the World Health Organization declared smallpox a thing of the past — the first disease humankind eliminated. It had been considered one of the five most deadly diseases in world history, along with cholera, plague, yellow fever and typhus. The attention then shifted to immunizations and battling tropical illnesses. Diseases such as polio, measles and tuberculosis were killing about 5 million children worldwide and disabling an equal number. Malaria was still a major killer in Africa along with African sleeping sickness, leprosy and leishmaniasis.

In 1973, the U.S. Center for Disease Control ranked Oklahoma low for its rate of immunization for polio (44th nationally), rubella (40th) and rubeola (51st). Among children ages 1 to 4, the percentages ranged from 30 percent inoculated for rubella to 55 percent against polio.

"These figures indicate that pre-schoolers are seriously un-immunized in Oklahoma. Cases of both rubella and rubeola already have been reported in several counties and more can be expected. Parents would see that their children receive immunizations either through public health facilities or their private physician," said David Adcock, director of immunization for the state health department, *Tulsa Tribune*, Jan. 19, 1973.

In August 1976, an infant in Kellyville died and four other children were hospitalized in an outbreak of whooping cough. About 30 children who came into contact with those children were treated with an antibiotic to kill the bacteria and lessen complications. The baby, Randy Dale Hallemeier, contracted the disease from brothers and sisters.

"We think it's pretty well contained. It's important for us to emphasize that these children weren't immunized," said Dr. Armond Start, communicable disease control director for the state health department, *Tulsa World*, Aug. 1, 1976.

Reports of under-vaccinated children led to a movement to require children have updated vaccinations before entering school. In 1975, a Tulsa survey showed 33 percent of pre-school children, between the ages of one to about six, were not adequately immunized. Nationally, there was a decrease from 84 percent of pre-school children receiving a polio vaccine to about 60 percent. In Tulsa, about 66 percent of preschoolers had been given a polio vaccine in 1973. That year, about 69 percent were immunized for measles, 69 percent for rubella and 79 percent for diphtheria.

In 1976, a change in Oklahoma law required parents inoculate students in the first through 12th grades. Required were: Four doses of the oral polio vaccine, four doses of DPT or diphtheria, whooping cough and tetanus vaccine, one dose of measles or rubeola vaccine and one dose of rubella or German measles vaccine. It was put into place after several measles epidemics ran through the schools. Compliance was strong, with about 80 to 88 percent vaccination rate. Soon, concern was rising about the younger children.

"Parents appear to be more concerned with complying with the law than with protecting their children's health. Although the law is being met, parents are neglecting their preschoolers — and it is with the younger children that these diseases can be most dangerous. We haven't yet seen an increase in disease because of the few immunizations, but we're sitting on dynamite. If one of these diseases is introduced into the community, we could have an epidemic. There was an epidemic of diphtheria a few years back in Texas, and that's real close," said Dr. George Prothro, *Tulsa Tribune*, Oct. 29, 1974.

A Divisive Issue

One of the most significant court decisions affecting medicine occurred with the 1973 U.S. Supreme Court decision in Roe v. Wade that legalized abortion. The lead-up to that decision highlighted the opinions of local and state doctors on both sides of the issue. By the time of the ruling, all states surrounding Oklahoma allowed for access to abortion, some in limited cases. Oklahoma's only exemption was to save the life of the mother. The ruling stated the decision in the first three months is left to the woman and physician; the second three months allows for states to regulate the procedure in ways reasonably related to maternal health; and the last three months states can place the most onerous restrictions except to protect the life or health of the woman.

In June 1970, the American Medical Association passed a policy that approved abortion for social and economic reasons as long as it is in the best interest of the woman's health. The conference tackling the issue was described as "possibility one of the most tense questions they had." Dr. Ed Calhoon, of Beaver, Oklahoma, president of the Oklahoma State Medical Association was staunchly against abortion.

"Under no condition will I appoint a panel of physicians to be concerned strictly with abortion. Certainly the AMA's position has been a bit liberalized in application to the states where the laws are more liberal. But it's still a matter of law in the states. I am not personally in favor of more liberalized abortion laws. I will not support abortion on request, and I believe there's enough laxity of our morals now." — Dr. Ed Calhoon, president of the OSMA, July 19, 1970.

In July 1971, the head the OU School of Medicine's gynecology and obstetrics department wrote an editorial in the OSMA Journal arguing the state has not kept up with the advances in science. Dr. James A. Merrill stated the original purpose of the laws against abortion was to protect women against morbidity and mortality, which no longer existed. He argued the laws created a class difference, with wealthier women able to pay for illegal procedures or go to states with legalized abortion, while poor women could not. Dr. Merrill stated childbirth contained more health risks than abortion and, overall, access to birth control needed to be increased.

In August 1971, offices of the Comprehensive Family Planning and Therapeutic Abortion Association were set up in Stillwater, Norman and Oklahoma City to direct women with unwanted pregnancies to states where the procedure was legal. Representatives estimated about 400 Oklahoma women a year underwent illegal abortions. Planned Parenthood reported in 1972 getting about 100 inquiries a month about abortion services.

Dr. Max Deardorff, a Tulsa obstetrician and gynecologist, spoke in public about a need to repeal the state's abortion laws and promote the use of contraceptions.

"I have had a sharp change of feelings regarding abortion. The enormity of the problems of unwanted pregnancies and especially the number of botched abortions cannot be ignored." — Dr. Max Deardorff, *Tulsa Tribune*, Aug. 5, 1971.

At the state Capital before the U.S. Supreme Court decision, doctors were called by lawmakers to present testimony in bills that would have reformed the law.

"I think the fetus is only being attacked because it is defenseless. The fetus is an actual person. This is another phase in the life of a human being. The fetus is due the respect of a human being, like you and I," said Dr. Adolpt Vaumen, chief of staff for Hillcrest Medical Center, *Tulsa World*, April 8, 1971.

The OSMA president in 1971, Dr. Lucien M. Pascucci, a radiologoist in Tulsa, was also against changing the laws. "The unborn child has the right to live. When we start losing our regard for life, in the future we may be tempted to bypass the onerous task of caring for the mentally retarded and the aged and ill," said Dr. Lucien Pascucci, *Tulsa World*, Oct. 18, 1971.

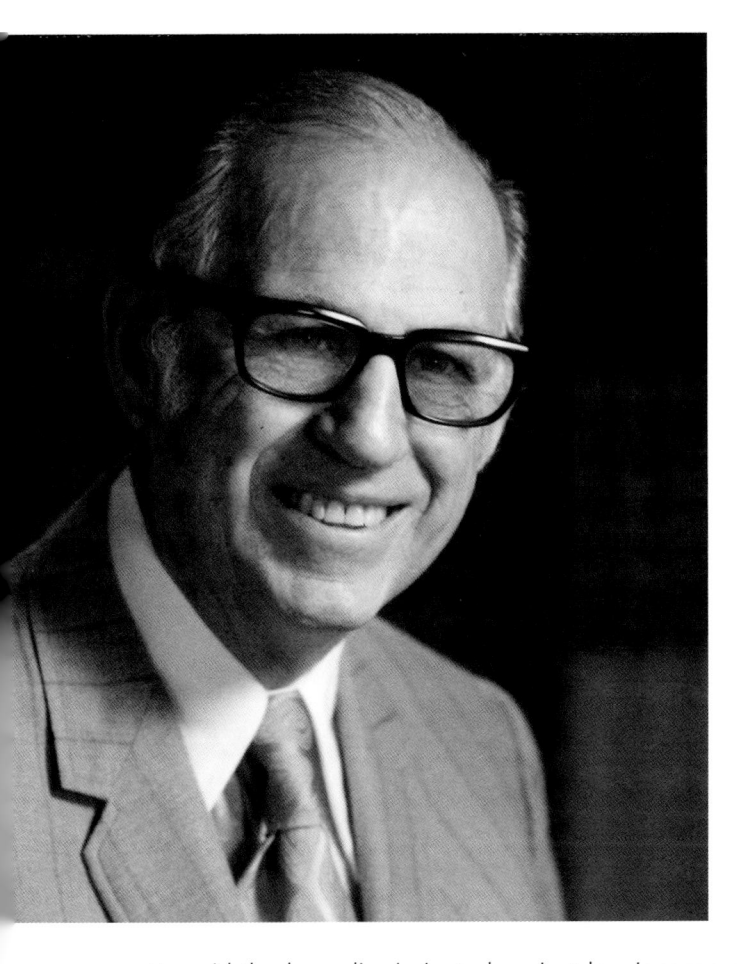

Dr. Lucien M. Pascucci.

"For people with means, it is no great problem, though they live in Oklahoma, if they decide they want to terminate a pregnancy. It is the disadvantaged people of this state who are discriminated against by the present Oklahoma laws. I walk a thin line every day, trying to stay inside the Oklahoma law and to serve the people who come to me in pain. Not the least of these was a 14-year-old girl whose mother deposited her on my doorstep and walked off, leaving the girl to work out her problems with what assistance I could give." — Jackie Longacre, executive director of Planned Parenthood, *Tulsa World*, Oct. 18, 1971.

In October 1972, Dr. Donald L. Cooper, director of Oklahoma State University's student hospital clinic, said a state survey of physicians showed that 51.5 percent supported repealing or adding more exemptions in the law. At a meeting of the Modern Oklahomans for Repeal of Abortion Laws, he called abortion the "least worst" solution in some cases. He said the laws discriminated against low-income women.

In the midst of the back-and-forth, law enforcement continued to arrest and prosecute doctors, nurses, staff and patients involved with abortion services. Some of the procedures were conducted under clandestine circumstances. The cases were all eventually dropped after the Supreme Court decision.

- In November 1970, Tulsa police made arrests in a suspected "abortion ring." Taken into custody were William Robert Cloud, former administrator at Doctor's Hospital in Okmulgee, Lola Rose Adams and Charles D. Fetter. During the trial in April 1971, a female police officer spoke of what she experienced going undercover as a women seeking an abortion in Tulsa. She made contact through Dr. W.J. Bryan Henrie of Grove, who had served a 25-month prison sentence for manslaughter and abortion in the death of a Tulsa housewife. The officer said arrangements for a $450 abortion were made through a series of phone calls and was told to meet at a parking lot near Yale Avenue and 32nd Street. She was taken to a home on the 1900 block of S. Riverside

Drive, where she was told to put on black-out sunglasses to enter. Once inside, she signaled to officers for the arrest. One staffer said she was the eighth pregnant woman they saw that day, including a 14-year-old girl who came with her mother. The case was stalled when defense attorneys challenged the constitutionality of the state's abortion laws and Roe v. Wade was accepted to be heard by the high court.

- In March 1972, a noted Tulsa obstetrician was arrested with two other men in a raid on a home facility near Lake Keystone used to conduct abortions. Dr. Elmer Malcolm Stokes was arrested along with David Stuart Taylor and Fetter, who was on bond from his earlier arrest associated with an abortion. The clinic had eight furnished rooms with a bed and television and a surgical room. The facility had been under construction for 19 months. The raid included sheriff's officers from Pawnee County, Tulsa police detectives, Tulsa County District Attorney S.M. Fallis and Tulsa County Medical Examiner Dr. Robert Fogel. Dr. Stokes had been a member of the Tulsa County Medical Society and Southern Hills Country Club and served as a governor's appointee on a 1961 mental health board.

- In 1969, Dr. Virgil Jobe in Oklahoma City was convicted of performing an abortion on a teenaged girl. He was sentenced to five years in prison but remained free pending appeals.

A *Tulsa World* series in February 1972 profiled women who had obtained illegal abortions in Oklahoma and legal procedures out-of-state. For those who went to New York, it cost $325 for one woman and $50 for another, plus the travel. To obtain an illegal abortion in Tulsa, a married mother of three reported being picked up by two men at her home and blindfolded as she sat on the floorboard of a car for the one-hour drive. She remained blindfolded through the procedure and on the ride home, also while on the floor of the vehicle.

After the Supreme Court decision, lawmakers passed legislation in April 1973 to become more in line with the federal case. One year after the decision was handed down, Reproductive Services opened in Tulsa to perform abortion procedures. The procedures were also being held in at least one physician's office and at the clinic, Statewide Clinic, Inc. Physicians and nurses were staffed at each location. No Tulsa hospitals performed the procedure.

In the ensuing years, various bills have been passed by lawmakers restricting abortions including parental consent, extensive patient questionnaires, waiting periods, mandated ultrasounds and revoking physician licenses. Some measures have withstood legal challenges and some have not. In nearly every Oklahoma legislative session, a bill is introduced that places restrictions on or outlaws abortion.

An opinion in the principles of medical ethics of the American Medical Association states it does not prohibit a physician from performing an abortion "in accordance with good medical practice and under circumstances that do not violate the law." The American College of Obstetricians and Gynecologists supports the availability of reproductive health services for all women and is committed to improving access to abortion. The OSMA takes no position on abortion, though it occasionally makes a statement on specific legislation. ■

CHAPTER 9
(1980 - 1989)

Changing Health Practices

AirEvac for
St. John Medical Center.

The boom of the oil days was destined for bust. That happened in 1985. The number of homes on the market doubled, the population leveled, city sales tax fell and some banks went under. The city worked to diversify its economy and looked to natural gas and new technologies as an answer. Interestingly, the largest employer was American Airlines, which reached more than 7,000 in staff that decade. Rockwell International also expanded during this time.

Two major floods — in 1984 and 1986 — caused the city to invest more than $500 million in mitigation and dam projects.

Much of the shopping, entertainment and new homes had shifted to the south of the city. Rock acts like Cheap Trick, The Pretenders, Hall and Oates came through Tulsa. Country musicians such as George Jones and Hank Williams Jr. made stops as well. The ORU Mabee Center hosted entertainers such as Barry Manilow while other venues from the Cain's Ballroom and Brady Theater offered space. Punk and underground sounds were heard at places like the Crystal Pistol Saloon and SRO.

In medicine, the AIDS epidemic changed health and social practices while technology ushered in better emergency communication systems. Going from no medical schools to several placed stress on the system at a time when the economy turned, and hospitals struggled with finances.

TOO MANY SCHOOLS

With three medical schools in the city, the Tulsa County Medical Society appointed a special committee to study its effects. After 16 months, a 150-page report was released and unanimously endorsed by the board of directors. While the recommendations were voluntary, the leadership had confidence the schools would be receptive. The most significant point was a call for a freeze in class sizes at all Tulsa medical schools and residency programs.

Arkansas River in Flood.

"Sufficient physicians are being graduated by Oklahoma's medical schools to meet present and anticipated statewide demands, including requirements for a growing population," the report states, *Tulsa World*, Nov. 24, 1981.

Other conclusions and recommendations:
- Existing ambulatory teaching clinics at the schools should be restructured to serve indigent patients exclusively, and the costs borne by government agencies responsible for such care.
- ORU's City of Faith "should assume exclusive responsibility for the care of indigent patients from outside the state of Oklahoma which it has attracted."
- The OU-Tulsa Medical College should continue its present format as a two-year school of medicine.

- It is not practical for the OU-Tulsa Medical College and the Oklahoma College of Osteopathic Medicine and Surgery to combine or share facilities or faculty.
- Tulsa's medical schools should work together in developing and coordinating programs of continuing medical education for graduate physicians and allied health care personnel in Tulsa County.
- Tulsa County Medical Society should establish a liaison committee to work with the three schools in a continuing study of physician manpower, paying particular attention to the impact the number of graduates has in Tulsa County.

Members of the study committee were Drs. John R. Alexander, Lenard Poplin, George H. Kamp and Victor L. Robards Jr.

The Rise and Fall of ORU's City of Faith

Huge red and white ribbons representing prayer and medicine were unfurled over the heads of nearly 10,000 people in attendance of the opening of the City of Faith Medical and Research Center on Nov. 1, 1981. Founder Oral Roberts tied the ribbons together in bows. Country music star Barbara Mandrell sang the national anthem.

"I welcome you to something that seems very small in our big world. It's exactly like God gave it to me," Oral Roberts, *Tulsa World*, Nov. 2, 1981.

By the mid-80s, the vision Oral Roberts had for a triumvirate of graduate schools — medical, dental and law — were falling apart. The first to fold was the dental school, announced in 1985. Dr. James Winslow, vice president of student affairs, said no student out of four graduating classes has gone into full-time mission programs. It would continue offering dentistry residencies in foreign mission posts.

ORU's City of Faith Groundbreaking.

"The reason that graduates are not going to the mission field is that the average indebtedness of our graduates is $35,000 per student. When a student graduates, he has no means to pay off his debt unless he goes into private practice, and this precludes his going into mission work. Without students going into mission fields, which is what Mr. Roberts told his supporters at the outset, we have not been able to raise enough support to continue the dental school in its present format," said Dr. James Winslow, *Tulsa World*, June 22, 1985.

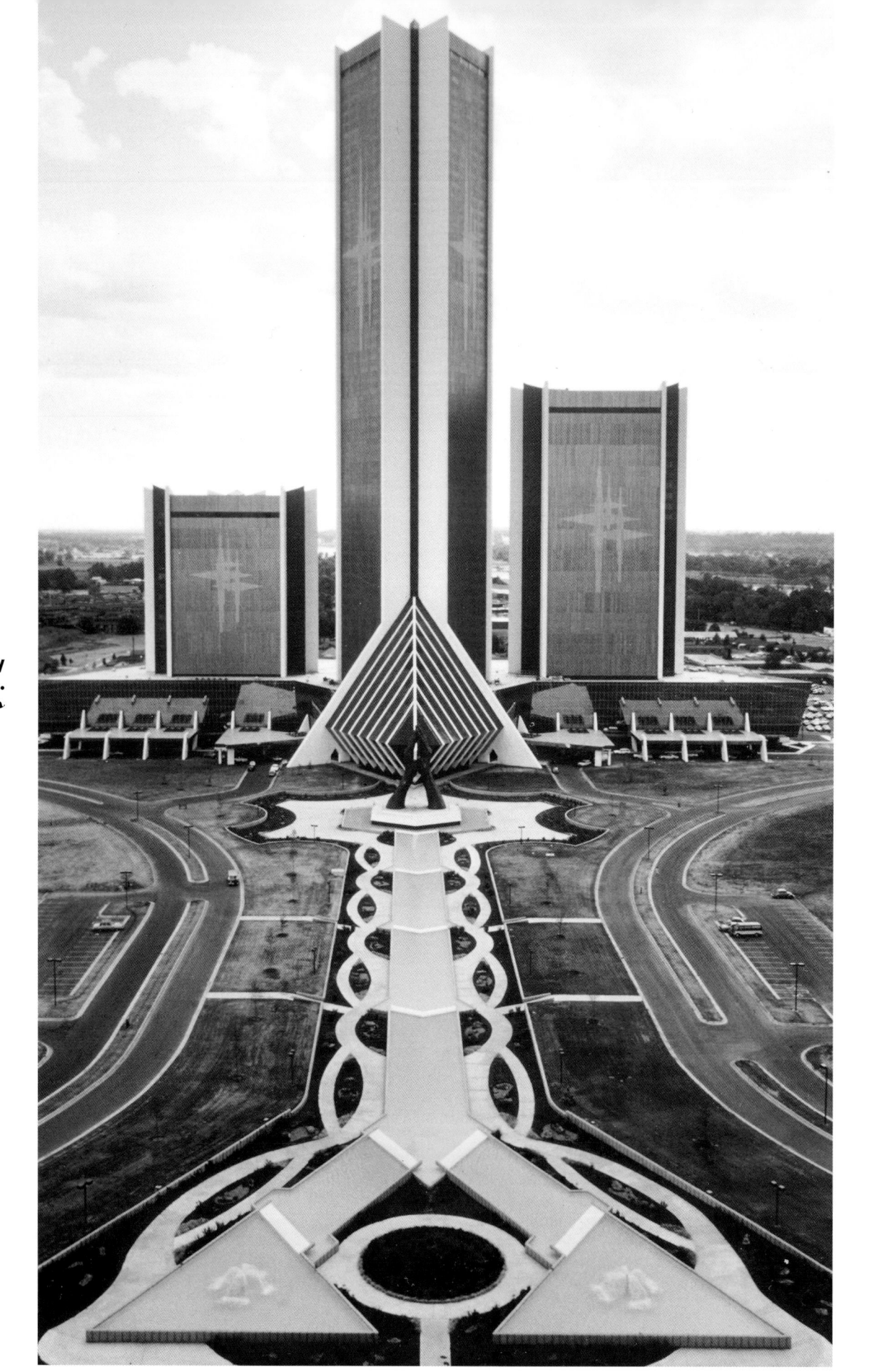

ORU's City of Faith.

In November 1985, Roberts announced the transfer of the law school to CBN University in Virginia Beach, Virginia. The Christian Broadcasting Network was led by fellow televangelist Pat Robertson. When the law school ended, Roberts vowed no more closures or transfers would occur.

On Nov. 3, 1985, Roberts made national pleas on his televised service for money and patients for the City of Faith stating the hospital "now is at the point it could be lost." He stated the facility was drawing about 500 patients a day, needed a minimum of 600 patients to break even and really needed 800 a day.

The City of Faith was featured at the center of a 60-story building in a three-tower complex with space for 777 beds. It opened with 294 beds. In addition to the under-utilization by patients, it also put accreditation into jeopardy. Crucial to the continued accreditation of any medical school is the access students have to sufficient patient-care experiences.

"So, I'm facing a real problem. If we don't have 100 more patients in a matter of days, per day in the clinic, we're in a position to lose part or all of our medical school," said Oral Roberts, *Tulsa World*, Nov. 5, 1985.

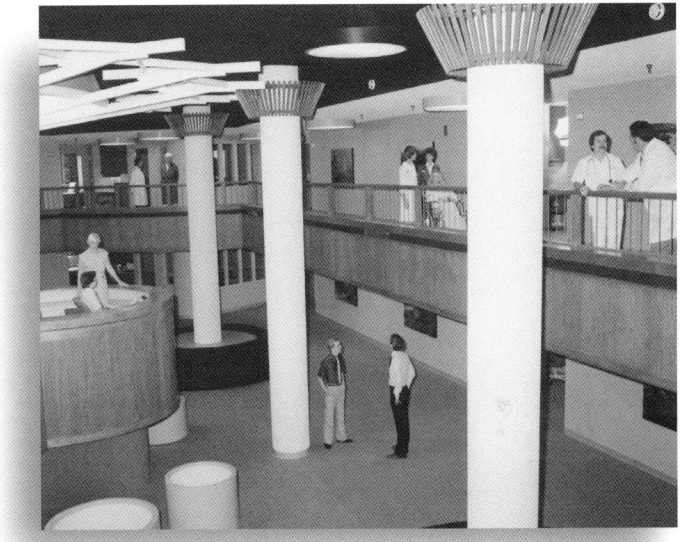

Interior of City of Faith Hospital.

In March 1986, Roberts announced God would "call Oral Roberts home" if he didn't raise $8 million to provide full scholarships for students attending the medical school. The goal was to raise $100 million to benefit the needs for the City of Faith operations.

"Oral is a very intense person. He believes that if he doesn't succeed in fulfilling God's will, he will be in disobedience to God's command. He feels very much that his life is on the line," said Dr. Jan Dargatz, vice president of creative development for ORU, *Tulsa World*, Jan. 6, 1987.

In April 1987, Richard Roberts announced $8 million had been donated for the medical missions. However, it was not enough to save the school, research center and hospital. On Sept. 13, 1989, Oral Roberts announced the closing to students, faculty and alumni during a chapel service. The congregation gasped, and a few students wept.

"I prayed today that I would not cry. I've cried all the tears in my soul," said Oral Roberts, *Tulsa World*, Sept. 14, 1989.

The school and center were $25 million in debt. About 600 employees at the City of Faith lost their jobs with 100 faculty members and 147 medical students also affected. The City of Faith complex would be retained and leased. Revenue was to be placed in the university's endowment fund. The medical students were assisted in transferring to other universities, and many faculty were hired by other institutions or started their own practices.

Doctors' Hospital Sold

In the early 80s, several suitors approached Doctors' Hospital about buying the institution. In May 1983, hospital officials confirmed it intended to sell the 221-bed facility to American Medical International of Beverly Hills, California, for a profit of $23 million to $25 million. It was the nation's second-largest hospital chain with hospitals in Claremore and Lawton. Louis Levy, attorney for the board of directors for Doctors' Hospital, said 10 percent of the AMI income goes to charity care, allaying fears it would not pick up indigent cases. Sale price of the hospital was $39.3 million, with a $10 million mortgage and other loans and liabilities being paid off.

The profit from the sale was used to create the Doctors' Foundation of Oklahoma, automatically becoming one of the top 10 largest foundations in Oklahoma. The mission is to support medical, research, education and welfare projects in the community. Twelve of the original founders served on the foundation's trustees.

AMI sold Doctors' Hospital and 36 other hospitals, including those in Claremore and Lawton, in May 1988 through an Employee Stock Ownership Plan.

Rising Hospital Costs

> A report released in 1987 found four of six Tulsa hospitals suffered financial losses. Hillcrest Medical Center, Osteopathic Hospital, Doctors' Hospital and City of Faith Medical and Research Center collectively came up more than $20 million short in balancing their budgets.

Called one of the most severe budget crunches in the past 30 years, hospitals took a scalpel to their budgets late in the decade. Institutions turned to pay cuts, shortened work weeks, voluntary furloughs, layoffs and hiring freezes to control expenses.

Administrators stated the crisis started about 1982 as federal officials slashed payments in the reimbursement program Diagnosis Related Group, which is what Medicare used to set its rates. It was based on the diagnosis, not the service. Under this system, hospitals were told how long a patient should be in the hospital and the set rate for a procedure or disease. Medical officials said this did not take into account complications, severity of a patient's illness or more up-to-date methods of care.

The nation's insurance companies and the alternative-delivery systems of health maintenance organizations (HMO) and preferred provider organizations (PPO) followed the government's lead by setting the same guidelines. HMOs allowed a person to choose a primary care physician from a network of local providers, who would then refer to in-network specialists or hospitals if needed. PPOs allowed a person to visit any in-network physician or provider without first getting a referral.

"Right now, we don't have a medical care-financing process at the federal level — we have a budget reconciliation process. And if the federal government doesn't stop trying to balance the budget across the back of the nation's hospitals, the inevitable end result is that health care will suffer. Patients will suffer. It has become so routine to hear politicians harangue about trimming the fat from the budgeted amount for medical care. So health-care providers cut fat and cut fat, but while no one was watching, the knife slowly started to carve away at the meat and muscle of our health-care system," said John C. Goldthorpe, Hillcrest Medical Center chief executive officer, *Tulsa World*, March 22, 1988.

The complicated nature of the various insurance plans prompted physician offices and hospitals to hire administrative assistants trained to handle the paperwork. At St. John Medical Center in February 1986, it became the "pre-admission" policy for all non-emergency procedures. The goal was to take the surprise out of the patient hospital bill. The hospital programmed its computer system with every insurance plan in the area. When a patient was pre-admitted, the insurance information was reviewed for any unknown requirements. This system has become common among U.S. hospitals and medical facilities.

"Physicians can no longer put patients in the hospital and assume they will be covered, and we found patients just often do not know what their policy covers," said Dr. Vic Robards, chief of the St. John medical staff, *Tulsa Tribune*, March 19, 1986.

Problems serving the indigent population were being felt at hospitals years before the oil bust. In December 1981, Hillcrest Medical Center began referring poor patients in non-emergency situations to other medical facilities in an attempt to hold down costs. St. John Medical Center also informed patients that less expensive care could be obtained from private physicians, the health department or other clinics. The other hospitals did not have a screening for indigent patients. Reimbursements from Medicare and Medicaid covered about 92 percent of the cost of care, with the difference made up among the private patients and insurance companies.

By August 1998, as a protest to what administrators called a disparity between Medicaid payments to Tulsa and Oklahoma City hospitals, Hillcrest Medical Center closed its emergency room to trauma patients for 30 days. The Oklahoma Osteopathic Hospital suspended emergency treatment of some trauma patients at the same time, citing personnel reasons. Saint Francis Hospital and St. John's Medical Center remained open.

"Hillcrest is angry. We're not going to lighten up on this," said Ira Schlezinger, Hillcrest vice president of strategic services, *Tulsa Tribune*, Aug. 18, 1988.

In November 1988, Hillcrest re-opened its emergency room to trauma patients after the Oklahoma Department of Human Services agreed to increase the amount the state pays for a day's care for Medicaid patients. Saint Francis and Hillcrest received retroactive raises.

A report released in 1987 found four out of six Tulsa hospitals suffered financial losses. Hillcrest Medical Center, Osteopathic Hospital, Doctors' Hospital and City of Faith Medical and Research Center collectively came up more than $20 million short in balancing their budgets.

To shore up costs, hospitals started paying attention to daily costs such as energy and bedsheets. In 1984, Hillcrest Medical Center cracked down after it was discovered the facility lost $86,145 the previous year to lost linens. This included $17,000 in scrubs, $15,000 in bed sheets, $11,000 in blankets and $6,000 in diapers. The hospital installed a new materials management system and considered bar coding. St. John Medical Center put energy-saving protocols in place that led in September 1984 to the designation as the No. 1 participant in a national program administered by the U.S. Department of Energy. The hospital won six grants from the federal agency in the 5-year program. From 1980 to 1984, St. John Medical Center saved $2 million in energy costs through measures such as tower cooling, high-efficiency motors, computerized controls of utility systems and items such as storm windows, reduced lighting and timers.

911 Emergency Phone System Launches

A minute after midnight on May 1, 1980, Tulsans had the ability to call three memorable numbers for any emergency. It had actually been in operation for about two weeks to work out the ticks. This simplified system had been more than a decade in planning.

In the mid-60s, Tulsa officials began considering the notion, which was a national movement. Cost was the biggest consideration.

Sheriff Dave Faulkner: "I'd be glad to help look into it, but you have to think about the money."
Police and Fire Commissioner Bennie Garren: "I'm not against it; I think it has a lot of merit. We'd have to know who is going to pay for it and how it is going to be supported."
Tulsa Police Chief Jack Purdie: "I don't think we can tie the sheriff's office, the FBI and the police in on one line, but I think the public is entitled to one number for city emergency services such as police and fire."
Dale Olsen, Southwestern Bell district manager: "This is going to be a tough job for whoever tackles it." — *Tulsa Tribune*, Feb. 17, 1966.

In 1968, the American Telephone and Telegraph Co. made an announcement that Americans would be able to call for emergency crews with one universal number in "a few years." A *Tulsa Tribune* story predicted it would take "perhaps two years" to have it up and running in the city.

"Under the plan, dialing 911 would reach a central switchboard where every emergency service in a metropolitan area would be represented. Trained personnel would summon the proper type of help immediately — police, firemen, doctors. Emergency calls could even be made from public telephones — without the need of a coin." — *Tulsa Tribune*, Jan. 12, 1968.

More than 40 different emergency numbers existed in Tulsa and six surrounding cities. Those included police, fire, ambulance, sheriff and highway patrol. These varying numbers throughout not just the city, but also the nation, attracted attention of Congress, which sought avenues for municipalities to obtain the 911. The Oklahoma delegation had differing opinions on a 1967 resolution that would officially state Congress favors "one uniform nationwide fire reporting number and one uniform nationwide police reporter number."

Congressman Tom Steed: "When people need to make an emergency call, they don't think very well. It would be simpler for everyone concerned if we had a universal number."

Congressman John Jarman: "It makes sense. I'm just shooting from the hip, but it looks like something worthwhile."

Congressman James V. Smith: "It seems to me that it is a good resolution, if there is no opposition from local municipalities. Local folks might think of it as regimentation if it gives them no right to choose."

> More than 40 different emergency numbers existed in Tulsa and six surrounding cities.

> To save a life, To stop a crime, Dial 911.

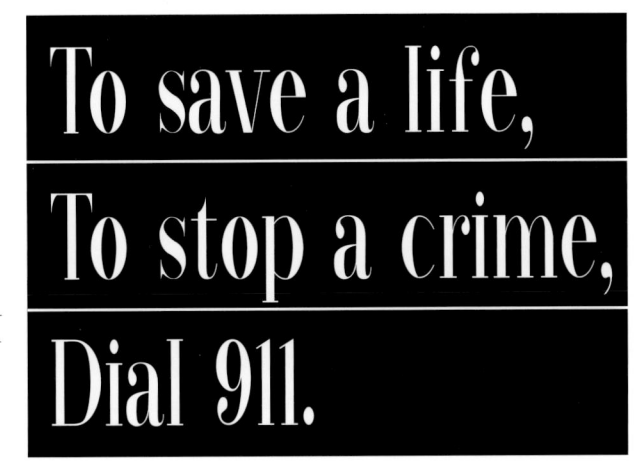

Congressmen Ed Edmondson: "It has always been my understanding that the national practice, to call police, is to dial the operator and ask for help. Let's look at the telephone book. It says, 'dial the operator in any emergency.' I'd like to know what's wrong with that procedure. I think the resolution certainly will be given very careful consideration."

Congressman Page Belcher: "Ordinarily, people just dial zero."

Senator Mike Monroney: "It looks like it would be a very fine thing if all municipalities would have a common emergency code. Of course, we couldn't compel municipalities to adopt a common code because of state's rights."

Senator Fred Harris: "It would be a very simple method for calling for help." — *Tulsa Tribune*, Oct. 2, 1967.

A Tulsa feasibility study in 1978 stated implementing a 911 system linking police, fire and ambulance would cost about $957,000 with operating costs of about $71,000 per month. It also warned that some system may slow emergency response times. In 1978, the Tulsa County Medical Society Auxiliary conducted a telephone survey about the community support for the system and found 90 percent backed the 911 number. Of those in support, 78 percent stated they would pay a 25-cent charge a month on their phone bills for the service. In the Tulsa mayoral election that year, Jim Inhofe campaigned with implementing a 911 system as one of his promises. After his election, Inhofe pushed for the service. Southwestern Bell estimated a system would cost $15,000 to install and $2,500 a month in equipment rental. Personnel costs were estimated at a high of $4,000 a month.

"In the middle of the night, especially on something like a prowler call, it's a lot easier to dial 911 than our regular (7-digit) police number. A lot more citizens seem to be trying it out on weekends," said Tulsa Police Sgt. Ron Ryan, *Tulsa Tribune*, May 16, 1980.

The public education campaign was explaining what constituted an emergency and what information to provide. Officials described it as a situation in which life or property was in immediate danger. Callers were asked a brief description before being transferred to the correct department, which then needed an address and name and nature of emergency.

In a 1982 *Tulsa Tribune* story, operators discussed the problems with the high number of non-emergency calls through the perspective of the Broken Arrow system. In one week in Broken Arrow, 126 non-emergency calls and 17 legitimate emergency calls were made to the 911 system. During rainstorm and tornado sirens, people would call to ask about the weather and sometimes intoxicated people called to talk.

"I don't think people know what an emergency is. People call when a bicycle is stolen. I had one woman call on the 911 line and ask for the number of the library. A lot of kids call and play on it. You can tell right away. Sometimes, they say 'I have an emergency.' Other times they ask if my refrigerator is running," said Annette Wood, Broken Arrow Municipal Center receptionist, *Tulsa Tribune*, Sept. 29, 1982.

Within the first six months, problems arose. Between 30 percent and 60 percent of calls were either put on hold or abandoned by the caller. Operators were swamped and there was no room to add staff. The equipment could not differentiate between emergency and routine calls. Each call was answered as it came in.

In January 1982, the Houston-based research firm Bernard Johnson, Inc., found the Tulsa system outdated in its technology and recommended replacing it. The suggested system would pinpoint calls and reduce response time by routing directly to departments. The estimated cost was $697,744 with a monthly cost of $32,126, which City and Fire Commissioner Roy Gardner called "a hell of a lot of money." He also questioned several criticisms of the report. Instead, the city came up with a different solution.

Even before the report, city officials were working on ways to fix the complaints. A new office was located to house the 911 operators to improve working conditions and morale. It allowed for more staff to be hired. In February 1982, a computer system contracted by the telephone company was in place to separate the types of calls. The latest technology of tracking an address of an incoming call was being investigated. By March 1982, an analysis showed that 80 percent of all 911 calls were answered on the first ring and 100 percent on the second.

"It's taken months of constant pushing, but Tulsa's system works — even toll-free from pay phones — and includes neighboring communities. All was accomplished with little expense other than the nine additional employees hired. Our 911 system has been fixed, but there can always be improvements." *Tulsa World* editorial, March 7, 1982.

Emergency Vehicles In Air

Tulsa Life Flight was established in September 1979 with an agreement between Saint Francis Hospital and Hillcrest Medical Center to primarily serve the rural area in northeastern Oklahoma. Studies showed the mortality rates in rural Oklahoma were 30 percent to 50 percent higher because of not having access to a major hospital. But, it also had a contract with Emergency Medical Services Authority, which oversees emergency services within the Tulsa city limits. Cost of a ride on Life Flight was $75 per flight plus $4 per mile and any supplies used. A Life Flight from Muskogee to Tulsa averaged about $285 in the first year.

"Having worked as an administrator in rural Oklahoma, I know of the inordinate delays that can occur. It isn't uncommon to have a five-hour delay between an accident and definitive treatment. And, I can't help but think it results in permanent damage or worse," said Kenneth Hagar, Saint Francis Hospital assistant administrator, *Tulsa World*, Sept. 9, 1979.

In its first two weeks of operation, it was only called into service four times. For several months, it averaged about one flight a day. However, by its first anniversary celebration, the service reported 418 flights, according to its first director, Mike Sulzycki. The Astar 350 helicopter was leased from Aviation Medical Services. It was based at Saint Francis Hospital with helipads at both institutions. Admittance to any other hospital was handled through ground transportation.

Life Flight Taken in the 1980s.

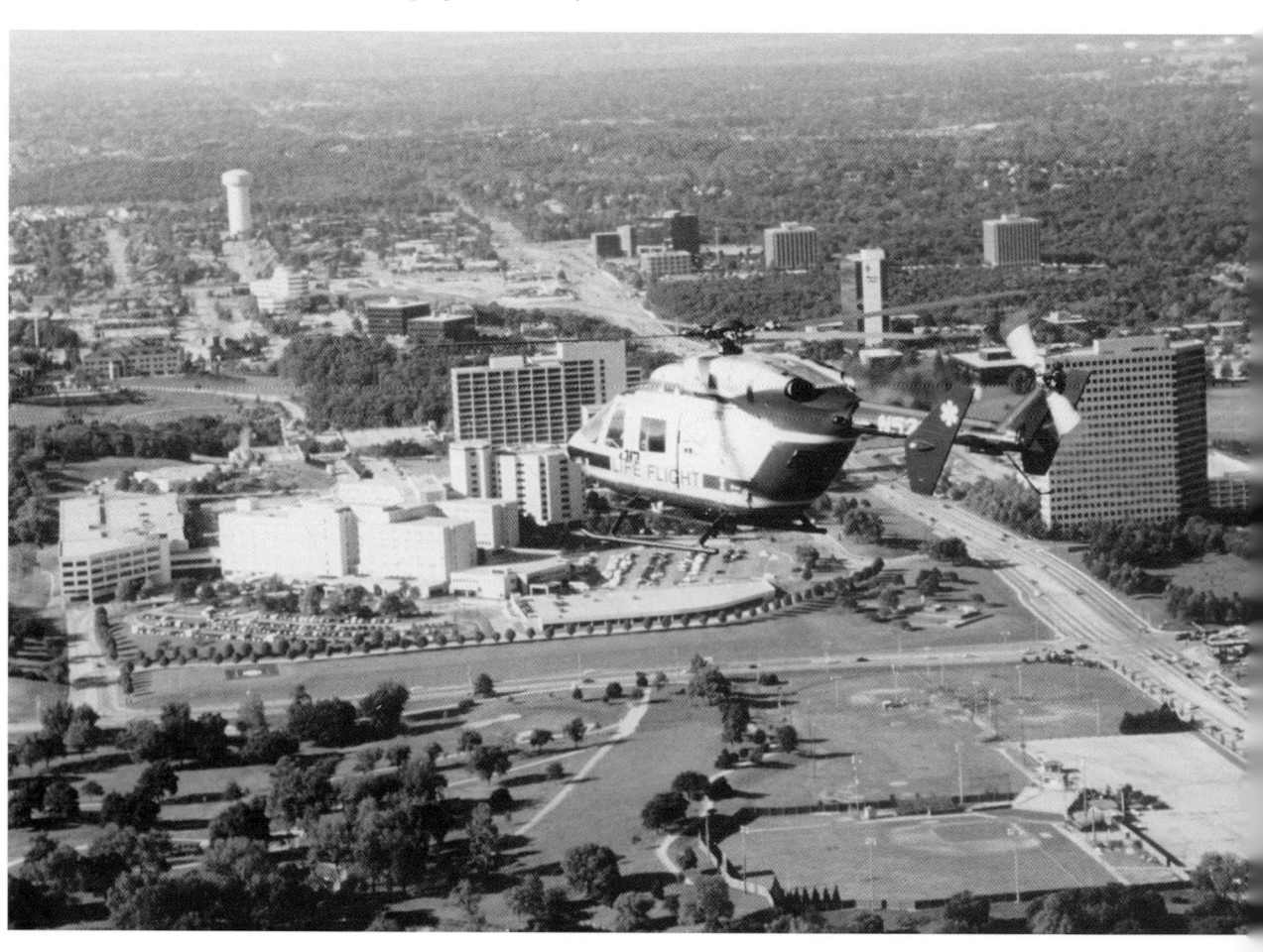

"This kind of thing had never been done before in Oklahoma. It took a tremendous amount of work and education to let people know we were here and show them what we could do for them. We don't have any statistics that tell us how many lives we have been able to save. But, we have had doctors tell us that a certain patient would have died if it hadn't been for us. And a vast majority of our calls have truly been emergencies," said Life Flight Director Mike Sulzycki, *Tulsa Tribune*, Sept. 12, 1980.

At the Oct. 7, 1979 dedication, it featured dignitaries from both Hillcrest Medical Center and Saint Francis Hospital.

From Hillcrest: James D. Harvey, president of the hospital; G.W. Davidson, chairman of the board of trustees; Walter H. Helmerich, member of the board of trustees; and Archie Lawrence, chaplain. From Saint Francis: Sister Mary Blandine, administrator; Henry Zarrow, member of the board of directors; and the Rev. Joseph W. Howell, chaplain. Also attending were Dr. Robert G. Tompkins, chairman of the Tulsa Life Flight Operations committee, Police and Fire Commissioner Jack Purdie and Gene Thaxton, manager of telecommunications at the Oklahoma Department of Public Safety.

The Tulsa Life Flight Operations committee included Dr. Robert G. Tompkins, Dr. James R. Culp, Dr. Steven Landgarten, Dr. Daniel E. Miller, Dr. John Sacra, Dr. C.T. Thompson, Kenneth Hager, Margaret Hinds and nurses Dorothy Doll, Sandra Downie, Susan Herron and Jan Talbott. Herron was the flight nurse supervisor, and the flight nurses were Linda Fields, Steve Ludiker, Cinda Mammen and Jim Murphy. Alternate nurses were Randy Foster, Judy McClendon and Mike Taylor. Pilots were Doug Drury and Joe Trudo.

Dr. Robert Tompkins, the chairman of the Life Flight Operations Committee.

By its fourth anniversary in September 1983, Tulsa Life Flight had become the fifth busiest air ambulance service in the nation. Many rural communities had raised money to build helipads for its residents to use the service. In 1986, it logged 1,903 flights and celebrated its 10,000th flight in January the following year — a premature baby transferred from McAlester. About 65 percent of patients were taken to Saint Francis Hospital and Hillcrest Medical Center. St. John Medical Center received about 25 percent of patients, and the rest went to the Oklahoma Osteopathic Hospital.

"The importance of Life Flight, however, can't be measured in numbers alone. It's value is in saving lives — not only to Tulsa but to most of northeastern Oklahoma." — *Tulsa World* editorial, Jan. 5, 1987.

In December 1986, an announcement was made about the formation of another citywide air ambulance service called AirEvac. It was an agreement between Hillcrest Medical Center, St. John Medical Center and the Oklahoma Osteopathic Hospital. Life Flight was to continue operating independently

Continued on page 156

A New Epidemic

The AIDS and HIV epidemics rushed in changes to medical practices, sexual behavior, classroom health instruction and panic, at least in the beginning.

U.S. physicians began reporting new cases of AIDS (acquired immune deficiency syndrome) to health authorities in 1981. Because it was first recognized within the gay, male community, it did not receive great attention in the initial phases and spawned myths and hysteria. The first story written about the disease in the American media was on May 18, 1981, in the gay publication *New York Native* by journalist Lawrence Mass. The U.S. Centers for Disease Control had been gathering information on the outbreak of clusters of deaths and illnesses among gay men. Within a few years, media across the country were writing about the disease as it spread to the greater population.

"Several recent polls show a majority of Americans aren't knowledgeable about the disease. The sheer numbers of cases, and the horrible deaths of AIDS victims have created a kind of hysteria and panic among some groups in this country."
— *Tulsa World*, Sept. 27, 1987.

The medical explanation for AIDS: The human immunodeficiency disorder virus (HIV) attacks the white blood cells that protect a body from infections. This suppression of the immune system makes people with HIV vulnerable to illnesses not threatening to others. It is transmitted through blood, semen, genital fluids and breast milk. Those must come into contact with a mucous membrane, damaged tissue or directly injected in the bloodstream.

The first case of a person with AIDS reported in Oklahoma was in January 1983, which was the first year Oklahoma required reporting. Four years later, 101 cases were reported with 28 of those in Tulsa County. It jumped to 209 cases by January 1988. By the end of December 1988, there were 507 people with AIDS living in Oklahoma with 143 in Tulsa County. The state required reporting of HIV starting in 1988.

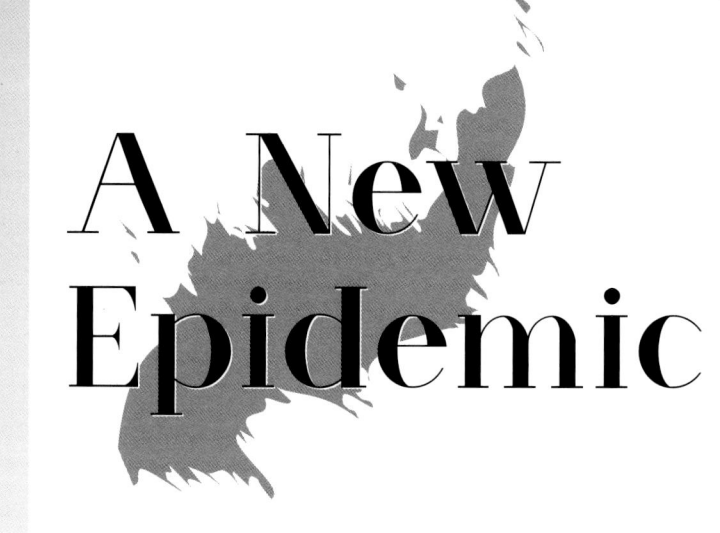

The average AIDS patient in Oklahoma during the mid-80s had a life expectancy of 3.8 months after diagnosis. Much of this was from not being tested to receive a diagnosis before the final stages of the disease. About 70 percent of people who contracted the disease died within two years and 93 percent died within the three years.

Oklahoma responded with advisory councils, task forces and new and failed legislation. In 1987, the Legislature passed a bill to require all convicted prostitutes be tested for HIV. If positive, the person would be required to give the names of clients under oath. It was vetoed by Gov. Henry Bellmon, citing public health officials who doubted it would lower the infection rate and the unconstitutionality of forcing a person to testify. In June 1987, the Department of Corrections went ahead with the mass testing of its prisoners for HIV and AIDS — only one of four states at the time to have tested its entire population. The results found that 41 inmates — less than 1 percent of the prisoner population — tested positive for the AIDS antibodies.

Wagoner Public Schools dealt with a parent revolt and court's orders when it was discovered an 8-year-old with the HIV virus wanted to enroll in school. The boy, a hemophiliac, contracted the disease during one of his blood clotting treatments. The family believed they were telling the school of the boy's medical condition in confidence, but the information was leaked. A lawsuit was filed by parents to keep the boy out of school. Wagoner County District Judge Bill Bliss ruled in November 1987 that the boy had a right to an education and must be allowed to enroll. U.S. District Judge Dale Cook reaffirmed the court's ruling in December 1987.

School districts, including Tulsa and Broken Arrow, created policies on accommodating students with AIDS and HIV, which included confidentiality and reviewing each on a case-by-case basis. Private schools followed with policies reflecting those in public schools.

In April 1987, Gov. Henry Bellmon approved a bill mandating AIDS education in school, focused on how to avoid contracting the HIV virus. The law required students to receive AIDS prevention information at least once between the 7th and 9th grades and again at least once between their sophomore and senior years. State education officials developed a curriculum guide to meet standards set out by the state health department.

Local districts created curriculum review committees, which then emphasized that prevention would focus on abstinence. In some cases, the health departments rejected classroom materials for portraying inaccurate information.

Oklahoma passed the first AIDS policy in May 1987, drafted out of the Governor's Task Force on AIDS under the direction of Hannah Atkins, Gov. Bellmon's secretary for social services. It banned any discrimination against a person with AIDS or HIV.

"Discrimination of any employee, including those who suffer from a contagious disease, cannot be tolerated. The dangerous epidemic AIDS poses even greater problems for victims and their employers. I am pleased that the state of Oklahoma is setting an example for other employers in establishing a policy and procedures that protect the afflicted, their co-workers, the employer and the general public," stated Gov. Henry Bellmon, May 28, 1987.

While a cure remains elusive, treatments to improve immunity and slow down the virus have come onto the market. The U.S. government first approved a treatment in 1987 with AZT (azidothymidine), which reduces the replication of the HIV virus. When AZT became available, it was in limited production only to doctors for patients meeting specific medical guidelines. Many other potential drug treatments were hung up in the government bureaucracy of research and unavailable or too costly. When AZT was made available, a Tulsa AIDS patient reported that the drug cost about $850 a month.

"Tulsans with the disease are taking it upon themselves to learn about new drugs and alternative treatments, sometimes before their doctors. But many experimental drugs are available only through controlled studies at various test sites across the country. Some Tulsa AIDS patients say they are forced to fight for a spot in such a study to obtain the drugs they feel they need to boost their failing immune systems. Others travel to Mexico, where some of the drugs are available over the counter. Some even resort to homemade variations of drugs available here – remedies cooked on a stove or prepared in a kitchen sink." – *Tulsa World*, Aug. 23, 1987.

Another Tulsa patient described going with a group to Mexico to buy rivavirin and isoprinosine, which are anti-viral drugs. Yet another told a reporter he made "work-alike" versions of AIDS remedies in his kitchen. Holistic treatments such as acupuncture and deep tissue massage were also used.

"My doctor just believes what he's read in his medical book. I know we have to wait until different things are approved –

Continued on following page

they have to do tests. But I guess as human beings, we're all looking for that magic pill. When I first got sick, I didn't even know what was available. But I learned. Here I am, I've had (pneumocystis carinii pneumonia) three times, and I'm not dead. There's a lot of hope. I'm buying time with AZT. I'm buying time until something else comes along," said a Tulsa AIDS patient, *Tulsa World*, Aug. 23, 1987.

Even though the health department offered testing for the virus, Tulsa physician Dr. Dan Fieker was among a group of doctors creating a laboratory for anonymous testing with a charge of $50. People were given a number for results, and those with positive tests were given referrals for places to get services. Confidential AIDS Testing Center was opened by another group of physicians in February 1986 for anonymous testing for a fee of $40.

"We believe there is a significant patient population that is concerned about potential exposure to the AIDS virus, but who may be reluctant to go to his or her family physician or to the Tulsa City-County Health Department to be tested," said Dr. Dan Fieker, *Tulsa World*, Feb. 24, 1987.

The health department offered anonymous testing but required an appointment with a counselor for the testing and post-testing to get information. It was found that 30 percent of people never return for results. It was a frustration for health officials to have information for follow ups.

"Right now, I don't have access to figures that would indicate what the problem is. We don't know if these 30 percent represent 65-year-old grandmothers who come in, receive an hour of counseling and realize that they aren't at risk of contracting the disease and so never return for the test results. We don't know if these are individuals in a high-risk group who don't return because they don't want to know the answers. We need to find out who isn't coming back and why they aren't coming back," said Dr. Ralph Wooley, director of the Tulsa City-County Health Department, *Tulsa World*, Aug. 28, 1987.

As education spread along with the virus to diverse populations, the health department and other testing centers began to fill up. The state health department began requiring the reporting of names and addresses of people who tested positive for the AIDS virus, which drew pushback from medical officials and legal experts. Some attorneys were suggesting people use fake names and addresses when going for testing. Dr. Jeffrey A. Beal, a Tulsa internal medicine physician, testified before a Congressional human resources panel criticizing such state policies. He stated patients often wait until "full blown symptoms" manifest and that the closest experimental treatments for patients are more than 500 miles from Tulsa. He told the story of a Tulsa executive who came to his office "blue and gasping for breath" three days before his death: "He chose death instead of exposure."

"It is my belief that three factors are at fault for these devastating survival statistics: fear of discrimination, financial hardships and non-existent treatment options. The result of this mandatory reporting will not only facilitate ongoing discrimination, but will deter further voluntary testing," said Dr. Jeffrey A. Beal, *Tulsa World*, April 29, 1988.

Health care workers began wearing gloves, goggles and protective clothing during work. The CDC in April 1986 released guidelines for medical officials to wear the gear when they may be extensively exposed to blood or bodily fluids. Tulsa police and firefighters also adopted policies to wear protective clothing in certain circumstances. Most physicians and hospitals immediately adopted the recommendations.

The CDC stated transmission to a medical care worker was "minuscule," citing numerous studies.

"I don't think anyone's too hysterical yet. Sometimes you can't help but get blood all over you. If a patient is dying, you want to help him. You don't ask him what he's dying of. I have a husband and a son. I certainly don't want to be getting AIDS and bringing it home. I think it's a fine line between being cautious and being paranoid," said Patrice Mounger, Tulsa paramedic, *Tulsa Tribune*, Aug. 10, 1987.

The Tulsa AIDS Task Force, led by Bill Pierson, director of the sexually transmitted diseases program at the Tulsa City-County Health Department, held fundraisers to raise money for a home for people in the advanced stages of AIDS-related illnesses.

"What's more, you've got to realize that these people are so ill they cannot work. When they get a diagnosis of AIDS, that generally means they lose their job and their health insurance. For so many AIDS patients, the diagnosis also means they lose their friends and family. They have no job, no insurance, no friends and no money. You can't imagine just how alone these people are," said Kevin Gabel, spokesman for the Tulsa AIDS Task Force, *Tulsa World*, Nov. 14, 1986.

The Catholic Diocese of Tulsa opened St. Joseph Residence in January 1988 as a home for men with AIDS who had nowhere else to live. It was not a medical facility, but a shelter. Addresses for the homes and shelters for people with AIDS and HIV were not released at the time, citing concern for safety.

Private businesses were encouraged to develop AIDS policies and educational programs for employees.

The Tulsa City-County Health Department set up an information center and hotline for questions about AIDS and HIV in February 1988. The center was housed at its main office at 4616 E. 15th St. It was prompted by the nearly 3,500 calls about the disease to the agency in the previous year. The agency launched its AIDS hotline in April 1988.

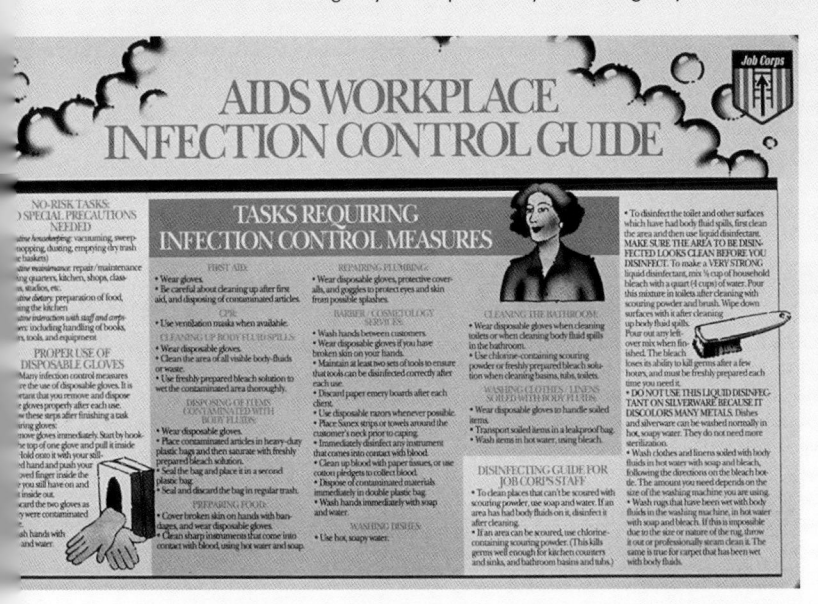

"There are a lot of people running scared about the disease, and they really shouldn't be," said Glenn Burnett, director of health information and education of the Tulsa City-County Health Department, *Tulsa Tribune*, Feb. 18, 1988.

The case numbers continued to increase, with 2,290 cases of HIV and 1,682 living cases of AIDS in Oklahoma as of June 1999. By the end of 2014, there were 6,332 people living in Oklahoma with the AIDS virus, and the state ranked 24th in the country in the number of new diagnoses.

In 1991, Tulsa CARES was founded to provide a coordinated approach to health care and social services to people with AIDS or HIV. The nonprofit provided case management to help find health care, housing, mental health services, nutrition and updated research information. In 1998, the nonprofit HOPE (Health, Outreach, Prevention, and Education) testing clinic was founded to provide testing and referral services for HIV and sexually transmitted diseases. The AIDS Coalition of Tulsa, under the administration of the Community Service Council of Tulsa, is another supporting organization. The Oklahoma State Department of Health releases an annual nearly 200-page HIV/AIDS resource guide filled with locations for medical services, legal needs and social supports.

with Saint Francis Hospital. Efforts to expand Life Flight to the other hospitals failed, which led to the change. The move led to a lawsuit filed in April 1987 by Hillcrest Medical Center against Saint Francis Hospital over the division of property, with the use of the name Life Flight at issue. Hillcrest argued that since the partnership establishing Life Flight had dissolved, then the assets needed to be divided. A settlement was reached by the end of the month. It allowed Saint Francis Hospital to continue using the name.

Getting Shots

In 1983, Oklahoma suffered through a whooping cough epidemic with 330 cases reported, making it the worst outbreak in 30 years and making up more than 15 percent of all whooping cough cases in the nation that year. Children were disproportionally affected, with 60 percent of cases between the ages of 6 months to 6 years. One-third of all patients required hospitalization. The U.S. Public Health Service released a study about the outbreak the following year with this conclusion:

"Low immunization levels in children appear to have been a major factor associated with this outbreak. Three or more doses of DPT (the vaccine) prevent disease in approximately 80 percent of the recipients."

It was a statistic that continued to dog the state. In 1988, it was found that 60 percent of 2-year-olds in Tulsa County were not immunized against seven dangerous diseases.

Editorials pressed for changes.

"Is it ignorance or just taking too much for granted? When it comes to health, Oklahomans may be guilty of both. Science and immunology virtually wiped out smallpox, whooping cough, diphtheria, tetanus and polio in this country and pharmaceutical companies are turning their attention to delivering these vaccines to remote reaches of the world. But in Oklahoma, a survey of health departments in the ten most populous counties showed that only 40 percent of all 2-year-olds had received immunizations against seven prominent childhood diseases. That is a disgrace... Sadly, the biggest problem might be parents who take good health for granted." — *Tulsa World*, editorial, Aug. 10, 1988.

"Many parents of 2-year-olds today are too young to remember the frightening days of iron lungs and polio wards. Perhaps that fact explains why 60 percent of 2-year-olds in Tulsa and nine other counties in the state have not been immunized against polio and seven other dangerous diseases. Perhaps it is time for parents to inquire of their parents and grandparents about the days of diphtheria or polio's crippling reign. A vivid description might convince a mother or father that quieting a screaming 2-year-old, who is incensed after being stuck in the bottom, is worth the pain." — *Tulsa Tribune*, editorial, Aug. 11, 1988.

A push to keep refining vaccines was boosted with the 1986 National Childhood Vaccine Injury Act, which was placed in the federal Omnibus Health Bill. It came from work of a group calling itself the Dissatisfied Parents Together, or DPT. It established a no-fault compensation system financed through an excise tax on the vaccines. People who could show injury from an inoculation could receive funds to cover medical expenses up to $250,000. It also required that physicians tell parents of all possible side effects and keep records of any reactions.

"It is unarguable that more damage would be done to children by disease if vaccination programs were dropped. And, however small a percentage, those who were injured by the nationally mandated vaccines must be compensated in some way. Turning their grief into action, these DPT families have provided guidance and leadership in solving this problem." *Tulsa World* editorial, Nov. 10, 1986.

Drug Culture

The use of illegal drugs, including prescription medication, started hitting its zenith by the early 80s. The National Council on Drug Abuse in 1975 found the No. 1 choice of substance among drug abusers was Valium, a sedative for seizures and anxiety disorders known as diazepam in its generic form. That decade sounded the alarm on abusing prescription medications especially when taking with alcohol. By the mid-70s, local medical officials launched public awareness campaigns aimed at pregnant women. Dr. Martin Greenberg, chairman of the department of newborn medicine and director at the Eastern Oklahoma Perinatal Center at Saint Francis Hospital, stated at least one baby a month was born at a Tulsa hospital addicted to substances inherited from the mother. If the baby survived the withdrawal, the child may have had health problems or could have returned to a home of a parent addicted to substances.

"Drug abuse hit Tulsa later than some other sections of the country, and we may just be beginning to witness the tragedy of what a mother's habit can do to the innocent newborn," said Dr. Martin Greenberg, *Tulsa Tribune*, Oct. 31, 1975.

In 1979, Tulsa Public Schools participated in a radio program with KWGS in conjunction with National Public Radio examining drug abuse in schools. TPS had suspended 97 students grades 7 through 12 the previous year for drug use and 64 students for alcohol abuse.

"For anyone to say there is no problem is utterly ridiculous. But what we see at school may not be the full extent of the problem," said Dr. Wayne Bland, director of TPS junior highs, *Tulsa Tribune*, July 21, 1979.

By the mid-80s, it was apparent substance use has become more pervasive among 18- to 30-year-olds. A national survey found half had smoked marijuana and one in five used cocaine.

"Young Americans are experimenting with drugs far more than their counterparts did in the heyday of the drug counterculture of the 1960s and early 1970s." — *Tulsa World*, June 23, 1985.

First Lady Nancy Reagan launched a "Just Say No" campaign targeting youth, and parents started paying attention to possible signs of substance abuse. At a Tulsa Parent-Teacher Association's Task Force on Drug Abuse in 1981, Dr. Bob Block, of the University of Oklahoma-Tulsa Medical College quoted from a 1972 article he wrote in a pediatrics journal stating no harmful effects of marijuana had been proven, "Unfortunately, it's 1981, and that is no longer the case." He spoke about the drug dulling the senses and brain function with marijuana use.

"Kids in Oklahoma don't know beans about drugs, although they sure think they do. They'll talk about drugs, and their misinformation is incredible. The extent of their information is also incredible, but they're about 10 years behind. The drug of the late 70s and early 80s is alcohol and not beer. You're going to see a lot of alcohol, a lot of marijuana, some contaminated stuff such as PCP, a lot of medicine chest drugs, some LSD, some cocaine," said Dr. Bob Block, *Tulsa Tribune*, Aug. 28, 1981.

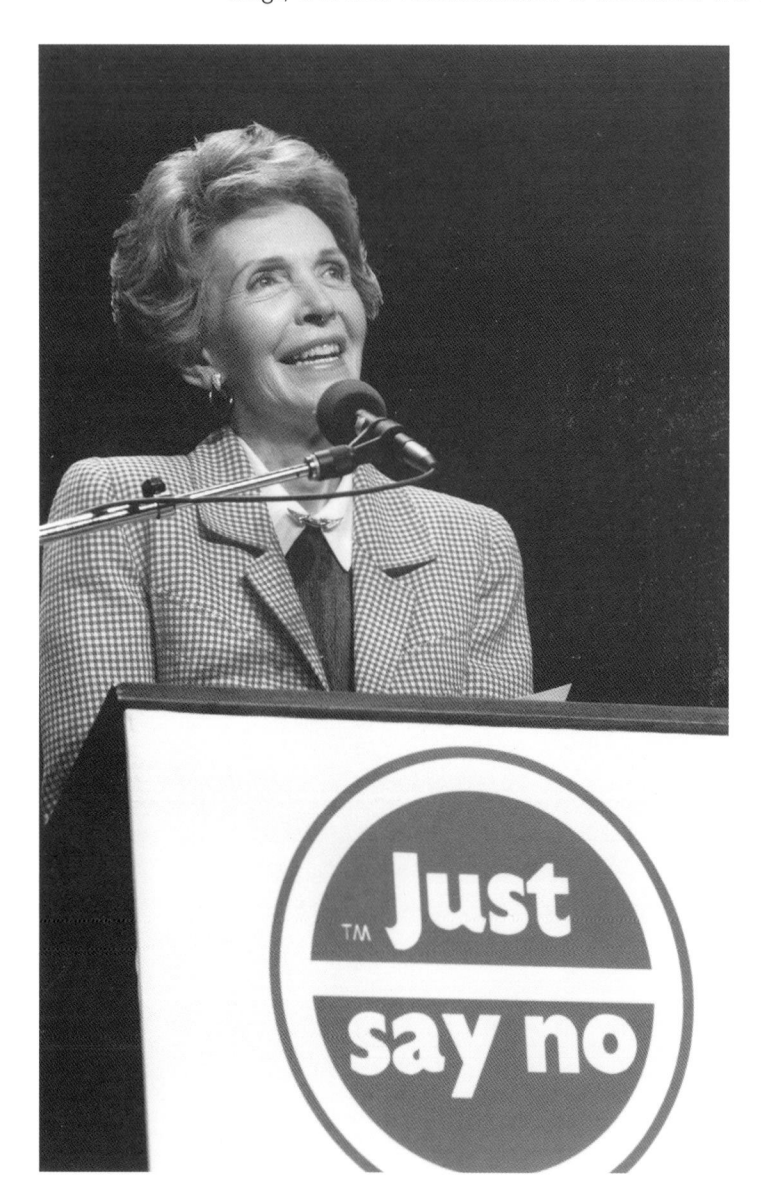

Support groups and treatment programs sprang up across Tulsa and the region to deal with issues of addiction. Some were self-help such as Alcoholics Anonymous and Narcotics Anonymous. Treatment programs such as the Palmer Drug Abuse Program were founded with endowments from foundations and donations. Some groups specialized with populations including the Women's Treatment Center, Salvation Army and HOW Foundation rehabilitation centers. Programs evolved into in-patient treatment, which provided about 30-day intensive services, along with out-patient care and self-help support groups.

"These groups are there because the need is there. So there are an awful lot of people in Tulsa who have problems with drug or alcohol abuse or both, and they need programs of this kind to help put their lives back together," said Allan Gates, director of Hillcrest Medical Center's outpatient treatment program.

Private businesses started offering employee assistance programs. Alcohol and drug abuse ranked with family problems as reasons for reduced employee productivity. The loss for a company shows up through increased absences, increased insurance claims and decrease in job performance. Hospitals and the Tulsa Council on Alcoholism Inc. were managing the programs for companies.

Mrs. Reagan Speaking at a "Just Say No" Rally in Los Angeles.

"I'm amazed at the turnaround in corporate attitudes just in the past year. EAPs are a double-edged sword. They are as good for the company as for the employee," said Dave Pynn, director of the St. John's Medical Center's chemical dependency and employee assistance services, Tulsa Business Chronicle, Aug. 6, 1984.

Law enforcement officers began training physicians and nurses on the scams that addicts and drug rings played to get prescription drugs, including falsifying diagnosis documents. The Oklahoma State Bureau of Investigation began investigating these types of frauds in 1975. At the end of the 80s, six state agents, one federal agent and eight investigators from the state regulatory boards were assigned to monitor every hospital, pharmacy and clinic in Oklahoma. Because this was an impossible task, law enforcement relied heavily on health professionals to be alert to prescription fraud.

"State drug agents say that while their war against drugs includes battles against marijuana growers and drug chemists, a significant part of Oklahoma's street drug traffic is legitimately manufactured pharmaceutical drugs. Investigators say Oklahoma is a popular target for criminals who divert legitimate drugs onto the black market. They say well-organized rings, often from other states, con Oklahoma doctors out of narcotics prescriptions or persuade state pharmacies to fill forged prescriptions. Oklahoma attracts rings from states that have stricter record-keeping requirements on drug prescriptions." — *Tulsa World*, Feb. 15, 1988.

As addiction and mental health needs began to take more of a toll on medical services, it set the stage for laws tightening access to certain categories of drugs. Technology would make it easier to track with databases and online communication.

FERTILITY

Twins born on Dec. 15, 1983, at the Hillcrest Infertility Center to Van and Deborah Lyda were the first born in Tulsa after conception through in vitro fertilization. The 23-year-old mother had Levi, 5 pounds 2 ounces, and Lucy, 4 pounds and 1 ounce, after a complicated pregnancy and labor five weeks premature. The babies were being cared for in the special care nursery and expected to be healthy. They were the fourth set of twins born after in vitro fertilization in the nation.

The couple previously had a 5-year-old daughter, conceived naturally. Deborah Lyda experienced health problems requiring the removal of her Fallopian tubes. For their next pregnancy, the couple turned to the infertility center, which was the fifth center of its kind in the U.S. The in vitro fertilization process involves retrieving eggs from the mother's ovaries, fertilized with the father's sperm in a laboratory, left in an incubator for two or three days then transferred to the mother's womb. Four embryos were transferred into Deborah Lyda, and two developed.

"We definitely wanted more kids, but there was no way she could be pregnant naturally. And it was really worth it," said Van Lyda, *Tulsa Tribune*, Dec. 16, 1983.

A couple having trouble conceiving a child approached fertility specialists Drs. J. Clark Bundren and J.W. Edward Wortham Jr., in 1984 when the physicians were serving as co-directors of the Hillcrest Infertility Center, later renamed Hillcrest Fertility Center. The woman went through four surgical procedures to retrieve her ova, or eggs. The eggs were fertilized with her husband's sperm and returned to the woman's womb. However, some fertilized eggs on the fourth procedure were withheld and frozen. For 11 months, one of those eggs stayed frozen before being transferred to the mother's uterus.

On May 4, 1987, a girl was born at Hillcrest Medical Center, becoming the first baby born in Oklahoma by the in vitro fertilization and frozen embryo process.

Up to this point, only five babies in the U.S. had been born through this process. The first child in America conceived and born through in vitro fertilization was Elizabeth Carr on Dec. 28, 1981, in Norfolk, Virginia. Internationally, 14 such babies had been born in England and Australia, but the U.S. lagged after the procedure was caught up in a controversy over ethics and restricted federal funds.

**Intracyto-
plasmic
Sperm
Injection**
 ❧

Oklahoma's first child through in vitro fertilization/frozen process was only referred to by her first name in the media — Darla. Her parents asked for their names to be withheld. The infant was delivered by Dr. Richard Dixon, an obstetrician-gynecologist, about five weeks premature. He had been the woman's physician for years before she sought treatment at the fertility clinic. Pediatrician Dr. Robert Hudson attended the Caesarean-section delivery.

Darla's birth took a complicated journey. Her conception occurred in October 1985, and her parents intended for implantation in early 1986. But in January 1986, Dr. Bundren and Wortham were fired from their positions over a business disagreement. Three couples were caught in the middle of the dispute between Hillcrest and the doctors because they had frozen embryos stored at the center. Unable to reach an agreement where the doctors could complete the embryo implants, Hillcrest offered to arrange and finance trips for the couples to alternate fertility centers in the U.S.

The embryo that would become Darla and her parents were taken to Good Samaritan Hospital in Los Angeles for specialist Dr. Richard Marrs to finish the procedure. Because of her prematurity, Darla was transferred to the intensive care unit at St. John's Medical Center to receive respiratory therapy. She was released a few weeks later. Her parents spent about $20,000 in the quest to have Darla.

"Just take one look at her and you'll see why I say she was worth it all. She's absolutely beautiful," said Darla's mother, *Tulsa World*, May 15, 1987.

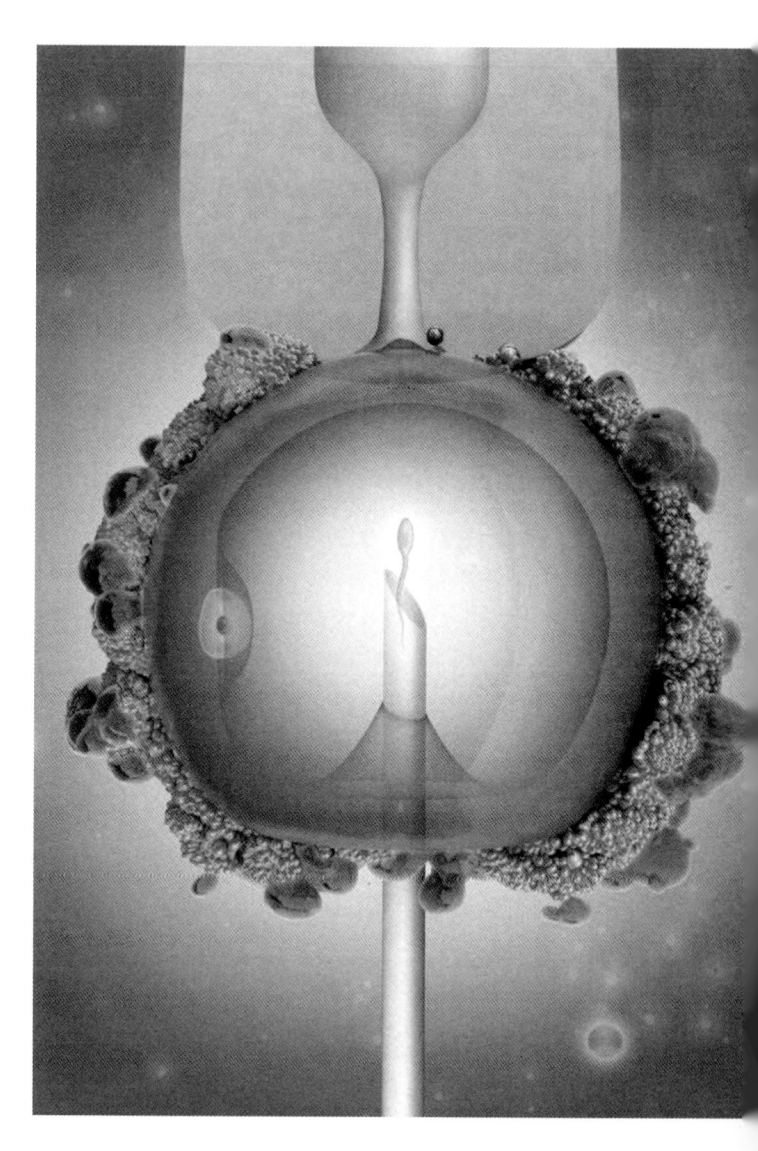

IVF represents about 1.5 percent of U.S. births, or more than 61,000 babies, a year, according to 2012 data from the Society for Reproductive Technology. Each IVF cycle costs about $12,400 on average in the U.S. with an overall chance for a baby at about 1 in 3, depending on the age of the woman. For those younger than 35, rates are more than 40 percent but it drops to 10 percent per cycle for women older than 42. Physicians performed about 113,000 cycles in 2003 and increased to more than 165,000 in 2012.

WEIGHTY ISSUES

Two in-patient treatment programs for eating disorders opened at two Tulsa hospitals in the summer of 1984. A 10-bed section opened at Saint Francis Hospital, and Hillcrest Medical Center started a 20-bed program. Both had a focus on anorexia and bulimia, which was estimated to affect about 4 percent of the population in an eight-county area. As research emerged to treat the disorders as a mental health issue, the programs were designed to combine psychological, nutritional counseling and outpatient services.

"A lot of the group therapy will deal with the feelings of women and on the social pressure and emphasis on being thin. They will work on being more assertive and handling anger. It won't just be who binged the most. That will be de-emphasized in favor of what caused the underlying problem," said Dr. Donald Inbody, medical director of the Saint Francis program, *Tulsa World*, June 21, 1984.

In the ongoing research on obesity and weight loss, Hillcrest Medical Center participated in a Harvard University study of the Optifast program. In the mid- to late-80s, those programs were medically supervised, protein-sparing, modified fasts used in combination with behavior modification, exercise and nutrition counseling. Results of the study, which included Tulsa patients, showed that weight loss decreased obesity-related symptoms such as high-blood pressure and diabetes.

"Likewise, the medical risk of obesity-related diseases such as diabetes, arthritis, hypertension and a whole host of other complications diminish significantly with a modest weight loss. The research demonstrates that in order to lose weight and not gain it right back, at least nine months of active involvement in a weight treatment program is necessary," said Dr. George Blackburn, Harvard Medical School associate professor of surgery and study's chief researcher, *Tulsa World*, Dec. 2, 1987.

Hillcrest expanded its HELP program, which was dedicated to healthy living, in 1983 to include smoking cessation, weight management, stress control, heart health and fitness. The Saint Francis Hospital's "Wellness Program" also grew that year in the facilities at the Williams Professional Building and the second floor of the Physical Performance Center. Both hospitals offered the services to corporations, citing data on the business savings by having a healthy workforce.

"Hospitals are more committed to a health care delivery system. We have recognized we are truly a part of the total picture instead of just an illness care system," said Scott Serota, administrator of ambulatory and support services at Hillcrest Medical Center, *Tulsa Business Chronicle*, Nov. 21, 1983.

Plastic Surgery

The decade saw a large increase in elective cosmetic surgeries nationally and in Tulsa as people sought to nip and tuck away their physical flaws. Plastic surgery had been around since the turn of the century, with a 1916 landmark paper in the *Journal of the American Medical Association* by Dr. John Staige Davis of Johns Hopkins Hospital describing the role of plastic surgery within the medical field. The first issue of the *Journal of Plastic and Reconstructive Surgery* was issued in July 1946 and board certification was in place by 1950. The Korean War brought advances in the field including internal wiring techniques for facial fractures and the use of rotation flaps to correct skin injuries and deformations. In the 60s, plastic surgeons were gaining momentum in the medical field with one appointed to Surgeon General in 1969 and another winning the Nobel Prize. The decade also brought along silicone, which ended up being a staple in cosmetic surgery.

In the 80s, an economic boom and public awareness of cosmetic surgery brought the surgeries to the masses.

Tulsa physicians were offering all nationally available cosmetic and reconstructive surgeries by the end of the decade. About 30 percent of surgeries were reconstructive, such as removing scars, burn injuries or breast augmentation after cancer surgery. The rest were a combination of elective and reconstructive.

"(The percentage) is increasing because of general public acceptance of cosmetic surgery. Now you seldom hear the term 'vanity.' People talk more in terms of self-improvement. It's very worthwhile to make yourself look better and feel better, and all the money people spend on clothes, makeup and hairstyles is no different than the money spent on cosmetic surgery," said Dr. Palmer Ramey, *Tulsa Tribune*, Jan. 8, 1987.

One advance that plastic surgeons utilized was an imaging profile synthesizer. This technology could show patients a realistic picture of the result of facial reconstruction surgery. The procedures used photographs of the patient, then displayed the computer-generated changes based on the type of surgery. These imagers were already in use by dentists and cosmetologists.

Many procedures were performed in doctors' offices, which saved patients money. Hospitals were used when general anesthesia was necessary or the doctor had an at-risk patient. Nationally, plastic surgeons were frontrunners in ambulatory surgery with an average of 75 percent of procedures on an outpatient basis.

While women composed most of the patients, men seeking elective plastic surgery began to pick up in the 80s. Tulsa was no exception.

"Men are more interested in their overall physique and are more concerned about appearance. This is evident in the popularity of jogging. There are cosmetics for men, hairstyling, designer clothing, and, with that, comes the interest in cosmetic surgery," said Dr. Paul A. Howard, *Tulsa World*, July 15, 1984.

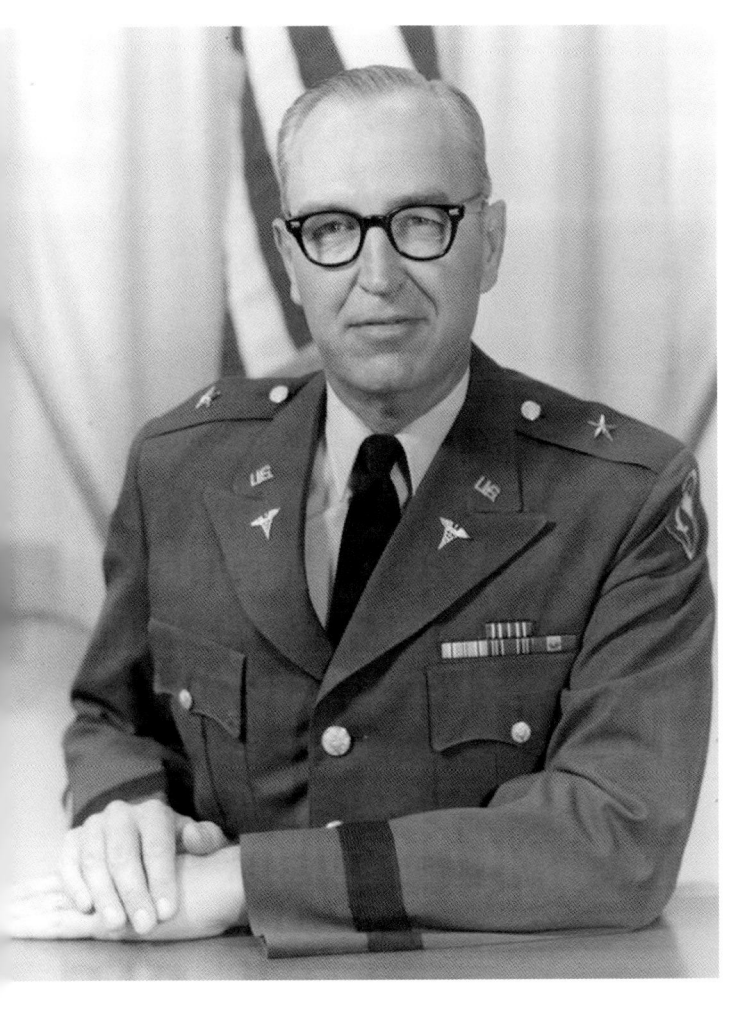

One of the most popular surgeries was a blepharoplasty, or eyelid surgery. Physicians said people in the south and other places with hot weather are more exposed to the sun, causing wrinkles with age. Rhytidectomy surgery, a type of facelift, was also commonly requested to correct a droopy neck. Younger people were most interested in nose reshaping.

"Women are often proud of having cosmic surgery and can't wait to go out and tell their friends. Men are more secretive," said Dr. Paul A. Howard, *Tulsa World*, July 15, 1984.

As the decade ended, Tulsa cosmetic surgeons reported between 15 percent and 20 percent of their practices were men.

"Ten years ago, that percentage would have been closer to 1 or 2 percent. People are more aware of appearance, especially men in corporate and executive position. They're more concerned with looking young and successful. It has a lot to do with competition. With the business world expanding and more competition in corporations and society, I think it's going to be more popular every year," said Dr. Thomas Dodson, *Tulsa World*, July 11, 1988.

Dr. Hal B. Jennings, a Plastic Surgeon who Served as Surgeon General of the U.S. Army.

Having knowledge about the motivations and expectations of patients was integrated into the practice of cosmetic surgeons.

"We don't just take everyone who comes in and say 'We'll do whatever you want.' I like people to have an idea of what they would like improved instead of saying, 'What do you think I should have done, you're the doctor.' That indicates to me that maybe they haven't put as much thought and effort into their decision as I'd like them to. It's hard to define in words what makes a good candidate. That's where the psychology of plastic surgery practice comes into play," said Dr. Palmer Ramey, *Tulsa Tribune*, Jan. 8, 1987.

Kidney Transplants

Hillcrest has the third oldest kidney-transplant program in the state. By the mid-80s, kidney transplants had become almost common at Hillcrest Medical Center. Dr. Alistair Paton performed the first such transplant in January 1973. By July 1, 1984, the hospital had conducted at least 185 kidney transplants, which was the accepted treatment for patients — particularly among children and young adults — with end-stage renal disease. The average age of patients starting dialysis was in the mid-50s, which was also the upper age limit for transplant eligibility.

The success rate for kidney transplants increased with the discovery of cyclosporine, which controls and depresses a body's natural immune reaction. Also, the use of blood transfusions before the procedure helped condition a body to better accept foreign cells by producing antibodies to fight organ rejection. The cost of a kidney transplant was about $40,000, which was lower than other organ transplants and about the same as a year of dialysis.

Research and Technologies

Hospitals started to increasingly join national research studies and acquire modern equipment in a quickly changing world of technology.

In February 1984, Tulsa ophthalmologist C. William Simcoe performed a cataract surgery with at least 2,000 doctors watching from around the globe. It was believed to be the first world-wide satellite transmission to broadcast live from Tulsa. Dr. Simcoe extracted cataracts and implanted three synthetic lenses on three patients at St. John Medical Center as physicians in 20 North American cities watched on closed-circuit television. As Dr. Simcoe operated, he fielded questions from the witnessing doctors. The event was sponsored by Cilco, a manufacturer of Simco-designed instruments and flexible plastic lenses. The video system was created by Tulsan Leon Rollerson and included a visual of the microscope images seen by the surgeon. New York producer David Fox handled the technical broadcasting details.

"This is great. You pick up new techniques by watching other surgeons. Sometimes it's the smallest thing, but it can sometimes solve a big problem," said Dr. C.W. McClure, an Oklahoma City surgeon, *Tulsa World*, Feb. 5, 1984.

At Saint Francis Hospital, doctors participated in studies involving drugs to help brain damage from strokes, blood clotting and cancer. In 1988, neurologists Drs. Harvey Blumenthal, Ord Mitchell and Michael Haugh oversaw a study on the calcium-blocking drug Nimodipine, which was developed as a high-blood pressure medication. The drug was given to eligible patients within 24 hours of the onset of a stroke. Doctors were interested to see if the drug would block the toxic amounts of calcium flowing into brain cells when the oxygen flow is interrupted. This and other research evolved Nimodipine away from its original intent to the more common usage in treatment for complications of subarachnoid hemorrhage (a form of cerebral bleed). That same year, the hospital's oncologists and hematologists entered a study of a human protein — erythropoietin — for use in cancer treatment. Anemia is a major side effect of drugs used in chemotherapy, and it was discovered this naturally occurring protein was key in delivery of red blood cells to the body. Another key discovery came through DNA research, which allowed the possibility of producing a body's chemical in bigger amounts. The use of erythropoietin became a part of the options for cancer treatment but remains under ongoing studies.

"Only in the past few decades have doctors begun to unravel the complex chemical language of the body. By analyzing the body's chemicals — often present in minute quantities — they are learning how these molecules 'communicate' with cells." — *Tulsa World*, Dec. 8, 1988.

Saint Francis Hospital's oncologists and hematologists in 1987 took part in national research of tPA, tissue plasminogen activator, to treat pulmonary blood clotting. It was the third leading cause of death in the U.S. The hospital and the University of Oklahoma Health Sciences Center had participated in 1986 in research that found tPA successfully dissolved clots in coronary arteries in stopping heart attacks midstream. Dr. William McEntee of Cardiology of Tulsa, Inc. oversaw Tulsa's portion of that study.

"Each minute we can trim from the time the chest pain begins until we began giving the drug means less damage to the heart muscle. The goal of the drug isn't to do away with angioplasties or bypass surgeries. If we can keep the artery cleared for 21 hours, that gives us 21 hours in which to determine how we can best treat this patient," said Dr. William McEntee, *Tulsa World*, July 22, 1986.

The extension of the tPA research was to determine if it was effective in eliminating blood clots forming in the deep veins of the leg and lung.

"Standard treatment is to give heparin, an anti-coagulant that will prevent the clot from growing

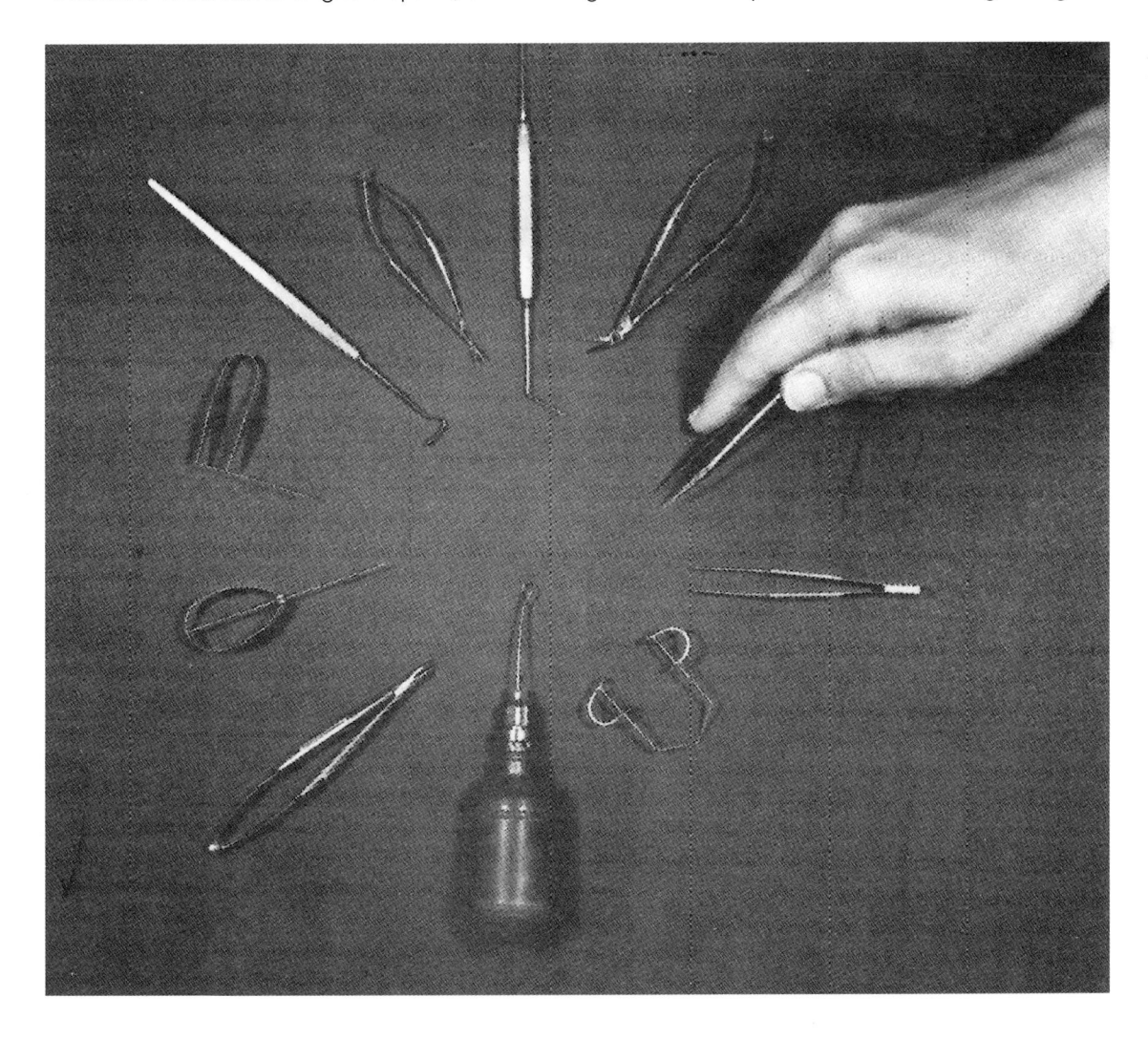

A Sampling of Instruments Invented by Ophthalmologist C. William Simcoe.

and will eventually promote (breaking up of the clot). Unfortunately, the average length of time to dissolve the clot is about seven days. During that length of time, the valves in the leg veins can be damaged or destroyed," said Dr. Alan Keller, oncologist/hematologist with Cancer Care Associates, *Tulsa World*, July 5, 1987.

tPA is currently used with diseases featuring blood clots, such as pulmonary embolism, myocardial infarction and stroke. The most common use is for ischemic stroke.

Lasers, called "scalpels of light," were able to shed light on even a hemorrhoid to make surgery more tolerable for patients. The advancement of this tool was put to use by Dr. Haskell H. Bass Jr., a St. John Medical Center colon and rectal surgeon, in hemorrhoidectomies in 1986. The use of a laser in hemorrhoid surgeries reduced the time a patient could return to work from 14.5 days to 3.2 days.

"The result is that the patient has less bleeding, less swelling, less pain and is able to return to work much sooner, requiring much less medication. Because the laser cuts through such a finer plane than the scalpel, the surrounding tissue isn't harmed. Because the laser coagulates the small blood vessels at the site, the surgery is virtually bloodless. Also, it is very difficult to sterilize the tissues of the colon area using conventional means, but the laser essentially sterilizes the surrounding area, preventing infection risks. Even with a laser, you have to have the proper training to be able to do the surgery correctly. A laser is only as good as the hands that hold it. A laser doesn't make a good surgeon," said Dr. Haskell H. Bass Jr., *Tulsa World* Aug. 22, 1986.

St. John Medical Center became the first hospital in Oklahoma to gain approval for a kidney-stone crusher, which was a machine using a high-energy shock wave to pulverize kidney stones. In October 1984, the Oklahoma Health Planning Commission approved the $1.6 million machine. Now, Shock Wave Lithotripsy is the most common treatment for kidney stones in the U.S, according to the National Kidney Foundation.

Because of the technological advancements and costs associated with medical care, patient expectations became an issue. Saint Francis Hospital participated in a three-year national study sponsored by the Emergency Medicine Foundation, funded by the W.K. Kellogg Foundation, on how to hold down emergency room costs. It was believed that doctors and nurses may have been ordering expensive tests out of routine rather than medical necessity. A patient education policy was implemented at the hospital on June 1, 1983, to explain why a procedure would not be necessary.

"It has been coming for some time that medical technology is outstripping the humane side of medicine. We are in favor of patient education time rather than testing for all our assumptions… When you look at health care as part of the total gross national product, any way you can impact on it without compromising quality health care should be done. The nation may not be able to afford all this technology," said Dr. John Sacra, Saint Francis Hospital medical director of emergency services, *Tulsa World*, June 8, 1983.

CHAPTER 10
(1990 - 1999)

Transforming Health Care

Dean Kayse Shrum, M.D. with OSU-CHS Medical Students.

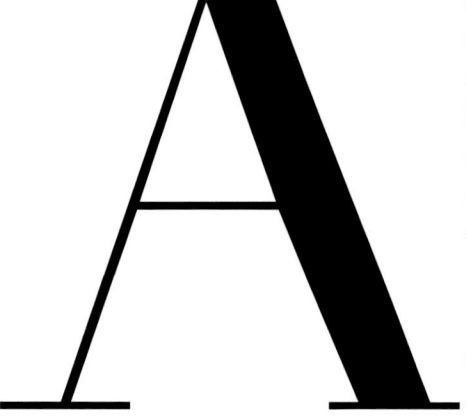

As medical technology and treatments advanced, the 90s ushered in the big business of delivery and management of medicine. Hospitals merged, closed and expanded based on several economic influences through a mix of non- and for-profit companies. Medicare and Medicaid changes led to alliances among medical institutions to better care for low-income, elderly and disabled patients.

It was also a time of healthier lifestyles as people stopped smoking and paid more attention to mental health. The aging population was leading to more brain research and concerns about retirement living. It was also a time to eliminate the historic gap between allopathic and osteopathic medicine.

Question of Over Saturation

As the decade opened, six hospitals operated in the city as the question hovered over whether the bed availability had reached a saturation point. The difficult 80s showed that no one facility could meet the needs of an entire region. There were a total of 3,195 beds, led by Saint Francis Hospital with 935 beds followed by St. John with 754.

"Basically, Tulsa is overbedded. I don't see how everybody can survive in this environment. I think it's becoming much more keen, more cutting edge. One of my daily challenges is to make sure the programs we implement here are not duplicated elsewhere in the community. There is so much competition. A lot has to do with ego. If one facility has a lithotripter, another wants a lithotripter. It's not because the consumer demands it. It's like you can't let somebody else get a competitive advantage. Overall, I think there will be struggles. I don't see how Tulsa can be an island that is different from the rest of the country," said Jerry Rothlein, president of Children's Medical Center, *Tulsa World*, Jan. 21, 1990.

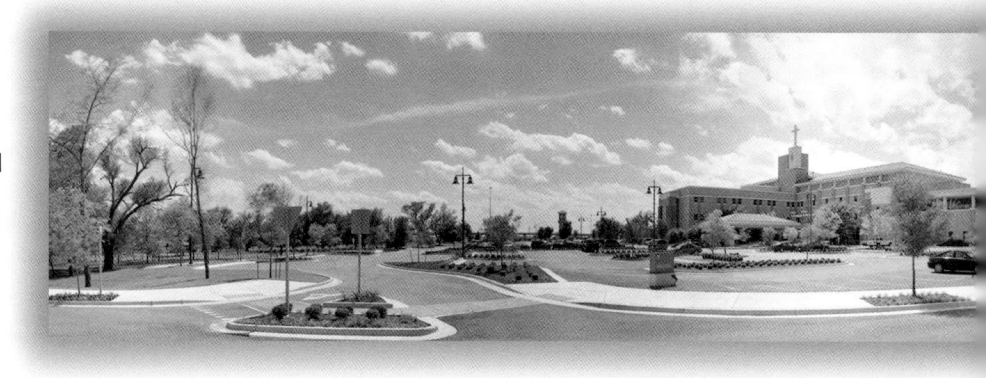

Saint Francis South.

"If you were starting today, you might not build as many (bed spaces). But would it be better to have them all in one big hospital? I don't think so. I don't think we have too many beds," said John Goldthorpe, president of Hillcrest HealthCare System, *Tulsa World*, Jan. 21, 1990.

In foretelling the business transactions — both failures and successes — are summed up by Doctors' Hospital Executive Director Jack Olpin. The hospital would be among those to experience closure in the next decade.

"Tulsa is an overbedded community, as many are. Health care in the '90s is going to see some definite crises. I think we're going to see a lot more sharing in the future. I concede there were problems two years ago, but there has been a fantastic turnaround," said Jack Olpin, *Tulsa World*, Jan. 21, 1990.

The era saw the rise of marketing among hospitals. This tactic was almost non-existent before the 90s.

Tulsa Regional was a leader in this with the launching of an advertising campaign in 1990 featuring physicians on the job. There were three television ads, and the doctors were paired as the following: Drs. Michael Eimen and Terry Grewe, Drs. Robert Lawson and Kenneth Calabrese and Drs. Ernest Pickering and Edwin Berger. Newspaper ads centered on Drs. James Marshall, Robert D. McCullough II and Robert Nebergall.

In 1992, the hospital aired a television ad with former patient Mike Barnum and his wife, Paula. Barnum had suffered a heart attack and was successfully treated with angioplasty to open a clogged artery. The piece included many of the people who were part of the treatment including registered nurse Phyllis Cotham and Drs. Michael P. Carney and Arthur Wallace Jr.

"We've become very aggressive in terms of marketing. We will maintain an aggressive marketing posture, " said James MacCallum chief executive officer of Tulsa Regional Medical Center, *Tulsa World*, Jan. 21, 1990.

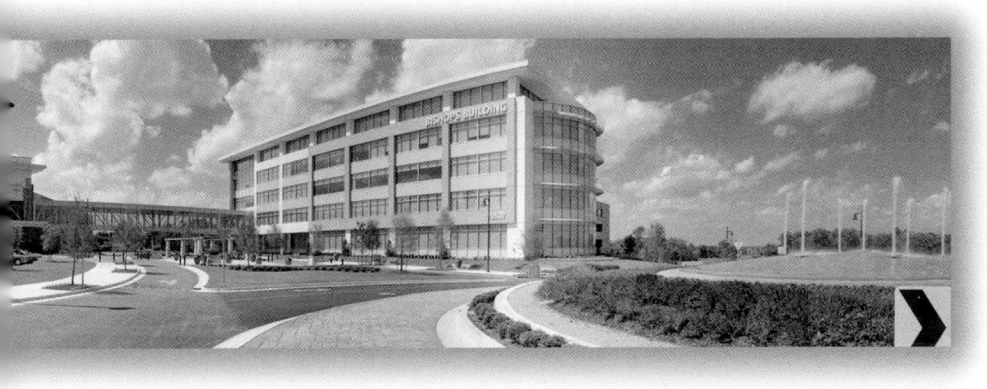

HILLCREST CREATES THEN DISSOLVES MERGERS

The first major move by Hillcrest Medical Center was taking over Children's Medical Center in 1993 and moving services to its main campus. A year later, it was announced Hillcrest and Tulsa Regional would sign a memorandum of understanding with the intent to consolidate both institutions under one parent corporation.

"We'll see these mergers going on and on. As the business of medicine becomes much more oriented to the bottom line, that's exactly what will happen," said Dr. Harold Brooks, dean of the University of Oklahoma College of Medicine in Tulsa, *Tulsa World*, Oct. 20, 1994.

This was largely prompted by the Legislature's move in 1993 to convert the $1.1 billion Medicaid health-care program for low-income people to managed care in an attempt to save money. The Oklahoma Health Care Authority was created to revamp and administer Medicaid. Health maintenance organizations were able to bid on contracts to provide care to Medicaid recipients. Saint Francis Hospital and St. John Medical Center teamed up with Mercy Hospital and St. Anthony Hospital in Oklahoma City to form Community Care, an HMO.

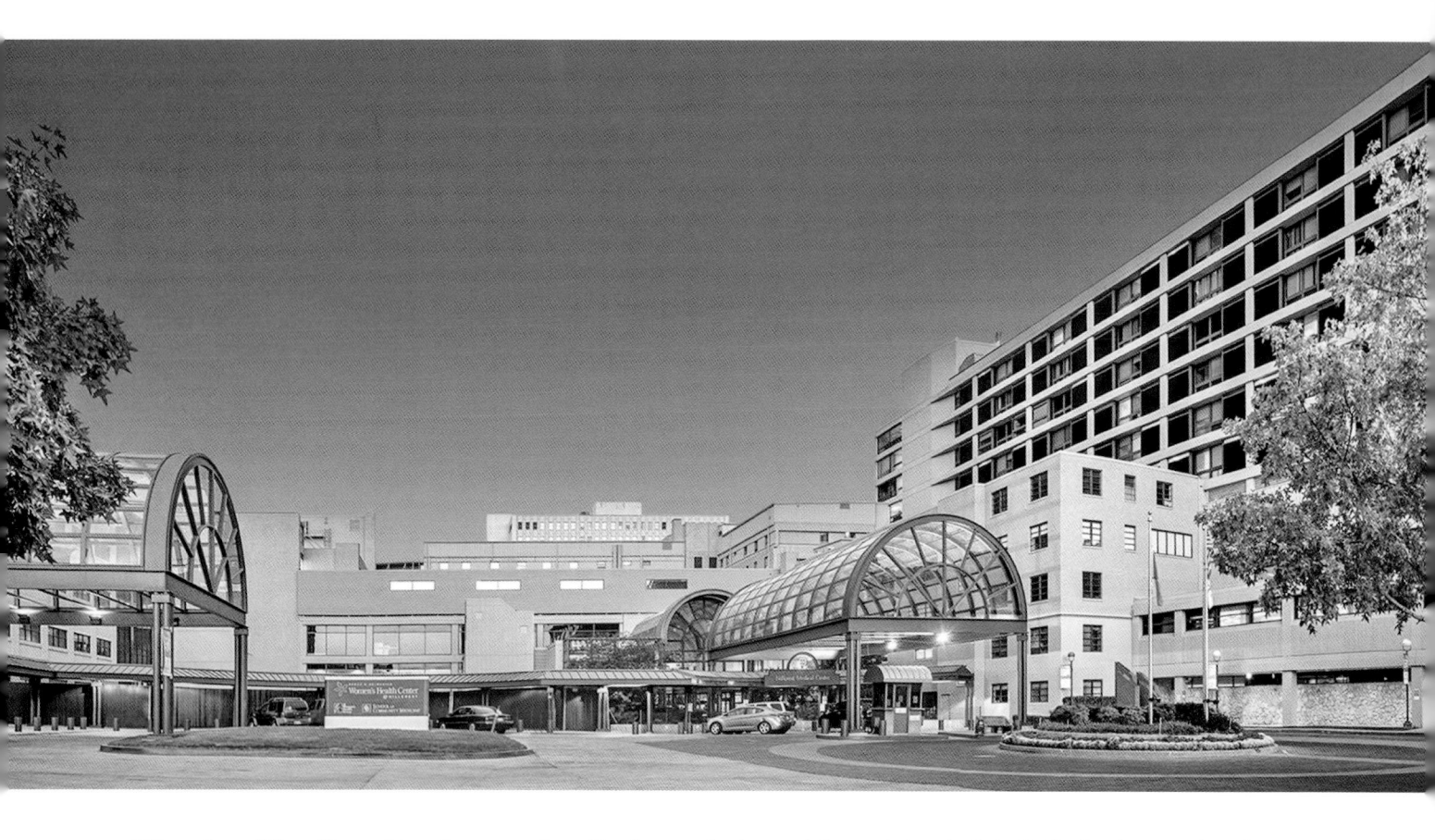

Hillcrest Medical Center at 1120 S. Utica Ave.

"We will combine the strengths of both organizations while retaining their individual values and traditions. By reconfiguring current services and reallocating existing resources, we will lower costs, broaden our geographic area of service and provide greater access to quality health care throughout eastern Oklahoma," said Donald A. Lorack Jr., Hillcrest president, *Tulsa World*, Oct. 20, 1994.

In addition to its main campus and Tulsa Regional, Hillcrest by the end of the decade had acquired 60 specialty clinics; three long-term care facilities; hospitals in rural areas, such as Cushing and Fairfax; and SouthCrest Hospital, which was a joint venture with Dallas-based Triad Hospitals Inc.

Then, financial woes began plaguing Hillcrest with a significant slope starting in 1998. In July 2000, Moody's downgraded Hillcrest's bond rating to Ba1, which signaled a higher risk for investors and could make funding difficult. It had an operating loss of $100.3 million. Hillcrest put up the Children's Medical Center campus for sale in June 2000, moving services to Hillcrest and Tulsa Regional Medical Center. It sold Doctors' Hospital and its share of SouthCrest to get out of debt.

In August 2004, the Nashville, Tennessee-based Ardent bought the Hillcrest Healthcare System, including the main campus and Tulsa Regional, for a little more than $300 million. Ardent began in 1993 and was originally known as Behavioral Healthcare Corp. because it had six behavioral health facilities in its system. As it acquired other medical institutions, it changed its name to Ardent Health Services in 2001.

Among the first moves after the purchase, Ardent began construction on the $55-million Bailey Medical Center in Owasso. It committed to invest $100 million into the Hillcrest system within the first five years of ownership. In the first year, it spent more than $42 million in programs and increased care to uninsured patients by $6 million, bringing the annual total to $38 million.

In the first year, Ardent and Oklahoma State University presented a plan to the state Legislature to lease Tulsa Regional Medical Center to the state. It was not approved, but a joint legislative commission was created to study possibilities for the hospital.

SOUTHCREST OPENS, DOCTORS' CLOSES

After two years of planning, the doors to SouthCrest Hospital opened on May 3, 1999, at 8801 S. 101st East Avenue. The five-story, 153-bed facility cost about $60 million and was a project of Hillcrest Health System and Columbia HCA/Healthcare. Before it opened, Triad Hospitals was spun off from Columbia/HCA as an independent company. SouthCrest opened as a joint venture between Hillcrest and Triad. Pacific Group provided day-to-day management. Anthony Young was named the first president and chief executive officer of the hospital.

An open house attracted more than 7,000 visitors, and residents responded by using the facility. The first baby born in the hospital was Taylor Naome Hancock, born May 3, 1999, at 6 pounds, 2 ounces and 19 inches long.

"We had an excellent opportunity to have our daughter be the first baby born at this beautiful, brand- new hospital. Of course, we jumped on it," said Jason Hancock, *Tulsa World*, May 4, 1999.

The area had a projected growth of 15 percent over the next five years. By 2000, it was expected that 33 percent of the metropolitan area would be living within a five-mile radius.

"The design of it is just very unique in the sense you can pull up to the front door and walk straight in. It's not like you have to go find a parking space at a large distance. It should be very convenient and very easy to get around. The fact that there are so many people in that part of town, it's just another alternative to what has been there," said Jerry Rothlein, senior vice president at Hillcrest, *Tulsa World*, Feb. 2, 1999.

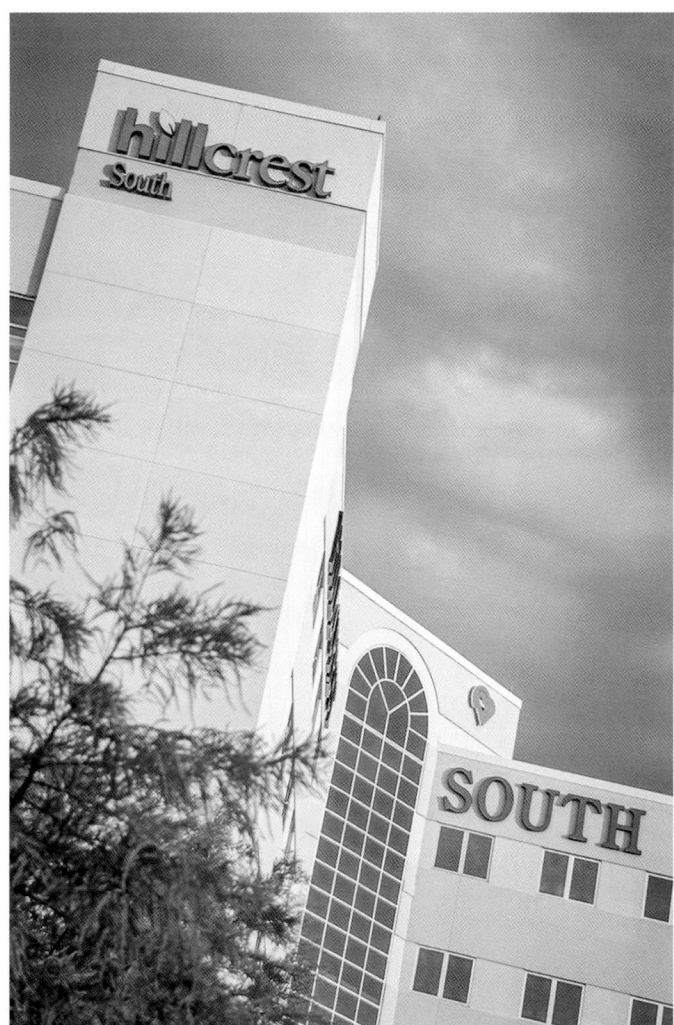

Hillcrest South Hospital.

Financial problems at Hillcrest HealthCare System led to selling its share of SouthCrest for $44 million to the Dallas-based chain Triad Hospitals, making it the sole owner. The hospital's name, employees and policies remained unchanged.

Triad was a publicly traded company on the Nasdaq. When the deal was made, the company was listed as being the third-largest hospital-management company in the United States.

"Triad is a growing company with a bright future and has the resources to continue to support and be a part of the south Tulsa community. I would rather have a for-profit hospital in the community because they pay taxes, which go right back into the community," said SouthCrest CEO Anthony Young, *Tulsa World*, Jan. 2, 2001.

While one hospital opened, another closed. After nearly three decades, Doctors' Hospital sold in 1995 to become affiliated with Hillcrest HealthCare System.

In November 2000, officials announced the closure of Doctors' Hospital and the layoff of 170 of the facility's employees. Those layoffs were of non-medical staff — manager, secretaries and clerical workers. Services at the hospital including obstetrics, psychiatric care and pediatrics were relocated to Hillcrest and Tulsa Regional Medical Center.

At the time of its closure, Doctors' Hospital had 209 beds, 615 employees and a medical staff of 290 physicians.

A legacy to the physicians who founded the facility is the Founders of Doctors' Hospital Foundation. The founders used the sale of the property to establish a charitable organization. It had net assets of about $36 million in 2015. It supports a variety of community needs and programs including those at the University of Oklahoma College of Medicine at Tulsa, American Red Cross and the Gathering Place urban park.

Tulsa Regional Medical Center Grows into OSU Medical Center

The decade started out strong for the Oklahoma Osteopathic Hospital, which was renamed Tulsa Regional Medical Center in 1989, with expansions and a healthy bottom line. By the close of 1992, the hospital's indebtedness had been refinanced at historic low levels of interest. It announced a $14 million construction project including a new four-level ambulatory care center and emergency medicine complex. About $10 million of the budget came from the issuance of $20 million of new tax-exempt bonds. The Tulsa Regional Medical Center Foundation launched a major fund-raising drive.

In 1991, it bought the historic McBirney mansion to be remodeled and turned into an eating disorders center for the Los Angeles, California-based Rader Institute. By 1995, the center was no longer affiliated with the hospital and had relocated to another property in south Tulsa. The mansion was vacant and put up for sale the following year.

The nonprofit hospital was purchased in 1996 by Columbia/HCA of Nashville, Tennessee. It was a short-lived venture after the company became embroiled in a federal fraud investigation. That led

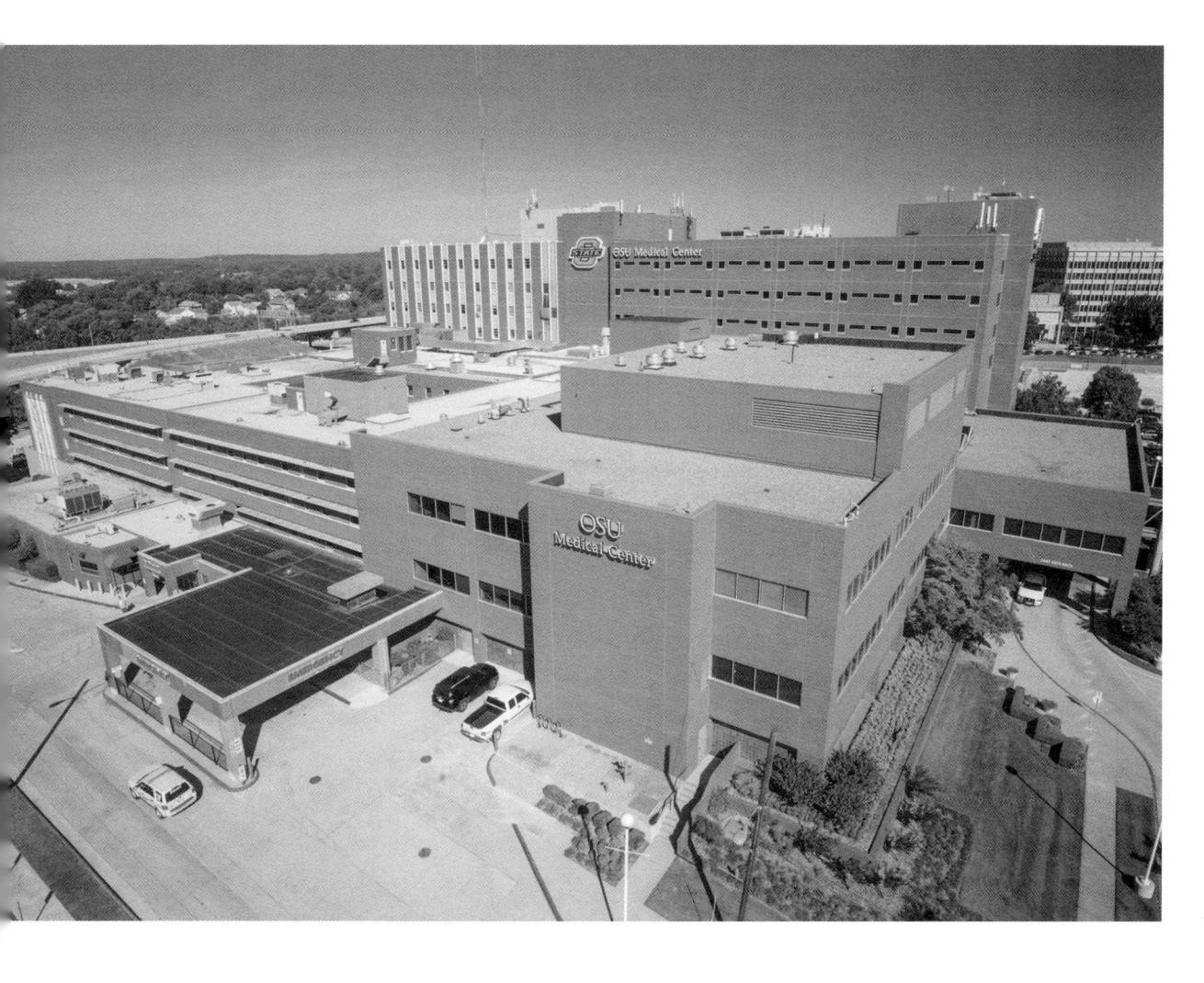

OSU Medical Center.

to guilty pleas and fines reaching $1.7 billion. The crimes involved top executives engaged in scams of fraud and kickbacks.

The hospital had merged with Tulsa-based Hillcrest Medical Center, which was a nonprofit. But, the Ardent Health Services bought it in 2004. The company nearly closed the building for lack of funds. The city formed a trust in 2009 to take over the hospital, which had become affiliated with Oklahoma State University. In November 2006, it officially became the Oklahoma State University Medical Center. That year, the hospital signed a 50-year academic agreement with the OSU Center for Health Sciences to become the permanent teaching hospital. The relationship is overseen by the OSU Medical Authority.

Saint Francis Health System Emerges

Moving into the 21st century, Saint Francis Hospital developed a master facilities plan. The hospital had grown to include several institutions including its main 276-acre campus, Warren Clinic, Laureate Psychiatric Clinic and Hospital, the Children's Hospital and Saint Francis Hospital South.

Warren Clinic was the largest physician practice in the state with locations in 10 Oklahoma communities including Tulsa, Broken Arrow, Owasso, Coweta, Jenks, Sand Springs, Stillwater, McAlester, Vinita and Haskell.

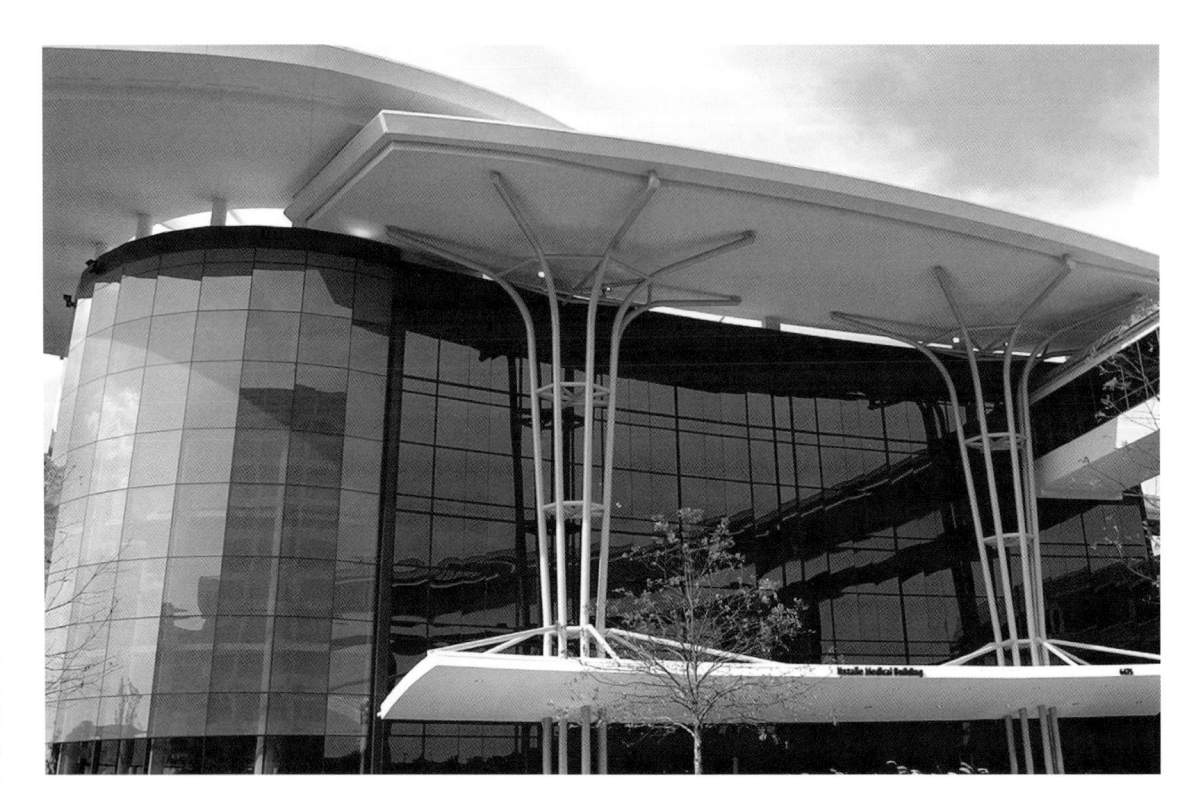

Saint Francis Natalie Medical Building.
ะ๖

In 1995, the facility established The Children's Hospital at Saint Francis, but it would take another decade before ground was broken on a separate facility. The Children's Hospital was founded as a regional center providing specialized pediatric and intensive care.

"We developed our Master Facilities plan as a way to respond in a proactive, tangible way to patient and physician requests for more convenient parking, easier access to services and more customer-friendly features. Any new construction we undertake is really based on our vision and mission as a health provider," said William E. Weeks, president and CEO of Saint Francis Health System, *Tulsa World*, Dec. 15, 1999.

The master facilities plan included:
- The main campus to add a 5-story building with six outpatient surgery suites, 40 physician offices, outpatient physical therapy, radiology and laboratory services; and, a sky bridge linking two covered parking garages to the hospital and the Warren Medical Building.
- Broken Arrow campus expansion of a 5-floor building adjacent to the hospital, new outpatient diagnostic center and exterior renovation.
- The opening of a new comprehensive heart center with a 110-space covered parking garage.
- Renovation and expansion of the Women's Center. Expansion of the trauma emergency center including a minor emergency center.
- Expansion of the endoscopy suites.
- A second MRI suite.
- Expansion of The Children's Hospital urgent care center.
- Renovation of the pediatric oncology facility.
- The Saint Francis breast center expanded.

- The existing Saint Francis shuttle service extended to the campus medical office buildings.
- Construction of Montereau in Warren Woods, a continuing care retirement community. The 37-unit community has a combination of independent living units, assisted living units and skilled nursing beds on 172 acres.

By the mid-decade, the system had doubled its outpatient visits and employed a staff of about 3,800 employees. By December 1999, it had 730 physicians and 6,600 employees.

"When you truly care for the people you serve, it means providing expensive services that no patient could ever afford or live without. Every choice we make, every service we add, every insurance contract we sign, we do with our mission in mind. These long-range plans will help us to be prepared to serve the needs of the community by ensuring that we have the necessary capacity and technology available to our physicians and staff. As the community grows, we will continue to expand into areas that best fit our patients' needs and wishes.

"If you look around the country, many hospital systems have seen a steady decline in patient volumes while Saint Francis has experienced the opposite effect. Our surgeries, outpatient procedures and overall hospital admissions have been rapidly increasing over the past few years. I think this can be attributed to the excellent quality of our physicians and the dedicated and caring nature of our staff," said William Weeks, *Tulsa World*, Dec. 15, 1999.

First Woman Chosen as Chief of Staff

During the golden anniversary of the Oklahoma Osteopathic Hospital, Dr. Beverly Mathis, D.O., was elected chief of staff of Tulsa Regional Medical Center. She became the first woman to hold this position among Tulsa's four major hospitals.

Interestingly, Dr. Mathis is the granddaughter of Dr. C.D. Heasley, one of the founders of the Oklahoma Osteopathic Hospital, which became Tulsa Regional in 1989.

Dr. Mathis, a board-certified nephrologist, is a Tulsa native and graduate of Edison High School. She attended Drury College and the University of Oklahoma, where in 1973 she received a bachelor's degree of health. In 1981, she graduated from Oklahoma State University-College of Osteopathic Medicine.

At the time of her election, she was in private practice and assistant director of dialysis at Tulsa Regional.

In 2000, Dr. Mathis was named Physician of the Year by the Osteopathic Founders Foundation. Each year, this honor is bestowed on a doctor, chosen by their peers based on extraordinary service to patients, community, osteopathic profession and education of young osteopathic doctors. It has been awarded at the annual Winterset Ball.

Relationship Mends Between Allopaths and Osteopaths

For at least a decade, the Tulsa County Medical Society had been advocating to open membership to the osteopathic physicians. Prompted by the Tulsa group's push, in 1998, the state medical association made a rule change, and Tulsa began taking applications from practitioners of osteopathic medicine.

"Our time has come. M.D.s and D.O.s over the last several years have worked closer and closer together. This is going to be sensitive to some people. As with any degree of change, and certainly in dealing with two historically separate professional organizations, there may be individuals in both camps who have some reluctance or some concerns," said Paul Patton, executive director of the Tulsa County Medical Society, *Tulsa World*, May 10, 1998.

The membership change reflected the education changes in osteopathic medicine. Up until the early 80s, most graduates of osteopathic colleges went straight into medical practice after completing a year of internship. Unlike allopath physicians, they were not required to enter a residency program for further training.

However, by the mid-80s, M.D.s and D.O.s faced the same admission requirements for medical school, completing four years of basic medical education and passing comparable state licensing examinations. Both kinds of doctors are licensed to perform surgery and prescribe medication in all 50 states.

Many osteopathic physicians perform their residency through an M.D. program. In 1999, at the University of Oklahoma College of Medicine, nearly 21 percent, or 30 out of 145 residents, were osteopathic doctors.

Alzheimer's Tangles.

When the membership was opened, M.D.s and D.O.s were already working side-by-side in medical groups, clinics, managed-care plans and hospital staffs.

"Almost all other states long ago have allowed osteopathic membership in the state medical association or societies. It became illogical that we should be separate groups," said Dr. William Geffen, pediatrician and president of the Tulsa County Medical Society, *Tulsa World*, May 10, 1998.

Treating the Older Brain

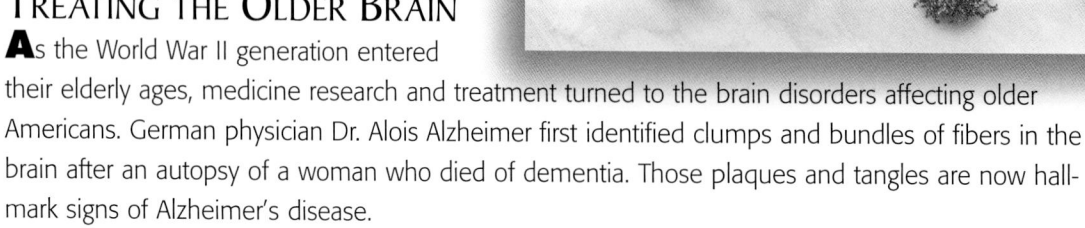

As the World War II generation entered their elderly ages, medicine research and treatment turned to the brain disorders affecting older Americans. German physician Dr. Alois Alzheimer first identified clumps and bundles of fibers in the brain after an autopsy of a woman who died of dementia. Those plaques and tangles are now hallmark signs of Alzheimer's disease.

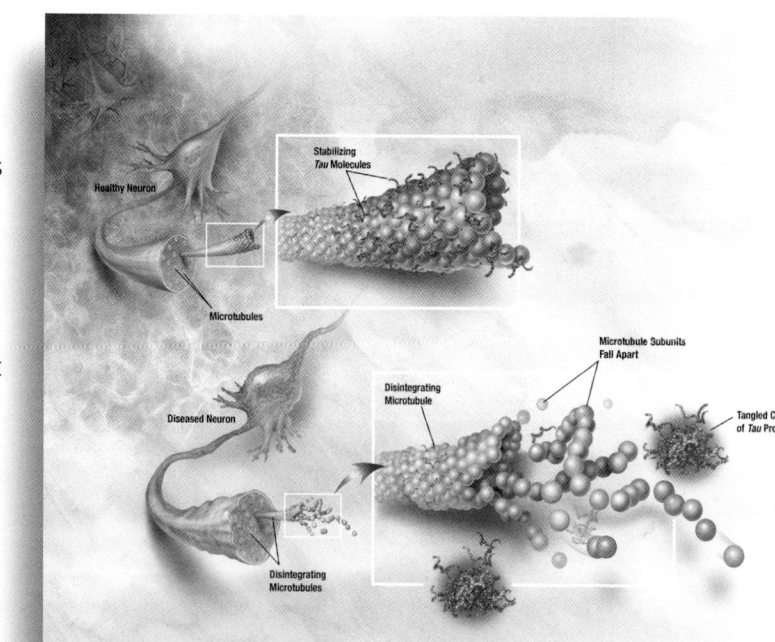

No cure exists, but advances are being made in diagnosing and managing the disease and behaviors such as agitation, delusions, anxiety and wandering.

By the end of 1999, Alzheimer's was the most common cause of dementia in older people, affecting about 70 percent of total dementia patients. As the new century was about to begin, about 4 million U.S. residents were diagnosed with Alzheimer's or associated dementia. Generally, the disease strikes people older than 65.

"Really, in the last three or four years, we have focused on management and treatment of Alzheimer's more than in the previous whole decade. There is just a tremendous amount of information coming out on Alzheimer's," said Dr. Insung Kim, associate professor of medicine with the University of Oklahoma College of Medicine-Tulsa campus, *Tulsa World*, Sept. 27, 1999.

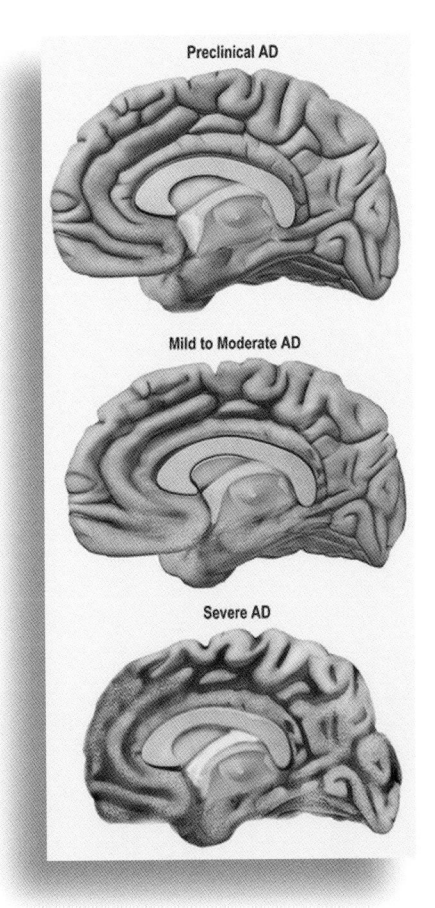

Among some of the emerging treatments in the 90s:
- Vitamin E, an antioxidant, was found to possibly help salvage or preserve brain cells. A study published in April 1997 in the *New England Journal of Medicine* showed that high doses of vitamin E improved a patient's functional level and delayed the need for institutionalization.
- Estrogen, a female hormone, had already been thought to protect women against heart disease and osteoporosis. Studies were emerging to indicate women using estrogen reduced their risk of dying from Alzheimer's disease by 50 percent.
- Nonsteroidal anti-inflammatory medications such as ibuprofen, often prescribed for heart disease, started in clinical trials for possible protective effects against dementia.
- Memory pharmaceuticals came onto the market to temporarily improve brain functions. Those include donepezil (Aricept), rivastigmine (Exelon) and galantamine (Razadyne), which have become commonly prescribed cholinesterase inhibitors. Some medications — such as tacrine, known by the trade name Cognex — were initially thought to have promise but were discontinued in the U.S. due to safety concerns.

Brain Affected by Alzheimers.

In 1999, the Alzheimer's Center of Tulsa opened at 1027 E. 66th Place to house up to 24 residents with individual bedrooms and bathrooms. It cost about $3,995 a month. The Oklahoma State University College of Osteopathic Medicine served as the facility's medical director. The center eventually changed hands, but an industry of memory care facilities developed.

Gov. Mary Fallin issued an executive order in 2015 instructing the Oklahoma Department of Human Services to review and revise a state plan created in 2009 to address Alzheimer's and dementia. The report, released in February 2016, had a wide-ranging set of recommendations such as requiring all related legislation first go through the DHS long-term care division, establishing a state research fund, offering tax breaks for caregivers forced to leave the workforce and creating a student loan forgiving program for medical students sub-specializing in geriatrics. Other concerns were GPS tracking of patients and education of staff in memory care facilities.

By 2015, people diagnosed with Alzheimer's or an associated dementia disorder rose to 5 million Americans — or one in three senior citizens. It became the sixth leading cause of death, costing about $236 billion. In Oklahoma, about 62,000 residents had Alzheimer's or dementia, and that is expected to reach 76,000 by the year 2025.

Laureate Psychiatric Clinic and Hospital.

The state had about 220,000 unpaid family caregivers, who gave about 252 million hours of care valued at $3.1 billion annually.

"Alzheimer's disease is crushing the American health care-system while putting significant financial constraints on families that are left in its wake. The financial toll is only equaled by the physical toll, both for those with the disease and those who are caring for them," said Mark Fried, president and chief executive office of the Alzheimer's Association's Oklahoma Chapter, *Tulsa World*, April 13, 2016.

MENTAL HEALTH EVOLUTION

The decade brought about the shift in the way Tulsa treats people with mental health disorders, embracing the notion of supported housing, community health treatment, parity in mental health insurance coverage and criminal justice diversion programs.

History has not been kind to people with mental health needs, with generations facing incarceration in large institutions and treatments including ice baths, electroshock and brain surgeries. The 1930s influence of Sigmund Freud brought talk therapy into vogue. Chemists in the 50s and 60s discovered medications, such as lithium, which showed success in managing erratic behavior. The 1960s birthed a movement to deinstitutionalize mental health care in favor of community housing, though it was slow to spread. The largest problem was a lack of infrastructure — housing, caseworkers and support services. As research showed community treatment and housing were preferable, mental health institutions experienced bulging populations.

Oklahoma officials made efforts in the late 70s to add more community health centers and homes so people with mental health disorders could move out of the institutions. Then, the bottom fell out of the state's economy with the oil bust of 1982. Plans that had been set in motion the previous decade to improve the mental health system halted. In Tulsa County, officials had been warning of problems to come.

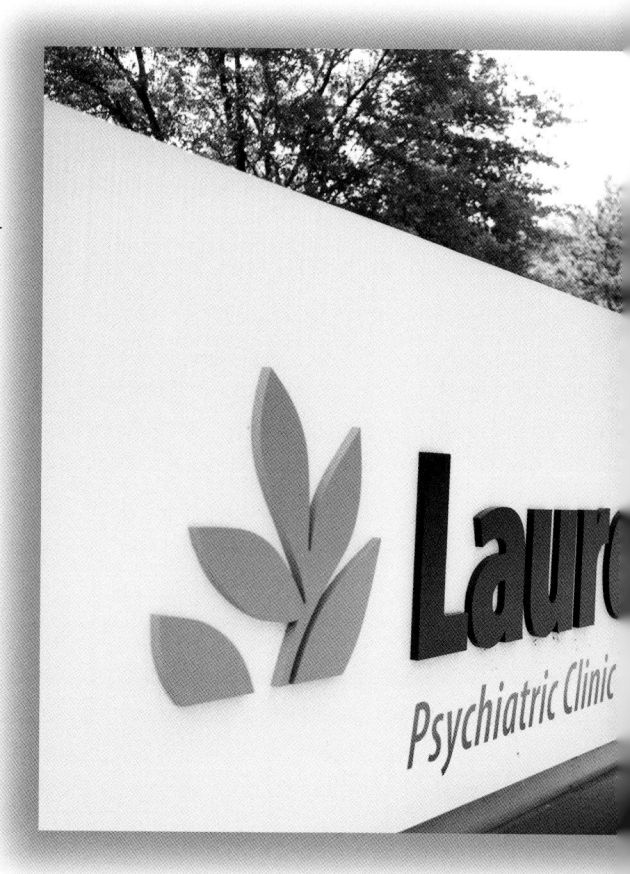

"We need someone interested in doing something for the care and rights of mental patients. The attitude now is, unless you're personally involved, who gives a hoot?" — Tulsa County District Judge M.M. McDougal, *Tulsa World*, March 14, 1976.

In 1978, J. Frank James, head of the state Department of Mental Health announced an initiative to build more community-based housing for people with mental health disabilities. Four years later, the economic crash hit. In 1983, the agency used its reserve fund to make up for declining allocations. For the following three years, $25 million more was slashed. It canceled plans for new construction and grants to community mental health housing services and reduced funding for drug and alcohol counseling programs. By 1986, caseworkers reported having 120 cases on average compared to the 40-client caseload nationally. The mentally ill homeless population had increased, and families were not able to afford private pay. Oklahoma had 21 community mental health centers with 66 satellite offices. Until the financial bust, the state had been showing some improvements. When the progress stopped, James said the problem was the failure of the state to fund and develop the community plans.

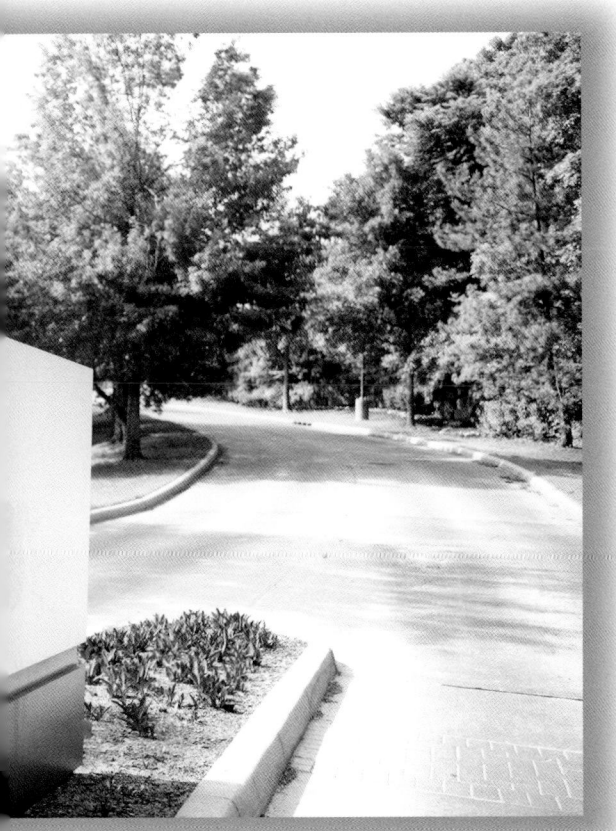

"The highly visible problem of homelessness and its connection to deinstitutionalization have led many state leaders to conclude that the entire movement was a miserable mistake. Deinstitutionalization... may have failed, but the community mental health movement has not," said J. Frank James, *Tulsa Tribune*, Nov. 18, 1986.

A sharp increase in homelessness in Tulsa in the early 90s led to the establishment of the Homeless Services Network through the Community Service Council of Tulsa. The nonprofits working with homeless people and people with mental illness asked for the network to serve as a clearinghouse for needs in the community. It continues to be the coordinating organization for the various programs in the city. Philanthropists, businesses and faith organizations play a crucial role in supporting the projects.

In 1990, a Tulsa Mayor's Task Force for Homelessness was formed. In 1995, a federally mandated study of the city's housing needs showed 1,569 Tulsans without a home.

"The study also shows that mental illness, alcohol and drug abuse or a combination of the two were blamed for the homelessness of 91 percent. Domestic violence and AIDS-related illness were the causes for 9 percent. The study also showed that more than 16,000 additional people in the area were at risk of homelessness. Tulsa leaders were not surprised that mental illness and drug abuse played a major role in homelessness." — *Tulsa World*, Jan. 22, 1996.

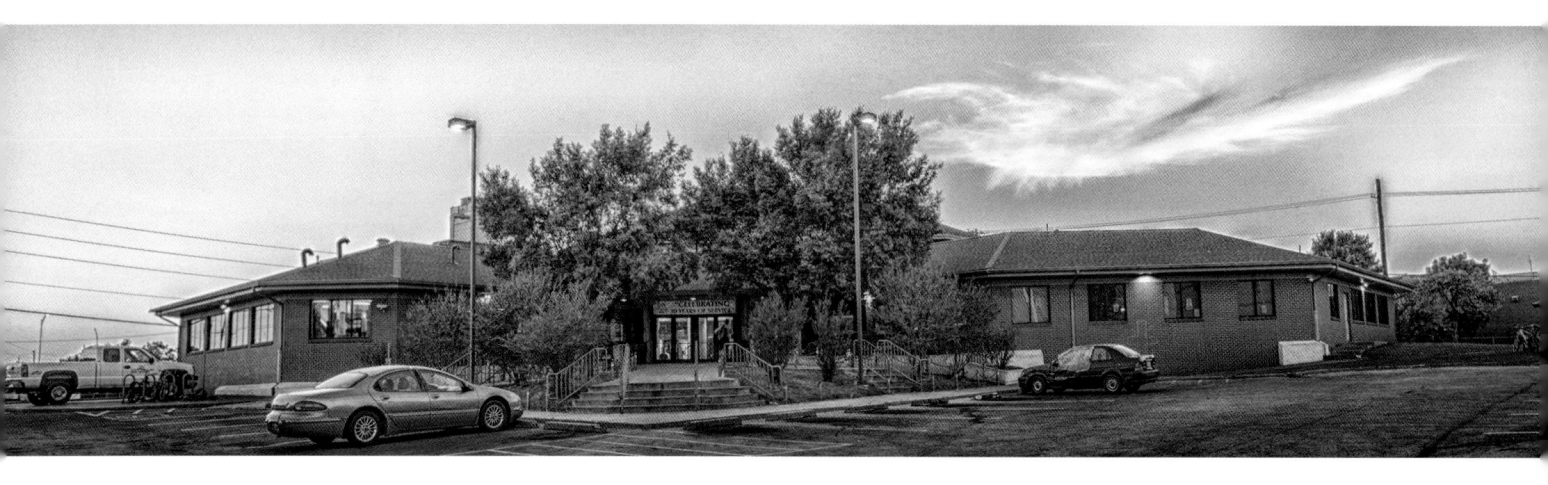

Tulsa Day Center for the Homeless.

Part of the problem was not having a place during the day for homeless people to gather and receive social support. In 1986, the Tulsa Metropolitan Ministry opened a 4,000-square-foot shelter in a warehouse and added a night shelter for the most at-risk in 1990. The family foundations of Henry and Anne Zarrow and Jack and Maxine Zarrow donated the land at 415 W. Archer Ave. to open a permanent shelter. The families have continued involvement with philanthropy to benefit homeless and mentally disabled people. In October 1994, the Tulsa Day Center for the Homeless dedicated a new 24,000-square-foot facility. On June 1, 1999, the Tulsa Metropolitan Ministry Day Center became the Tulsa Day Center for the Homeless.

Its opening was controversial for the community, with residents offering different opinions on where homeless people should live, shared Sister Sylvia Schmidt, executive director of the Tulsa Metropolitan Ministry, upon the center's opening.

"This has not always been an easy problem to deal with. But the religious community came upfront and said we have to respect the dignity of the homeless. They have it tough enough anyway. This facility will improve their quality of life because of its passion and care and will prevent more serious problems from happening that confront other urban areas," said Sister Sylvia Schmidt, *Tulsa World*, Oct. 30, 1994.

The shelter provides case management, health services and connection to mental health services. The medical clinic provides free health care from volunteer nurses and physicians. It is estimated at least 40 percent of clients have a mental illness. Typical cases seen at the clinic are diaper rashes on newborns, wounds, diabetes and blood sugar tests, headaches, cold relief, staph infections, bronchitis and dehydration. In 2013, the Day Center's medical clinic received the Dr. Rodney L. Huey Champion of Oklahoma Health award from Blue Cross Blue Shield honoring this unique service.

Other shelters operating in the 90s were at the Salvation Army, John 3:16 Mission and the Tulsa County Social Services Shelter. The nonprofits work in concert to avoid duplication and are members of the city's homeless network.

Recognizing a lack of housing for people with mental health disorders, the Mental Health Association of Tulsa sought to change that. The nonprofit formed on Dec. 1, 1955, as the Tulsa County Association for Mental Health and remains an affiliate of the National Mental Health Association. The early decades focused on providing volunteers at the Eastern State Hospital in Vinita and supporting groups for depression and suicide prevention. In 1988, the mission shifted after the United Way granted funding for the nonprofit to establish the Housing Task Force, which developed a strategy for building safe and affordable housing for people impacted by mental illness and homelessness.

In 1990, through the efforts of employee Bill Packard, the nonprofit obtained a $483,000 grant from the U.S. Housing and Urban Development. The next year, Walker Hall opened at 17th Street and Baltimore Avenue as a 12-bed apartment building for people with mental health disabilities. Case managers made sure residents were seeing their physicians, staying on medication and being connected to jobs or training, if clients were able.

"Walker Hall will plug the gap between coming out of the hospital and living independently. Many who live independently become isolated. They have no support. They quit taking their medication and the cycle starts again... Our vision and commitment for housing started in the late '70s and early '80s. There were a number of false starts. Since we are an advocacy group, not a direct service provider, we worked to get other agencies to do something. But nothing was being done. Our commitment is really to people who are vulnerable to ending up homeless," said Judy Leaver, executive director of the Mental Health Association in Tulsa, *Tulsa World*, Sept. 15, 1991.

Since then, housing through the mental health nonprofits has expanded to 24 apartment complexes, with more than 1,400 units, to serve more than 2,600 tenants with varying levels of mental health needs. Tulsa's mental health housing has become a national model by the U.S. Interagency Council on Homelessness, HUD, the U.S. Department of Veterans Affairs and the U.S. Substance Abuse and Mental Health Services Administration.

Illustration of brain regions studied in mental illness.

In 1994, the inaugural Zarrow Mental Health Symposium launched with "The Many Faces of Mental Illness," hosted by the Mental Health Association. It provided continuing education for mental health practitioners, featuring the latest research on mental health treatments. It has grown to attract more than 800 attendees becoming one of the largest behavioral health conferences in the region. The nonprofit has presented three national conferences, the latest being the "2016 National Zarrow Mental Health Symposium — Ready for Zero: Innovative Solutions for Housing and Recovery."

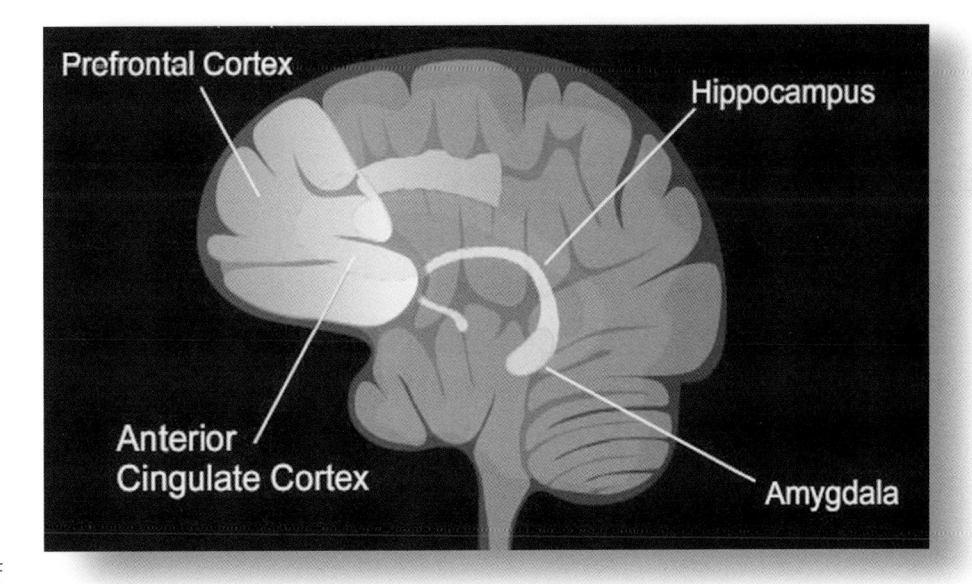

In 1995, the Tulsa Mental Health Association created the Jail Diversion Task Force, bringing together

Children's Advocacy Center, formerly the Justice Center, is a national model for the multi-disciplinary team approach to child abuse investigation and prosecution.

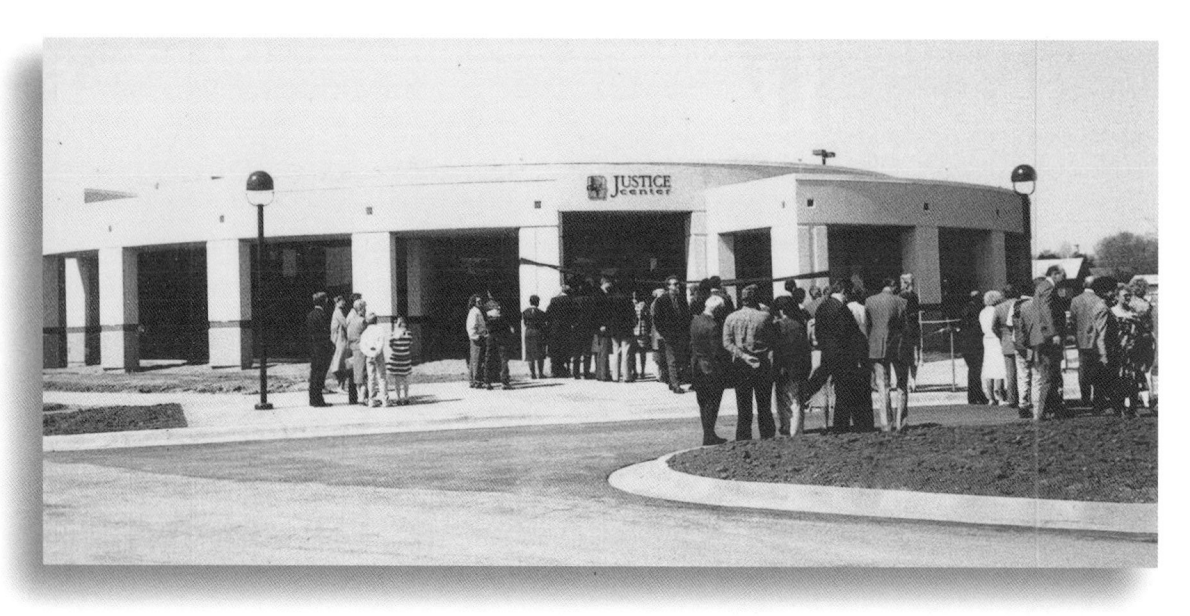

law enforcement, court officials and treatment providers to examine the problem of non-violent criminal defendants with mental health needs entering the judicial system. At its first meeting, members outlined some of the problems. The task force co-chairman, John Walsh, who was a member of the Oklahoma Sheriff's Association, said jail was a "dumping ground" for people with mental illness. No guidelines existed for officers to know how to handle situations with people in a psychotic state or where to turn for available resources. It was estimated at least 900 people with mental illness passed through the Tulsa Jail in 1994.

"Jails are there to control. They're not designed to give treatment. Unless you can identify the population, you don't have a way to get a handle on it," said John Walsh, *Tulsa World*, Sept. 8, 1995.

The task force work led the 2014 Special Service Docket in Tulsa District Court. It connected defendants to treatment. For those participating in the program, court costs were waived, and they remained out of jail. It also inspired the state mental health prison diversion efforts and judicial reforms. The group also advocated for better services while in jail, which led to the construction and opening of a mental health pod in 2016.

Several hospitals established programs in psychiatric care, including one at Doctors' Hospital for patients older than 55. Tulsa Regional added to its existing adults and child psychiatric care. St. John expanded its child psychiatrist services. Saint Francis transferred its child mental health beds to the Laureate Psychiatric Clinic, which was established in 1989.

By the end of the decade, lawmakers were grappling with the problem of inequality in mental health insurance coverage. Some policies excluded coverage for mental health disabilities or set higher deductibles for mental health treatment and medications. In 1999, the Oklahoma Legislature passed the "partial parity" bill, which required insurers to provide coverage to severe illnesses such as schizophrenia and bipolar disorder. Congressman John Sullivan, who represented Tulsa in the Second District, was a leading proponent of a federal parity bill. He appeared in Tulsa with Congressman Patrick J. Kennedy, D-Rhode Island, in 2007 to host a congressional field hearing on the issue.

"Doctors spoke of insurance companies rejecting their pleas for extended stays for suicidal and mentally ill patients. Families related problems finding mental health services for their children. Public officials laid out a vast amount of statistics. Business leaders explained how mental health coverage leads to more productive workers. Several people testified that insurance costs do not increase with mental health and substance abuse coverage," *Tulsa World*, Sept. 21, 2007.

"This is a civil rights issue. This country has always been about opening up opportunities throughout its history. This is another chance to open up opportunities to people who have been marginalized," said Congressman Patrick Kennedy, *Tulsa World*, Sept. 21, 2007.

"Mental health is a problem. It is so big, we cannot continue to brush it aside. There is a stigma, and it needs to be ended. The brain is part of a body like anything else and should be covered like anything else," said Congressman John Sullivan, *Tulsa World*, Sept. 21, 2007.

In 2008, the Mental Health Parity and Addiction Equality Act passed as part of the bailout of the U.S. financial system. Congress required insurance companies to provide coverage equally to mental health and other biological disorders. In 2010, the Affordable Care Act defined mental health and substance abuse treatments as one of 10 essential benefits. The measures reversed years of discrimination in healthcare insurance coverage.

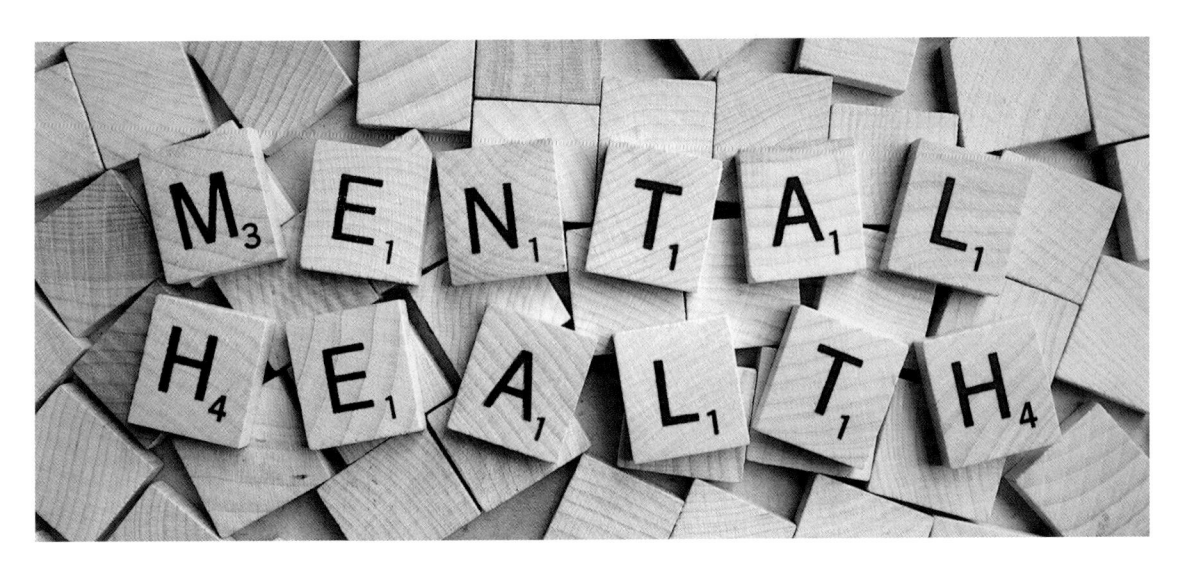

LANDMARK REPORT SHOWS ALCOHOL ABUSE

In a report deemed both "shocking" and "not surprising," the Oklahoma Department of Mental Health and Substance Abuse Services determined in September 1999 that alcohol was the most abused drug in the state, and about 130,000 residents needed treatment. It was the largest research project conducted in Oklahoma examining alcohol abuse.

"I take it as more evidence of how widespread the problem is, that people can look around them and see how much of a problem it is. They see it in their families, their co-workers, their friends," said Dr. Warren Dickson, project manager for Oklahoma's mental health department, *Tulsa World*, Sept. 23, 1999.

Dr. Robert W. Block

For most of his career, the Tulsa pediatrician specializing in child abuse and neglect heard the question, "How can you do this work?"

"How can you not?" he replied.

Dr. Robert "Bob" Block revolutionized the diagnosis and treatment of abused and neglected children. He was appointed as the first chairman of the American Board of Pediatrics subboard on child-abuse pediatrics (2006-2009) and holds the No. 1 certificate granted in the sub-specialty of child-abuse pediatrics.

The sub-specialty focuses on the forensic investigation of injuries that could meet the criteria of child abuse. These specialists are called in for consultations, which includes a review of the tests and analyses of other sub-specialists who have treated the child. They work with prosecutors on determining if child abuse occurred. Then, months or years later, child-abuse pediatric specialists offer legal testimony on behalf of the medical team that cared for the child.

"Not all children will have the opportunity to become adults, but every adult was once a child. The experiences and opportunities afforded to each of us in our early years, both positive and negative, have a long-term impact on our health and development and create a substantial imprint on the adults that we one day become. Pediatricians today are caring for and protecting the beginning of health for a child's entire life span, especially for vulnerable children who are victims of abuse or neglect. In order to optimize the health and well-being of our entire society, we must not view children and their welfare as isolated individuals or events, but instead recognize that children's physical and mental health must be addressed as the beginning of health across the entire life course," said Dr. Bob Block, U.S. Senate committee hearing testimony, Dec. 13, 2011.

After receiving his medical degree from the University of Pennsylvania, Dr. Block became interested in child maltreatment during his residency training at the Children's Hospital of Philadelphia between 1969 and 1972. He joined the faculty of the University of Oklahoma College of Medicine in Tulsa in 1975, serving as the Daniel C. Plunket chairman of the department of pediatrics.

As an educator, Dr. Block was nominated for the Aesculapian teaching award six times, winning on three occasions. He was awarded the prestigious Stanton L. Young Master Teacher Award, an OU Presidential Professorship, the Parker J. Palmer "Courage to Teach" Award by the Accreditation Council for

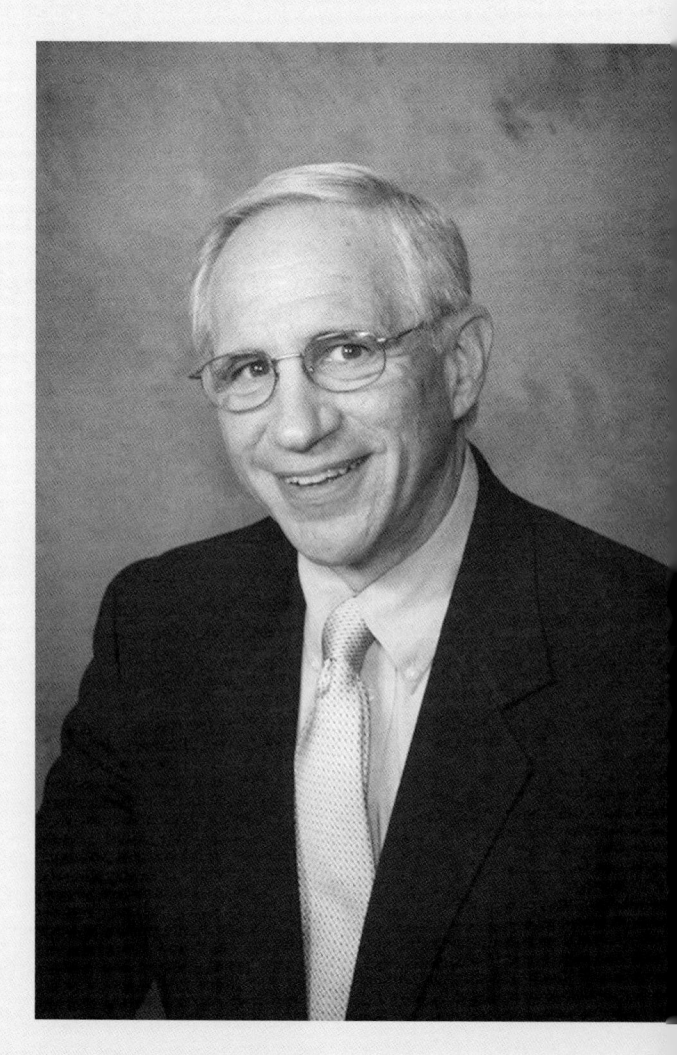

Graduate Medical Education and the Ray Helfer Society Award for his work in the field of child abuse.

As a physician, he has risen to become the most renowned expert in child abuse and neglect pediatrics and president of the American Academy of Pediatrics for the 2012-2013 term. Dr. Block served as president and board chairman of the Academy on Violence and Abuse and the U.S. Advisory Commission on Childhood Vaccines.

By creating child-abuse pediatrics as a medical sub-specialty, it allows for more organized clinical field research and support for pediatricians testifying in court in these cases. It is targeted for pediatricians and emergency-room doctors who are often on the front-line of care.

Dr. Block was appointed Oklahoma's first Chief Child Abuse Examiner in 1989 and served in that role until October 2011. He was past chairman and member of the Oklahoma Child Death Review Board from 1992 to September 2011. He has been a member of the medical team for the Tulsa Children's Advocacy Center and served as president and member of the board of directors for the Child Abuse Network.

He received the Award for Outstanding Service to Maltreated Children by the American Academy of Pediatrics and, in 2001, named one of the "Best Doctors in America."

Dr. Block's work dovetailed into the emerging research of brain development in young children, particularly in stressful homes and situations.

"We're learning so much about early childhood environments and the influence they have on health throughout the lifespan... how the brain responds to stress hormones, so even if you're not abused, if you live in poverty and acrimony with your parents so the family isn't stable that triggers things that may not be reflected until you are 30 to 40 or 50 years old," said Dr. Bob Block, *Tulsa People*, November 2011.

Dr. Block has been married for more than 42 years to his wife, Sharon, who is a retired science teacher and registered nurse. The couple have two daughters, Erika and Andrea, and have two grandchildren. He has since retired but continues to consult on cases.

Since 2006, OU-Tulsa has employed the area's only child-abuse specialists. Tulsa has two — Dr. Sarah Passmore and Dr. Michael Baxter.

After being a leader in child abuse pediatrics for decades, the university and hospital where Dr. Block conducted much of his work created a fellowship to continue his research. His influence can be traced directly to the program.

In December 2015, an agreement was reached between Saint Francis Hospital and the OU-Tulsa School of Community Medicine to expand the specialists and services provided for children who are abused. A key part of that was the establishment of a child-abuse pediatrics training fellowship through OU-Tulsa funded by Saint Francis. Dr. Lauren Conway was the first fellow in the sub-specialty training program.

It is the only such fellowship in Oklahoma, and it will continue to provide training and research in the sub-specialty of child-abuse pediatrics. ■

It found about 5 percent of the state's population abused alcohol, and 1 percent abused other types of drugs. When breaking down the demographic, 66 percent of homeless people abused alcohol and 52 percent of people with a mental illness had alcohol addictions. Among prisoners, 26 percent were alcoholics.

"It's important to note that the alcohol abuse is prompted by these sad circumstances, not the sad circumstances by the alcohol abuse. Now, I know some people with argue with me about that," said Dr. Warren Dickson, *Tulsa World*, Sept. 23, 1999.

SNUFFING OUT SMOKING

It was a 1979 brawl in a Tulsa County Courthouse that gave the first significant victory to non-smokers in Oklahoma.

Attorney Gerald D. Swanson carried a lighted cigarette onto a public elevator despite a state law and city ordinance against smoking in specific public places, including elevators. One of two plainclothes detectives, J.L.R. Brown, told him to put out the cigarette, and Swanson refused.

"Gerry said something: 'What are you going to do about it, anyway?' And the man said, 'I'm going to arrest you.' I thought they were just having a jawing match. I stepped off the elevators and had gone about 10 steps when I heard a rumble," said attorney Marion Dyer, *Tulsa World*, Aug. 3, 1979.

Witnesses said the officer grabbed the wrist of Swanson, who allegedly took a swing at the detective. The two officers then wrestled him to the ground before making the arrest. Swanson was exonerated on the assault charge in municipal court and pleaded no contest to the charge of taking the lit cigarette into the public elevators. But, his attorney Ed Parks gave notice he intended to challenge the constitutionality of the anti-smoking laws.

> **The year 1963 has the highest cigarette consumption on record...**

"It's ludicrous. It has no meaning. It cannot be fairly enforced, and it has nothing to do with the health and welfare of city government. This rinky-dink law was passed without any thought to rhyme or reason," said attorney Ed Parks, *Tulsa Tribune*, Dec. 8, 1979.

The Oklahoma Court of Criminal Appeals refused to overturn the fine levied against Swanson for violating the smoking ban. He still challenged the ban based on the fact he was only holding the lit cigarette and not actively smoking. Also, he asserts the city did not have the power to punish the violation of a "public nuisance" as a criminal offense, and the ordinance was "vague and uncertain." The court disagreed with Swanson's argument in a 2-1 decision.

The war against smoking was considered to have officially launched on Jan. 11, 1964, when the U.S. surgeon general released a landmark report. It stated clearly and specifically what Americans already knew:

Smoking will kill you. A *New York Times* article quoted defiant smokers who said they weren't going to quit, citing their "strong lung" and enjoying pleasures of life. The year 1963 has the highest cigarette consumption on record, with 46 percent of adults smoking an average of 4,345 cigarettes a year.

Some smokers did stop immediately, with cigarette use dropping 3.5 percent from 1963 to 1964.

Studies were ongoing for decades. With each one, it furthered the case against tobacco use. With each one, the tobacco industry released its own reports claiming no direct link between smoking and cancer.

In 1982, the annual U.S. Surgeon General report on smoking was devoted to the associations between smoking and specific types of cancer. It showed smoking was a major cause of cancer of the lung, larynx and esophagus and a "contributing factor" in bladder, kidney and pancreatic cancer. It also described lung cancer as a "largely preventable disease," stating that 85 percent of lung cancer deaths could be avoided if Americans never smoked. Lung cancer had been the leading cause of death in American males since the 1950s.

By the mid-80s, harms of second-hand smoking, sometimes called "passive smoking," started to emerge. A 1984 study from the nonprofit Studies on Smoking found women whose husbands smoked cigarettes died of cancer at nearly twice the rate of those whose husbands didn't smoke. A similar study had been released three years earlier in Japan. The *New England Journal of Medicine* published several articles about the impact on children in the homes of smokers, including a 1983 Harvard University study about the stunted growth of children's lungs. Some research focused on tobacco's impact on women, such as a 1983 report from the Boston University School of Medicine showing women smokers younger than 50 were five times more likely to die of a heart attack. Research also showed smoking connected to other illnesses, such as the flu. The Dow Chemical Co. report found in 1974 that its employees cost the company $657,146 in smoking-related illnesses. The use of low-nicotine and low-tar cigarettes did not reduce heart attacks and other diseases.

Insurance companies took notice and began structuring different packages and rates for smokers and non-smokers. A 1979 study of insurance customers found death rates among smokers were more than twice as great and some causes, such as respiratory cancer, ran as much as 15 times higher.

"I can't believe, in the face of these statistics, they're not going to sit up and take notice. The mortality patterns are so different that they cannot ignore them... We've studied the difference between smokers and non-smokers for 15 years and now we're absolutely convinced," said Michael J. Crowell, vice president and chief actuary for State Mutual Life Assurance Co. of America, *Tulsa Tribune*, Oct. 22, 1979.

These led to a movement among cities and states to crack down on smoking use in public. Arizona was the first state to pass a ban on smoking except in certain areas. The law passed in 1973 and applied to elevators, indoor theaters, buses, libraries, concert halls and art museums. The chief opposition to the Arizona law was Democratic Senator floor leader Harold Giss, who argued against it while smoking a cigarette, calling the measure "an invasion of privacy." A month later, he died of a heart attack at age 67.

"(We) must in the near future provi smokers a psychological crutch and

The president of Philip Morris wrote in a 1964 internal memo.

Minnesota was the first state to pass a law requiring separate areas for smokers and non-smokers in all shared enclosed public places. It became a model. Nebraska passed a nearly identical law in 1981 with Utah, Michigan, several California cities and Washington, D.C. following quickly. A sticking point during the 80s bans was restaurants.

"The pervasive attitude is to leave people alone to do what they want to do," said State Rep. Cleta Deatheridge, D-Norman, *Tulsa World*, Dec. 2, 1982. Deatheridge had attempted several times to amend the law to include eating establishments.

Oklahoma's smoking restrictions left out restaurants until 1987. That law exempted the legislature, bars, bowling alleys and restaurants seating less than 50. It was also an unusual law in that it forbade public places to go smoke free, instead requiring an established smoking section. Tulsa International Airport created smoking sections in 1988.

Tulsa City Hall implemented a smoking ban in 1987. The Tulsa Fire Department started hiring only non-smokers in 1986, which was the same year it offered voluntary cessation programs. Some businesses voluntarily offered non-smoking options. The Middle Path was the first restaurant in Tulsa to establish a non-smoking section. It set aside 19 tables in 1978 for non-smokers. In 1982, two floors of the Excelsior Hotel were deemed as non-smoking.

"We decided that enough people had inquired about it to give it a try. The results have been really gratifying. Those floors fill up first," said Judy Wallis, Excelsior Hotel marketing and communications manager, *Tulsa World*, Dec. 2, 1982.

Some workplaces banned smoking in employee areas. Tulsa's Satellite Syndicated Systems, a cable and satellite communications company, put such a policy in place in the early 80s.

"I have always had a sinus reaction to smoke, it really affects the way I feel and work... But beyond that, about three years ago, I saw a report about the cost to companies of a smoking employee. Obviously it affects the smokers' health, and I have first-hand experience of the effect it can have on people in the smoke-filled environment, not to mention the other costs involved, including cleaning of drapes and furniture, even the window," said Edward L. Taylor, president and chief executive officer of Satellite Syndicated Systems, *Tulsa World*, Oct. 21, 1984.

Tulsa County jurors began complaining about smoke-filled rooms, prompting a remodel.

some answers which will give self-rationale to continue smoking."

"Any more, since smoke has become such a naughty thing, people are real concerned about this type of thing. There's no smoking on courthouse elevators and no-smoking signs in courtrooms, so I guess the jury assembly room shouldn't be an exception," said Presiding District Judge M.M. McDougal, *Tulsa Tribune*, Sept. 3, 1981.

As efforts to curb tobacco use continued, concerns also rose about the marketing to young people. The Tulsa School Board banned student smoking in 1987. Teenage girls outpaced the boys when it came to smoking rates in the mid-80s. The trend held true in Tulsa.

"Smoking has been glamorized by the media. Smoking helps some girls cope with adjustments to adolescence and to sexual demands. Their level of anxiety is high, and adolescents are experiencing more pressures than they used to. Some kids go without lunch to buy cigarettes," said Richard Palazzo, program director of Street School, *Tulsa World*, March 5, 1984.

A leading proponent of the ban in Tulsa was Dr. Dan Brannin, an oral surgeon and member of the Tulsa City-County Health Department. He led a committee to look at banning smoking in most public places. He was also the past president of the American Board of Oral and Maxillofacial Surgery. He said the vast majority of his cancer patients were smokers, but also had concern for non-smokers, who:

"... Had over the years just come to accept smoke as a part of life — that when you were with friends and associates, you would be exposed to their smoke. But as the evidence proved more and more clearly the dangers of passive smoking. I think it is necessary to protect those non-smokers from the damage they could sustain simply by being around smokers. At the same time, I think the smoker has gotten a raw deal. The smoker doesn't try to create a problem for anyone else. The smoker doesn't even want to smoke. Polls show us that over 70 percent of the smokers want to quit, and 35 percent will try to quit every year. I will not accept the image of a 'zealot' on this issue, nor will I accept the portrayal of this ordinance proposal as an attempt to punish the smoker," said Dr. Dan Bannin, *Tulsa World*, March 15, 1987.

In 1995, California was the first state to enact a statewide smoking ban. Between 2004 and 2007, a trend took hold with states enacting stricter smoking bans. In 2009, Oklahoma's Clean Air in Restaurants Act created a rebate program to incentivize restaurants to close smoking rooms and become smoke-free. The bill also created the Oklahoma Certified Healthy Communities Act and Oklahoma Certified Healthy Schools Act. In 2012, Gov. Mary Fallin approved an executive order banning the use of tobacco on all state grounds.

The 90s brought about historic class-action lawsuit settlements against the tobacco industry. Oklahoma was the 14th state to file a suit against the tobacco industry to recover tax dollars lost in treating smoking-related illnesses. Oklahoma Attorney General Drew Edmondson was one of eight attorneys general to serve on the negotiating team. He was convinced by the mounting evidence that the tobacco companies lied to the public. Court documents showed that companies used attorneys and public relations firms to hide and spin information.

Chemicals were added to amp up addictive qualities, and youths were targeted as replacement users. The president of Philip Morris wrote in a 1964 internal memo:

"(We) must in the near future provide some answers which will give smokers a psychological crutch and a self-rationale to continue smoking."

In 1998, 46 states entered into a master settlement agreement. Four states — Florida, Minnesota, Texas and Mississippi — had settled their cases separately. The agreement projected to pay Oklahoma about $2 billion during the first 25 years of the settlement. In 2000, voters approved a state constitutional amendment to place part of the settlement payment into an endowment trust fund. The Tobacco Settlement Endowment Trust has a five-member board overseeing investing of the funds and a seven-member board of directors oversees spending from the trust in five areas: Research for combating cancer and tobacco-related diseases, tobacco prevention and cessation programs, health programs with an emphasis on children, health programs connected to schools and health programs for senior adults.

By 2002, an executive director and state office were established. The first project created a tobacco "quit line" to provide information, self-help materials and counseling to Oklahomans wanting to stop using tobacco products. Two years later, the board started the Communities of Excellence in Tobacco Control program to give grants to entities working to prevent and end tobacco use. In 2011, Oklahoma Health officials announced that for the first time, the state had more former smokers than current smokers.

About $77 million has been paid into the trust as of 2015, and about $47 million is available for the board to use. Of the funded programs: 38 percent goes to prevention programs; 26 percent to obesity, physical activity and nutrition programs; 20 percent to research; 7 percent to grant management support; 3 percent to emerging opportunities; 3 percent to evaluation and 3 percent to administration.

In 2014 — 50 years after the landmark U.S. Surgeon General report — Oklahoma's smoking prevalence had fallen to 21 percent. Between 2001 to 2014, cigarette sales fell by 1 billion packs and smoke-free households increased to 83.7 percent from 54.9 percent.

Oklahoma ranked 45th in overall health status, according to the 2015 United Health Foundation rankings. Oklahoma was also ranked 40th in adult smoking, 6th-highest in obesity and 3rd-highest in cardiovascular deaths.

Heart Transplant

On Sept. 17, 1993, a former Hale High School football coach received the first heart transplant in Tulsa. Jim Smith, 56, had heart problems during the past decade with heart attacks in 1984 and 1992, which resulted in a quadruple open heart bypass surgery. He suffered from ischemic cardiomyopathy, known as heart failure. At the advice of Dr. C. William McEntee, Smith decided to seek a heart transplant.

"The doctor said I had three months to live. At first I was scared to death. But the more and more they explained everything to me about a heart transplant, the more comfortable I felt with the idea. You always think it's someone else that it should happen to, not yourself," said Jim Smith, *Tulsa World*, 1994.

Smith was given priority by the Oklahoma Organ Sharing Network due to his worsening condition. At the time, about 30 percent of those needing a heart listed with the network died while waiting on a donor. Saint Francis had been approved in July 1993 as a heart transplant center by the United Network for Organ Sharing.

Within 22 hours of Smith going on the network's list, a 37-year-old who died of a stroke donated the heart and several other organs. After Saint Francis Hospital was notified Smith would receive the heart, a team jumped into action. Cardiothoracic surgeon Dr. Robert Phillips Jr. performed the surgery with assistance from Drs. James Whiteneck and Charles Berry. The attending cardiologist was Dr. Douglas Ensley.

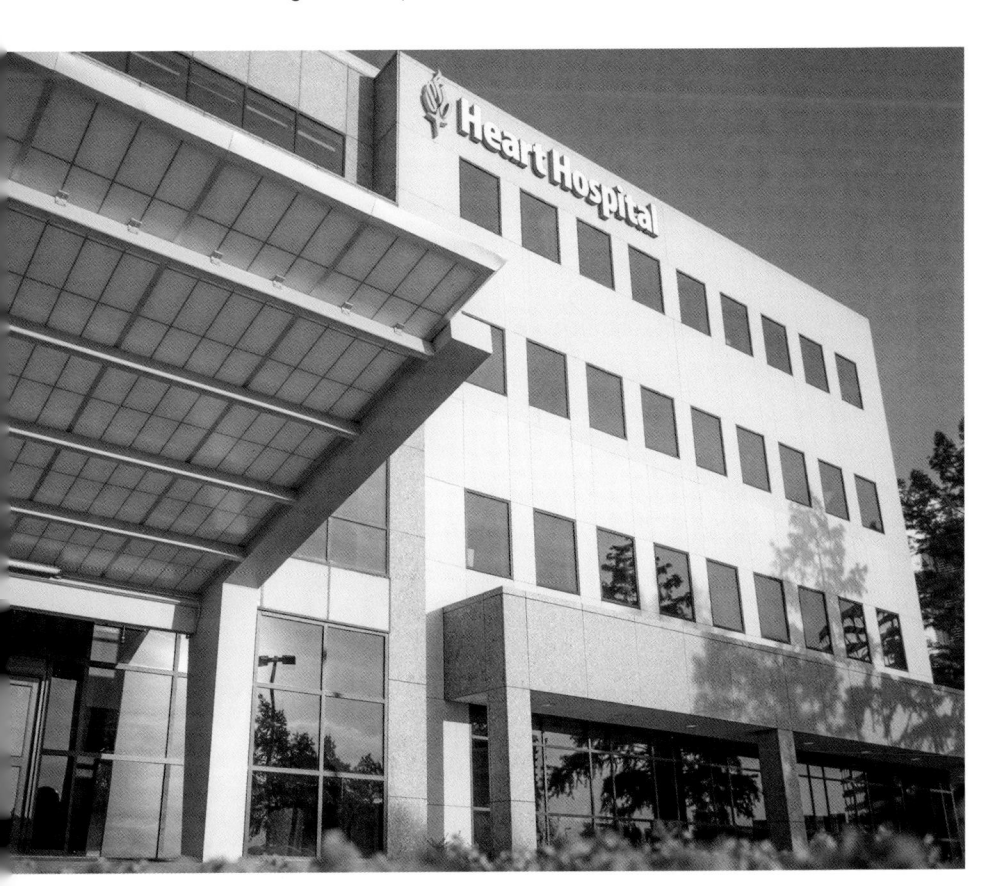

Smith was released after two weeks and resumed his exercise as a golfer. He had retired from McDonnell Douglas in 1993 and began working as a volunteer with the National Kidney Foundation and the Tulsa Heart Transplant Center. He died on Nov. 24, 1994.

Saint Francis launched a coronary care program at its medical facility near Broken Arrow in March 2004. It moved the expanded program — the Heart Hospital - to its main facility in 2008.

Saint Francis South Heart Hospital.

Saint Francis Hospital stopped performing heart transplants in 2008 after a policy change in heart distribution by the United Network of Organ Sharing. Starting in August 2006, the network offered hearts from donors to patients in a 500-mile radius deemed most urgent. Previously, donor hearts within Oklahoma were offered to in-state patients first. After the change went into effect, more than 50 percent of Oklahoma donor hearts were sent out of state. This put the hospital's Medicaid and Medicare reimbursement for the procedure in jeopardy. The federal government required a minimum of 10 heart transplants a year to get reimbursed, and Saint Francis Hospital had been averaging about 8 transplants annually. In addition, advanced treatment for heart disease reduced the need for transplants, and insurance companies had been increasingly referring Oklahomans to out-of-state clinics.

Tulsa-area residents needing a new heart traveled to Oklahoma City or out-of-state. Saint Francis continued its services for follow-up treatments.

"We very much regret that their program has closed. We think they provided an excellent service for the Tulsa community and that part of Oklahoma," said Dr. David Nelson, chief of the heart-transplant medicine division at the Nazih Zuhdi Transplantation Institute at Integris Baptist Medical Center in Oklahoma City, *Tulsa World*, Feb. 22, 2008.

Between 1994 and 2008, the Saint Francis heart-transplant program performed more than 140 transplants. Currently, more than 2,000 people undergo heart transplants each year in the U.S. with about 3,000 patients on a waiting list.

STATE OF HEALTH

As the new century dawned, physicians were taking up the cause for better overall health. In March 1999, Oklahoma was listed in a national report as the only state in the nation to experience a decline in health status since 1990. It came from ReliaStar Financial Corp, which ranked the state 44th in health status, down from 27th a decade earlier.

Leading causes of death were heart disease (34 percent), cancers (22 percent), injuries (7 percent), stroke (7 percent) and chronic obstructive pulmonary disease (5 percent).

Causes were high rates of smoking, poor nutrition, lack of exercise and poverty, which led to high uninsured rates. People in poverty tended to stay away from doctors and medical care until a crisis required an emergency room visit. Oklahoma had traditionally been listed in the top 10 states for highest rates of uninsured.

"On average, compared to the rest of the nation, Oklahoma is a poor place to live if you want to live a long time, if you want to avoid premature death, and if you want to live your life with unnecessary disability. We're not going to turn this thing around until the leadership in the state... really faces these facts," said Dr. Gordon Deckert, the immediate past president and spokesman for the Oklahoma State Medical Association, *Tulsa World*, March 4, 1999.

CHAPTER 11
(2000 - 2016)

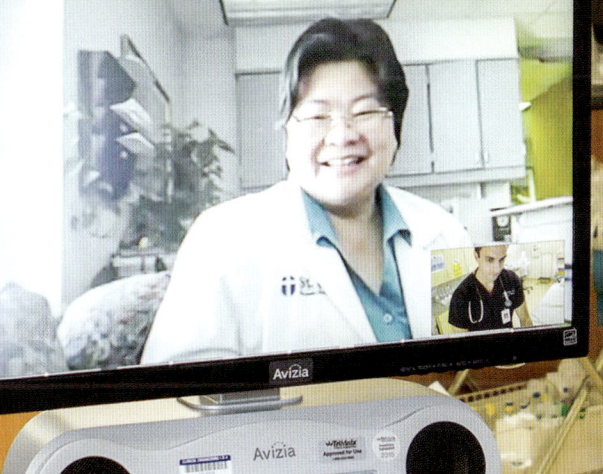

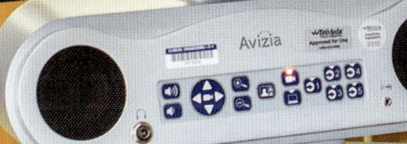

Moving into a New Era of Medicine

St. John's telemedicine technology.

The age of technology ushered in a sea change for business, medicine, industry and everyday life. Ease of Internet communications allowed for faster research and information sharing. This included the sometimes helpful, sometimes frustrating online medical websites patients use to gain knowledge. It also changed the business end of health-care delivery with the use of electronic medical and health records. Medical tools brought about a functional MRI to track brain cells and robotics to minimize invasive surgeries and recovery time for patients.

In 2000, a draft of the human genome map was released to the public giving people an opportunity to read information kept in a human body's 23,000 genes. It has been a cornerstone for discovering new treatments, cures and therapies.

At the same time, costs were soaring, nearly 18 percent of Oklahomans were without health insurance and medical schools were evolving to keep up with the demands. The new era would bring more niche care within hospitals, coordinated Tulsa medical school options and efforts to expand health insurance.

Affordable Care Act

The most significant — and polarizing — federal health reform of the modern era was the Patient Protection and Affordable Care Act, colloquially called Obamacare after President Barack Obama. It was passed and signed into law in March 2010. It was a comprehensive bill containing numerous provisions such as prohibiting the denial of coverage for pre-existing conditions, establishing minimum standards for insurance coverage, setting penalties for not having health coverage, increasing subsidies for low-income people and creating an online marketplace to compare and buy insurance policies. It did not replace private insurance, Medicare or Medicaid. Among the details, it allowed for more coverage of contraceptions, free prevention services for procedures such as mammograms and colonoscopies and a requirement for restaurants to have nutritional information available.

The law became a bitter partisan feud. The U.S. Supreme Court found most of the legislation constitutional in June 2012 but made state participation in Medicaid expansion optional.

Gov. Mary Fallin, a Republican, was sworn in as governor in January 2011 to work with a Republican-controlled legislature. The following month, Oklahoma was awarded a $54.6 million Affordable Care Act "early innovator" grant to build a state health-insurance exchange. In April 2011, Fallin was joined by Speaker of the House Kris Steele and Senate Pro Tem Brian Bingman to say the grant was to be rejected. Oklahoma Attorney General Scott Pruitt joined other Republican state attorneys general in filing lawsuits. Oklahoma-based Hobby Lobby and four private Oklahoma colleges (Oklahoma Wesleyan, Oklahoma Baptist, Southern Nazarene and Mid-America) challenged the birth control requirement. In November 2012, Gov. Fallin announced the state would reject expanded Medicaid funding and the creation of a state health-insurance exchange.

"If we tried to do our own state exchange, myself and other governors across the nation believe it's in name only because in the end it would be the Obama administration that would approve it. It does not benefit Oklahoma taxpayers to actively support or fund a new government program that will ultimately be under the control of the federal government, that is opposed by a clear majority of Oklahomans, and that will further the implementation of a law that threatens to erode both the quality of the American health care system and the fiscal stability of the nation," said Gov. Mary Fallin, *Daily Oklahoman*, Nov. 19, 2012.

The Oklahoma Policy Institute estimated an Oklahoma Medicaid expansion would have extended insurance coverage to about 150,000 people, or 1 in 5 of the state's uninsured. Most of those patients fell into a gap between earning too much for traditional Medicaid but not enough to qualify for subsidies to purchase health insurance on the online marketplace.

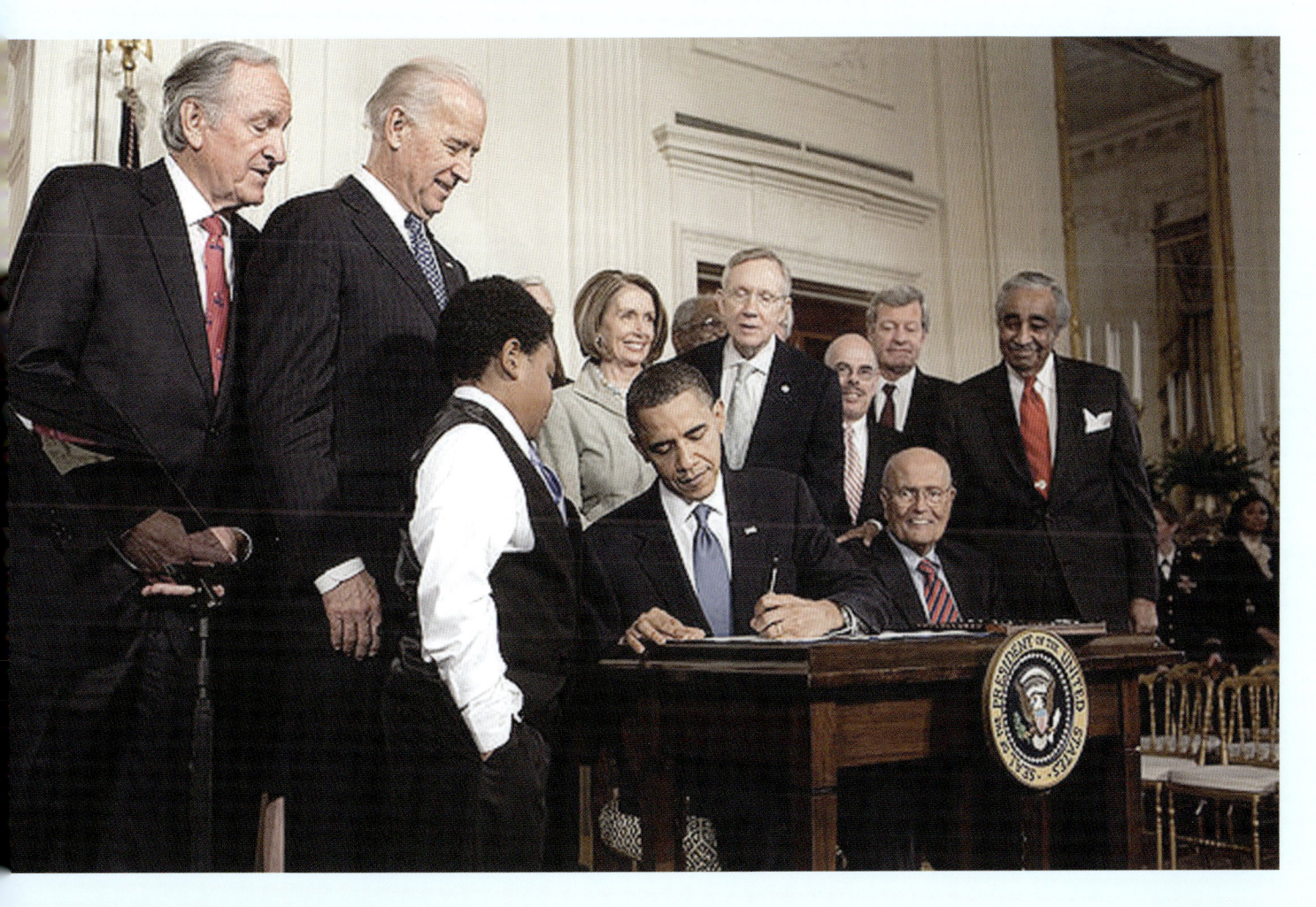

The state also promoted its Insure Oklahoma program, which provided state subsidies to eligible low-income workers. In 2015, about 18,000 Oklahomans were in the program.

"I am absolutely astounded that in a state with the level of health disparities that exist that we have leadership that says things like, 'We don't need federal money; we can take care of our own.' If that were true, then we wouldn't have infant mortality, obesity, diabetes, cardiovascular issues that are

President Obama Signs the Affordable Care Act into Law.

astounding in America in 2011. And yet we object to federal investment," said John Silva, chief executive officer of Morton Comprehensive Health Services, *Tulsa World*, Oct. 2, 2011.

Critics of the law say it drives up costs of medical care delivery and restricts choices for patients. When insurance rates were expected to increase in 2016, Oklahoma's deputy commissioner of the Oklahoma Insurance Department cited:

- Medical cost inflation averaged between 6 percent to 9 percent;
- Companies made inaccurate cash flow estimates for 2014 and 2015;
- Prescription drug costs were higher than estimated; and
- Companies underestimated how much treatment Affordable Care Act consumers would seek once getting insurance.

"The big story is, rates are going up. They didn't get the numbers right in 2015. They were guessing. Every carrier I talked to had lost money," said Mike Rhoads, deputy commissioner of the Oklahoma Insurance Department, *Oklahoma Watch*, July 10, 2015.

> "About 15 percent of the state's population did not have insurance, above the national rate of 12 percent. Of Oklahoma children younger than 17, about 9 percent did not have health coverage."

In June 2015, the U.S. Supreme Court ruled to protect the subsidies received by qualifying people buying coverage in the exchange. In Oklahoma at that time, about 80,000 Oklahomans received health coverage using these federal subsidies.

Facing a more than $1.3 billion state revenue failure in 2016, the legislature directed agencies to make across-the-board cuts. The Oklahoma Health Care Authority announced a possible 25 percent rate reduction in Medicaid, prompting a unanimous vote by the executive committee of the Oklahoma State Medical Association urging members to consider dropping out of Medicaid.

"We are fully aware this will create an access-to-care crisis for rural residents, vulnerable seniors, the disabled and the nearly 60 percent of Oklahoma babies born under Medicaid. But a 25 percent rate cut, combined with previous cuts that had already been made in recent years, will leave many of our members with little choice. This situation is simply unsustainable for most medical practices and will endanger many rural health-care settings," said OSMA President Dr. Woody Jenkins, *Tulsa World*, April 4, 2016.

"We're to the point where the provider rates are going to be cut so much that providers won't be able to survive, particularly the nursing homes," said Republican state Rep. Dr. Doug Cox, *Associated Press*, May 16, 2016.

"We are nearing a colossal collapse of our health care system in Oklahoma. We have doctors turning away patients. We have people with mental illness going without treatment. Hospitals are closing, and this is only going to get worse this summer if the Legislature does not act immediately to turn this around," said Craig Jones, president of the Oklahoma Hospital Association, May 16, 2016.

The Health Care Authority avoided the reductions after the Legislature found ways, including the use of one-time funding and restricting tax breaks, to stave off the deeper cuts.

In May 2016, Gov. Fallin said elected leaders were considering a proposal from the Oklahoma Health Care Authority called the "Medicaid rebalancing" model. The law allows states to tailor plans with approval from the federal government. Oklahoma's proposed alternative plan touts to lower the number of Medicaid recipients, reduce the number of insured and create a health savings piece to reward participants for healthy lifestyle choices. The Legislature failed to get the needed tax increase on cigarettes during the session for the up-front costs. It also got pushback.

"The plan is simply Obamacare Medicaid expansion rebranded. As conservatives concerned about fiscal responsibility, we urge lawmakers to reject it. The rebalancing scheme is a policy that expands the scope and size of the federal government and increases dependency on government programs. It removes one more state barrier that separates us from a single-payer system in the United States," states an editorial written by former Republican Oklahoma U.S. Sen. Tom Coburn and attorney Larry Parman, former Oklahoma secretary of state and commerce secretary, *Daily Oklahoman*, May 15, 2016.

As of January 2016, 31 states and the District of Columbia have adopted the Medicaid expansion, 16 states — including Oklahoma — rejected it and the rest are discussing a model that would pass federal compliance.

By the end of November 2015, Oklahoma had 126,115 consumers enrolled in an insurance program through the federal marketplace. Of those, 79 percent qualified for an average tax credit of $206 a month. About 15 percent of the state's population did not have insurance, above the national rate of 12 percent. Of Oklahoma children younger than 17, about 9 percent did not have health coverage.

Physician Shortage

As the new century dawned, Oklahoma faced a critical shortage of doctors, particularly in rural areas. In February 2011, the state was ranked as the most access-challenged in terms of health care by the *New England Journal of Medicine*.

The highest concentrations of physicians were located in Oklahoma City and Tulsa while western and southeastern areas had few doctors and even fewer specialists. For every 100 Oklahomans, there were 2.13 physicians, from a low of .17 in Coal County to a high of 4.11 in Oklahoma County.

The state had more than 200 Health Professional Shortage Areas, which were official designations of not meeting the national standard of one physician per 3,500 residents. Those areas were located in 66 of Oklahoma's 77 counties.

In Tulsa, there was a health disparity among sections of the city with the lowest life expectancy among residents in neighborhoods with the fewest doctors.

Among the issues contributing to the shortage were: Medical schools not increasing class sizes, residency slots being difficult to find and doctors choosing other states to practice. Also in the mix was the growing cost of medical school, expected rise in insured patients with the passage of the Affordable Care Act and an aging population. By 2030, nearly 1 in 5 Americans will be older than 65 and the 85-and-older population will more than triple by 2050. The average age of a physician in 2011 was 54, and 1 in 4 doctors was older than 60.

Of the Oklahoma medical students doing their residency in state, about 80 percent stayed in the state.

"The only way to get people to go to rural Oklahoma is to recruit them from rural Oklahoma," said James Hess, chief operating officer with the OSU Center for Health Sciences, *Tulsa World*, Oct. 2, 2011.

By 2015, Oklahoma had the eighth lowest number of physicians providing patient care per capita, according to a report from the Association of American Medical Colleges. Primary care providers represented about one-third of the shortage.

OU medical students in action.

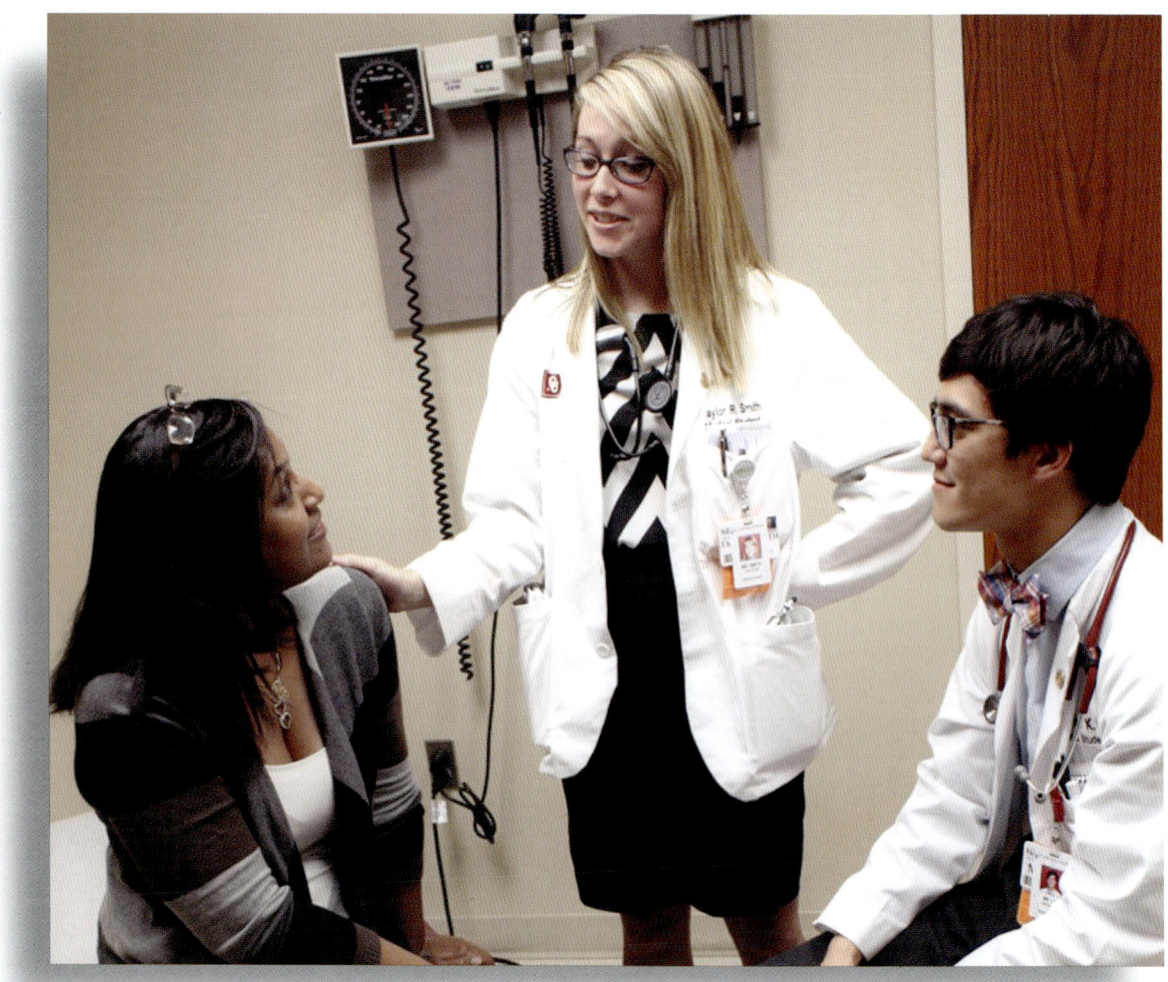

Tulsa Medical Schools Expand

Starting in August 2015, doctor of medicine students could complete their four years of medical education in Tulsa through the University of Oklahoma-University of Tulsa School of Community Medicine. In the first class of 28 students, Anadarko native Matthew Abbott explained health care in small towns.

"There are 6,000 people and, I think, two to three doctors. The math does not add up. You can see there is a great need for doctors in these rural communities. I really wanted to be a part of this. It is revolutionary because it is easy to probably get involved with the medical system and not see any changes to it. But if we really want to serve people, I think we have to be willing to say maybe this isn't the best option we have and maybe there are better things we can do to help them," said medical student Matthew Abbott, *Tulsa World*, Aug. 24, 2015.

A goal of the program is to reach under-served populations. The education involves doctors learning about the social determinants of health of the community to find ways to bring better access and affordability to care.

Tandy Education Center at OU-SCM.

"Many times, being able to help people is more than just giving them medicine; it's understanding where they come from. This is a great opportunity to take a cadre of medical students and educate them in that fashion from day one. Health care all across the country is moving very rapidly to a model of population-based health care, which is that physicians and other health-care providers try to take care of whole communities rather than just individual patients as they walk in the door. The School of Community Medicine is really ahead of its time because it's based on that principal," said OU-TU School of Community Medicine Dean Dr. James Herman, *Tulsa World*, Aug. 24, 2015.

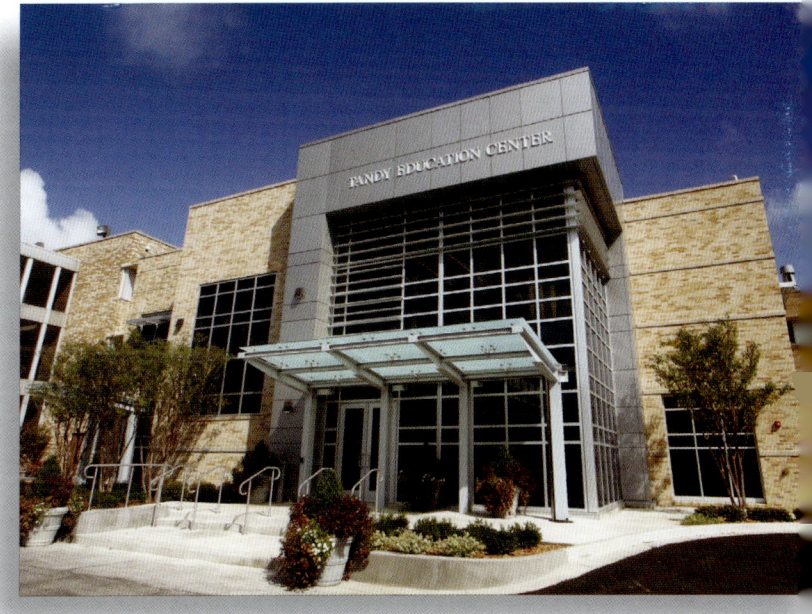

The School of Community Medicine is housed in a $6.4 million, 16,000-square foot facility — called the Tandy Education Center — at the OU-Tulsa Schusterman Center at 41st Street and Yale Avenue. It includes state-of-the-art simulation and training facilities, including 10 exam rooms, two inpatient intensive care/emergency rooms and a furnished model apartment for simulation training, four interview rooms, two debriefing rooms, a multipurpose training room and student lounges. It was funded with a grant from the A.R. and Marylouise Tandy Foundation of Tulsa.

"These are two flagship universities in this part of the country, and when you bring them together, you can do some extraordinary things at a time when America really needs it. The amount of money spent on health care needs to be rethought, and bringing these different partners together allows you to do that," said Dr. Gerald Clancy, dean of the TU College of Health Sciences and vice president of health affairs, *Tulsa World*, Aug. 24, 2015.

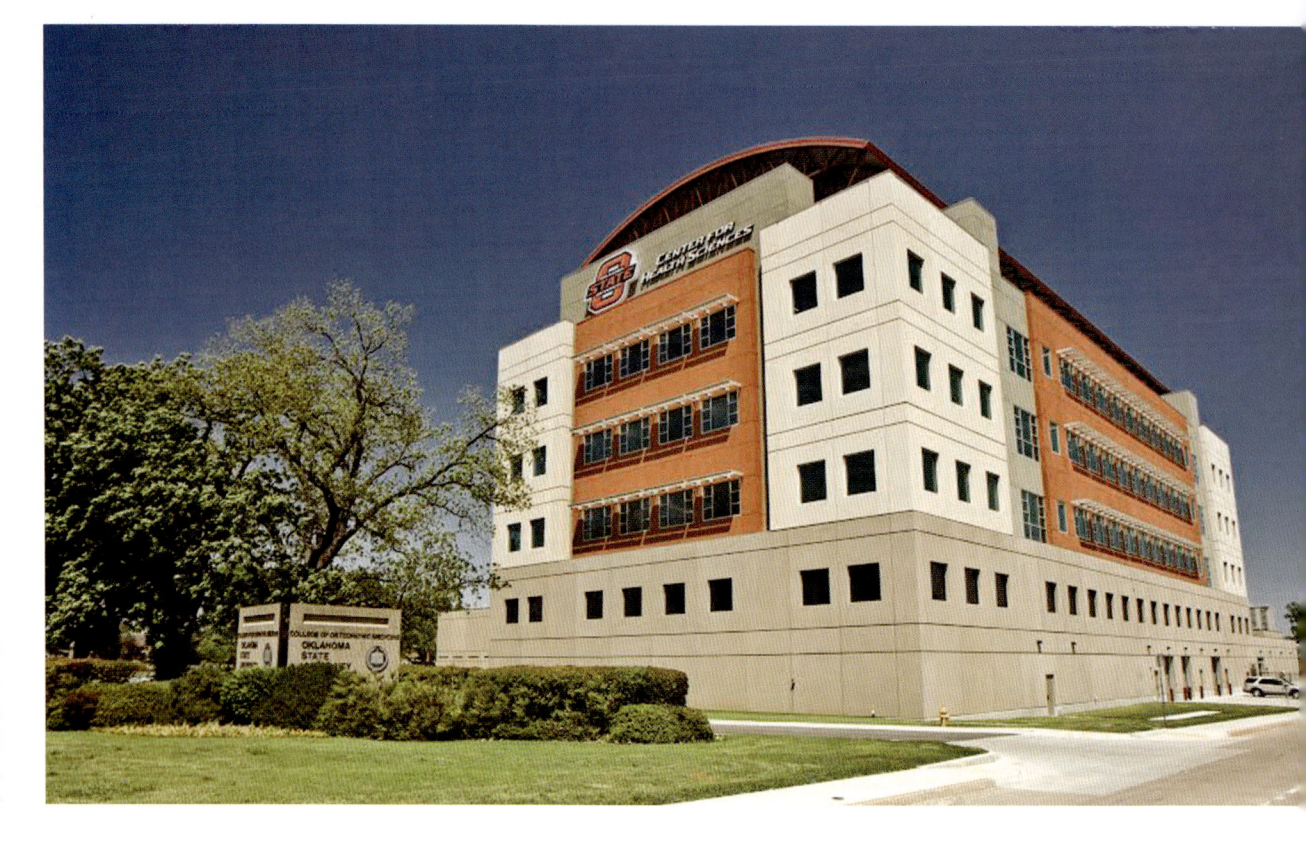

OSU Center for Health Sciences Medical Building.

After the establishment of the Oklahoma State University Medical Center in November 2006, the osteopathic school began to grow and stability was shown in the former Tulsa Regional Medical Center, renamed the OSU Medical Center. It is the largest osteopathic teaching center in the U.S.

Construction began on a four-story, $45-million medical, academic and simulation center at the west campus, 1111 W. 17th St. It will include a hospital simulation center, clinical skills lab and space for classrooms, lectures and conferences. A 223,000-square foot, five-story parking garage is part of the project. Designed by Dewberry Architects, it is set to open in 2017.

"Medical education has just changed so much over time, and it's more technology-driven," said Dr. Kayse Shrum, OSU-CHS president, *Tulsa World*, March 31, 2015.

Among additions to the curriculum was an intensive course on obesity starting in 2015. Obesity medicine became a subspecialty in 2013 and a national movement took hold to incorporate obesity into medical school education. Oklahoma had the sixth highest rate of obesity in 2015 at 33 percent of the population. The concept of obesity medicine focuses on proper nutrition, physical activity and behavioral changes.

"It really takes all of us — both here in the medical profession and those out in the community — to come together to address such a complex disease because it does require complex solutions. This really puts us on the cutting edge nationally because there are very few medical schools that have any curriculum in obesity medicine, and the ones that do, it tends to be very minimal and elective. The complications of obesity are so extensive — diabetes, heart disease — it impacts the quality of people's lives and longevity. In

Oklahoma, we really have a disproportional level of obesity and diabetes and heart disease, and our providers often haven't been well trained in obesity medicine," said Colony Fugate, director of the OSU Family Health and Nutrition Clinic, *Tulsa World*, Jan. 8, 2016.

Mental Health Care

This era brought about a mental health crisis for Oklahoma. By 2013, Oklahoma ranked No. 2 in the U.S. for prevalence of mental illness. The state was also No. 9 in percentage of adults with a dependence on drugs or alcohol, and No. 5 in percentage of adults with suicidal thoughts. About 70 percent of adults needing services were not receiving it, and 40 percent of youths needing mental health services were not being served. Between 700,000 and 950,000 Oklahomans needed mental health or substance abuse services.

The state could not keep up with demand. An array of services were developed to reach the underserved in mental health and substance abuse addiction. That included a push for more psychiatrists, community sentence courts and team-based, home-health approaches.

In 2015, the Oklahoma Department of Mental Health and Substance Abuse Services approached the OSU Center for Health Sciences to partner on a psychiatric residency program. The university obtained funding and accreditation for five students to begin residencies on July 1, 2016.

The new psychiatric residency program is meant to provide relief for the shortage of mental health physicians in the Tulsa area and to make a dent in the long-term problems created by a lack of psychiatrists statewide. The only other residency programs are through the OU School of Community Medicine Department of Psychiatry and two in the Oklahoma City area.

"That comes up with really very few spots for Oklahoma in general. So a lot of our future psychiatrists are leaving the state for training and they're not coming back. We just don't have enough spots to train future psychiatrists and on the other hand, there's not enough psychiatrists in Tulsa," said Dr. Jason Beaman, chairman of the department of behavioral services at OSU-HSC, *Tulsa World*, March 14, 2016.

To reach among the most difficult and unstable populations are PACT teams, or Program of Assertive Community Treatment. It was developed in the 80s as a team approach to care by surrounding a patient with a support team, available 24 hours a day, seven days a week. Services are brought to the client, rather than depending on patients making it to an office for appointments. The team includes doctors, nurses, social workers and a peer counselor. While each team costs about $10,000 per client per year, the annual savings in health care costs starts at about $15,000.

Seventeen of Oklahoma's 77 counties have at least one PACT team.

In Tulsa by 2016, three PACT teams existed — one based at OU-TU School of Community Medicine (called OU-IMPACT, or Oklahoma-Integrated Multidisciplinary Program of Assertive Community Treatment) and two at the nonprofit Family & Children's Services. Together, those served about 275 people. A study by OU-Tulsa researchers a few years earlier found that another nearly 700 Tulsa residents could be eligible for services, but not enough slots were available.

"By the time they get to us, it's pretty serious, and they have few social supports and are showing a lot of symptoms of psychotic episodes. Often, they do not like the health-care system. The health-care system has failed them. It takes a long time to build the relationship, at least six months to a year," said Dr. Erik Vanderlip, psychiatrist and family-medicine physician managing the OU-IMPACT team, *Tulsa World*, Aug. 30, 2015.

For decades, teams struggled to provide holistic care — mind and body — because different doctors handled different health issues. The communication and funding were handled separately by psychiatrists and the primary care doctor. It was left up to the patient to coordinate care. This led to patients getting better mentally but not physically. Most people enrolled in a PACT team were suffering from high cardiovascular disease.

"They are dying at 55 from strokes, heart attacks and other cardiovascular events. The real things that are killing them are cardiovascular reasons. Many smoke like chimneys. But there is high blood pressure, diabetes and cholesterol," said Dr. Erik Vanderlip, *Tulsa World*, Aug. 30, 2015.

That changed with the Affordable Care Act, which enhanced traditional community mental-health services to allow for better primary care coordination. These government-defined services were called "health homes," and PACT teams were included. Even when Oklahoma turned down Medicaid expansion for individuals, federal funding was made available to programs featuring health homes.

The OU-IMPACT team was included in a statewide initiative called Health Homes to coordinate better primary care for their clients. After a six-month evaluation of the program, it found improved physical health factors such as cholesterol screenings, blood pressure and diabetes maintenance. In 2015, members of the American Psychiatric Association completed a position statement calling on psychiatrists to do a better job of managing the physical health conditions of their patients along with their mental-health needs.

"We are creating a psychiatric hospital, but in their homes. You can't just discharge someone from the team for missing an appointment or not following all the rules. Once they are part of the team, we are responsible for them. We find them wherever they may be," said Dr. Erik Vanderlip, *Tulsa World*, Aug. 30, 2015.

HEALTH DISPARITIES

In 2006, Tulsa learned that a 14-year gap in life expectancy existed between residents who lived in the north and south neighborhoods of the city. The comprehensive report was prepared by the Lewin Group, a national health care and human services consulting firm. For years, arguments about the disparity and lack of resources in north Tulsa and in pockets of west and east were based on observation and scant statistical information. The report provided the data and proof of the problems. These areas had the fewest doctors and medical facilities available. In north Tulsa, there was one physician for every 26 doctors practicing in midtown.

Broken down by ZIP codes, those with the lowest life expectancy were in 74126, 74106, 74116 and 74127. These neighborhoods also contained the highest percentage of racial minority groups and reflected the highest concentrations of poverty and unemployment. Residents in the 74126 were arguably in the worst area in the state, with the shortest life spans. That area had no doctors, hospitals or any type of health service. The boundaries are roughly from 36th Street North, north to 86th Street North and from just west of Peoria Avenue to North 100 West Avenue.

A patchwork system of mobile medical units and health clinics in stores and schools sprouted to meet the need. These included OU-Tulsa with a Sooner Schooner II mobile health clinic, OSU Health Sciences Center with a Dr. Pete mobile telemedicine clinic and Wal-Mart stores with several Redi-Clinics.

"I can tell you that the initial response to our clinics was that we are meeting a need. The clinics provide more access and more affordability for our customers. We don't look at our clinics as a replacement for primary care, but as a supplement," said Wal-Mart spokeswoman Deisha Galberth, *Tulsa World*, May 22, 2008.

Good Samaritan Health Services was another mobile health unit providing care to the underserved in Tulsa. The medical mission was founded in 1999 by Tulsa physicians Drs. John Crouch and Mitch Duininck, who were affiliated with the Oral Roberts University Medical School before it closed. By 2014, the mobile mission had expanded to three trucks serving about 650 people a month in primary care and chronic disease management. The 74126 ZIP code was among the consistent stops made by the mission.

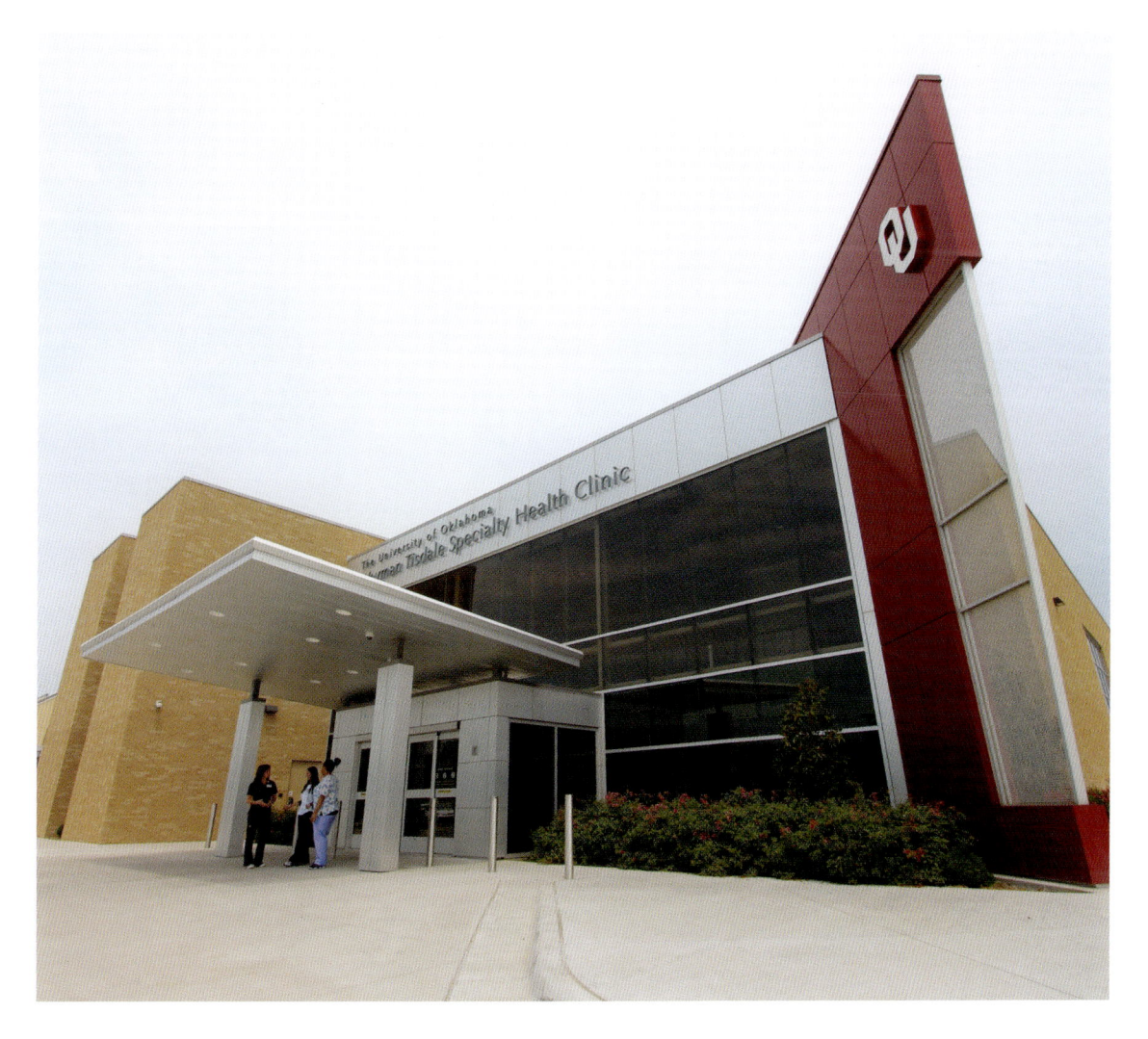

The University of Oklahoma Wayman Tisdale Specialty Health Clinic.

"That particular ZIP code has the ignominious reputation of being the worst ZIP code for premature death. Much of that we understand is because of their limited access to health care. We are overwhelmed in Tulsa. We don't have a hospital for the indigent. Hospitals are so glutted with indigent patients. In all of our locations, we're seeing a large number of working poor and a growing number of people from rural areas. Many are embarrassed to come. What health care resources we do have become overwhelmed very quickly. The need is great," said Lynn Hersey, operations manager for Good Samaritan Health Services, *Tulsa World*, May 22, 2008.

While these were credited for helping provide some medical care, officials warned it was not a replacement for a primary care physician or well-equipped facilities.

Dr. John Crouch and the Good Samaritan Mobile Unit.

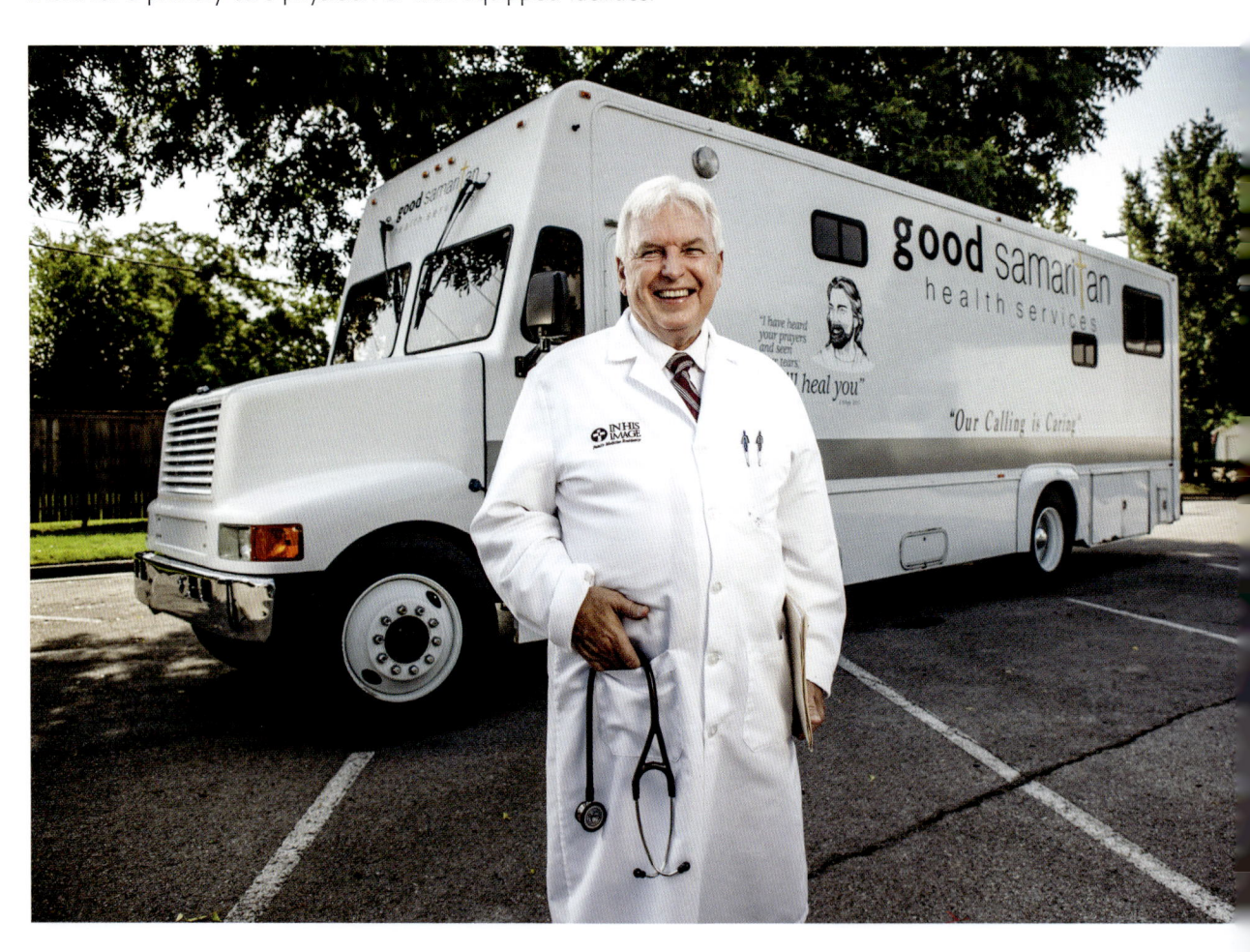

"Mini-clinics certainly play a role in acute care. It's not a bad fix. These short-term clinics really don't have a role in helping with the long-term care of chronic patients," said Dr. Gerald Clancy, president of the OU-Tulsa Medical College, *Tulsa World*, May 22, 2008.

To address the disparity, several steps were taken.

In August 2012, OU Wayman Tisdale Specialty Clinic opened at 36th Street North and Hartford Avenue. The $20 million facility was to give residents access to specialties and locate more physicians in the area. It is named after the Booker T. Washington High School standout, who went on to become a college basketball star at OU and played 12 years in the NBA. Returning to Tulsa, Tisdale then embarked on a music career, becoming a renowned jazz musician. He died in 2009 due to complications of cancer. Half the clinic's funding came from public sources: $6 million from the Oklahoma Legislature and $4 million from the Oklahoma City-based University Hospitals Authority and Trust. About $10 million in private funding was donated by the George Kaiser Family Foundation, the Morningside Healthcare Foundation, Saint Francis Health System, St. John Health System, the Anne and Henry Zarrow Foundation and the Helmerich Foundation.

By March 2014, it had added 11 specialty services and saw about 1,000 patients a month, with demand growing. That month, construction began on a $1.8 million expansion for 20 more exam rooms to accommodate 200 to 300 more patients. It included a 1,500 square-foot education center, which opened in December 2014. It houses the Wayman Tisdale Foundation, which was established to focus on health education and help people afford prosthetics. The foundation was inspired by Tisdale after his right leg was amputated in 2008 due to complications of bone cancer and after he was fitted with a prosthetic. He wanted the foundation to assist others unable to afford the technology. The center also houses his memorabilia.

"We ought to measure ourselves not by military power, economic power, but also by the power of

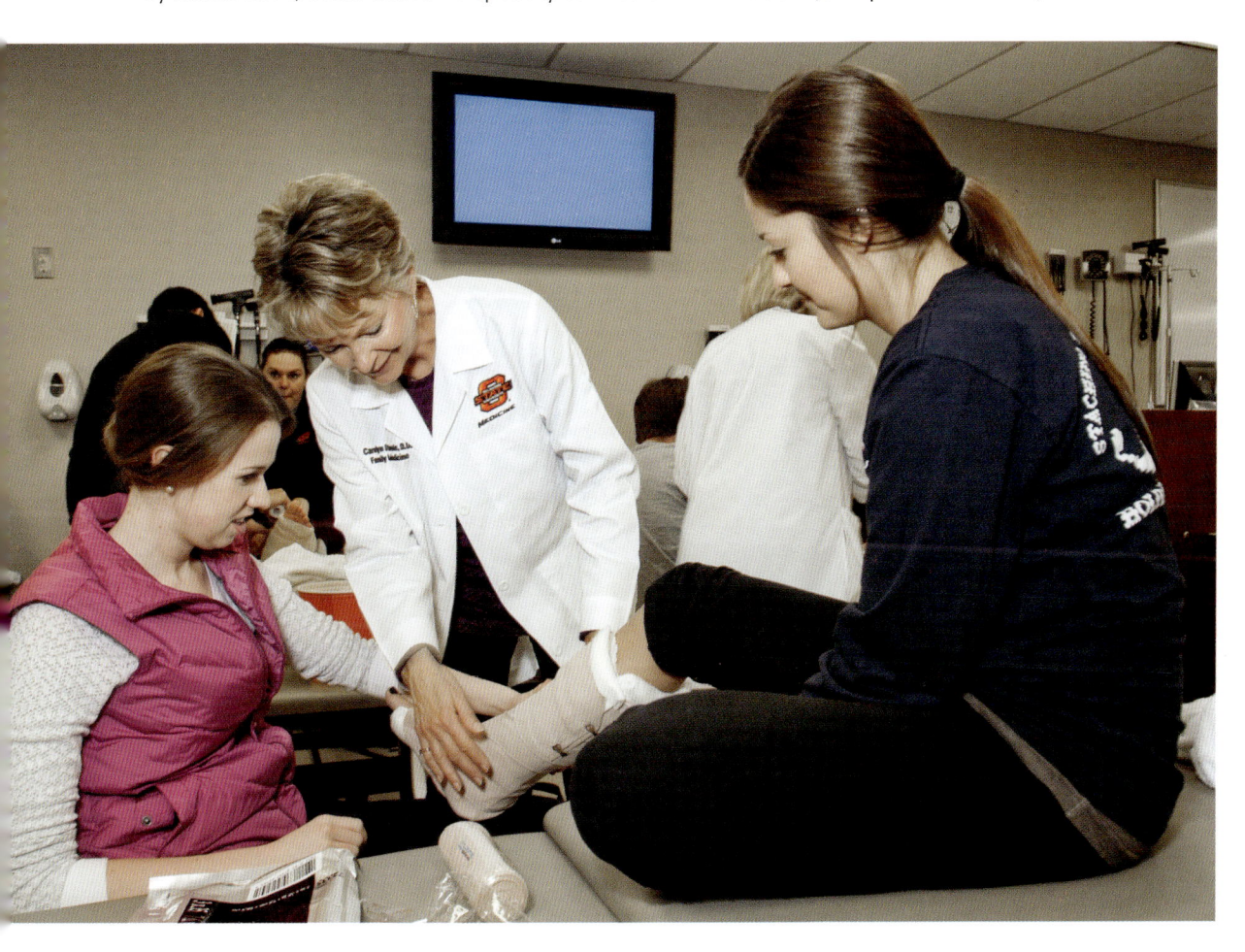

OSU-CHS Casting Lab.

kindness. How we treat each other reveals as much or more about ourselves than anything else. That's what's so special about this clinic," said OU President David Boren at the clinic's dedication, *Tulsa World*, Dec. 3, 2013.

In total, more than $46 million in public and private funds were spent in health-care facilities in north Tulsa. In addition to the OU Wayman Tisdale Specialty Health Clinic, other new or expanded facilities were, $15 million in Vision 2025 funds for Morton Comprehensive Health Services, $10 million for the Tulsa Health Department's North Regional Health and Wellness Center as well as investments in Crossover Health Services and the Hutcherson YMCA.

OSU Telemedicine Bus.

Within 10 years, north Tulsa had the Wayman Tisdale's Specialty Clinic, Westview Pediatric Clinic, Crossover Clinic, Greenwood Healthcare Specialists for Women, Hillcrest Pregnancy Center and Catholic Charities.

The University of Tulsa announced in 2015 its inaugural class of the Albert Schweitzer Fellowship, which is a national program to develop future leaders in health through service projects addressing the root causes of health disparities. Tulsa was the 14th city to host the fellowship program.

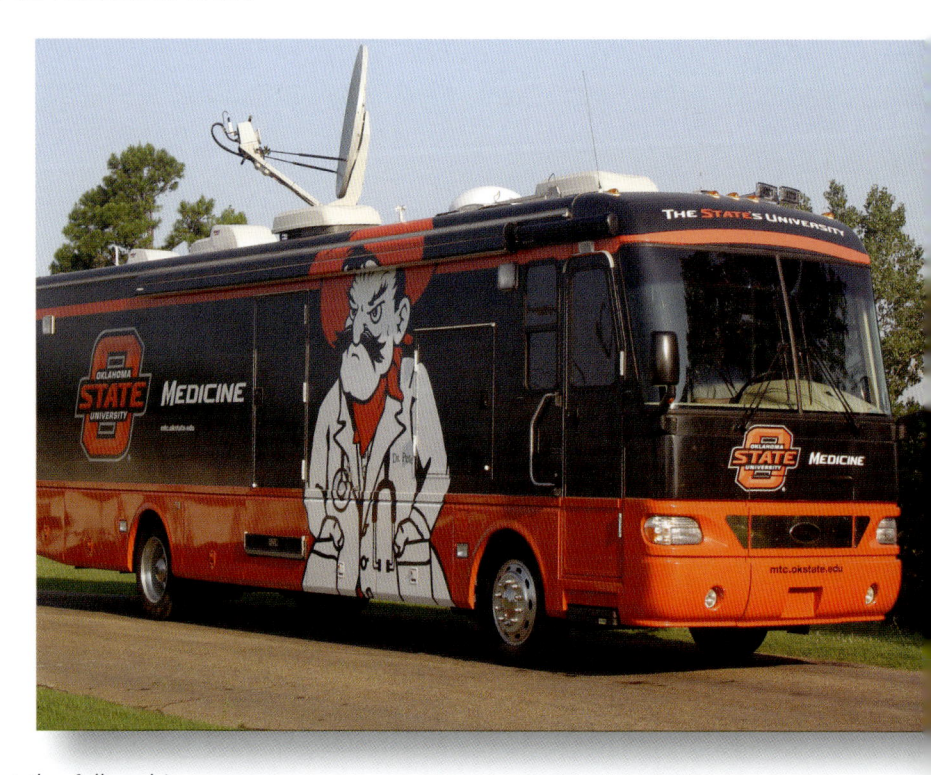

The fellows were named from TU, OU, OU-Tulsa and the OSU Center for Health Sciences. The class included aspiring physicians, clinical psychologists, occupational therapists and social workers. The projects last one year. Among the first projects were teaching weekly nutrition education classes at low-income schools, assisting Latino patients to manage chronic diseases, helping veterans reintegrate into society and connecting patients to community resources.

"When the year is over, our goal is to have a cohort of professionals who are committed to addressing health inequities in Tulsa. The other dream for the program is that our fellows are well-versed in the specific issues addressing various populations in Tulsa and that they have the relationships that they need to continue to address those issues. We're mostly looking for individuals who are deeply interested in understanding health inequities in Tulsa and have a real drive to do something about them," said Rachel Gold, director of the Tulsa fellowship chapter, *Tulsa World*, March 12, 2016.

The first class included Tim Nissen, Danielle Zanotti, Vanessa Garcia, James Scholl, Shannon McBeath,

Michael Sutton, Zach Giano, Olivia Shadid, Meredith Wyatt, Paul Abbey and LaTasha Lucas.

The Tulsa City-County Health Department, in partnership with OU-Tulsa and the George Kaiser Family Foundation, followed up on the Lewin report. In September 2015, the "Narrowing the Gap" report found the efforts had decreased the gap between the worst and best ZIP codes for life expectancy from 13.8 years to 10.7 years. On one end of the spectrum was 74126 with a median household income of $25,191 and life expectancy of 69.7 years. The other end was 74137 with a median household income of $81,322 and a life expectancy of 80.4 years.

The 74137 boundary runs from South 81st Street to South 121st Street and Sheridan Avenue west to the Arkansas River.

"This was a multi-sector response to the fact that we have this huge disparity in the city of Tulsa and Tulsa County... that what ZIP code you live in had a great impact on how long you actually live. When you have a 14-year gap, I think everyone found that reprehensible and unacceptable," said Bruce Dart, executive director of the Tulsa Health Department, *Tulsa World*, Sept. 3, 2015.

The report examined all ZIP codes in the county and found improvements in 16 counties, with the greatest jump in the 74126.

"Almost everywhere in Tulsa, including the best ZIP code, mortality stayed about the same over 10 years, so obviously everything we've done in that ZIP code has made a difference," said Monica Basu, senior program officer with the George Kaiser Family Foundation, *Tulsa World*, Sept. 3, 2015.

The efforts brought about a public awareness of other societal issues.

"The No. 1 reason a patient doesn't get to me is not because they forget. It's because of transportation issues. There are a lot of communities that wouldn't want to talk about this. They'd try to push it to the side because it doesn't look good. Instead, everyone responded to it and there was a willingness to act," said Dr. Gerald Clancy, dean of the TU College of Health Sciences and vice president of health affairs and former president of OU-Tulsa Medical College, *Tulsa World*, Sept. 3, 2015.

By July 2016, efforts to lessen the disparity were extended to social determinants of health. The Tulsa City-County Health Department launched an initiative to bring together entities to work on a plan with measurable outcomes to address economic sustainability, education, social cohesion and neighborhood and environmental conditions.

"We realize that when you're trying to improve the health of a community that ensuring the residents have access to health-care services and primary care is a slice of the pie, but it probably accounts for 10 to 15 percent for what is truly needed for the community, so you have to look at these other factors. Ultimately, we want to create a culture of health where individuals have everything they need within the confines of the community they live," said Reggie Ivey, Tulsa Health Department chief operating officer, *Tulsa World*, July 5, 2016.

Rise of Physician Assistant and Nurse Practitioners

One of the side effects of health-care reform was the growing need for more mid-level practitioners such as nurse practitioners and physician assistants. These health-care providers work alongside physicians in the daily work. Physician assistants can prescribe certain medications, and some states allow for the same responsibilities as doctors.

The Affordable Care Act included physician assistants in the definition of primary care doctors. The law encouraged innovative health-care delivery, often emphasizing a team-based approach. In 2010, Oklahoma had about 1,100 physician assistants, who made about 3.6 million visits the previous year. The largest specialty — at about 95 percent — was in emergency medicine.

Physician assistants receive the same training as a doctor, but less time in that training. Usually, a PA gets about 30 months of post-graduate education before joining a practice or hospital. Doctors often instruct patients to treat PAs as physicians. PAs can spend more time with patients to establish relationships, giving more access to health-care providers.

"They're absolutely invaluable as a partner. I look at them as an extension of my practice," said Dr. Charles Foulks, chairman of the department of internal medicine at the OU-Tulsa School of Community Medicine, *Tulsa World*, Feb. 2, 2014.

Nurses got concerned about what was viewed as an attempt to restrict patient access. The Coalition for Patients Rights was an advocacy group formed to promote the work nurses could do outside the direct supervision of doctors. Oklahoma had about 900 nurse practitioners in 2011, and most had a doctorate. About 90 percent of all nurse practitioners accept Medicare and Medicaid, and about 20 percent practice in rural areas.

"We are actually trained to provide care across the spectrum. We all collaborate and talk about patients and what we need to do. And that's where health care needs to go. We need physicians, we need PAs, we need nurse practitioners to take care of all the sick people in Oklahoma," said Mindy Whitten, a nurse practitioner at the Warren Clinic and legislative chair for Oklahoma Nurse Practitioners, *Tulsa World*, Oct. 3, 2011.

Heart Hospital Emerges

In 2008, the Oklahoma Heart Institute became part of the Hillcrest Medical Center in its plan to construct the largest freestanding hospital in the state dedicated to cardiovascular services. The 181,100-square foot, 104-bed Hillcrest Heart Pavilion opened in January 2009 near 11th Street and Utica Avenue. The heart institute had practiced at Hillcrest since 1986 as a separate entity.

The $64 million Hillcrest Heart Pavilion houses all of Hillcrest's cardiovascular services, including a cardiovascular diagnostic center, a 24-bed cardiovascular intensive care unit, a heart failure center and an education center.

By 2012, the heart institute expanded to Hillcrest Hospital South, Hillcrest Hospital Claremore and Bailey Medical Center in Owasso. It had maintained its relationship with SouthCrest Hospital.

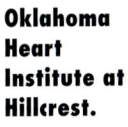

Oklahoma Heart Institute at Hillcrest.

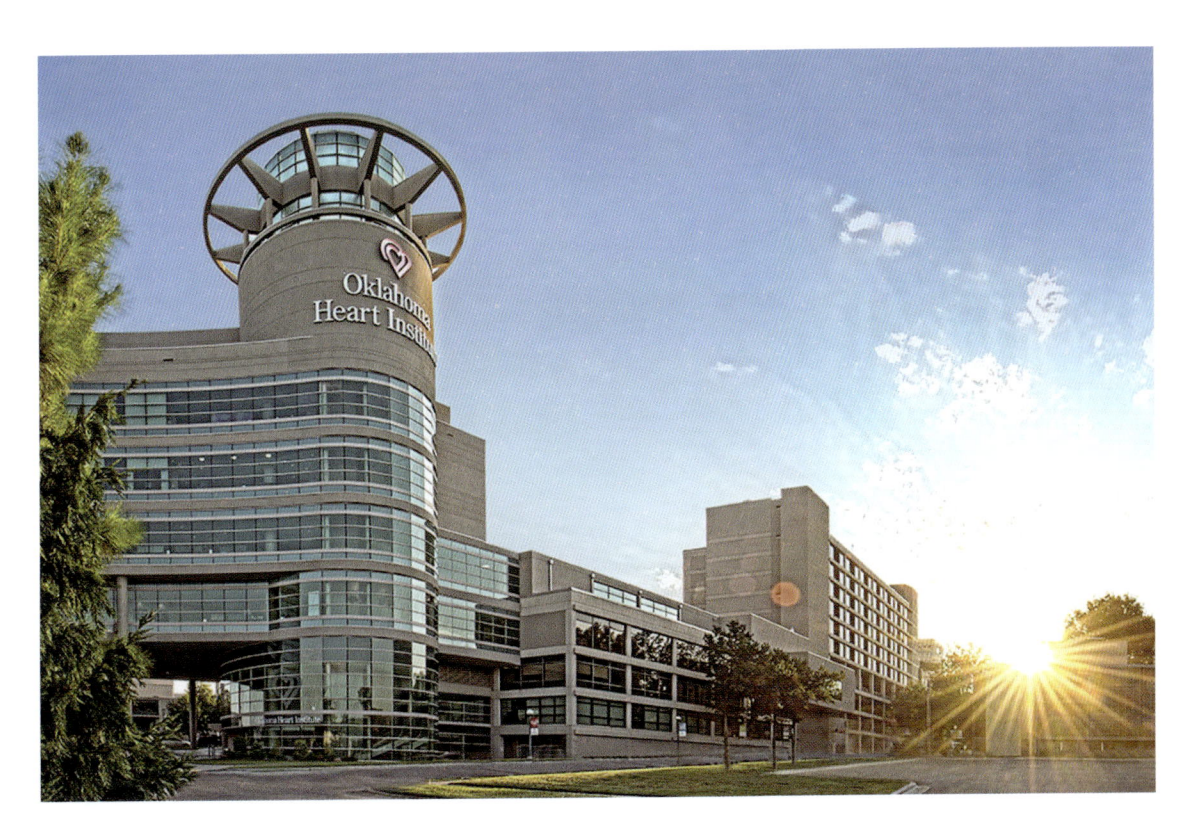

"It will be the largest cardiovascular MRI center in the country. We will have a large prevention program and the latest imaging, which allows less invasive diagnostic testing. Nobody should have to leave Tulsa to get the best cardiac care available," said Oklahoma Heart Institute president Dr. Wayne N. Leimbach, *Tulsa World*, April 22, 2008.

Advancements in technology led to a cardiology renaissance, particularly as it related to patients who had multiple heart surgeries or were unable to survive invasive procedures. New tools, such as 3-D mapping, allowed surgeons to navigate through blood vessels and the heart making surgery possible. Ablation therapy helped doctors isolate pathways causing hearts to skip or produce extra beats to determine the cause. The Impella catheter gave patients with only one functioning blood vessel an option other than a heart transplant. It is a type of mini heart pump that creates blood flow while blockages are cleared from the single blood vessel. People suffering from blood clots could be treated with the Trellis catheter rather than traditional blood thinners. The catheter removed clots by inflating balloons on either side and vacuuming it away.

The Oklahoma Heart Institute was the area's first hospital to offer the Transcatheter Aortic Valve Replacement procedure for those living with diseased aortic valves once considered inoperable. This is targeted to people needing a heart valve replaced but cannot handle open heart surgery. Dr. Kamran Muhammad was recruited to Tulsa to perform those procedures.

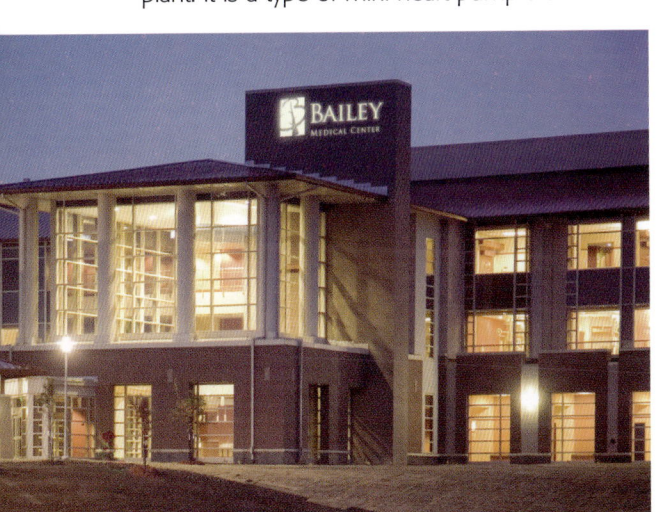

Bailey Medical Center in Owasso.

"You used to watch people die. Now you can do something for them," said Dr. Wayne N. Leimbach, co-founder of the heart institute, *Tulsa World*, Feb. 28, 2014.

In 2015, Oklahoma had the third-highest death rate due to cardiovascular diseases, and heart disease was the No. 1 killer of Oklahomans and stroke the fifth cause of death to state residents.

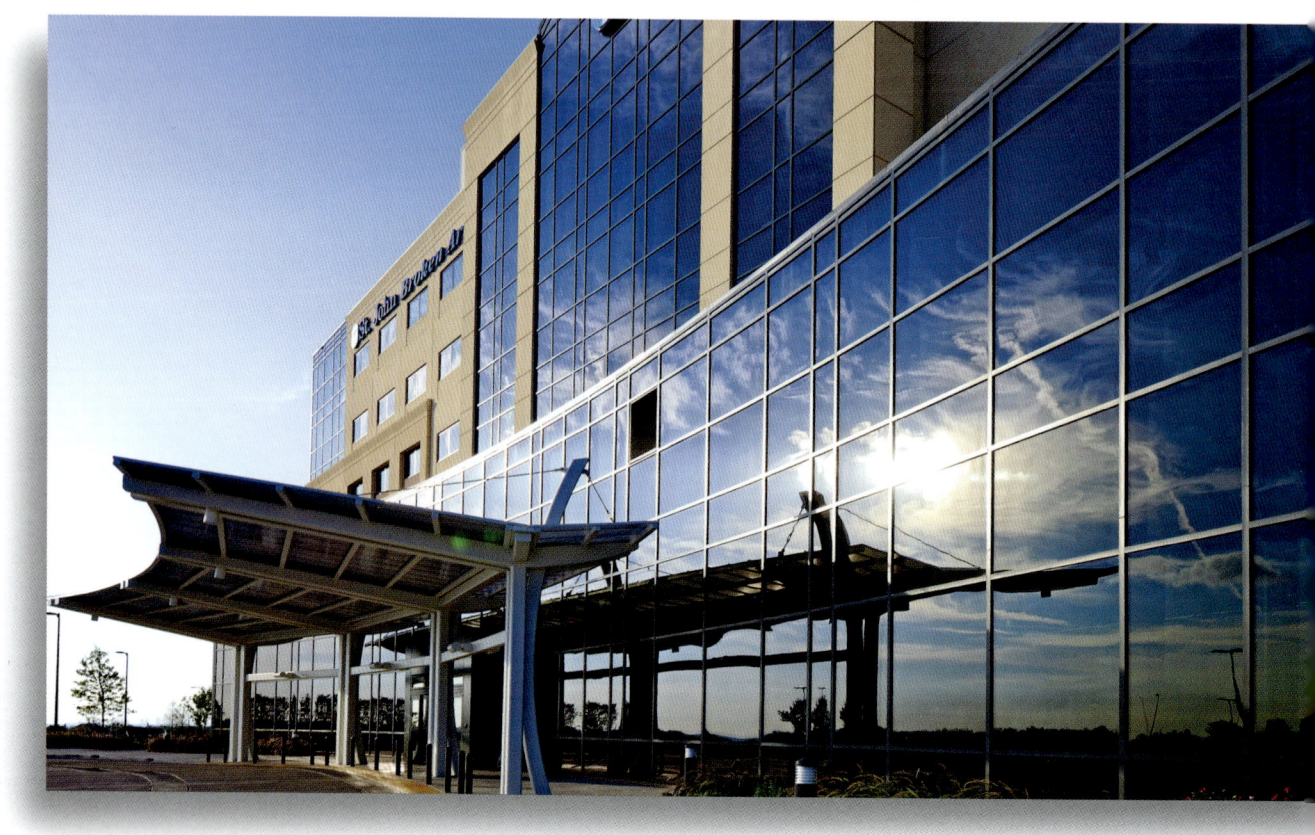

St. John Broken Arrow.

ADDITION OF PRIVATE, SPECIALTY HOSPITALS

While three hospitals dominated the Tulsa landscape — St. John Medical Center, Hillcrest Medical Center and Saint Francis Hospital — private facilities were created to fill in certain niches.

Oral Roberts University had been leasing space in its CitiPlex Towers, 2408 E. 81st St., since 1995. By 2001, Cancer Treatment Centers of America in Tulsa and Hillcrest Specialty Hospital were operating in the facility. In June 2001, Orthopedic Hospital of Oklahoma opened in 70,667-square-feet of newly constructed space in the building.

OHO Chief Executive Officer Don Burman said the hospital was created in response to patient demand. Local doctors invested into the launch of the institution that included a 22-physician founding board. The Board included orthopedic surgeons from Central States Orthopedic Specialists and Eastern Oklahoma Orthopedic Center, neurosurgeons Drs. John Marouk and Karl Detwiler and physicians from Associated Anesthesiologists.

About 150 staff — nurses, medical technicians, therapists and administrative employees — worked in the hospital. Reconstructive surgery, total hip and total knee replacement surgery, treatment of spinal disorders, sports medicine, repair of complex fractures and hand injuries and other orthopedic treatments were offered. It featured a therapeutic swimming pool and in-patient rehabilitation beds.

"We have a single-minded approach to orthopedic medicine. If that's all we do, then by definition we should see that expertise passed on to our patients," said OHO CEO Don Burman, *Tulsa World*, May 30, 2001.

The hospital expanded in 2006 with the addition of 10 general surgeons and again in January 2008 when Urologic Specialists of Oklahoma joined. In March 2007, it changed its name to Oklahoma Surgical Hospital.

In 2002, Tulsa Spine and Specialty Hospital opened at 6901 S. Olympia Ave., which was north of a budding new development between U.S. 75 and the Arkansas River. The 80,000 square-foot facility was built on 54 acres to accommodate future growth. The 21-bed facility focused on elective surgeries to fix medical issues such as ruptured disks, degenerative arthritis of the spine, slipping vertebrae and spine tumors.

Investors included 12 pain-management doctors and neurosurgeons. It employed 65 people including nurses, aides, scrub technicians, radiology personnel and housekeeping. The caseload for a nurse was up to four patients.

"We can offer a level of attention, care and empathy that the big hospitals are having trouble giving," said Dr. David Fell, neurosurgeon and one of the hospital's founders, *Tulsa World*, Sept. 22, 2002.

Critics of the private hospital trend argued that those would admit only insured patients who need profitable elective operations, which left full-service hospitals with uninsured patients and expensive procedures. Founders of these institutions countered by saying the competition forced large hospitals to compete on price and service.

"It's good for the businesses who have to pay for health care and good for patients because they can get more specialized care more economically," Fell said. "It's just bad for the big hospitals because they have to learn to compete." — Dr. David Fell, *Tulsa World*, Sept. 22, 2002.

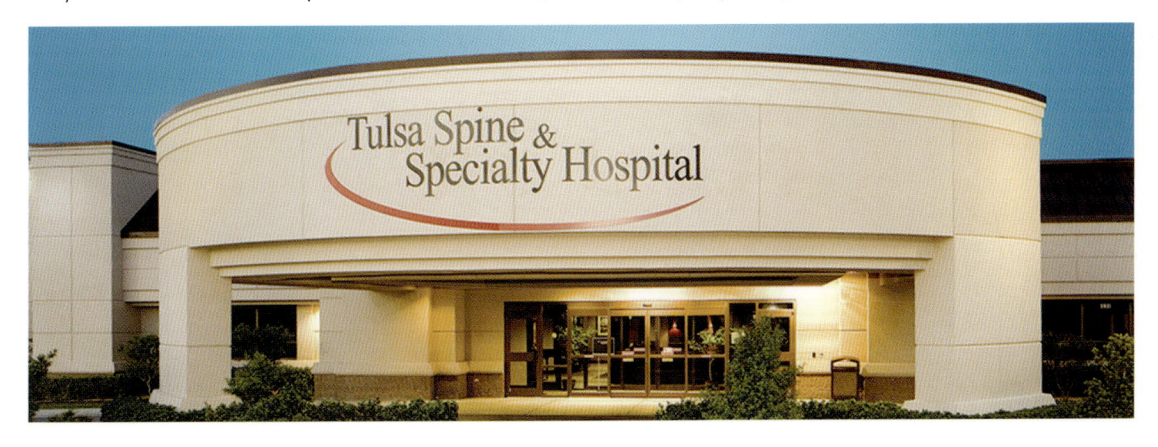

Tulsa Spine and Specialty Hospital.

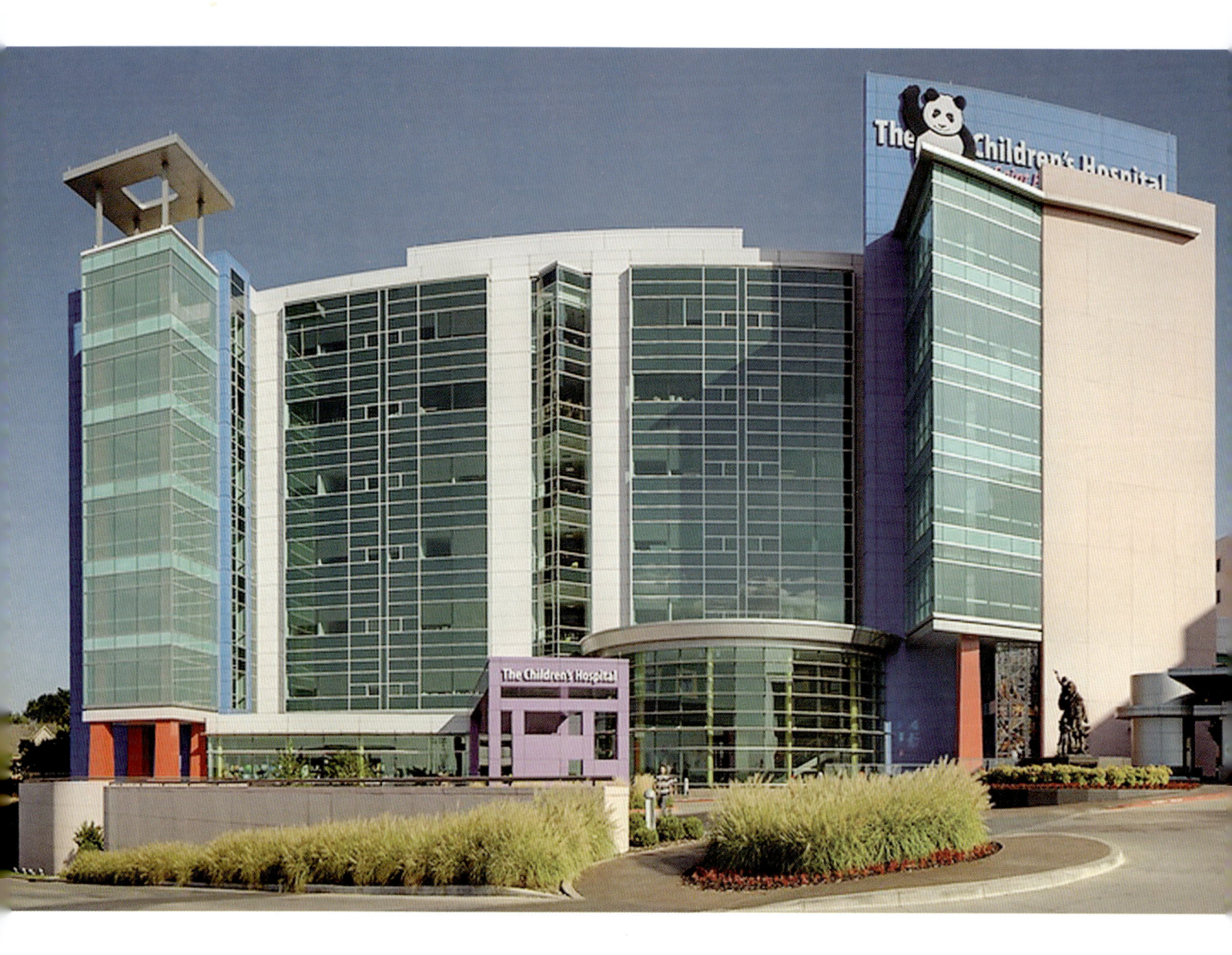

Saint Francis, The Children's Hospital.

Birth of the Children's Hospital

For decades, children received specialty care scattered at different hospitals and facilities. In 2000, a group of Tulsa pediatricians emerged to change that system to find a home for a comprehensive children's hospital. The Tulsa Coalition for Children's Health formed as an advocacy group, attracting support and dues from nearly all the city's 100 pediatricians. Dr. Dawn Mayberry served as president for the organization. She said the motive for the hospital was to increase the quality of care for children. A hospital would centralize services, attract subspecialists and encourage research.

A first round of discussions with the hospitals found support but no interest in being the home for such a facility. A grant paid for an assessment of children's services by the Katz Consulting Group.

"It told us we had a unique pediatric community. We had private doctors, had academic doctors and some were hired by institutions. We had a very different model. Most cities had academic doctors at a freestanding children's hospital associated with a university. It also showed our population was big enough to support most subspecialists. It validated what we knew," said Dr. Dawn Mayberry, interview, July 25, 2016.

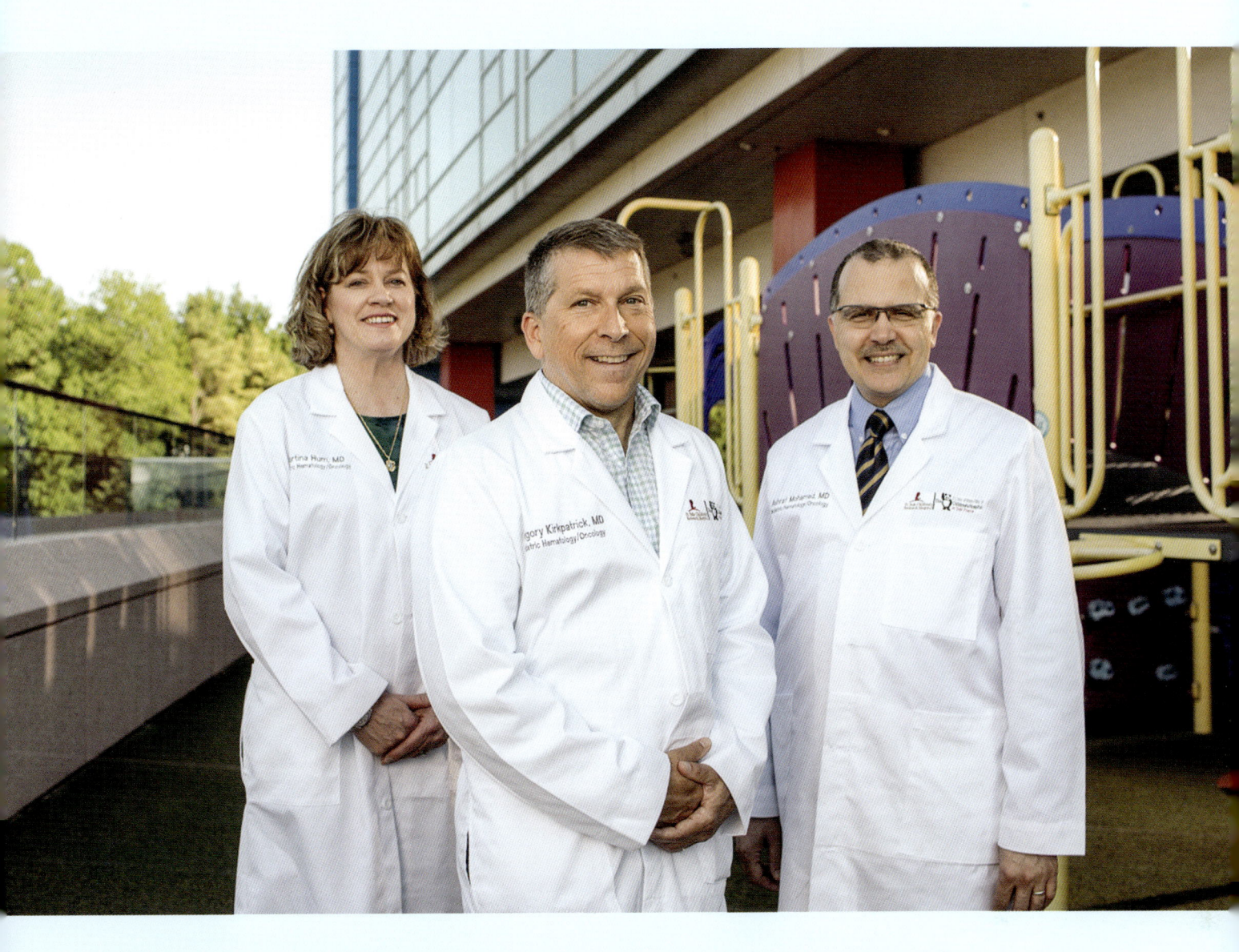

While the assessment was being conducted, a change in administration occurred at Saint Francis Hospital. A meeting in 2003 between representatives of the Tulsa Coalition for Children's Health and Jake Henry Jr., president and CEO, and John-Kelly Warren, chairman of the board, ended with promise for a possible new facility.

"It was a whole different atmosphere from Saint Francis, and we discussed the model of a children's hospital within a hospital rather than a freestanding hospital. (Henry) felt like we had unity in the pediatric community for this, and that gave them more incentive to move forward," said Dr. Dawn Mayberry, interview, July 25, 2016.

Saint Francis officials worked with OSU Center for Health Sciences and OU-Tulsa to ensure pediatric residents would be at the new hospital. The children's coalition group worked with hospital officials to determine what types of specialists and procedures were most in need.

In February 2005, Saint Francis broke ground for a $56 million children's hospital located on the north-

The Children's Hospital at Saint Francis, St. Jude Oncologists.

> **"The Children's Hospital at Saint Francis is the first St. Jude Children's Research Hospital affiliation in Oklahoma and the most western location."**

east side of the existing hospital. It had its own parking garage and entrance off 61st Street. The 104-bed, 155,000-square-foot, five-story facility opened in 2007.

Unlike the rest of the hospital's pink facade, it had a more modern glass design by the Ritchie Organization and featured a panda on the exterior. The design of the rooms kept families in mind, equipping them with space for parent overnight stays, access to showers, coffee makers and refrigerators.

"Having the family there and involved in a child's care is important to getting well. Older hospitals didn't take into account families staying with children and being part of their treatment plan," said Dr. William Banner, director of The Children's Hospital, *Tulsa World*, Feb. 8, 2005.

In August 2014, the pediatric services expanded as part of the hospital's $206 million in projects for the entire facility. It included a pediatric emergency center with 25 treatment rooms, separate waiting rooms and entrances, and child-friendly lighting and decorations. It had a heated and covered ambulance bay with space for 14 ambulances and a room for EMSA staff to take a break or fill out and file reports.

In May 2016, St. Jude Children's Research Hospital announced it would house its eighth national affiliate clinic in Tulsa through a partnership with The Children's Hospital at Saint Francis. The Children's Hospital had already been providing care for childhood cancers and other life-threatening diseases. The clinic would bring the St. Jude research and resources to the physicians practicing at the hospital. This was the first St. Jude affiliation in Oklahoma and the most western location.

Children receiving treatment at the St. Jude Affiliate Clinic at The Children's Hospital fall under its funding model. Families will never receive a bill from St. Jude for treatment or related travel, housing or food. Another benefit for patients is the access to research. Children will have less waiting time for cutting-edge treatment. Research from St. Jude laboratories will go directly to its patients. It took a nearly 2-year vetting process for the Memphis, Tennessee-based facility to make the decision.

"This is not an in-name-only affiliation. It is not a marketing agreement so we can put a marquee that might suggest more than it produces. Indeed, our clinic is now an extension of the world leader in pediatric cancer research and treatment right here in Tulsa, in northeastern Oklahoma. It's a fairly selective process. There are only seven other affiliate clinics, so we feel honored to be chosen to be one. It gets the most cutting-edge care into this community at a much faster rate," said Jake Henry Jr., president and CEO of Saint Francis Health System, *Tulsa World*, May 20, 2016.

St. Jude is credited for improving the worldwide childhood cancer survival rates from 20 percent in the 1960s — when it was started — to about 80 percent in 2016.

"I think this affiliation will be a game-changer for pediatric cancer care in the state of Oklahoma," said Jake Henry Jr., *Tulsa World*, May 20, 2016.

CHAPTER 12

(Epilogue - The Future)

Forcasting the Future of Medical Care

Artistic Illustration of a Density Map of the Enzyme B-galactosidase.

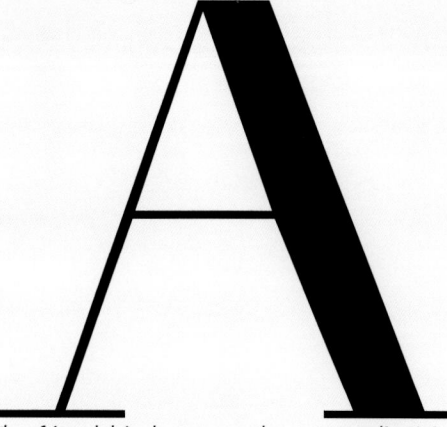

At lunch one day in June 2016 at a Tulsa retirement home, 86-year-old Dr. James Coldwell was visiting 90-year-old Dr. Robert "Bob" Endres, handing him the latest copy of the *Journal of Clinical Lipidology*.

"Oh, I got that one," said Dr. Endres.

The two then spoke about an article in another journal on the latest brain research among Alzheimer's patients.

"Since I've been here, I've had more interest in the aging brain," Dr. Endres said with a laugh.

The friendship between the two pediatricians started more than 60 years earlier at Washington University Children's Hospital in St. Louis, where the Oklahoma natives met and completed their medical training in pediatrics.

Dr. Endres returned to Tulsa and spent his career in the Tulsa Children's Clinic private practice. Dr. Coldwell followed a few years later to serve as chief of pediatrics at Children's Medical Center, which cared for children with special health needs.

"He has more knowledge of most of the weird stuff in town. If there is a strange disease, Jim will know it," said Dr. Endres.

When the two started their pediatric work in Tulsa, only about 18 pediatricians were practicing in the city. They spoke of that time being a tight community of doctors. This group formed the Oklahoma chapter of the American Academy of Pediatrics, electing Dr. Dick Russell to represent the state at the national convention in 1978. The organization published "The OK Pediatrician" newsletter and started a pediatric colloquy attracting national speakers to Tulsa.

"The changes taking place in medicine today rely on having the backing of an institution. The old-time doctor who is on call, goes to the ER, stitches up lacerations and holds office hours is all gone. Now, you are an office doctor, subspecialist or pediatrician at a hospital or institution. It's totally different. That's not a bad thing though," said Dr. Coldwell.

"But, research and treatment of some of the rare diseases is vitally important. The maintenance of such programs is impossible without better funding and support from large institutions. We were doing that at Children's Medical Center and did good work."

The doctors share an unending natural curiosity about medical science. Their conversation is not so much about the past but about modern and future possibilities. They recall when only three pediatric subspecialties existed — hematology, neonatology and cardiology.

"Now there are more than 20 pediatric subspecialties. That's where we're going," said Dr. Endres.

What lies ahead in Tulsa County medicine will come from the forward-thinking minds of doctors, physician assistants, nurses and others invested in finding a better health-care system.

Dr. Dawn Mayberry, a pediatrician, was in the generation after the retired doctors and was a founder of the Tulsa Coalition for Children's Health, which sought a children's hospital. She sees the rise of telemedicine to reach rural and under-served populations as a plus for health care.

"If we can't bring in people with specialties to areas, then we need to be more aggressive in telemedicine. We can sit at a computer with a patient in Tulsa and have a consultation with an expert in Houston for advisement. This creates more of a partnership," said Dr. Mayberry.

"The technological advances in surgery have been huge. The pharmaceuticals have become better and more effective. There are going to be more options and more awareness among the public."

Dr. Rachel Gibbs, obstetrician and gynecologist, steered her career away from delivering babies and into robotic surgery. A device like the da Vinci robot helps physicians treat conditions from cancer to heart disease. The physician sits at a nearby computer console — rather than at the operating table — to view real-time images of the patient. Robotic arms, one with a camera, manipulate the instruments guided by the nearby physician.

This eliminates physician fatigue during surgery; the instruments have a wider range of motion; visibility with 3-D imaging is better; and the less invasive procedure significantly cuts down on recovery time. The incisions are smaller, resulting in less blood loss and pain.

"It's a different mindset," said Dr. Gibbs. "You depend on your scrub nurse and surgical assistants at the bedside. It's more of a team approach rather than the doctor doing things separately."

These types of tools are making more surgeries available on an outpatient basis, said Dr. Gibbs. The advancements of early detection and diagnosis are making treatments more effective. Vaccines, such as Gardasil, may lead to great reductions in cancer in the coming decades, she said.

Simulated Surgery Using the da Vinci Robot Technology.

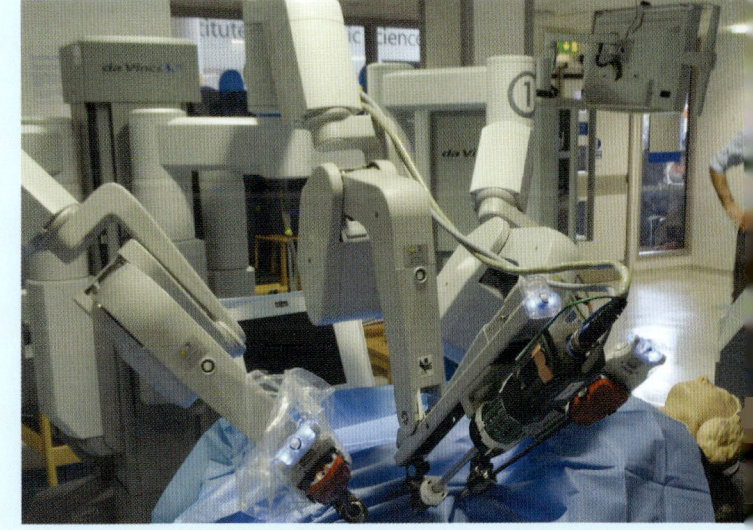

Retired neurosurgeon, Dr. David Fell, said his 1970s medical school training was heavy on diagnostic education. During his career at Neurosurgery Specialists in Tulsa, neuroimaging advanced with tools including CAT (computerized axial tomography) scans, PET (positron emission tomography) scans, MRI (magnetic resonance imagining) and the functional MRI. It shifted neuroscience medicine from figuring out what was wrong with a patient to finding better treatments and surgical techniques.

These types of jumps in knowledge and technology are reasons physicians and medical professionals engage in life-long learning.

"I had a doctor in medical school say, 'If you do the same operation the same way three years later, you are not evolving,'" said Dr. Fell. "There is a trend toward relying solely on imaging studies to make a diagnosis, and neglect of the taking of a good history and performing a careful physical examination."

The approach of integrating mind, body and spirit into health care will become more common, said Dr. Mitch Duininck, of Family Medical Care of Tulsa and president and director of In His Image Family Residency.

By knowing and addressing a patient's faith and physical needs, doctors can be more effective in practicing medicine, he said. It gets to the mental-health aspect of care.

"In the past, doctors would call a chaplain. Why not say to patients that a doctor is willing to pray with them? That's part of who the patient is," said Dr. Duininck. "It's not only about medicine and nutrition, but also counseling and the way a person practices his or her faith. It's a spiritual way. God touches people, and that's a whole-person approach to medicine. To me, medicine is more than going to pills, it's about the whole person."

Dr. Duininck has been part of many international mission trips with other Tulsa physicians, often in dangerous countries. He believes Tulsa will continue to have international medical missions to these Third World and disaster-ravaged regions.

"We consider it a calling. We are not doing this for the danger or adrenaline rush. People are in need and don't have medical care. We believe God loves everyone, and we know we are representing Tulsa when serving in these places," he said.

Through the efforts of Good Samaritan, which is the domestic mission arm of In His Image, pockets of poverty and uninsured in Tulsa are also receiving medical care. He believes community efforts will continue to bridge the gap of health disparities.

"It's unique in the way Tulsa is a very giving community," said Dr. Duininck.

Customer service will be emphasized in health-care delivery, said Dr. Kenneth Muckala, founder of Harvard Family Physicians. Aspects such as patient satisfaction surveys will become an important part of practices and institutions.

"That is from how we greet patients at the front desk to the bedside manners of doctors," said Dr. Muckala. "It's how we spend time. It's not about the amount of time that is spent, but it's the way the time is spent. It's a change in how quality of care is measured."

Retired physician, Dr. George Caldwell, said the lessons of the past can be a guide to the ongoing changes in health-care delivery. Dr. Caldwell was instrumental in establishing urgent care clinics and, as president of the Tulsa County Medical Society, passing legislation to protect patients and physicians.

"Any change we make has to be tied to access and quality to the patient. If it doesn't, we shouldn't have it," said Dr. Caldwell. "The bottom-line is always access and quality. We need to daily demonstrate that to the voting public."

Dr. Mitchell Duininck: Disaster Relief in Pakistan.

Back at the retirement home, Dr. Coldwell updates his old friend and fellow pediatrician about his latest work in the treatment of patients with phenylketonuria (PKU), which is a rare inherited condition resulting in a natural build-up of the protein phenylalanine. He continues to see patients who are newly diagnosed and those who have lived with the diseases for decades.

Just because a physician or nurse retires, doesn't mean the end of medical curiosity.

"If everybody and everything is alike, you don't learn. This gives a window to look through. It's a journey," said Dr. Coldwell.

Future Legacies

FUTURE LEGACIES

Tulsa County Medical Society

The Tulsa County Medical Society (TCMS) was established in 1907 as Oklahoma entered the union as the 46th state. Previously, the professional organization for physicians in the area was the Indian Territory Medical Association. In its nearly 110-year existence, the group has grown from a handful of doctors to more than 1,000 allopathic and osteopathic physicians and medical students.

Its mission: "To promote the art and science of medicine, foster ethical practices among members and unite the medical profession in promoting public health. To be the advocate for both physicians and patients, to support quality health care, to be a leader in health care reform and to sustain a continuing dialogue between the membership and the community in which we live and work."

Through the years, the organization has led countless projects to benefit the Tulsa community, ranging from aid in the aftermath of the 1921 race riot to the continued volunteerism in a drug distribution program for indigent patients.

TCMS provides administrative support for the specialty societies of The Oklahoma Section of the American Congress of Obstetricians and Gynecologists, the Oklahoma State Dermatology and Dermatological Surgery Society and the Tulsa County Obstetrical and Gynecological Society.

In 1931, The Alliance to the Tulsa County Medical Society was organized by Mrs. Hugh Graham. Members have been active volunteers at area nonprofits and raising funds for The Day Center for the Homeless, The Parent Child Center and the Tulsa County Medical Society Foundation.

The first major initiative by TCMS was the construction of St. John Hospital, which was a joint project with The Sisters of the Sorrowful Mother of New Jersey. Ground was broken in 1920 but the Depression delayed completion until 1926.

Members of TCMS decided to seek the creation of the nonprofit Blue Cross plan in 1940. Medical leaders in Oklahoma City and Tulsa agreed that $10,000 was needed to establish the hospital prepayment plan, and the city raising the money first would get the company headquarters. The office opened at the Tulsa Loan Building, 4th and Main streets, later that year. In 1945, the Blue Shield plan was created as a companion.

Polio became a public threat throughout the 50s and 60s, particularly for children. When the oral Sabin vaccine was made available, TCMS was among the leaders in a mass immunization project in 1963. Every member of the society participated. TCMS purchased $100,000 of the vaccine, and residents paid 25 cents per dose. No one was turned away, and some people paid more. In the end, the TCMS had a $104,000 surplus. Half the money was used to start a scholarship fund, and the rest was donated to charities.

When it came to medical education, TCMS hosted regular seminars, speakers, consortiums and other professional development opportunities. For nearly seven years, it also pushed for a medical school through a committee. The committee spent about $18,000 on a feasibility study, leading to the creation of the Tulsa Medical Education Foundation in 1971.

The foundation was formed with a board to include six members of TCMS and two each from Hillcrest Hospital, St. John Hospital, Saint Francis,

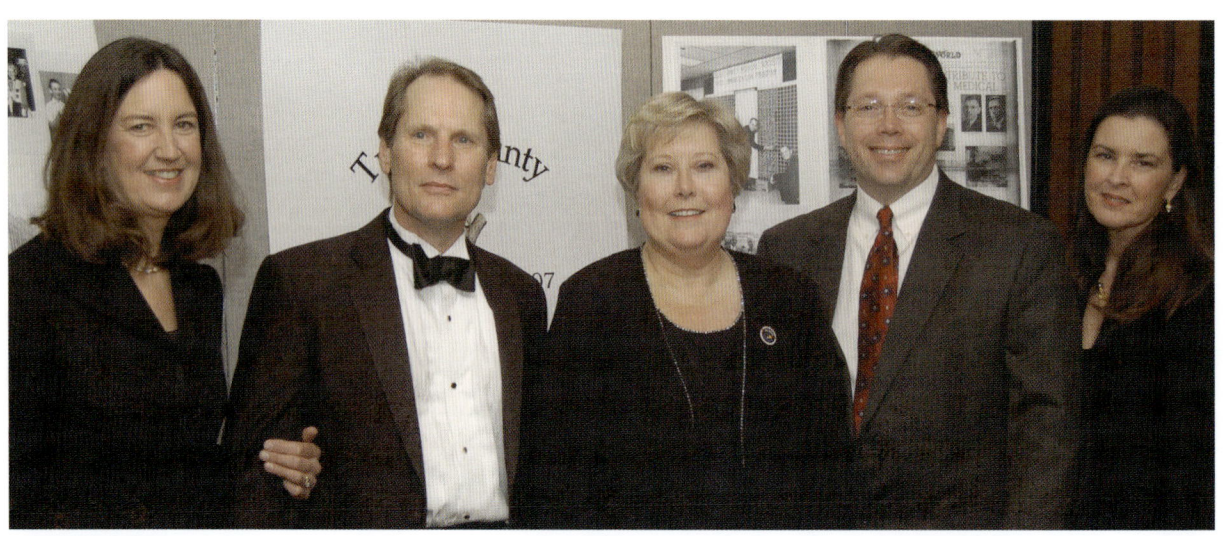

Kari Caldwell, Dr. George Caldwell (2007 TCMS president), Lt. Gov. Jari Askins, Dr. Daron Street (2006 TCMS president) and his wife, Debra Street.

FUTURE LEGACIES

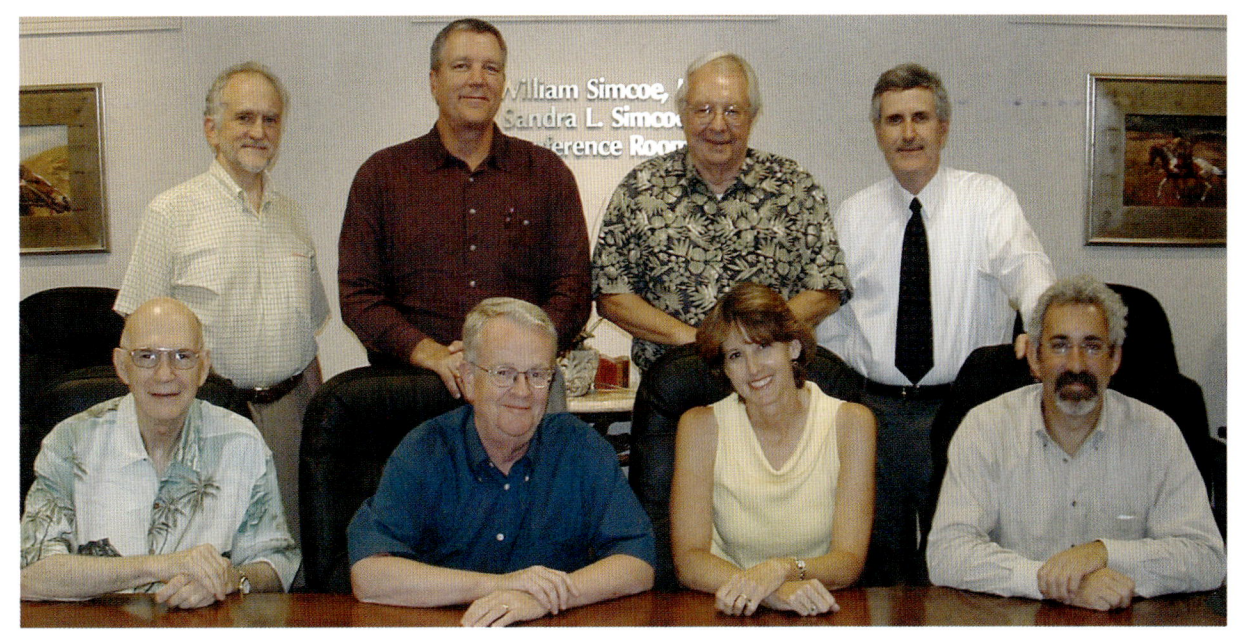

The TCMS Foundation Board members (seated from left) — Dr. Rollie Rhodes, Dr. John Minielly, Gail Gillock and Dr. David Nierenberg. (standing from left) — Dr. William Geffen, Dr. Lynn Frame, Dr. Gerald Gustafson and Dr. Brad Garber.

Doctors' Hospital and Children's Medical Center, two from Tulsa Chamber of Commerce and two from the University of Oklahoma Medical School. The following year, state law established a branch of the OU Medical School in Tulsa, where students could complete their final two years of training

In 1987, the TCMS Foundation, a tax-exempt, charitable organization was created to support the work of the organization.

Its mission: "Through the professional expertise and engagement of the Tulsa County Medical Society member physicians and Alliance, utilizing the prudent management of its resources, and with the help of donor funding, the Tulsa County Medical Society Foundation will develop, create and maintain programs in the Tulsa area designed for health promotion, health education, and disease prevention and treatment."

Starting in the late 80s, TCMS led discussions with the Oklahoma State Medical Association to open membership to osteopathic physicians. In 1998, the state bylaws were changed, and TCMS immediately began issuing memberships to osteopaths.

After 95 years, the TCMS started construction on its first permanent home.

From 1907 to 1937, it was located in the old Oklahoma Hospital, the Commercial Club, First National Bank, the Chamber of Commerce, the Ketchum Hotel, Municipal Hall (now the Brady Theater) and the Tulsa Hotel. From 1937 to 1963, the group was housed in the downtown Medical Arts Building then moved to the Utica Square Medical Center until 1986. Until the new home opened in October 2002, it was located on the fifth floor of the 2021 South Lewis Building.

The $1 million, two-story building at 5315 S. Lewis Ave. was built after 18 months of fundraising. A crucial part of the effort came from a 2-to-1 matching challenge for donations from former TCMS board president Dr. Wallace Hooser through his family's non-profit foundation.

TCMS launched the Recycled Medication program in 2004 after Dr. George Prothro, executive director of the Tulsa City-County Health Department sought a way to transfer unexpired, packaged medications from nursing homes to the county pharmacy for use to indigent patients. Oklahoma State University's Michael Lapolla led the research into the legality, cost savings benefits and model for such a program.

To allow for the program, state laws needed to change from the mandated disposal of unused medications. It took four legislative sessions and extensive discussions with nursing home owners, pharmaceutical suppliers, regulators, media and other groups to pass the necessary laws.

Once established, the Golden Oldies — a TCMS group of retired physicians and their wives — took charge of collecting the medications from long-term care, nursing facilities and delivering to the county pharmacy.

In 2012, the medication program reached the $10 million milestone after distributing 110,387 prescriptions to low-income Tulsa County residents. The amount is based on the average wholesale price. As part of the celebration, the county renamed the Tulsa County Pharmacy to the George Prothro, M.D., Pharmacy of Tulsa County. By December 2016, that value had climbed to more than $20 million and nearly 204,492 prescriptions distributed.

The most recent program established by the TCMS Foundation is Project TCMS, a program that coordinates referrals for non-emergent specialty care for

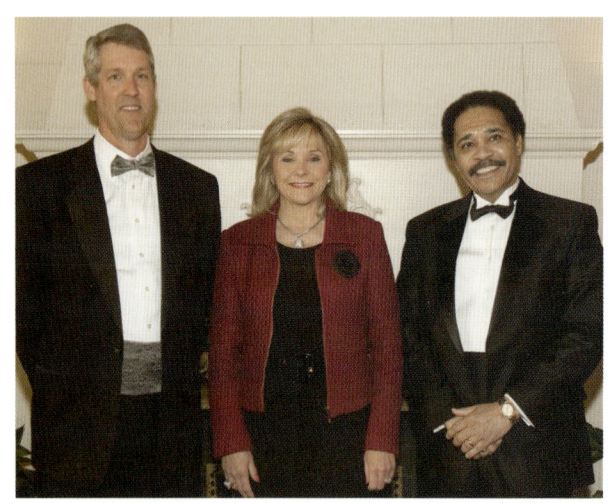

Dr. Jeffrey Galles (2011 TCMS president), Gov. Mary Fallin and Dr. David Harris (2010 TCMS president)

uninsured low income Tulsans. The program was developed in 2011 and implemented in April 2012. A total of over $3 million in donated care has been provided through the program, through a network of volunteers including 167 physicians, 12 hospital partners, 50+ healthcare vendors and 14 funding partners.

Dr. W. Albert Cook was the first TCMS president and a respected eye, ear, nose and throat physician based in the Medical Arts Building. He performed the first operation in Tulsa for cataracts, crossed eyes, mastoid and tonsils. In addition to his medical resume, he was also the first golf champion of Indian Territory and part of the Anti-Horse Thief Association.

The list of past presidents is an equally impressive roster of community leaders and advocates. The presidents were from different backgrounds and medical specialties, but they had as their central focus the advocacy for quality health care. This has been accomplished through legislative efforts and community education. Leaders recognize the need for a strong voice to promote the best practices and access to health care.

The presidents have worked in close concert with the executive directors of the organization: Lloyd Stone (1938-1941), Jack Spears (1941-1986), Paul Patton (1986-2008) and Mona Whitmire (2009 to present.) ∎

Oklahoma State Medical Association

The Oklahoma State Medical Association (OSMA) works hand-in-hand with the Tulsa County Medical Society. It is the statewide professional organization advancing physicians and advocating on public health issues of importance to their patients. Some 4,000 physicians, residents and medical students are members.

OSMA's physician leaders, staff and lobbyists promote pro-medicine policies to strengthen public health and improve our state's environment for physicians. They often thwart anti-medicine state and federal legislation and policy before it hits the public radar. When necessary, they rally physicians and the public to action, making the impact clear to those seeking to infringe on reimbursement, the scope of their practices or otherwise harmful measures. OSMA's proven intermediary services support physicians with insurance company challenges.

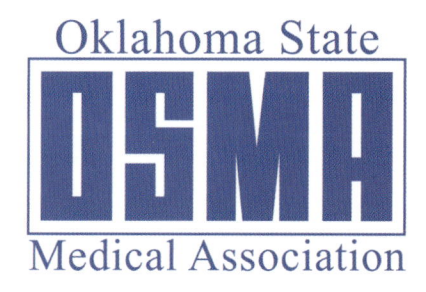

The Oklahoma State Medical Association also offers education and tools to physicians for leadership in their practice environments and medical community. Membership provides them continuing medical education (CME) at a cost well below market rates from the highest-rated source in the state (as accredited by the Accreditation Council on Continuing Medical Education). The latest to protect and advance their professions are also offered via weekly alerts on industry developments and a journal with peer-reviewed articles.

All physicians with an M.D. or D.O. degree who live in Oklahoma and are licensed to practice medicine in the state are eligible for membership in the Oklahoma State Medical Association and their affiliate county societies. United, Oklahoma's physicians assure their voices are heard and receive great benefits, never walking alone in their profession of healing. ∎

FUTURE LEGACIES

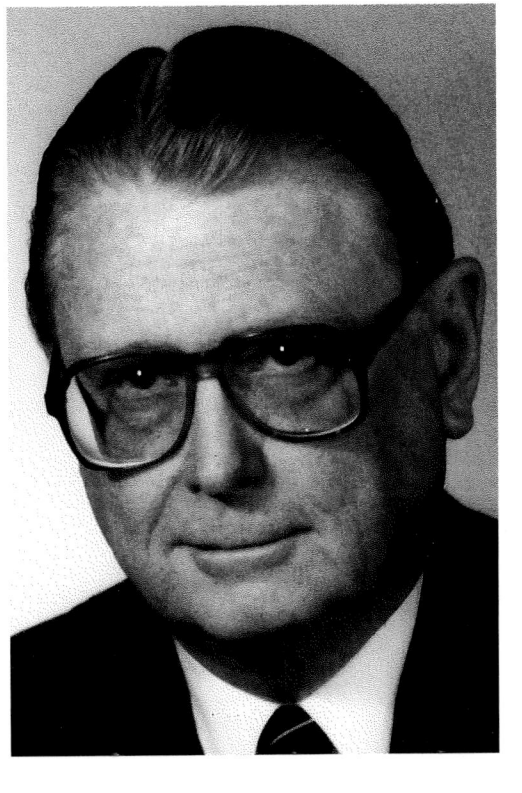

TCMS Executive Director, 1941-1986
Jack Spears, M.D.

Jack Spears led the Tulsa County Medical Society as its executive director through four decades of growth into the modern era, from 1941 to 1986. In his spare time, he became a nationally known film historian. Under his leadership, the medical society went from about 100 physicians to more than 1,000, with a shift from downtown practices to across the region.

"Tulsa went from a place where you could get good medical care to one of the Southwest's leading medical centers." — Jack Spears, *Tulsa World*, 1986.

A native of Arkansas, Spears arrived at the Tulsa County Medical Society in December 1941 after just a few months of serving as general manager of the Wagoner Chamber of Commerce. He had graduated from the University of Arkansas in June 1941. The medical society was located in the Medical and Dental Arts building at Sixth Street and Boulder Avenue. A person got to the office by going to the 11th floor then walking up a flight of stairs to floors remodeled from the original attic. It had a library, librarian and operated a medical credit bureau. Medical services were all located downtown.

"I knew absolutely nothing about the medical profession, but there was a great group of doctors," said Jack Spears, April 2, 2008, in an interview with Dr. Jerry Gustafson.

Spears and World War II arrived at about the same time. Of the 150 physicians in the county, about 40 doctors served in the war. He worked with a group of older physicians to meet needs on the homefront.

During the regular scientific programs held at the Mayo Hotel, several famous physicians spoke to society members. The events also served to benefit the Oklahoma Medical Research Foundation.

Among the projects during his leadership were the opening of the Red Cross Blood Center in 1949, the mass immunization of county residents for polio in 1963, the establishment of the University of Oklahoma-Tulsa medical school and the formation of a medical society scholarship fund.

A public relations maestro, Spears was involved in innovative communications programs such as long-running television and radio programs, community health fairs, a monthly magazine and other publications. The Oklahoma State Medical Association presented Spears its Distinguished Service Award in 1980 and named him an honorary member, at the time only the group's third such honoree, in 1989.

Spears was known to have a quiet, dignified style.

"I found the work fascinating, and I always loved Tulsa. And I can say with great sincerity that I like doctors. They're the salt of the earth." — Jack Spears, *Tulsa World*, 1986.

Spears was active in the Tulsa community over the years logging more than 40 annual fundraising campaigns for the Tulsa Area United Way. He served on boards such as the Tulsa Center for the Prevention of Child Abuse, Tulsa Medical Education Foundation, Tulsa County Public Health Nursing Association and the Arthritis Foundation of Eastern Oklahoma.

On the side, he managed to develop a reputation as a film buff and amateur movie historian, writing the books, *Hollywood: The Golden Era* and *The Civil War on the Screen*. He has been quoted or credited in more than 200 books or publications.

When Spears retired in 1986, he was the longest-tenured executive director of any medical society in the United States. He died on July 16, 2012, at age 92. ■

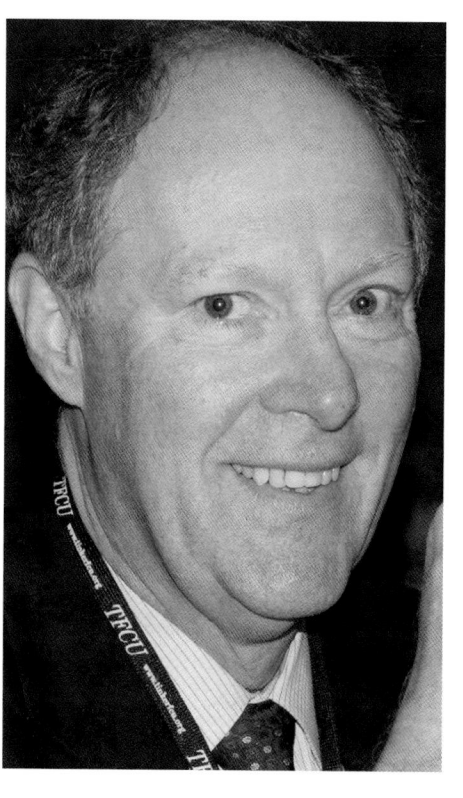

TCMS Executive Director, 1986-2008
Paul Patton

During an era of massive changes in the health care system, Paul Patton took the Tulsa County Medical Association into a more high-profile role by encouraging legislative actions, expanding membership and adding programming.

Mr. Patton grew up in Tulsa, graduating from Hale High School in 1963, followed by an undergraduate in journalism from the University of Tulsa in 1971 and a graduate degree in business from the University of Oklahoma. His college education was interrupted for two years to serve in the Army.

After graduation, he worked as the communications director for OETA. When Gov. George Nigh was elected, Mr. Patton ran the governor's office in Tulsa to cover northeastern Oklahoma activities. For two years, he worked in a Tulsa private public relations firm.

After being named as executive director of the Tulsa County Medical Society in 1985, Mr. Patton put an emphasis on marketing the work of the organization and becoming more involved with government affairs.

"Historically, doctors didn't need to be involved with political activities. But, during that time, the world would change dramatically for health care and certainly for doctors and practitioners. One of the things that changed was the realization they needed to be involved in government and legislative activities. Laws were being made that had a huge impact on practitioners, whether they had a hand in it or not," said Paul Patton, June 2016.

Mr. Patton worked with the board to raise money for a new facility and oversaw plans for the construction. While biking one day, he located the statue of Asclepius, the Greek god of medicine and healing, on a building being demolished in Utica Square. He arranged for it to be relocated at the entry to the new building.

"That was really exciting to build a building for our own use and for use in the community," he said.

The board embraced efforts to expand educational opportunities and health care access for the community. In some instances, changes in the delivery of health care made it more complicated, particularly for low-income and older patients to receive services.

To meet the needs, many of the programs initiated during that time are still providing assistance and support to the community. Some examples:

• The TCMS Foundation was established to provide non-budgeted financial support for community projects.
• Area free clinics were identified, and TCMS provided volunteer physicians to staff the clinics.
• A Committee on Concerns of Older Tulsans was created to address issues related to senior citizens. The VIP Program was an idea from the committee. It coordinated efforts for Tulsa physicians to identify and accept Medicare assignment for low-income patients over 65.
• A program launched to recycle unused prescription medications from area long-term care and nursing facilities, with retired physicians volunteering to pick up the drugs. It has expanded to collect medications from the public.
• Physicians increased participation in legislative issues regarding health care and medical liability reform.
• As part of the growing awareness of the changes in physician practices, TCMS altered its membership eligibility requirements and, for the first time, accepted osteopathic physicians as members.

"To sum up Paul — He stands for things he believes in and does not give up. That's a rare but very precious commodity in my judgement. We were very fortunate to have had him as executive director," said Dr. Wallace Hooser, 1999 TCMS board president, May 2016.

FUTURE LEGACIES

TCMS Executive Director, 2009-Present
Mona Whitmire

Providing a safety net for low-income patients and support for Tulsa-area physicians, Mona Whitmire continues to lead the Tulsa County Medical Society into the future.

Ms. Whitmire was named the executive director of the organization and the Tulsa County Medical Society Foundation after her predecessor, Paul Patton, retired in 2008.

One of her proudest initiatives is Project TCMS, which is a program started by the society's foundation in 2012. It connects low-income, uninsured Tulsa County residents referred from primary care clinics to volunteer specialty physicians. The services provided are at no cost to the patient and no reimbursement to the providers. Since its inception in April 2012, the program has provided over $3 million in donated care and services to the community. Ms. Whitmire credits Dr. Victor Robards, M.D., for having the vision to provide access to non-emergent specialty care for uninsured, poor Tulsans when he served as the TCMS president in 1976. She attributes much of the success of the 5-year program to the ongoing efforts of the TCMS Foundation Board.

Before being named as executive director, Ms. Whitmire worked as an associate executive director for the organization. She started her career at Tulsa Regional Medical Center (now Oklahoma State University Medical Center) in the medical staff office, where she worked for 20 years. This experience has given Ms. Whitmire 41 years of working with Tulsa-area physicians.

"I love my job and the physicians I have the opportunity to work with. I see all of the work they do outside of their busy medical practice to support our community and make Tulsa a better place to live and work, and I am inspired by their generosity," said Mona Whitmire, June 2016.

The many physicians who have worked with Ms. Whitmire have significantly influenced her life through their commitment to medicine, family and community philanthropy. Some of those include Drs. Marc Milsten, Gerald Gustafson, Rollie Rhodes, Lynn Frame, Todd Brockman, Jeffrey Galles, Eric Cottrill, John Hubner, David Harris, Peter Aran, Lynn Wiens, Steven Katsis, Jamal Siddiqui, Michael Haugh, John Minielly, William Geffen, David Siegler, Doug Stewart, Wally Hooser, Dan Fieker, Michael Weisz, and Jenny Boyer.

"These physicians and others who feel like family have shaped the course of my life, and I am forever grateful for their friendship," she said.

Working with medical students and residents is among the joys of Ms. Whitmire's job. In 2016, a mentorship program started to match medical students and residents with physicians to provide guidance during their medical training.

"Their enthusiasm and dedication to the goal of completing their education, training and practicing medicine is inspiring. The healthcare system is constantly changing and as an organization, we gain much momentum through the participation of medical students and residents," she said.

In recalling the centennial celebration of the Tulsa County Medical Society, Ms. Whitmire said the four employees — Patton, Tanya Luce, Janie Higgins and herself — had a combined total of 100 years of service to the organization. Joetta Cunningham, Kim Morris and Pam Oppelt now work alongside Ms. Whitmire.

"TCMS and the TCMS Foundation staff is simply THE BEST," she says. "Our wonderful staff is completely devoted to the mission of our organizations."

She is married to Mark Whitmire. When not working, they enjoy sports, traveling and spending time with their amazing children.

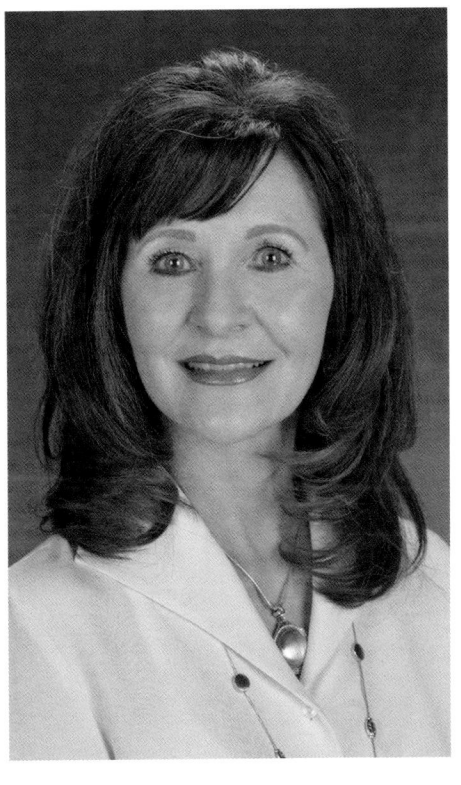

TCMS Associate Executive Director, 1985-2007
Tanya Luce

During the nearly 46-year career, Tanya Luce was a bridge between two long-serving executive directors and an integral part of building several successful programs with the Tulsa County Medical Society.

Born in Tulsa, Ms. Luce graduated from Edison High School and began work with the medical society in July 1962. Her first job was under Zelma Fink, manager of the society's Medical Credit Bureau. Together, the two collected delinquent medical bills from patients of most physicians in Tulsa County. After Ms. Fink's sudden death in the early 70s, the decision was made to close the credit bureau due to outside competition for that service. Ms. Luce was tasked with shutting down the program, then she became the secretary to Executive Director Jack Spears.

Known as a patient multi-tasker, Ms. Luce had an ability to listen to group discussions and follow through with an action plan. After Mr. Spears retired in 1985, she accepted the promotion to associate executive director under the newly hired Paul Patton.

"Mr. Patton and I assumed the responsibilities for supporting the TCMS physicians in every activity from continuing medical education, legislative, community services and social events, providing the avenues to promote their profession, while serving the Tulsa community," said Tanya Luce, June 2016.

Among her accomplishments as an associate executive editor:
• Organizing a credentialing service and verifying the credentials of physicians for area hospitals. This involved consulting on a software program and participating with other services nationwide.
• Helping to establish the Tulsa County Medical Society Foundation.
• Assisting in the drug recycling program, which gathered unused prescription drugs and transferred to the county pharmacy for distribution to low-income patients.
• Organizing a service aiding medical specialty groups with meetings and continuing education.

As a member of the American Association of Medical Executives, Ms. Luce traveled to various cities for continuing education. She worked with organizations — including Domestic Violence Intervention Services, Tulsa City-County Health Department and the Vo-Tech Medical Assistant program — in policies requiring and implementing smoke-free environments.

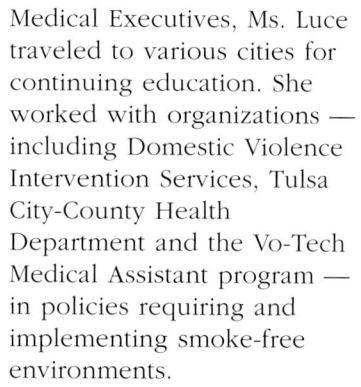

When staffing was needed to fill volunteer physician programs for free medical clinics and other community healthcare organizations, she handled the recruitment and scheduling. At the medical society, Ms. Luce was instrumental in the formation of the retired physician program, The Golden Oldies, and provided ongoing support.

Calling it "a most satisfying accomplishment," Ms. Luce had a hand in the planning and construction of the permanent medical society home at 5315 S. Lewis Ave.

"After almost 100 years, the medical society had its own home serving the physicians and community of Tulsa. During my tenure, TCMS was located in the Medical Arts Building at Sixth Street and South Boulder, Utica Square Medical Center, BOK Building at 21st Street and South Lewis prior to moving to its own building."

Ms. Luce retired on Dec. 31, 2007 and to care for her mother and disabled husband, both now deceased. As she looks back on her tenure, she describes it as "a very satisfying career."

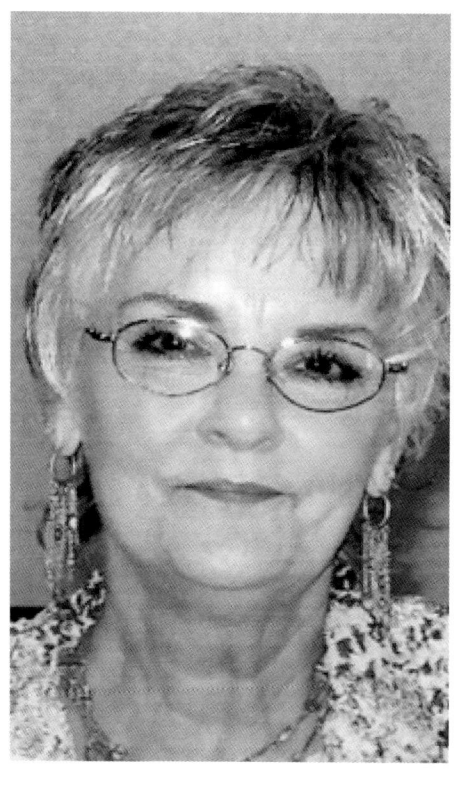

Aesthetic Surgery Institute of America

The Aesthetic Surgery Institute of America (ASIA) is dedicated to enhancing a patient's appearance and self-confidence. It is located in midtown and offers cosmetic surgical and non-surgical procedures in a beautiful, private setting.

The modern, all green facility was built to ensure patients have a pleasant and comfortable experience. Environmentally focused, the center is located in the former Carpet City building. Upon purchasing the iconic building, Dr. Nicole remodeled the building with an upscale, industrial-chic design reminiscent of Tulsa's celebrated Art Deco period. The facility is heated and cooled by an in-ground geothermal well field deep below the parking lot. No fossil fuels are used on site.

Dr. Nicole Patel attended the University of Illinois in Champaign-Urbana for her undergraduate studies, graduating Summa Cum Laude with highest departmental distinction. She completed her medical degree at the highly regarded Rush Medical College in Chicago before completing a five year general surgery residency in New York City at Mount Sinai Cabrini Medical Center. She was asked to be the administrative surgical chief during her final year.

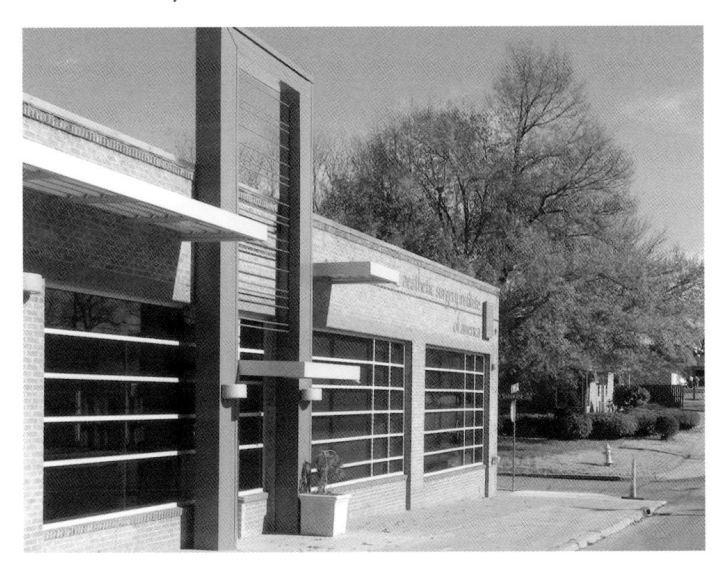

She subsequently completed a cosmetic surgery fellowship before starting Aesthetic Surgery Institute of America (ASIA). She is double board certified with board certification in general surgery by the American Board of Surgery and in facial and body cosmetic surgery by the American Board of Cosmetic Surgery.

Aesthetic Surgery Institute of America (ASIA) is focused entirely on elective cosmetic surgical and non-surgical procedures. Dr. Nicole's patients are healthy, procedures are elective, and the practice does not accept insurance.

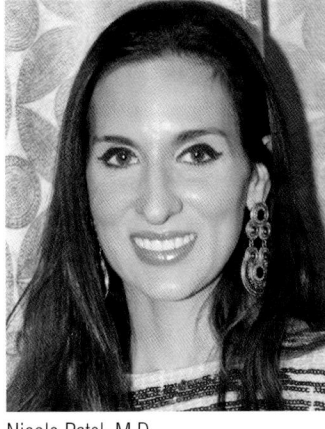

Nicole Patel, M.D.

Improving aesthetic appeal, symmetry, and proportion, and helping patients look and feel their best, are the key goals.

Devaluation of the profession is an ongoing concern because any licensed physician can legally perform cosmetic surgery, regardless of how they received cosmetic surgery training.

"Because most cosmetic procedures are performed in a surgical suite rather than a hospital, I feel it is going to be a challenge for the future. Unfortunately, some physicians are trying to make extra money by jumping on the cosmetic surgery bandwagon without the necessary training required for such procedures. They may not be aware of the risks involved or may not have the additional training to get to that point. They may get into coupon-type advertising and cheapen medicine," says Dr. Nicole.

Another challenge Dr. Nicole faces is the misnomer that cosmetic surgery is only for the wealthy. She says the majority of her patients are middle-income women dealing with issues related to childbearing and the natural process of aging.

Dr. Nicole specializes in natural facial rejuvenation through anti-aging skin care products, facial fat transfer, laser resurfacing, micro needling and various injectables. Body procedures include breast augmentation, lift and reductions, breast revision, and gynecomastia treatments. She also offers liposuction and laser liposuction, tummy tucks, body lifts, and labiaplasty.

She says, "Some patients may not require surgery. I don't like the look of 'operated faces' so I use skin care products, nonsurgical procedures, mineral makeup, and nutritional supplements to achieve the most youthful results."

Other non-surgical procedures include laser hair removal, wrinkle reduction, dermal fillers, laser treatments, micro-needling, platelet rich plasma, eyelash enhancement, and Venus treatments.

Marcel Binstock, M.D.

Dr. Marcel Binstock was born in Strasbourg, France, in 1935. At the outset of World War II, that city's population was evacuated in anticipation of impending hostilities. Thus began a journey of moves culminating in his family fleeing to Switzerland in 1943 to escape Nazi persecution due to their Jewish ancestry.

Shortly after their return to liberated France, he and his family immigrated to the United States in 1948, settling in Vineland, New Jersey, where he graduated high school. He then attended Indiana University, earning a degree in zoology. Subsequent to graduating from Pittsburgh University Medical School in 1963, he completed a one-year internship at Los Angeles County General Hospital.

The following three years were spent as a family physician for Kaiser Permanente in Los Angeles and as an emergency room physician for the city of Los Angeles. A chance encounter with a wounded ophthalmologist in the emergency room sparked an interest in that specialty. After completing a three-year residency at Georgetown University, he took a fellowship in retinal surgery at Baylor University in Houston.

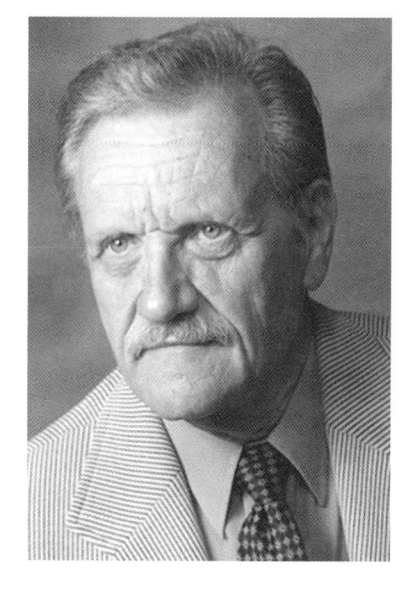

At the urging of a colleague, Dr. William Perryman, a descendant of Tulsa's founding family, he opened Tulsa's first retinal clinic in 1971. Known as Tulsa Retina Clinic Inc., it was situated at Hillcrest Medical Center for 20 years, then moving to the former Doctors' Hospital for the next decade.

In 2010, he retired, turning over the practice to two younger retinal specialists.

Reflecting on his professional career, he expressed deep gratitude for the fortuitous scientific advancements of the current era, and his ability to enlist them in the care of his patients. ■

Robert W. Block, M.D., F.A.A.P

Son of a pediatrician, Robert Block, M.D.'s pediatric career focused on advocacy, academics, and advisement especially regarding brain health.

"Because there's neuroscience not just advocacy, we know if we can protect the brain early on, it's less likely the child will experience health problems that come from the stress of neglect, abuse, poverty, and violence," he explains. "We pay more for putting stents in someone's heart rather than supporting brain health early on to prevent heart disease."

He attended Wesleyan University then medical school at the University of South Dakota and the University of Pennsylvania — where he graduated. He received residency training at Children's Hospital of Philadelphia then served three years in the military at Munson Army Hospital at Fort Leavenworth where he met Dr. Daniel Plunket.

In 1975, when Dr. Plunket was appointed chairman of the Department of Pediatrics at the University of Oklahoma's (OU) medical school in Tulsa, he recruited Dr. Block to help develop the department.

Dr. Block credits Tulsa's pediatric community, who incipiently volunteered their time to teach students and train residents, for helping to establish the department.

He consulted on developmental and behavioral issues including as a clinician in the At Risk program helping families with troubled mother-infant dyads. "The incidence of child abuse within that population was extraordinarily low — almost non-existent," he says of its success.

In 1988, he helped launch through OU, the Child Abuse Network, a multidisciplinary team at the Children's Advocacy Center — Oklahoma's first co-located facility helping abused children.

He was appointed Oklahoma's first Chief Child Abuse Examiner (1989). He's a pioneer of the Helfer Society that lobbied the American Board of Pediatrics to approve the new Child Abuse Pediatrics subspecialty. As chair of the new sub-board, he helped develop the subspecialty's certification standards and written examination.

He served as chair of the Committee on Child Abuse and Neglect of the American Academy of Pediatrics then became the Academy's President (2011-2012). As president, he was an ardent advocate of brain health. Now he serves as Professor and Chair Emeritus, Pediatrics and enjoys full-time retirement.

He and his wife, Sharon, have two daughters and three grandchildren. ■

Todd A. Brockman, M.D.

The roots of Todd Brockman, M.D.'s practice date back to 1955 when his father in-law, Dr. Robert Spencer, a comprehensive ophthalmologist, established his practice in Tulsa. Dr. Brockman married Dr. Spencer's daughter as undergraduate students at Texas Christian University. When he was attending medical school at the University of Texas in Houston, Dr. Spencer inspired him to pursue ophthalmology. Dr. Brockman went to Philadelphia for an internship at Presbyterian Hospital and residency at the University of Pennsylvania's Scheie Eye Institute.

He took over Dr. Spencer's practice in 1986 and collaborated with other doctors in the early '90's to form The Eye Institute, a hybrid of joint business office services and private practice. In 2000, he helped launch Eye Surgery Center of Tulsa, an ambulatory surgery center. A few years ago, he added ophthalmologist, Dr. Jamal Siddiqui, to his practice.

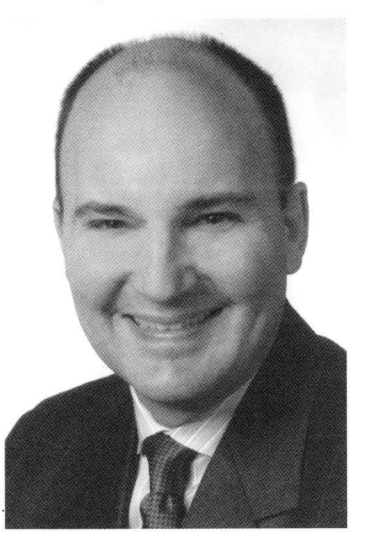

Ophthalmology is an ideal career for him — combining surgery with an office practice. "The bigger part of my day is interacting with patients." He advises young ophthalmologists to maintain an office practice along with performing surgeries, since "it's all about the people".

He has witnessed many surgical advances considering he was a senior resident when cataract surgery became an outpatient procedure. "The continuum of my career has progressed from big incisions taking the lens out in one piece, to ultrasound, and to laser for cataract surgery."

Dr. Brockman has served as president of the Tulsa Surgical Society, Tulsa County Medical Society, and Oklahoma State Medical Association. He is on the Board of Trustees for the state association and served as a two-term chairman. He's a clinical professor in ophthalmology at the University of Oklahoma School Of Medicine.

Albert Brownlee, M.D.

During his more than 40 years in practice, patients were like family to pediatrician and allergist Dr. Albert Brownlee, M.D. The 1950 Guthrie graduate attended Draughons Business College in Oklahoma City before entering the U.S. Army for two years. Upon return, he went to Central State University then was accepted into the University of Chicago School of Medicine, where he earned his degree in 1961.

Dr. Brownlee completed his internship and residency at the Mabee Children's Hospital in Tulsa. While there, he was featured in the Tulsa World newspaper for administering oral polio vaccines to nursing home residents and jail inmates in a county program. Then, he worked in family practice from 1963 to 1968 at the Guthrie Hospital, where he served as the chief of staff. He finished a residency in pediatric allergy at Children's Hospital in Oklahoma City.

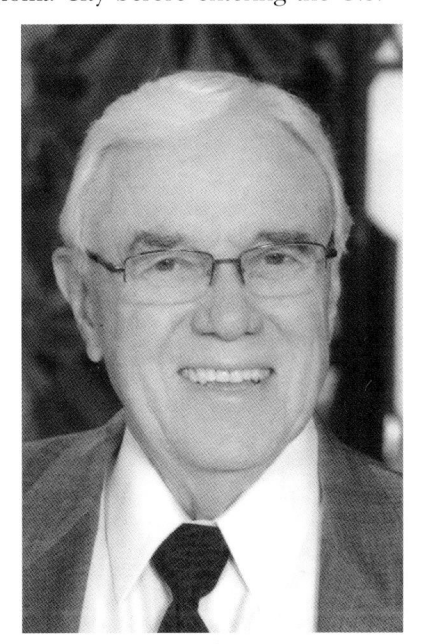

Returning to Tulsa, Dr. Brownlee joined other pediatricians at the Springer Clinic and later the Children's Clinic of Tulsa. In the early 80s, he left to start the solo practice, Children's Allergy Clinic. He retired in 2005.

In addition, he has participated in the Tulsa Medical Society's Drug Recycling program since its inception in 2004, volunteers at a church youth camp as its physician and served on the board of trustees for the state medical association.

Dr. Brownlee and his wife, Jerri, have been married for 63 years and have three sons, seven grandsons and three granddaughters.

Allergy Clinic of Tulsa

Excellence in patient care is the hallmark of the physician-owned Allergy Clinic of Tulsa (ACT), a value traced back to founder, Dr. Leon Horowitz, Tulsa's first board-certified pediatric allergist. In 1959, he opened a private practice at 21st and Yale. His medical assistant Jane Cowan worked with him from the start and retired from ACT as office manager fifty years later. The Clinic moved to the former Utica Square Medical Center before settling in the current office at 1727 S. Utica.

As the practice grew, Dr. Horowitz searched for a partner specializing in adult allergy. He met Dr. David Hurewitz by chance while attending an allergy conference in San Diego — Dr. Hurewitz was a Naval allergist — serving during the last two years of the Vietnam War — at Balboa Naval Hospital in San Diego. Although they had already talked on the phone, this meeting was the catalyst for Dr. Hurewitz to visit the Clinic at the time. He joined in July 1975, and the two allergists practiced together for almost twenty years.

A selling point for Dr. Hurewitz joining ACT was Dr. Horowitz tackled difficult cases. "At the time, many allergists only did skin tests and gave shots. I was trained to treat very sick people requiring hospitalization. Thus, Dr. Horowitz's practice was for me because he saw sick, challenging patients in his office and in the hospital." On occasion, they made house calls to evaluate patients' homes for allergens or follow up on those experiencing severe symptoms. Now, far fewer patients are hospitalized.

Dr. Horowitz was an excellent mentor committed to his patients. Today, some of his pediatric patients, now adults, are receiving care at ACT. One time, while in Colorado, he flew back to Tulsa to tend to a patient recently intubated — this made a lasting impression on Dr. Hurewitz. "Dr. Horowitz was a well-established physician. I benefited by his reputation and made my own," shares Dr. Hurewitz.

Dr. Hurewitz established his own reputation for patient care, evident by the awards he's received including "Best Doctor" by *Oklahoma Magazine* and *Tulsa People*. He treated every patient with compassion. "I always introduced myself, then said, 'I want you to tell me the story of your problem, so I can understand.' " He valued displaying humanity such as using personal touch, speaking in layman terms, and recording endearing facts about the patient.

Dr. Horowitz was a skilled diagnostician, spending quality time listening, taking detailed histories, and thoroughly examining each patient. When the OB/GYN practicing next door retired, Dr. Horowitz bought the physician's x-ray machine. Now, ACT has a CT Scanner and radiology onsite.

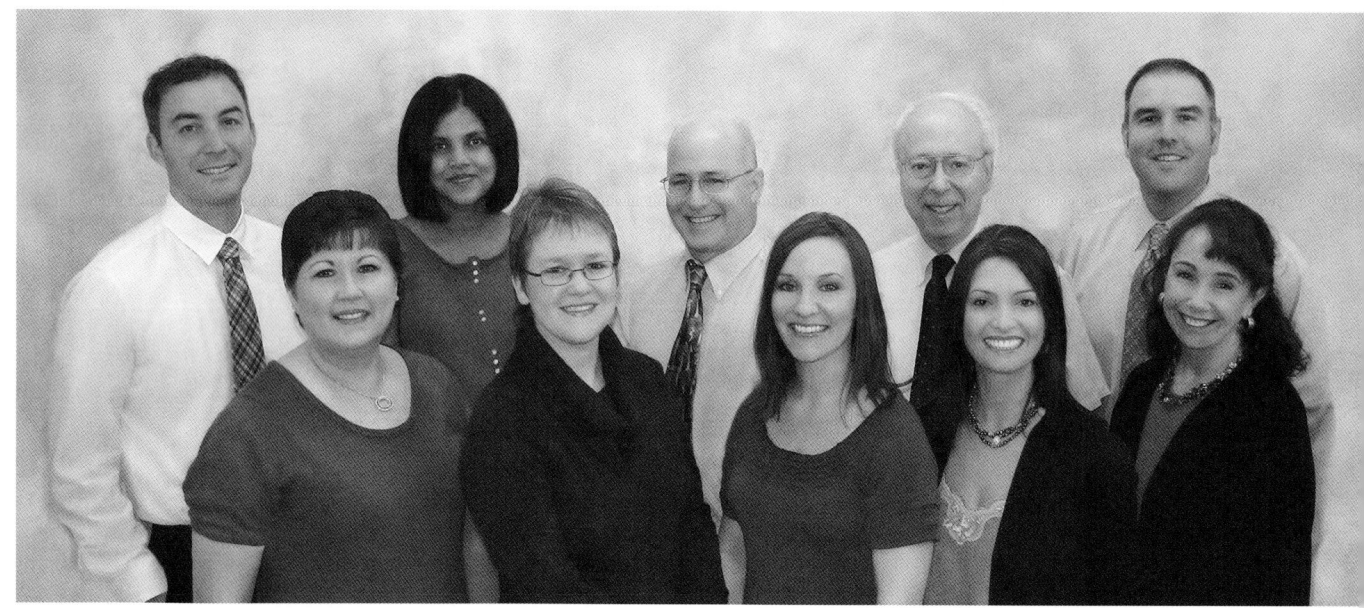

Front Row, L to R: Karen Arnold, ARNP, CNP, Dr. Kathryn Brown, Katie Sims, PA-C, Dr. Lodie Naimeh, Dr. Jane Purser.
Second Row, L to R: Dr. Timothy Nickel, Dr. Rumali Medagoda, Dr. James Love, Dr. David Hurewitz, Todd Coleman, APRN, CPNP.
(Missing in the photo is Erin Soulek, PA-C)

FUTURE LEGACIES

When Dr. Horowitz wanted to retire, he promised to stay until Dr. Hurewitz found a new partner. After a long search, he called Dr. Jane Purser who was practicing allergy in Los Angeles. She was highly recommended by the head of the department where she had trained. They had a brief conversation at which time Dr. Purser politely declined the offer, explaining that since her husband was a college Chemistry teacher, he needed a job also.

Serendipitously, shortly thereafter, Dr. Hurewitz treated the wife of a University of Tulsa (TU) chemistry faculty member. She shared TU was interviewing for a chemistry faculty position. Armed with viable information, he again asked Dr. Purser and her family to visit Tulsa and ACT.

"To find out that patients are the center of care and the staff have been with the Clinic for twenty-plus years, and are treated beautifully, I was so pleased," shares Dr. Purser, who joined ACT in 1993. Her husband received a faculty position at TU and is now tenured.

Dr. James Love, a pediatric allergist with a Ph.D. in Immunology, interviewed with Dr. Hurewitz, but visiting ACT sealed the deal: "They were so nice, honest, and caring about patient care — very old school. I thought this was the place I would enjoy practicing." He joined in 1996.

Dr. Lodie Naimeh visited ACT's booth at a job fair where she interviewed with Dr. Hurewitz. She joined in 2000 after visiting the Clinic, and Dr. Hurewitz found a job for her husband, a psychiatrist.

Raised in Beirut, Lebanon, Dr. Naimeh received most of her medical training through the American University of Beirut. She came to the United States for fellowship training in Pediatric Endocrinology then Allergy and Immunology at the University of Iowa Health Center.

Dr. Naimeh implemented several oral food challenge protocols soon after joining ACT. Dr. Naimeh currently provides oversight to ACT's Radiology Department. She's the medical/technical/quality director over ACT's MiniCat Sinus CT machine, the only device of its type in Northeastern Oklahoma. The services are accredited by the Intersocietal Accreditation Commission. Dr. Naimeh's role includes ensuring strict guidelines are adhered to in areas of patient radiation safety and overall patient care.

Dr. Timothy Nickel joined the Clinic in July 2004 after completing a fellowship in Allergy and Immunology at the University of Kansas. He was referred to the Clinic by his father in-law's physician.

Dr. Kathryn Brown joined ACT in 2007. She credits having been an allergy sufferer as a child with family members having components of asthma, sinus, and allergy as partial influence in pursuing this field. During her residency rotation in allergy, she could relate to patients, found the field interesting, and conducted research in allergy.

A Sri Lankan native, Dr. Rumali Medagoda received her medical school training in Sri Lanka, but came to Tulsa for pediatric residency training at OU's medical school where she rotated at ACT. During her Allergy and Immunology fellowship at the University of Texas-Galveston, a hurricane destroyed her department, causing the fellows to find other locations to train. Dr. Medagoda came to ACT for two months. After completing her fellowship, she joined the Clinic in 2010. "I'm around strong women with Dr. Naimeh, Dr. Purser, and Dr. Brown that I can look up to."

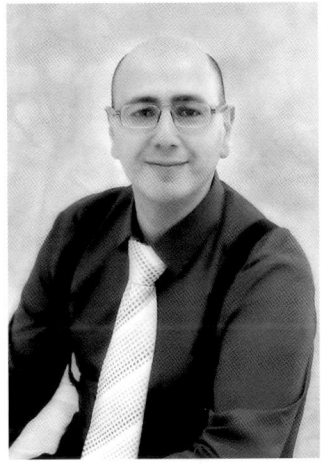

Dr. Ahmad Mourad, a Syrian native, joined in 2015. He graduated from the University of Damascus, but received his pediatric residency and Allergy and Immunology fellowship training in the United States.

With a multiethnic staff, the Clinic can facilitate patients from diverse cultures and languages including Spanish, French, Arabic, and sign language.

Whether the physicians were trained as pediatricians or internists, they treat children and adults in all areas of allergy, asthma, and immunology. Yet, each physician has a particular niche to elevate the practice.

Dr. Purser finds treating patients suffering from the worst cases of sinus disease and nasal polyps gratifying, along with those suffering from mastocytosis, anaphylaxis, latex allergy, and hives.

Dr. Love is one of the few oral immunotherapy specialists in the region — a treatment where children with a severe food allergy such as to peanuts, eggs, and dairy are orally desensitized and gradually introduced to the food so they don't experience an allergic reaction. ACT was the first in Tulsa to provide this therapy. "So far, we've taken over seventy-five children from very allergic to now eating those foods — that's very rewarding," he shares.

Continued on following page

Dr. Love's one of two immunologists in Oklahoma providing newborn screening for immune deficiency especially severe combined immunodeficiency (SCID) using the TREC test. This program started in Oklahoma in January 2015. Dr Love also enjoys teaching allergy and immunology to the medical students and residents rotating through ACT.

Dr. Nickel has taken over ACT's research program for Hereditary Angioedema (HAE), an orphan disease. "We have many patients with this condition. They're missing a special complement to the immune system resulting in leaky blood vessels and swelling," Dr. Hurewitz shares. ACT is a Center of Excellence for HAE. "The primary treatment is replacement of an enzyme inhibitor that's deficient in these patients. This treatment hadn't been approved by FDA in the US, even though it had been the standard of care in Europe for many years," Dr. Nickel explains.

Initially, when research trials began, Dr. Hurewitz was the first and only primary investigator in Oklahoma on new treatments of HAE. He participated in a team that infused medication in double-blind, placebo-controlled clinical trials and witnessed patients dramatically improve after treatments. When a pharmaceutical company invited him to Barcelona with other investigators to summarize data from all the studies, he discovered he was the first in the world to infuse their drug.

Dr. Brown offers expertise in drug allergies. During her residency training at Washington University (St. Louis), she learned from a mentor specializing in drug allergies. "I get the very complex cases that'll take a long time, but I'm glad to do it." She specializes in venom allergies — her mentor during her fellowship training at Johns Hopkins conducted most of the venom research.

Dr. Medagoda specializes in asthma, allergies, and eczema issues especially with pediatric patients. "I like that we're treating allergy and asthma and can see improvement. We treat children with immunotherapy, so they'll grow up without allergies as adults."

Tulsa's multi-ecological environment is difficult for allergy sufferers; yet, ideal for allergists to see a full spectrum of allergic responses. ACT, a member of a national pollen counting network, posts the daily pollen count on their website and provides this information to the city and *Tulsa World*, a service Dr. Horowitz started. This allows patients to identify if allergens are high and to know what steps to take to reduce exposure or to treat symptoms.

ACT provides additional information on social media. "We have a great Facebook page, and I post good articles there. It's being educated about the disease, so our patients can get accurate information and screen incorrect information," shares Dr. Medagoda.

The information available in the field of Allergy, Asthma, and Immunology is vast and dynamic with significant breakthroughs in the past decade. "The number of primary immune deficiencies we've been able to diagnose has increased ten fold every three to seven years. Now we have over 250 primary immune deficiencies with known genetic causes we can detect. That field's exciting and expanding rapidly — hopefully this will lead to better diagnosis and treatment therapies," Dr. Nickel explains.

The physicians at ACT work hard to not only stay current with the latest medical research in their field, but implement technological advances in their practice.

One advance is sublingual therapy for grass and ragweed pollen considered safer than injections. Another is an asthma treatment, "Recently, two new anti-IL-5 antibodies that block asthma have been approved by the FDA in the past months, so we have that available now," shares Dr. Nickel.

"We're entering the age of biologicals — genetically-engineered proteins, such as Xolair, that treat asthma by grabbing onto an allergy protein in the body and not letting cells use it. We have specialized antibodies and medicines available, not just simple prednisone inhalers we had years ago. Medicines are stronger, more selective, and better at taking care of individual disorders," shares Dr. Love.

Another advance the Clinic provides is immune replacement therapy. "When you're immune deficient, your body lacks type of markers to give the adequate immune response. We have a system where we infuse patients in our office with immunoglobulin to give them protection and teach them to do it subcutaneously at home," shares Dr. Naimeh.

The Clinic provides rapid dose immunotherapy where allergists can administer higher doses of immunotherapy quicker and get patients on the maintenance dose faster. Patients are receiving once-a-month maintenance dose within several weeks instead of within eight to twelve months. When the physicians can get patients on the maintenance dose, the treatment periods are spread out more.

Yet, the physicians are cautious advocates, not always immediately administering all the latest drugs. "You always have to balance the positive effects a medicine is giving with the unknown concerns that might come later. That's why, as a pediatrician, I try not to use too many medicines within their first year. I believe it pays to be hesitant to prescribe a new medicine until it has been tried on more patients than just small study groups," Dr. Love explains.

These physicians treat dermatological issues including atopic dermatitis, an allergic disease of the skin, and contact dermatitis, a reaction when the skin's exposed to a foreign substance.

Treating a variety of conditions, allergists have an interdependence with the primary care physician and other specialists including dermatologists, otolaryngologists, and pulmonologists. "Tulsa has an excellent collegial medical community. I always tell patients that it's virtually impossible to find a doctor in Tulsa who's not excellent," Dr. Love shares.

The physicians give back to the medical community. They're members of various medical societies including the American Academy of Allergy, Asthma, and Immunology and American College of Allergy, Asthma, and Immunology. When Dr. Love was President of the Oklahoma Allergy and Asthma Society, he helped Representative Jeanie McDaniel push legislation to provide epinephrine in schools.

The Clinic has a contract with OU-TU and Oklahoma State University's medical school (OSU-COM) and residency programs. "All of us have residents who rotate with us. The resident rotates with the physician who shares the same specialty in pediatrics or internal medicine," shares Dr. Naimeh.

Teaching medical students and volunteering free medical services are values rooted in ACT. Dr. Horowitz developed a free pediatric clinic at Hillcrest Medical Center through the former Tulsa Medical Foundation, treating patients and mentoring physicians-in-training. When OU opened its medical school here, Drs. Horowitz and Hurewitz developed and ran their pediatric and adult allergy clinics. Although Dr. Hurewitz retired recently, he's a volunteer clinical professor at OU-TU's medical school.

Dr. Purser serves as a faculty member at OU-TU's medical school, guest volunteer faculty at OSU-COM, and guest faculty member at In His Image, a Christian missions-based family practice residency program. "One reason why I give to teaching is because I wouldn't have been aware of this field unless I was taught by someone. I love to teach." She serves on medical missions trips to Guyana and recently, to Tanzania, and volunteers at OU's Bedlam clinic.

To facilitate their growing patient base including from out-of-state and surrounding rural areas, ACT

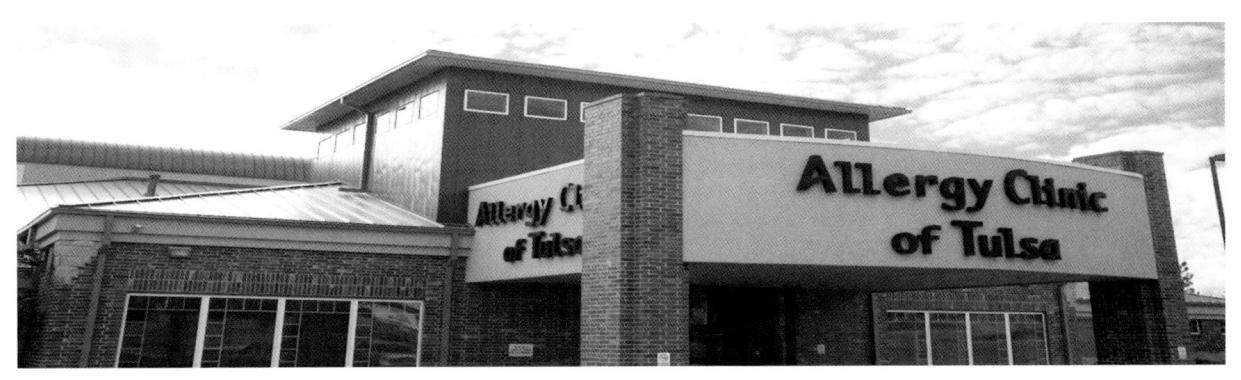

9311 S. Mingo Clinic

has five offices: at Utica, South Tulsa at Mingo, West Tulsa at Olympia, in Owasso, and Bartlesville. They have eighty-seven staff members including two nurse practitioners and two physician assistants. Every location has a lab for allergy injections, skin testing, and drawing blood. A compounding lab makes customized extracts at the Mingo office. They accept most insurance carriers including Medicare and Sooner Care.

"I experience great camaraderie here. We are all very open to trying therapies that'll benefit patients. There's no discussion where we say, 'we shouldn't offer this treatment because it's not financially lucrative.' We offer it because it's what patients need. The focus here is what's best for the patients," Dr. Brown shares.

Dr. Love credits Dr. Hurewitz for the culture of patient advocacy. "Dr. Dave has an amazing, servant mentality. He elevated patients to the pedestal they deserve and made sure no matter how long it took, he tried to fix every problem they had. We're happy to be working with each other and our staff's amazing. We're just happy people." ∎

George Caldwell, M.D.

Dr. George Caldwell worked in the political arena with the same skill as in Tulsa emergency rooms, urgent care clinics and prevention care programs for businesses.

As past president of the Tulsa County Medical Society and Oklahoma State Medical Association, Dr. Caldwell pushed for legislation regarding worker's compensation and access and quality of care. He served a term as president of the Oklahoma College of Occupational and Environmental Medicine.

"You cannot be a patient advocate unless you are politically involved," he says. "It is why I got involved in organized medicine."

After graduating from Carl Albert High School in Oklahoma City, he earned a bachelor's degree in psychology from the University of Oklahoma. Then, he spent about a year in northern California working as a social worker.

As the Vietnam War continued, he went into the Army and spent three months in active training followed by eight years in the Reserves, retiring with the rank of captain. Returning to OU, Dr. Caldwell completed a master's degree in public health and earned his medical degree in 1979.

Dr. Caldwell went into the specialty of emergency care and joined Emergency Care, Inc., a Tulsa-based medical group of about eight emergency room doctors, associated with Saint Francis Medical Center.

At Saint Francis, Dr. Caldwell headed up an occupational medicine service for private industry and helped establish the Health Club, which became the Health Zone. The service for businesses provided an analysis of on-site worker safety including a comprehensive review of human resource policies, environmental factors and employee practices.

"The way to save on worker's compensation is to prevent injury," he said. "You establish a culture of safety and reward safe behavior — not penalize the injured."

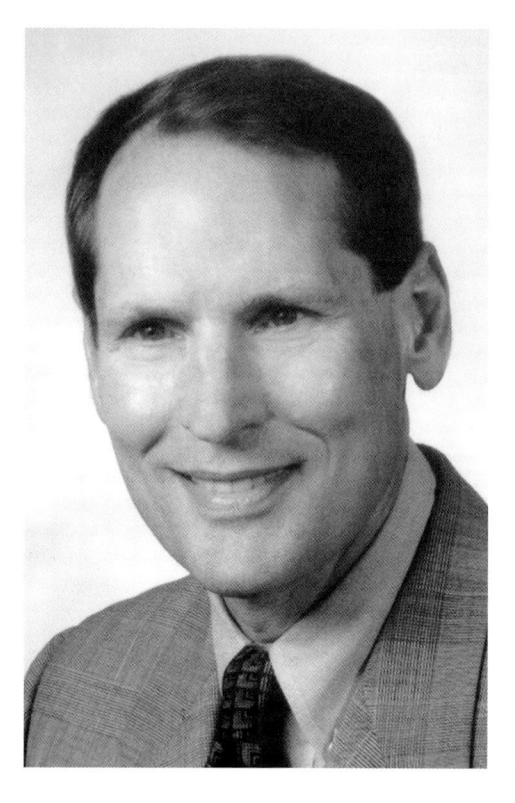

Dr. Caldwell's dedication to health prevention extended to the Health Zone, which transformed from therapeutic recovery center to a personal health facility. He served as the Saint Francis director of occupational health from 1986 to 2000. His time as an administrator set the stage for his work in politics and advocacy.

"As business practices changed and developed, I learned a tremendous amount from the professional administration of large organizations. Having that organizational sense demonstrated how to carry out a goal with the objective of an executive board in mind," he stated.

During his term in 2007, Dr. Caldwell was installed as the president of the Tulsa County Medical Society — its centennial year. The society retired the mortgage on its headquarters at 5315 S. Lewis Avenue and was awarded the national Daily Points of Lights for the society's medication recycling program. He also served as the president of the Oklahoma State Medical Association in 2011 and on the board for its health plan.

Political success was mixed, but he worked toward the tort claim exemption for physicians volunteering in clinics and a Medicaid expansion for children.

"We have no viable political platform that does not somehow benefit patients," he says. "Any change we make to the law has to be tied in with access and quality to the patient. If it doesn't, we shouldn't have it."

During this time, he was instrumental in founding two urgent care clinics as part of his medical group. "Access was the key and convenience to people who valued time," he said. The medical group dissolved and sold its businesses by 2014.

In 1981, Dr. Caldwell married his wife, Kari, a professional cellist, and the couple has two daughters, who are also accomplished musicians and singers.

Rodney L. Clingan, M.D., F.A.C.S.

In 2005, Rodney Clingan, M.D. became one of the first surgical specialists to join St. John's network as an employed physician. Since then, Dr. Mark Kiefer and Dr. Zachary Coburn have joined the growing practice.

Dr. Clingan's parents were nurses, exposing him to the medical field. He received his undergrad degree from Texas A & M University, performed research at Baylor (Houston) on the human genome project, and earned his medical degree from Texas Tech University. He received training in general surgery through the University of Oklahoma at St. John Hospital and colorectal surgery at the Greater Baltimore Medical Center.

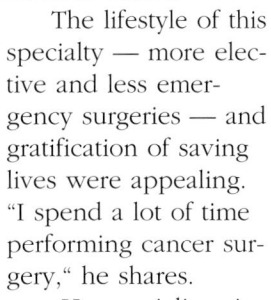

The lifestyle of this specialty — more elective and less emergency surgeries — and gratification of saving lives were appealing. "I spend a lot of time performing cancer surgery," he shares.

He specializes in performing minimally invasive surgery such as laparoscopy and robotics (advanced method) for colon resections and transanal minimally invasive surgery for removing rectal polyps. He's the first surgeon in Tulsa to perform InterStim sacral nerve stimulator placement for fecal incontinence treatment.

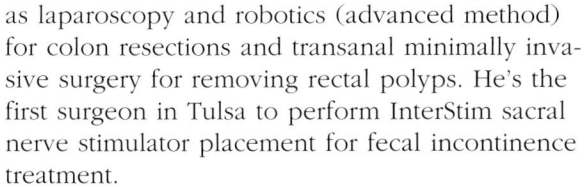

"When I started my practice, few people in Tulsa were doing laparoscopic surgery for colon resections," he explains about a contribution he helped bring to Tulsa. "When I returned from the completion of my training, the majority of my colon resections were laparoscopic."

Considering Tulsa a great community, he makes time to contribute. He was chairman of the Endoscopy Committee at St. John and currently serves as associate professor with the OU-TU School of Community Medicine. His wife has a law degree from The University of Tulsa, is actively involved in Spouses Alliance for the Tulsa County Medical Society and Oklahoma State Medical Association, and teaches exercise classes at St. John.

William R. Condrin, M.D., F.A.C.R.

A native of California, William Condrin, M.D. graduated from Santa Clara University for undergrad. He received his medical education from the University of Saint Louis (St. Louis, Missouri) in 1962 and internship and residency training through the National Naval Medical Center in Bethesda, Maryland. He was board certified in 1967.

He was chief of radiology at the Naval Air Station hospital (Jacksonville, Florida) and served a tour in Vietnam in 1969 and 1970. After ten years in the Navy, he returned to Jacksonville, practicing radiology for three years. Then he came to Tulsa, joining Radiology of Eastern Oklahoma, a private office practice founded by Dr. Bill Benzing in the 1960s and the first outpatient radiology service in Tulsa.

At one time, they had four offices in Tulsa — the most recent in the Kelly Building where they were the first tenants. They procured the first office CT scanner in Tulsa located in the Kelly Building where he worked for thirty years.

"Working with fellow radiologists, Dr. Paul Compton, Dr. Walter Gary, and Dr. Laura Lee, and interacting with the many physicians was very interesting and fulfilling." Before retiring in 2008, he joined Saint Francis's radiology group working in the Kelly Building and in the new imaging center. "Office practice of radiology is no longer possible in this day and age, which is very unfortunate."

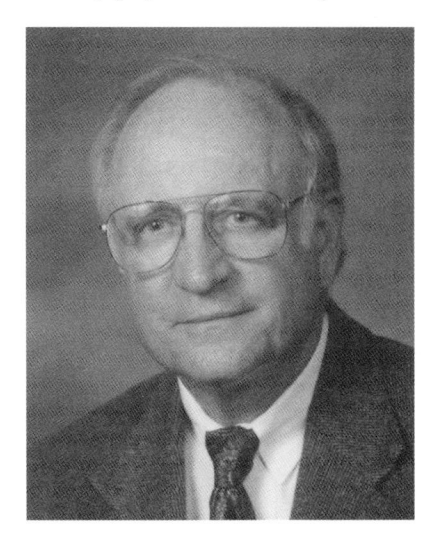

He was a member of the American College of Radiology, American Roentgen Ray Society, and Society of Nuclear Medicine. He served on the Jenks school board and was the physician for the Jenks varsity football team for ten years where his three sons played football. He currently helps with the Drug Recycling Program through the Tulsa County Medical Society.

J. Clark Bundren, M.D.

J. Clark Bundren, M.D., a pioneer of in-vitro fertilization technology (IVF), has participated in its evolution from the start of his over thirty-year medical career. From Bartlesville, Oklahoma, he is from a family of Oklahoma pioneers and explorers. His great-grandfather A.P. Wilcox was a postmaster in Enid, Oklahoma and participated in the opening of the Cherokee Strip in 1893 before statehood.

Dr. Bundren's role in IVF technology had its genesis when he was selected as a Sir Alexander Fleming Scholar at sixteen years of age. "We were working with cell culture systems as it related to better treatment for patients with malignancies and chemotherapy and immunotherapy," he explains regarding research he conducted through the Oklahoma Medical Research Foundation in Oklahoma City.

He received his undergraduate degree from Philips University, attended the University of Oklahoma College of Medicine, spending two years in Oklahoma City then finishing the last two years in Tulsa. His was one of the earliest graduating classes at the new Tulsa campus.

His emergence into IVF technology came in the late '70's when he was recruited to serve his Obstetrics and Gynecology residency and fellowship in Human In-Vitro Fertilization at Eastern Virginia Medical School (EVMS) in Norfolk. He was the youngest member of the Vital Initiation of Pregnancy Project led by professor, Howard Jones, Jr., M.D., a father of assisted reproductive technology in the United States, and Mason C. Andrews, M.D. In 1981, this team – including Andrews and Bundren —delivered the first baby conceived through IVF in the country. "I'm one of that small group scattered around the world that initially developed and made the technology successful and continually work on it today. That's been the focus of my career," Dr. Bundren shares. He was privileged to meet and deal with physiologist Robert Edwards, the 2010 Nobel Prize recipient in Medicine for his breakthrough in IVF technology, while working in Norfolk.

When members of the Tulsa medical community wanted this technology available in this part of the country, they recruited Dr. Bundren. He accepted a full-time position as an associate professor of Obstetrics and Gynecology at OU's medical school at the Tulsa campus. And he brought a few members from EVMS with him including embryology lab director, J.W. Edward Wortham, Jr., Ph.D. who still runs the labs in Oklahoma and the Fertility Institute of New Orleans. In 1983, Dr. Bundren and his team provided Oklahoma's first IVF baby conception.

As a pioneer of this technology, Dr. Bundren, from the beginning of his work, has faced a spectrum of opposition from religious and political leaders — including skeptics who didn't think this technology would work — but overcame them to continue advocating for women and couples suffering from infertility and reproductive issues. Through a landmark case at the Tulsa County District Court, he and his attorneys established the emerging trend of IVF facilities being run in privately-owned clinics instead of by hospitals so that the needs of patients, rather than hospital administrators and institutions, would be served.

This technology was already becoming heavily regulated before the first baby conceived through IVF in the United States was born. In 1978, Congress passed legislation preventing any National

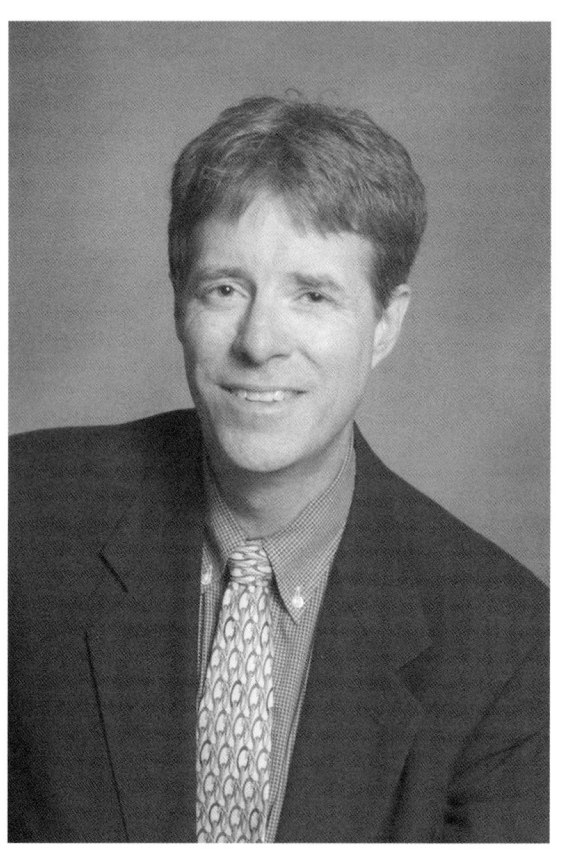

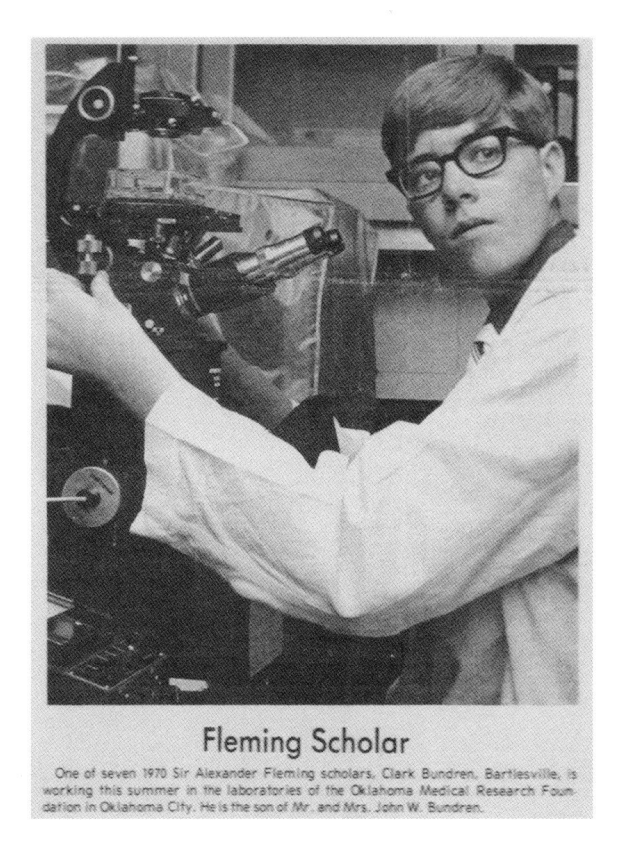

Fleming Scholar

One of seven 1970 Sir Alexander Fleming scholars, Clark Bundren, Bartlesville, is working this summer in the laboratories of the Oklahoma Medical Research Foundation in Oklahoma City. He is the son of Mr. and Mrs. John W. Bundren.

Institute of Health grants for IVF research; thus, any IVF funding for research could only come through private sources. Later, Ron Wyden, a congressman from Oregon, authored various national legislation regulating IVF clinics, labs, and other areas of this technology. Yet, pioneers like Dr. Bundren and his team pushed through the legislative restraints to make great strides in this area of medical care not only in the United States but in the international IVF community as well. "There are several principles used around the world that we developed through research projects early on in the 1980s in collaboration with the University of Tulsa," Dr. Bundren shares.

Unlike in the United States, some governments heavily support IVF technology. In Israel and Australia, where their governments provide mandated-IVF coverage, their utilization rates are at least double the utilization rates in the United States where only thirteen states have mandates for infertility coverage.

Yet, the procedures used in these countries are similar to ones practiced in the United States. Members of the IVF community meet regularly to discuss current events, latest breakthroughs, and modifications. "The systems are not run that differently if you are here, or if you're in Melbourne, Australia, or if you're in Paris, France," says Dr. Bundren about the close-knit global community. "We are all doing very similar things and getting similar results on our patients because we all work together and have for many years."

Through advances in technology and persistence of the physicians using this technology, the pregnancy success rates in this country have greatly improved. "At this present time, in most places around the United States, you can expect any good population of [IVF] patients to have almost half of the patients achieve a pregnancy in any given cycle," Dr. Bundren shares. The initial success rate was one pregnancy out of seven, then one out of five.

Dr. Bundren still serves as a full-time associate professor of Obstetrics and Gynecology at the OU-TU School of Community Medicine teaching residents and medical students. He provides gynecology and reproductive health services to patients and has privileges at various hospitals including Hillcrest, Saint Francis, St. John, and Tulsa Spine and Specialty Hospital. He works at the Bennett Fertility Institute in Oklahoma City. He has served as president of the Tulsa County Obstetrical and Gynecological Society. He is a member of the American Society for Reproductive Medicine and Society for Assisted Reproductive Technology.

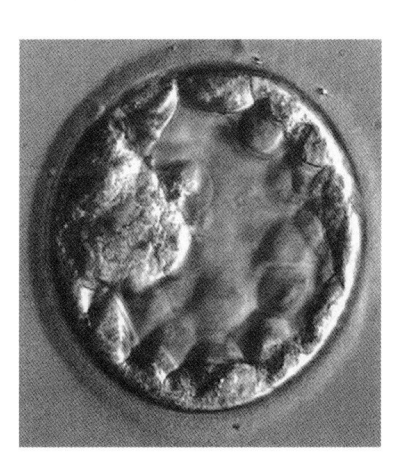

A Human Blastocyst

Bundren and his wife, Mary, a Tulsa attorney, have three children. His medical legacy continues: his daughter is an emergency medicine physician and his nephew is a medical student at Oklahoma State University.

Having committed over thirty years to developing and improving this technology, Dr. Bundren is proud of his work as a pioneer, knowing that he has helped many infertile couples. "That's why we work so diligently to try to improve cost effectiveness and success rates."

FUTURE LEGACIES

Dr. Frederick (Rick) Cohen, M.D.

Dr. Rick Cohen first came to Tulsa while in college in 1970 with his college roommate, Dick Ansteth, to visit his family, liked Tulsa and kept coming back. He was born in Japan and lived there through high school. His father went to Japan as part of the U.S. Occupation after World War II, and stayed for 27 years, a significant part of his family history. In high school, he decided to go into pediatric medicine because he not only loved children, but liked all the pediatricians and pediatric staff he worked with or encountered.

Dr. Cohen attended graduate school at Washington University in St. Louis, MO, and earned his Biology degree with honors, and conducted graduate research in prostaglandin biosynthesis, then completed the "Fifth Pathway" rotating internship at New York Medical College at St. Joseph Hospital in Stamford, CT. In 1980, he decided to make Tulsa his home, primarily because of the friendly people. He began his pediatric residency in 1980, followed by a fellowship in Academic Pediatrics, both from the University of Oklahoma-Tulsa Medical College.

Dr. Cohen is passionate about recognizing those who influenced him, and acted as role models and mentors, and most importantly and invaluable, was their caring attitude during training. Special thanks to Dr. Bob Block, program director/pediatric department at OU; Dr. Charlie Cooper, pediatric cardiology; Dr. Dan Plunket, Pediatric Chair at OU; and Dr. Subramania Jegathesan, to name a few.

Dr. Cohen has seen many changes in the pediatric field. He sees the value in the development of pediatric subspecialties, creating fields of focus, and positively impacting patient care. He has experienced the creation and emergence of electronic medical records (EMR) and is confident the continued development and refinement of EMR will enable doctors and patients to realize the benefits. Dr. Cohen is an advocate for additional funding for pediatric care, as it is essential for the health and well being of children.

Dr. Cohen is a Clinical Professor of Pediatrics at the University of Oklahoma-Tulsa School of Community Medicine, and thoroughly enjoys teaching future doctors. He has attended pediatric clinics in the past and currently continues to lecture to medical students. Dr. Cohen has served on the boards of the Tulsa Health Department and the American Heart Association, and been involved in various other committees and volunteer organizations. He has been a member of the Civil Air Patrol since 1986, is a pilot and the squadron medical officer.

One of the greatest compliments Dr. Cohen receives is when past patients outgrow his practice then bring their children back to him as patients.

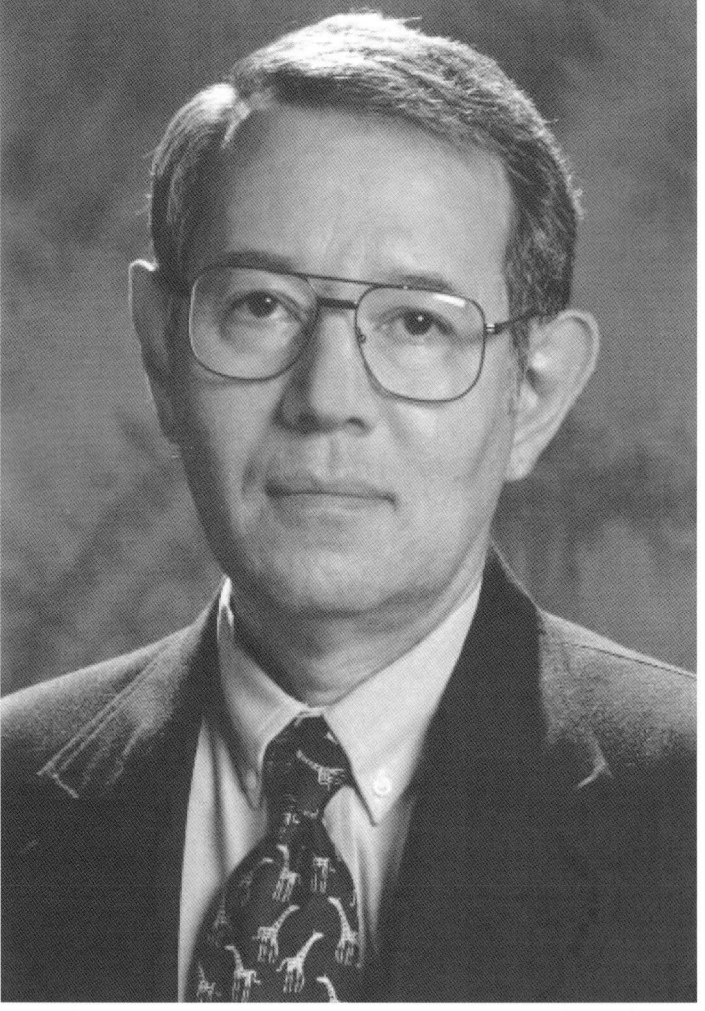

Max A. Deardorff, M.D.

Dr. Max Deardorff is the first in his family to study medicine. He decided that he wanted to become a doctor in the 7th grade when he wrote a paper for Mrs. Lee's social studies class at Woodrow Wilson Jr. High. His good friend's father was an orthopedic surgeon which provided him with additional inspiration along the way.

He received his medical degree from the University of Oklahoma School of Medicine in 1959. His internship with Hillcrest Medical Center began that year and led into his surgery residency from 1960 to 1961 and his OB-GYN residency from 1961 to 1964.

As soon as his residency was finished in 1964, he moved into private practice in Dodge City, Kansas. In 1969, he joined Drs. Mount and Maddox in Tulsa, Oklahoma, where he practiced for 25 years. In 1994 he joined the Warren Clinic, practicing another 15 years until he retired in 2009.

Deardorff has maintained memberships in the American Medical Association, American College of Obstetricians and Gynecologists, Oklahoma State Medical Association, Tulsa County Medical Society and Tulsa County OB-GYN Society. With the American College of OB-GYN, he served as president of the Oklahoma section and member of the District VII Advisory Council. As part of his time in the Tulsa County OB-GYN Society, he also served as President. He served on the board of directors at Saint Francis Hospital in the 1970s.

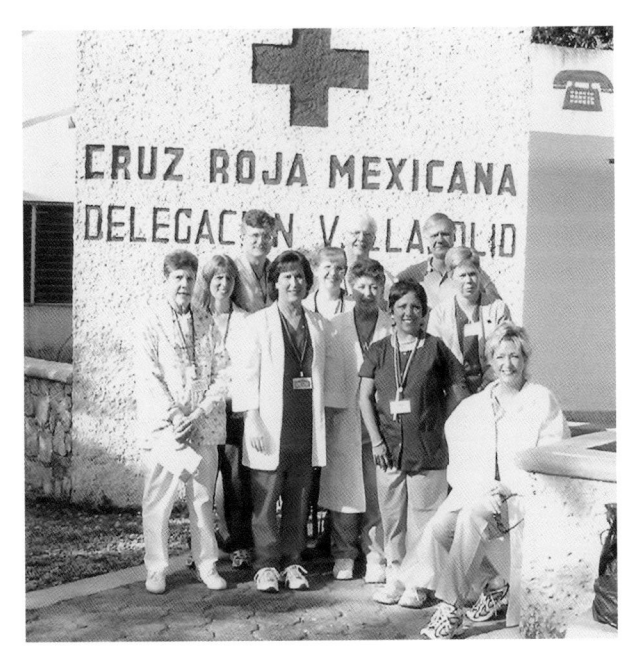

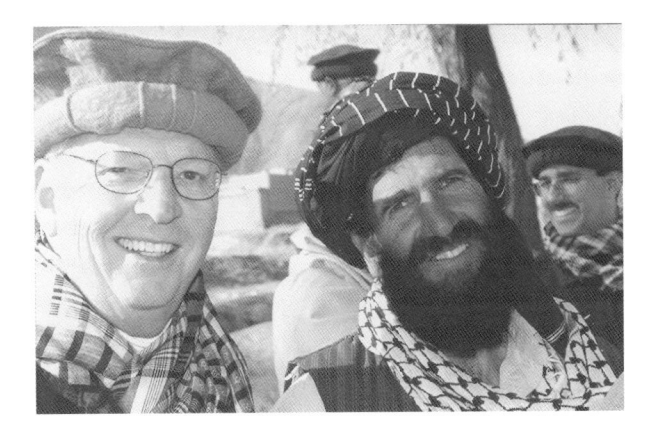

The three main hospitals in Tulsa (St. John, Saint Francis and Hillcrest) combined to form the Tulsa Medical Educational Foundation (TMEF). This was to supervise and coordinate the hospital-based residency programs. Dr. Deardorff served as president of TMEF. This organization evolved into the present Oklahoma University School of Medicine, Tulsa, where he obtained the title of Clinical Professor.

Out of all his accomplishments, he is most proud of serving in mission work. Through friends at his church, he and his wife Kay, a retired R.N., were introduced to volunteering for medical missions. He describes the experience as life changing, and has been on mission trips to locations throughout the world, including Russia, Croatia, Mexico, Nicaragua, Costa Rica, Brazil, and Afghanistan.

He says, "I went on three trips to Afghanistan in 2005 and 2006. I participated in seminars at Kabul University Medical School. Students ready to graduate had never worked with patients! The Taliban banned anything showing anatomy, even pictures in text books. Everything they learned was from lectures, memorizing everything. We bought some cow tongues and set up a workshop to teach them suturing techniques. They were so appreciative and eager to learn."

Two of his trips were to teach gynecologic surgery to OB-GYN and Family Practice Residents in the Cure Hospital, a Christian hospital in Kabul, and the outstanding teaching program in the country. There he worked with dedicated western doctors who were training those who would be the leaders in the country's climb out of the tragedy of the late 20th century and early 21st century.

One could summarize Deardorff's impact with the following words spoken by Dr. Lynn Frame, "Max taught me everything I know, but not everything he knows."

FUTURE LEGACIES

Eastern Oklahoma Ear, Nose and Throat (EOENT)

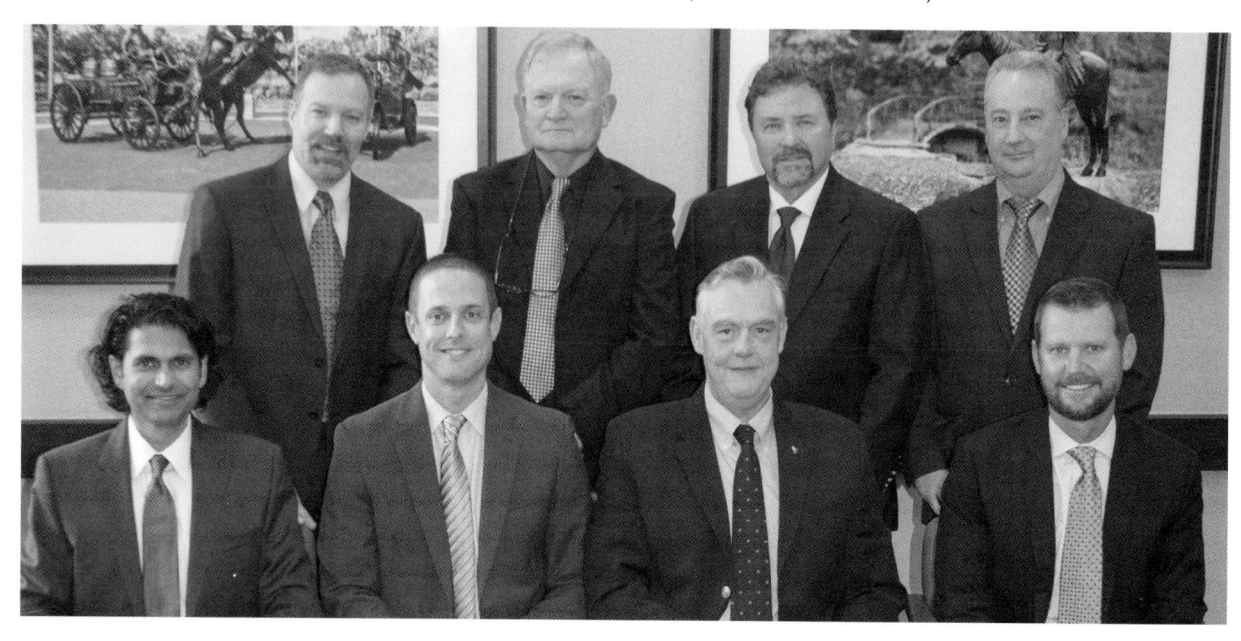

The mission of Eastern Oklahoma Ear, Nose and Throat (EOENT) has always been to provide the highest quality of professional care with integrity, respect and compassion.

In 1975 Dr. Rollie Rhodes with Dr. Charles Heinberg decided to establish an independent otolaryngology practice in South Tulsa at Saint Francis Hospital. From the beginning they based the practice on quality of care and compassion for their patients. In 1978 and 1979 respectively, Dr. Anthony Loehr and Dr. Robert Nelson joined the budding practice. In 1980 they expanded into their current office at 68th and Yale. They continued to grow by adding Dr. Stephen Brownlee in 1988, Dr. William Sawyer II in 1992, Dr. David White in 1994, Dr. David Hall in 2000, Dr. Atul Vaidya in 2003, Dr. Christopher Siemens in 2005, and Dr. Evan Moore in 2012.

Over the past four decades, EOENT has grown into the largest independent private ear, nose and throat clinic in the state of Oklahoma and has the only Board Certified neuro-otologist in the eastern side of the state. The physicians of EOENT practice at Tulsa Spine and Specialty Hospital, Hillcrest Hospital South, and Saint Francis Hospital's Main Campus and South campus. Over the years they have held medical staff leadership positions at all of these hospitals.

EOENT has provided quality care in all aspects of Otolaryngology since its inception. These include the sub-specialty areas of Neuro-Otology, Pediatric Otolaryngology, Endoscopic Sinus Surgery, Allergy, Head and Neck Cancer and Thyroid and Parathyroid surgery. Neuro-Otology deals with diseases of the ear and mastoid as well as dizziness and hearing loss. Pediatric Otolaryngology addresses the special problems that can occur in babies and children. EOENT runs a full Allergy clinic providing allergy testing and treatment and its surgeons are trained in complex sinus surgeries. Their physicians are also trained in the diagnosis and management of head and neck surgery patients. EOENT also provides comprehensive surgical management of complex benign and malignant thyroid and parathyroid tumors.

The physicians and employees of EOENT are very grateful to their loyal and faithful patients, who've entrusted them with their medical care over the past 40 years. According to Dr. Anthony Loehr and Dr. Stephen Brownlee, EOENT has been successful by building a business based on integrity, sound judgment and mutual respect for their patients and employees.

The physicians are anticipating a bright future and hope by continuing to provide quality medical care with compassion, so that the next 40 years will find EOENT providing the same excellent care for the people of Eastern Oklahoma.

Patrick Daley, M.D.

For more than 35 years, Patrick Daley, M.D., has operated one of the few solo pediatric practices in Tulsa. Citing his "excellent bedside manner" and known for laid-back style, he has been named No. 1 pediatrician by *Oklahoma Magazine* for several consecutive years.

Dr. Daley graduated from Oklahoma State University with a bachelor's degree in pre-med in 1974 and earned his medical degree from the University Of Oklahoma School Of Medicine in 1978. He was in the third class of the OU-Tulsa Medical College and completed his pediatric residency in Tulsa. He spent his final year of residency as the chief resident of pediatrics. After one year working in a group practice, Dr. Daley opened his own office, where he has cared for children ever since.

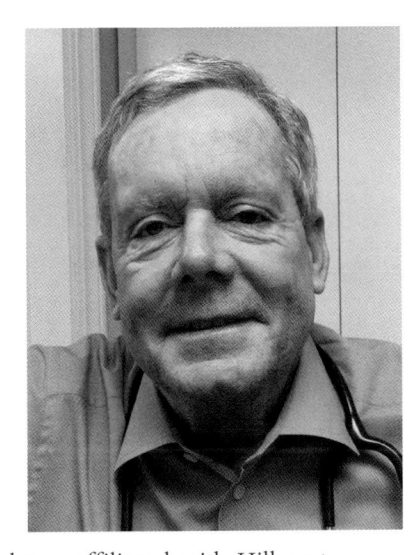

Dr. Daley has been affiliated with Hillcrest Medical Center and Saint Francis Hospital but has spent the most time with St. John Medical Center through several appointed positions. Among his roles at St. John Medical Center: Chairman of pediatrics, medical executive, executive credentials committee, pediatric intensive care unit committee, scan committee and medical education committee. He taught at Tulsa Medical College as a volunteer for five years and published a case review on opthalmia neonatorum. Dr. Daley is a member of Tulsa County Medical Society. For more than 18 years, he participated in the "doctor on call" segment featured during the noon newscast on a local television station. Dr. Daley has a civic interest in the Tulsa Boys Home. Throughout his practice, he voluntarily cared for residents of the Tulsa Boys Home when needed.

He is married and raised six children — Bill, John, Tom, Mark, Chris and Megan. He now has two grandchildren. Outside the office, Dr. Daley enjoys golfing, fly fishing and traveling with his wife.

E. Bradley Garber, M.D., F.A.C.S.

"The practice of medicine is an art, not a trade; a calling, not a business; a calling in which your heart will be exercised equally with your head."
SIR WILLIAM OSLER, M.D. 1849-1919.

Eugene Bradley Garber, M.D., F.A.C.S. is a Phi Beta Kappa graduate of the University of Colorado and AOA Graduate of Louisiana State University Medical Center. He served seven years in the U.S. Army Medical Corps and was the Chief of Otolaryngology at Landsthul Army Medical Center in Germany.

Dr. Garber completed a five-year Otolaryngology/Head and Neck Residency in Denver, Colorado and a two-year Plastic and Reconstructive Surgery Fellowship in Miami, Florida.

In 1973, during the first year of medical school, he married his high school sweetheart, Mary Christine Custar, and started a family.

He says, "My family has been my constant support, showing much love and encouragement, and enduring many sacrifices through this wonderful journey of education and medical practice."

Dr. Garber credits surgeon D. Ralph Millard, M.D., Chief of Plastic and Reconstructive Surgeon at the University of Miami as having a significant influence on his medical career.

"He instilled in me the principles of plastic and reconstructive surgery that have guided me through many difficult cases in the operating room," says Dr. Garber.

Dr. Garber is a member of several medical societies and is the past President of the Tulsa County Medical Society.

He says, "We are blessed to have a great medical community in Tulsa. Since establishing my solo practice in Tulsa in 1985, I have been fortunate to have worked with many excellent physicians, and I appreciate the trust they have given me in caring for their patients."

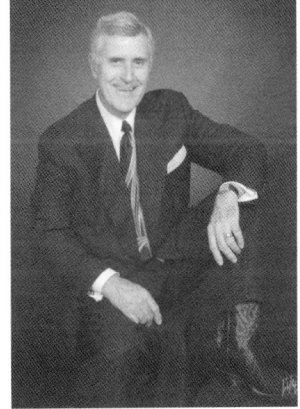

FUTURE LEGACIES

Charles A Farmer, M.D., F.A.C.E.P.

Hard-earned accomplishments and well-deserved accolades gird the 40-year span of Charles Farmer's medical career. In 40 years' time, a lot of life is lived as well. And rarely could someone's personal life and professional career intersect in such dramatic fashion as it did for Dr. Farmer within the walls of St. John Medical Center.

Charles (Bo) Farmer M.D., F.A.C.E.P., was born and raised in the small rural town of Dumas, Arkansas. After his sophomore year at Arkansas Tech University in Russellville, Bo married his college sweetheart, Sheri, and graduated two years later in 1967. He went on to receive his medical degree from the University of Arkansas School of Medicine in Little Rock in 1971, during which time he and Sheri had their first two children, Lori and Misti. While in medical school, he was elected to the AOA National Honor Medical Society.

After medical school, Bo moved his family to Tulsa to do a mixed medicine/surgery internship at St. John's Hospital. That February on the OB floor, coincidentally the same floor where he was rotating that month, Bo and Sheri joyfully welcomed their third child, Joli, into the world. Immediately upon her arrival, Bo and Sheri realized that she was missing her left arm. In that moment, celebration and sorrow intermingled together and foreshadowed a pattern that is inevitable when one is both living a life and establishing a career in the very same building.

The family moved again after Bo's internship to Pensacola, Florida, where Bo served as a Navy Flight Surgeon. After clocking more than 300 hours of flight time, he considered a career as a physician astronaut. Unfortunately, NASA had recently stopped accepting flight surgeons into the space program. While that was disappointing, the family time spent on the beautiful white beaches of Pensacola and the birth of their fourth child and only son, Chad, made their time in Florida memorable and fulfilling.

The Farmer family returned to Tulsa in 1975 for Bo to do a surgery residency, and shortly after that Bo and Sheri welcomed another baby, their fifth and final one, whom they named Kali. During this first year of residency, Bo's path took a dramatic and unexpected turn when St. John CEO Sister M. Therese Gottschalk asked him to serve as the Director of Emergency Medicine. After much thought and consideration, he accepted the position in January of 1977, and he served loyally and passionately as director for the next 34 years. So in a sense, he didn't choose Emergency Medicine, but rather it chose him.

Only six months into his 34-year tenure, however, Dr. Farmer received a life-changing phone call while he was finishing up a night shift in the Emergency Department. An overhead page summoned him to the nurses station for an urgent phone call. When he answered the phone, the person on the other end of the line told him that his oldest daughter, Lori, was found murdered that morning at Girl Scout camp. His friend and partner in the department, Dr. Lloyd Anderson, drove him home where he had to share the devastating news with his wife. Lori was five days shy of her ninth birthday.

As a husband and father of four living children, life dictated that he return to work in order to provide for his family. Day after day, he continued to see patients and take phone calls at the same place

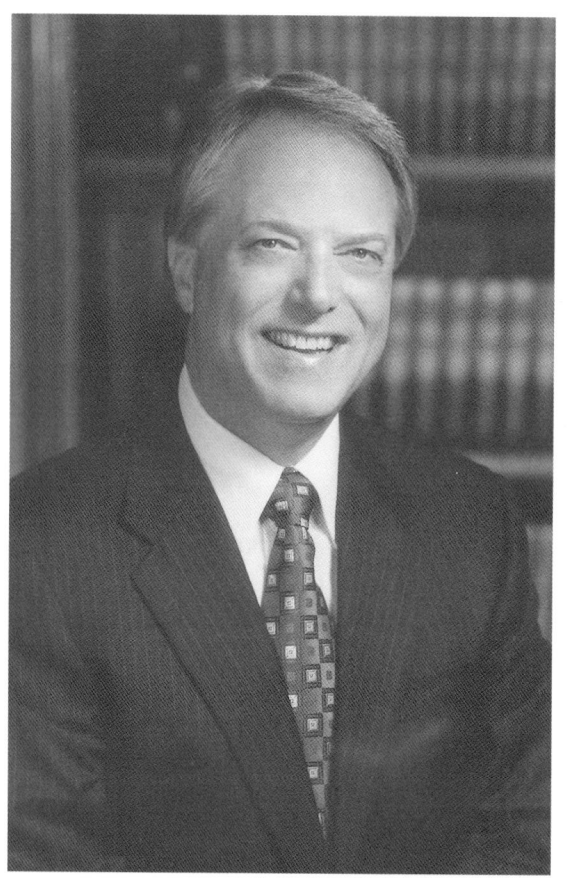

FUTURE LEGACIES

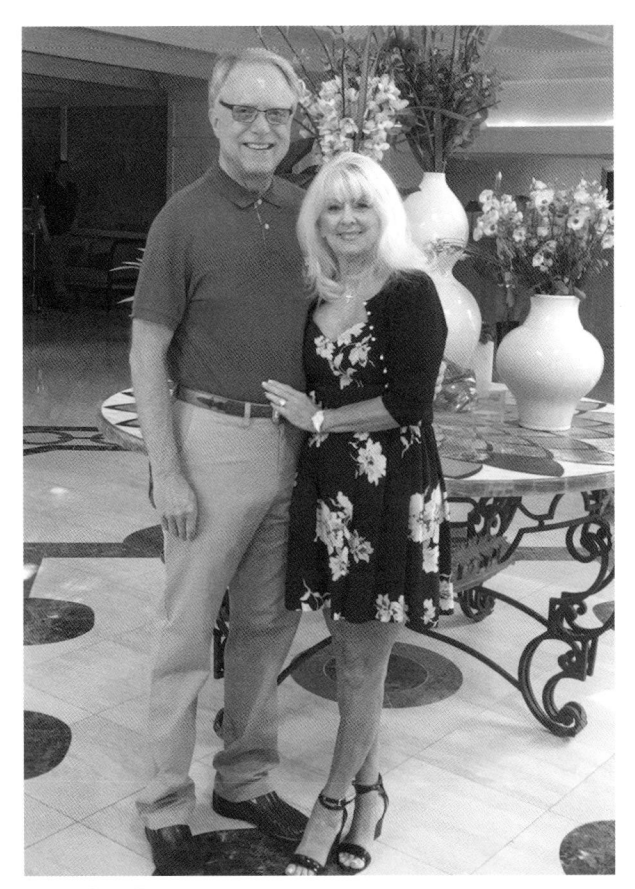

Bo and Sheri Farmer

where he learned his daughter had been killed. He also maintained his ED shifts and leadership positions throughout the ensuing criminal trial. Not only did he continue working through his grief, but he built a commendable career by providing exemplary medical care for his patients and innovative leadership for his colleagues over the course of several decades.

During Dr. Farmer's 40 years at St. John, he pioneered many advancements in medical care beyond his role as a physician and Director of the Emergency Department. He served on the Medical Executive Committee for 34 years, was the Director of Employee Health Service for 15 years, the Director of Hyperbaric Medicine for six years, the Director of the St. John Sapulpa Emergency Department for six years, and the Medical Director of the St. John AirEvac helicopter medical transport service. He was also instrumental in the initiative to develop the St. John Cardiovascular Institute and served as course director of the first St. John Cardiovascular Symposium. He was appointed to the Honorary Staff in 2002.

Continued on following page

Farmer Family Members in the Medical Field

Dr. Farmer's passion for and commitment to the practice of medicine was undoubtedly passed on to his children. His daughter Misti has achieved a notable career in medical ultrasonography and is now obtaining her master's degree in strategic leadership in order to further her career in ultrasound teaching.

Misti's son Chase Coates, Dr. Farmer's grandson, is a highly respected paramedic and supervisor with the Tulsa Emergency Medical Services Authority (EMSA) and he was recently honored with the prestigious "Star of Life" award. Chase's wife, Sarah, has her own ties to St. John where she works as an RN in the neurotrauma unit of the ICU.

Dr. Farmer's son, Chad, has followed in his father's pioneering footsteps by becoming one of the first physicians in the country to be fellowship trained in Palliative Medicine. Chad is now a nationally recognized physician in his specialty and he practices in Tampa and Pensacola, Florida, where he was born.

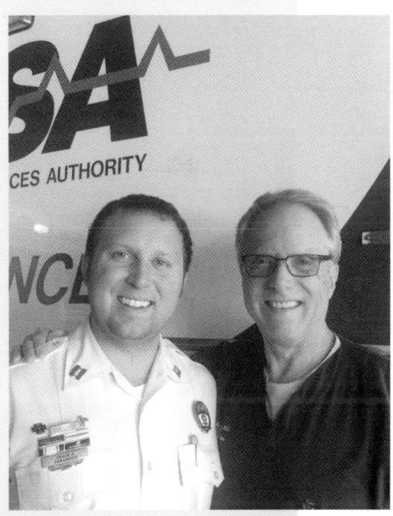

Bo Farmer with his grandson Chase Coates.

Dr. Farmer's daughter Dr. Kali Cole is a pioneer in her own right as the first female opthomologist to establish her own solo private practice in Tulsa. Kali's husband, Dr. Scott Cole, is a hematologist-oncologist with the Cancer Specialists of Oklahoma/St. John-M.D. Anderson Cancer Center.

Dr. Farmer's daughter Joli is not employed in the medical field, but she still maintains a connection to medicine through her husband, Todd Beasley, who is an anesthesiologist at St. John.

Bo is eternally grateful to his wife Sheri who is the rock on which his family is built. Her unending support, nurturing, guidance and encouragement have sustained the entire family throughout the years.

243

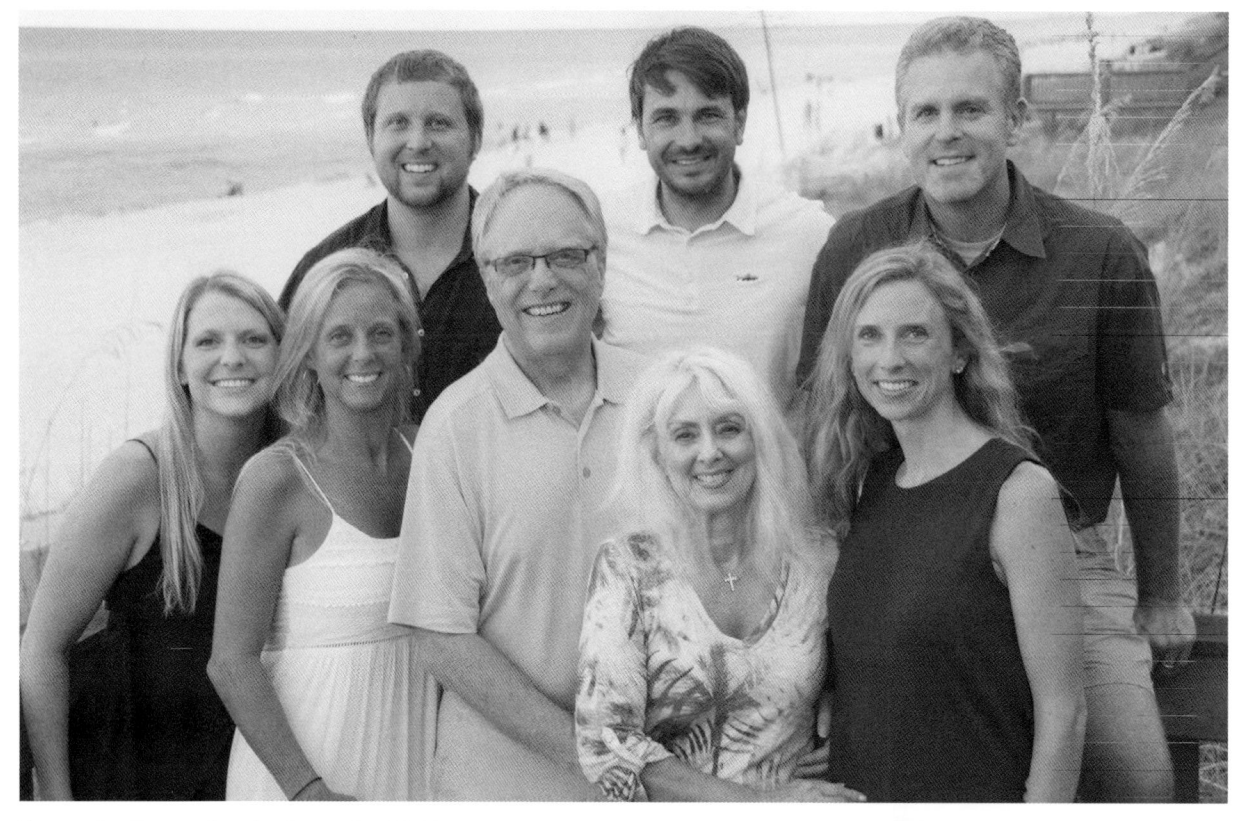

Farmer family members in the medical field
front row from left — Sarah Coates, Misti Shannon, Bo and Sheri Farmer, Kali Cole
Back row from left — Chase Coates, Scott Cole, Todd Beasley
Not pictured — Chad Farmer

Another large portion of Dr. Farmer's medical career includes his involvement in the Southern Medical Association which comprised 17 southeastern states and the District of Columbia. He served as Chairman of the Emergency Medicine Section, Councilor from Oklahoma, was on the Executive Committee and then ultimately was elected to serve as President of the organization in 2005.

Throughout the years, many personal events, both good and bad, brought Dr. Farmer back to his workplace. At these times, however, he was not the doctor but the husband, dad or grandad of the patient. He was full of joy, pride and nostalgia when several of his grandchildren were born at St. John, reminding him of when his own daughter was delivered there over twenty years earlier. When his children or grandchildren needed stitches or a cast, he was back at the ED he had just left hours earlier after finishing up a shift.

One of the most traumatic personal experiences the family faced at St. John was when Sheri was admitted to the ED with a kidney stone. In a matter of hours, her health rapidly deteriorated and she became septic. Sheri was moved to the ICU and,

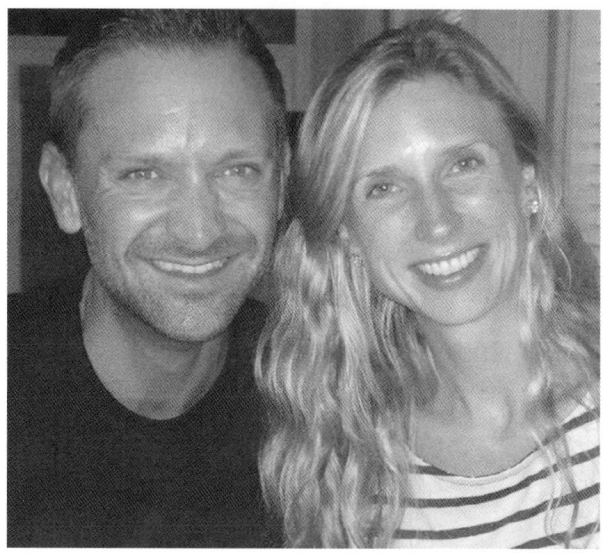

Bo and Sheri Farmer's physician children Chad Farmer and Kali Cole

with multiple organ systems failing, she was put on a ventilator for eleven days. Dr. Farmer would sit by her bedside for hours and then ride the elevator down a few floors to work his shift in the ED. Against all odds, Sheri survived. Once again, it was an unprecedented melding of his personal and professional life within the walls of St. John Medical Center.

Before Sheri's release from the hospital, Dr.

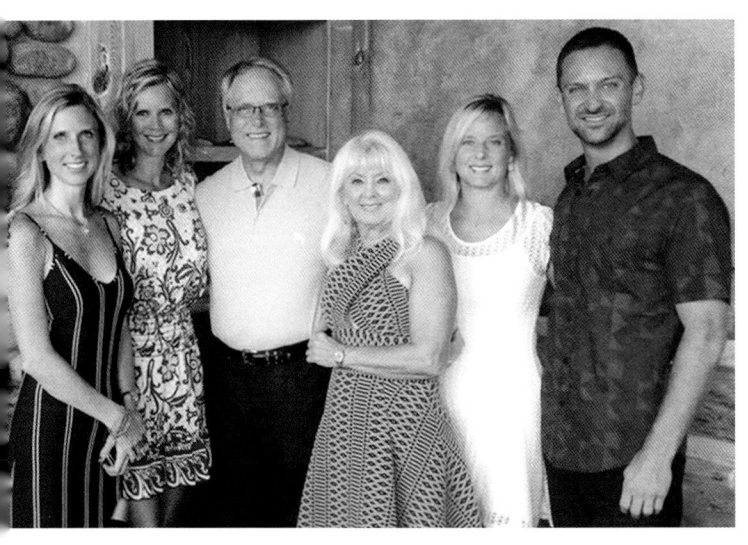

Celebrating Bo and Sheri's 50th wedding anniversary from left — Kali Cole, Joli Beasley, Bo and Sheri Farmer, Misti Shannon and Chad Farmer

Farmer attended one last Executive Committee meeting after retiring from his ED Director and Chairman positions. This time, however, he had his wife by his side. Together they were able to express their sincere gratitude to the St. John leadership and medical staff for the support they had received over the last 34 years and for the heroic efforts that had been put forth to save Sheri's life. Dr. Farmer stood before his longtime friends and colleagues and poignantly summarized his career at St. John's with this touching statement:

"You've heard of life and death stories. Well, it has occurred to me that mine is more a story of death and life. As you know, Sheri almost died a few days ago. The reason she is with me tonight is a combination of miracle and medical intervention. I am struck by the realization that the two most significant events in my life stand as bookends on each side of my career. At the beginning, my daughter was dead when she should have been alive, and now at the end, my wife is alive when she should have been dead. So as you see, it truly is a story of death and life and St. John, and all of you as my friends and colleagues, have been at the center of it all."

As a result of his many personal experiences and his professional influence at the hospital, Dr. Farmer's life and legacy will forever be entwined with both the past and the future of St. John Medical Center. Over the last 40 years, they have served and shaped each other in significant and beneficial ways that will leave a lasting impact on them both.

IN ADDITION TO HIS 40 YEARS OF SERVICE TO ST. JOHN,

Dr. Farmer has pioneered many advancements in emergency medicine locally, statewide and nationally including:

- Among earliest board certified emergency physicians
- "Fellow for Life" of the American College of Emergency Physicians
- Established two St. John Minor Emergency Centers, the first one being only the fifth such ambulatory urgent care centers in the country, with two of his partners
- Original Trustee of the Board of Tulsa's Emergency Medical Service Authority (EMSA) and continued working with the service for 32 years in several other positions including Chairman of Emergency Physicians Foundation, Chairman of the Medical Control Board and interim Medical Director
- Trained as one of the first physicians to be an instructor for Advanced Cardiac Life Support (ACLS), a new program at the time developed by the American Heart Association in 1978
- Affiliate Faculty and National Faculty member for ACLS in addition to being a representative to a national ACLS Standards Conference
- President of the Tulsa Chapter and the Oklahoma affiliate of the American Heart Association
- Medical Director of the St. John Paramedic Training Program
- Chairman of the Medical Advisory Committee of the first Tulsa Vo-Tech Paramedic Program
- Chairman of the of the Medical Advisory Committee of AirEvac, St. John's helicopter patient transport service
- Medical Director of AeroCare Medical Transport, Inc., the first fixed-wing air transport service in Tulsa
- Medical Director of AirEMS, a successor to AeroCare
- Vice-Chairman of the Oklahoma Trauma System Improvement and Development Advisory Council (OTSIDAC), a council formed by Governor Frank Keating to create a regional trauma system for Oklahoma

Family Medical Care of Tulsa, In His Image Family Medicine

When the Oral Roberts University City of Faith hospital and medical school closed in 1989, some physicians on its staff wanted to preserve the Christian-centered practice of medicine. For those doctors, board-certified in Family Medicine, this led to the formation of Family Medical Care of Tulsa, In His Image Family Medicine Residency, In His Image International, and Good Samaritan Health Services mobile medical outreach.

Dr. John Crouch was the chairman of the ORU medical school's department of Family Medicine at the time. By 1990, he and several doctors made the switch from the City of Faith to an affiliation with Hillcrest Medical Center, where the training program was based for over twenty years. In July 2011, the organization transitioned to St. John Medical Center.

Family Medical Care of Tulsa is the private practice arm of the training program. It moved in April 2014 into a new facility at 7501 S. Riverside Parkway. The building is equipped with three patient care pods, a centrally located physician teaching area, lecture and conference rooms, a walk-in clinic, Behavioral Medicine clinic, counseling offices, laboratory services, x-ray services, and administrative offices for In His Image and Good Samaritan. It has four satellite clinics (three in Tulsa and one in Okmulgee) located in low-income neighborhoods.

The Family Medicine training program is fully accredited by the Accreditation Council for Graduate Medical Education (ACGME). More than 270 physicians have graduated from the program and most stay in contact through the In His Image Alumni Association. While about 15 percent of residents are from Oklahoma, over 25 percent of graduates remain in northeastern Oklahoma to practice medicine. Of the graduates, about 18 percent are serving in long-term, international medical missions and another 15 percent are working in Indian Health Service and in other places with underserved populations. Many of the alumni who live in the United States are active in international medical outreach and medical education.

The international missions arm — In His Image International — often sends physicians to countries where people need medical help after national disasters or during times of political unrest. Teams have been sent to help after earthquakes, floods, tsunamis, and refugees fleeing terrorism. Of the graduate residents, about forty have done full-time medical missions in other countries. The ministry has helped establish eight international physician training programs to bolster medical care in countries of need.

In 1998, Good Samaritan Health Services was founded as a local mission to offer free medical care to the poor and uninsured or underinsured in Tulsa. Within a year, one site grew to several through the use of the first medical truck. In 2007, a second medical truck — a state-of-the-art, 63-foot tractor trailer — was added. Area churches provide

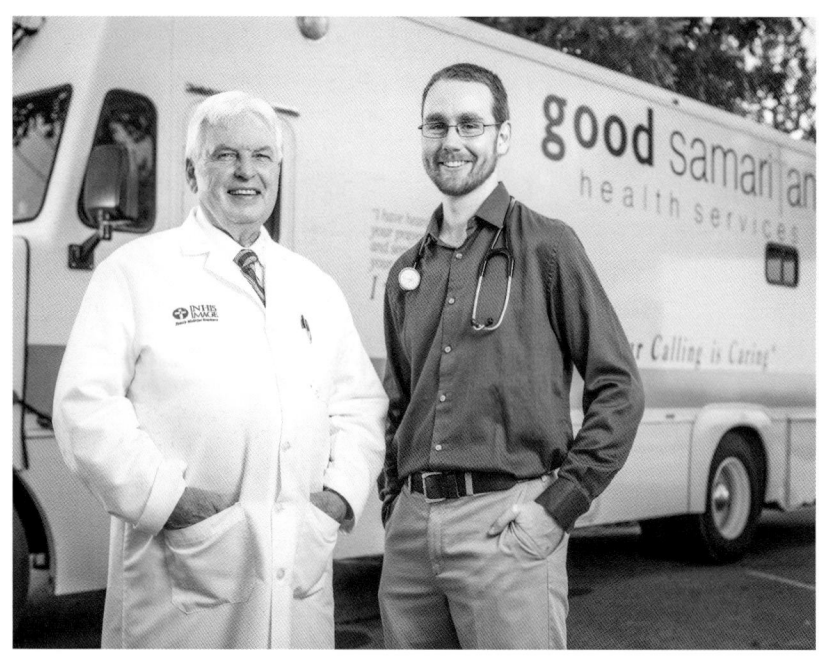

Dr. Crouch and a Family Medicine resident with one of our mobile medical vans.

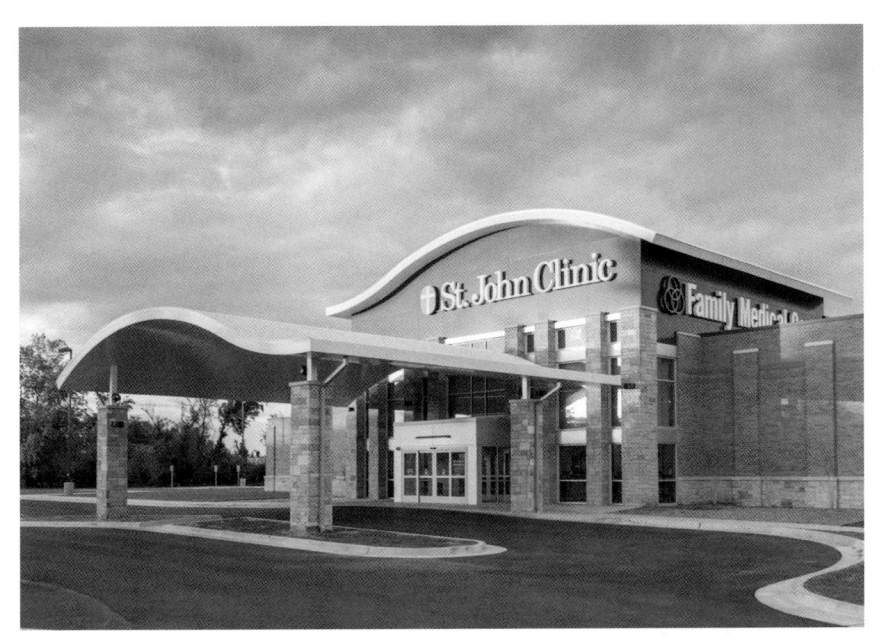

St. John Family Medical Care Clinic.

the facilities for patient check-in and volunteers for the clinic operations. Each month, the health service provides more than fifty free medical clinics to more than six hundred patients at fourteen sites. To provide the care, more than thirty physicians volunteer their time, and many of those are In His Image resident doctors.

THE FOUNDING PHYSICIANS OF FAMILY MEDICAL CARE OF TULSA AND IN HIS IMAGE

John Crouch, M.D., serves as President of In His Image International, the Founder and Executive Director Emeritus of the In His Image Family Medicine Residency Program, and President of Good Samaritan Health Services. He graduated from Southern Illinois University and the University of Illinois-Urbana in 1963. He completed his education at the Washington University School of Medicine. He served a tour as a medical officer and battalion flight surgeon in the U.S. Army during the Vietnam War, where he received the Bronze Star and Air Medal awards.

In 2001, Dr. Crouch was named Oklahoma Family Physician of the Year and was awarded the Educator of the Year the following year by the 18,000 member Christian Medical and Dental Association. He served on that association's board and as its President.

Mitchell Duininck, M.D., is currently serving as President and Director of In His Image Family Residency, overseeing about 22 faculty physicians and 36 resident physicians. He graduated from Bethel College in St. Paul, Minnesota, and earned his medical degree from ORU School of Medicine. Dr. Duininck has completed medical missions in many countries and has led disaster relief medical teams to Zaire, Honduras, Indonesia, Pakistan, Myanmar, and Iraq.

Edward Rylander, M.D., serves as Vice President of the Family Medical Care of Tulsa clinic and is a core senior faculty member of the training program. He graduated from Oral Roberts University with a Bachelor's Degree in 1981 and earned his medical degree from the ORU School of Medicine in 1985.

Frank Hamilton, M.D., Medical Director of Family Medical Care, received his medical degree at the University of Oregon Health Sciences Center in Portland, Oregon, and completed his internship and residency at the San Bernardino County Medical Center of Family Practice in San Bernardino in California. He is a member of the Christian Medical and Dental Association, Oklahoma Academy of Family Physicians, and the American Academy of Family Physicians.

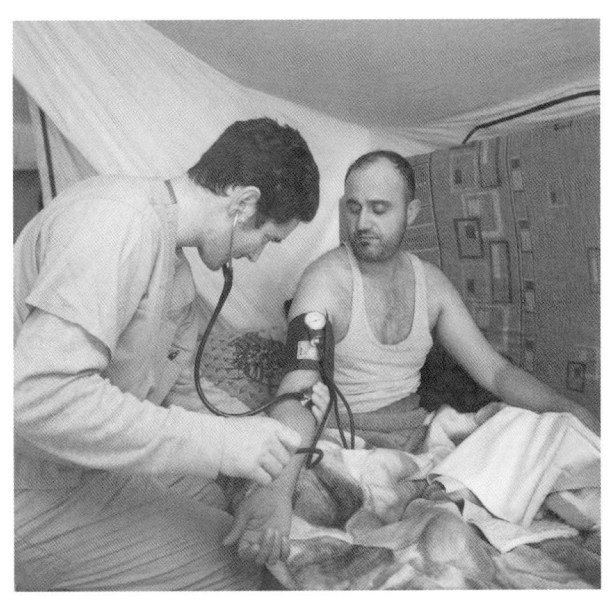

In His Image resident caring for a refugee in the Middle East.

Jeffrey L. Galles, D.O.

Jeffrey Galles, D.O. received his medical heritage from his nurse practitioner mother and chiropractor father. "Listening to them talk about health care and patients fascinated me." Four of his five siblings are physicians including Mark Galles, M.D. an internist with Warren Clinic.

Dr. Galles attended the University of Oklahoma for undergrad, then the Oklahoma College of Osteopathic Medicine and Surgery. His father and his family physician, James Turrentine, D.O., were influences for him pursuing an osteopathic education. He spent his one-year rotating internship at the Tulsa Regional Medical Center and internal medicine residency at the University of Iowa.

In 1992, Dr. Galles came to Tulsa, practicing at Utica Park Clinic (UPC) as an internist—a field that's ideal for him. "My relationship with patients allows me to manage more complicated illnesses because we can test different strategies together." With the continuity he creates with patients, he incorporates a holistic approach to patient care. "You listen to the patient, meet family members, and understand different perspectives of their health, genetics, and background. You incorporate those factors in a holistic approach to understand each patient's unique needs."

Dr. Galles has witnessed sweeping changes in health care throughout his career and cites the past three years as the most dynamic. He embraces the current trend of the primary care physician serving as a "medical gatekeeper" responsible for guiding patients through the complex healthcare system. "Patients now have more financial responsibility and physicians have a responsibility to guide them to appropriate, cost-effective care. I think patient-centered care benefits both the patient as well as the healthcare system as a whole."

Dr. Galles has served in various leadership roles at the Hillcrest HealthCare System (HHS) including Medical Staff President at Hillcrest Medical Center, current UPC Chief Medical Officer; he has chaired the Performance Improvement Committee at Bailey Medical Center in Owasso and the UPC Quality Improvement Committee. He also oversees the four-year CMMI Comprehensive Primary Care Initiative at UPC.

Dr. Galles is proud to have served his entire career at Hillcrest Medical Center (HMC) in Tulsa, OK. The origins of Hillcrest began in 1918 when nurse Dolly Brown McNulty founded Morningside Hospital and School of Nursing. In 1940, Morningside was renamed Hillcrest Memorial Hospital and twelve years later the hospital was renamed Hillcrest Medical Center. In 2004, Ardent Health Services purchased HHS, becoming a for-profit healthcare system. Currently, HHS serves Northeastern Oklahoma with four regional hospitals, three Tulsa hospitals, the Oklahoma Heart Institute, and UPC. UPC currently cares for over 50,000 patients a month. "When I joined the group, we had 35 physicians, and now we have almost 240 physicians and Advanced Practice Providers," he shares regarding HHS's growth.

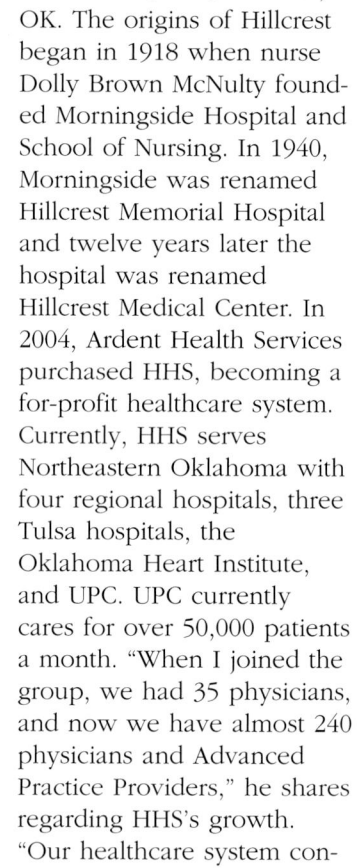

"Our healthcare system continues to grow and we continue to strive to improve the health care for the people of eastern Oklahoma."

Dr. Galles is active in the medical community. He served as chairman, board member, and first DO president of the Tulsa County Medical Society. He has served as clinical associate professor at OSU and OU-TU medical schools, provided volunteer physician services for Project Get Together, MyHealth Health Information Exchange, as well as the Tulsa County Health Improvement Organization (CHIO).

He and his wife, LuAnna, have two adult children.

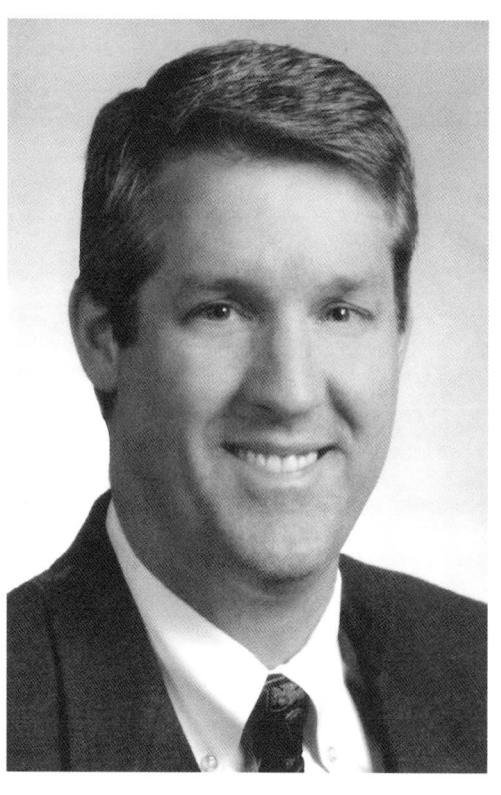

Robert Garrett, M.D., F.A.C.S.

Robert Garrett, M.D.'s work ethic began on a dairy farm in Tulsa, Oklahoma — a trait required for cardiovascular surgeons who work long hours, perform lengthy surgeries, and are available for emergencies. He attended the University of Oklahoma for premed and medical school education, Tulane University in New Orleans for residency training, and the University of Oregon Health Sciences Center in Portland for thoracic training.

He returned to New Orleans to start his practice. Two years later, he settled in Tulsa to join Dr. Robert Blankenship, Dr. Frank Fore, Dr. Bill Loughridge, and Dr. George Cohlmia at Cardiovascular and Thoracic Surgery. He credits these partners and other veteran cardiovascular surgeons for helping him establish a great foundation as a surgeon. "Dr. Fore and Dr. Blankenship are incredible partners. They're very hard working and take great care of patients — I learned a lot from them."

Dr. Garrett spent twenty-five years in private practice. Although he rotated to different hospitals including Hillcrest, Saint Francis, and Heart Hospital, he practiced predominately at St. John. For the past nine years, Dr. Garrett and his partners joined the St. John Health System — an arrangement he's satisfied with. He credits former CEO, Sister Therese Gottschalk, as a great influence in this decision.

He appreciates the changes in cardiothoracic surgery. "I've seen a great deal of modifications and changes in medicine, and certainly in technology, the procedures, and spectrum of what we do. I think most changes, especially since many are less invasive, have benefited patients a great deal." A few examples are inserting heart valves with catheters instead of performing open surgery, and using scopes and robotics for certain thoracic procedures. Yet, many issues such as heart and vascular disease require the traditional approach.

Another change he's witnessed is the regulation of physicians' hours — limiting work hours and number of calls. This regulation has increased the popularity of hospitalists and physicians preferring standard work hours. With fewer physicians entering cardiothoracic surgery training and many cardiothoracic surgeons retiring, there's a shortage: "By no means is this field dying, but fewer people are going into it because of the length of training and hours required." Other subspecialties can help with the load, but ultimately only cardiothoracic surgeons can perform certain procedures since they take a long time to master.

Yet, despite the strenuous lifestyle, Dr. Garrett loves his career and gives back to the medical community. He's involved in OU-TU's general surgery residency program primarily helping fourth-year residents. He's able to inject wisdom from years of experience, advising on various issues such as dealing with patients and loved ones, preparing patients for death, and handling the protocol of referring physicians.

He's a member of various societies including the Tulsa County Medical Society, Tulsa Surgical Society, Oklahoma State Medical Association, American College of Chest Surgeons, and Society of Thoracic Surgeons.

He credits his wife, Stephanie, and their three adult children, Tanner, Tyler, and Ellie, for playing a big part in everything he's accomplished. Despite a demanding career, Dr. Garrett always made his children's activities a priority.

As a native Tulsan, Dr. Garrett's pleased to practice here: "I think we practice medicine as well as any place in the country — there's essentially no major medical need that can't be handled here. Tulsa can be proud of its medical community with great physicians, hospitals, and a rich history."

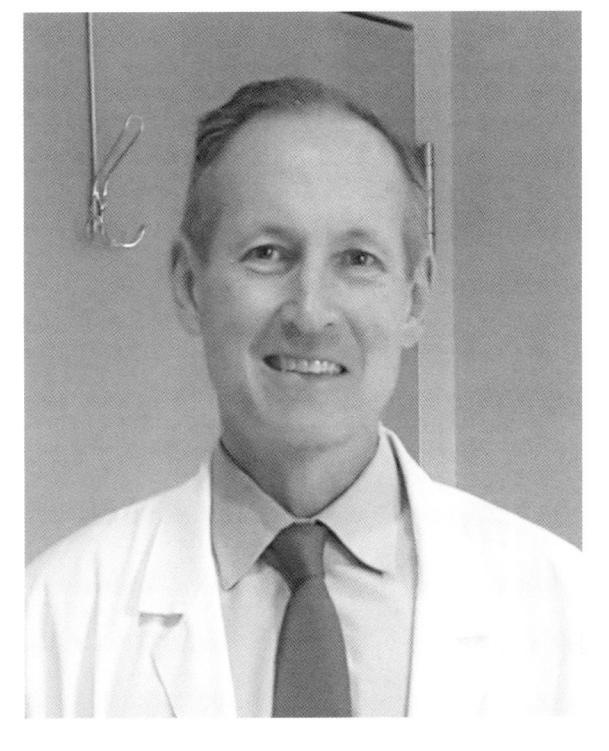

Rachel Gibbs, M.D.

Dr. Rachel Gibbs, M.D., native of Bentonville, Arkansas, worked as a nurse before earning her medical degree and specializing in cutting-edge, robotic technology in gynecological surgery. She graduated from Oklahoma Baptist University School of Nursing with a bachelor's degree in 1981 and cared for burn patients at Oklahoma Baptist Medical Center in Oklahoma City.

While on staff at the hospital, she earned her medical degree from the University of Oklahoma College of Medicine in Oklahoma City in 1987 and completed her residency in obstetrics and gynecology at the University of Arkansas College of Medicine. In 1991, Dr. Gibbs returned to Tulsa to join the Springer Clinic, which had been a physician-owned practice until its merger with Warren Clinic in 2006. She spent 22 years in obstetrics and gynecology before concentrating exclusively on surgery in 2013.

In 2009, Dr. Gibbs joined a small number of Tulsa doctors in completing training in the use of robotic technology in surgery. The device, controlled by surgeons at a console, is equipped with three-dimensional vision imaging and instruments with a wider-range of motion than other tools.

Dr. Gibbs' community involvement includes serving on the boards of the Tulsa Fetal and Infant Mortality Review Board, Call Rape and the Baptist Children's Home. She is married to attorney George Gibbs, and the couple have two sons.

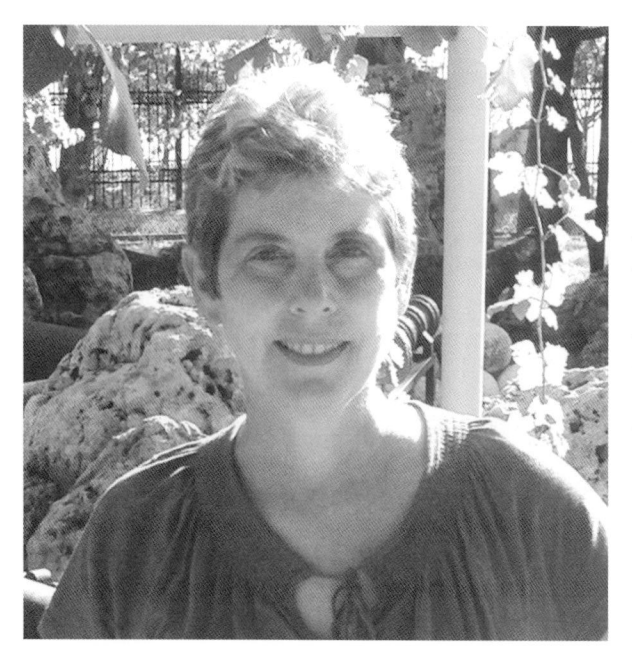

Roger V. Haglund, M.D., M.S.U.

Roger Haglund, M.D., son of Swedish immigrants, was educated at the University of Minnesota. He served in the Navy where he learned electronics, a skill for employment that financed undergraduate studies and allowed him to save the G.I. Bill for medical school. He had a general rotating internship in Seattle, then spent his four-year urology residency at the VA Hospital in Minneapolis. While working as Chief of Urology at this hospital, he also earned a Master of Science in Urology at the University of Minnesota.

In 1960, he joined Dr. E.N. Lubin in Tulsa and worked in private practice until retiring in 2001. Today, that practice has more than twenty urologists.

Throughout his forty-one years of urologic practice, he's witnessed many changes: "Better endoscopic operations, lithotripsy, renal transplantation and robotic procedures are of note." Tulsa's Renal Transplantation Program was started by Dr. Haglund, Dr. V.L. Robards, and nephrologists at Hillcrest Medical Center.

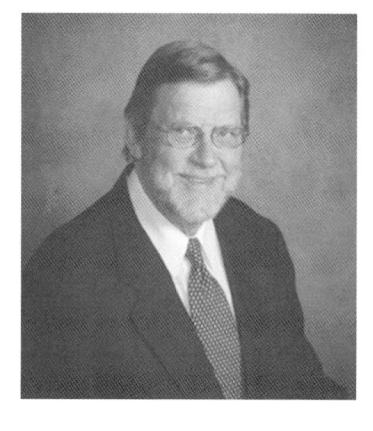

Dr. Haglund has served as President of the Hillcrest Medical Center staff, the Tulsa County Medical Society (when OU established the College of Medicine-Tulsa), Oklahoma Organ Sharing Network, South Central Section (SCS) of the American Urological Association (AUA), and American Association of Clinical Urologists. He received the prestigious Gold Cane Award from the AUA, a Lifetime Achievement Award in Urology from the National Kidney Foundation of Oklahoma, and a Distinguished Service Award from SCS of the AUA. He has the rank of Clinical Professor Emeritus at OU's College of Medicine-Tulsa.

He resides in Tulsa with his wife, Jacqui, who retired as General Counsel of Blue Cross Blue Shield of Oklahoma. His two daughters, Lisa Ann and Birgit Lyn, are M.D. physicians.

Harvard Family Physicians, P.C.

Harvard Family Physicians, P.C., was founded by Dr. Kenneth Muckala, M.D., as a family medicine practice in 1989. A 1967 graduate of the University of Minnesota Medical School, he had been a member of Springer Clinic in Tulsa and a long-time member of a Minnesota rural practice providing surgical and obstetrical care.

Dr. Muckala has continued on the concept set forth by the founders of the former Doctors' Hospital located near Harvard Avenue and 23rd Street, which was eventually sold. Five of the founders joined the Harvard Family Physicians through their retirements — Warren Gwartney, M.D., John Keown, M.D., Curtis Clifton, M.D., Emil Childers, M.D., and Joseph Salamy, M.D. The physicians were instrumental in securing a location for Harvard Family Physicians in a doctor's building adjacent to the hospital.

Dr. Muckala credits the staff for the clinic's growth and reputation, from front desk employees to the physicians along with his long-time administrators, Patrick Schwartz and Samantha Vu.

The new practice was joined by Dr. Paul M. Krautter, M.D., who graduated from Rice University and the University of Texas at Galveston. Shortly after, Dr. David Griffiths, M.D., arrived from Beverly Hills, California, after graduating from Stanford University and the University of Oklahoma College of Medicine. Dr. Robert Mahaffey, M.D., was added after having been a professor in the family medicine department at the University of Oklahoma in Tulsa; Dr. Robert Aikman, a prominent obstetrician and gynecologist joined in 1999. It is estimated he delivered at least 27,000 babies before his death to cancer in December 2009 at age 69.

The practice then expanded with the addition of Dr. Michael Foster, M.D., a professor of medicine at the University of Oklahoma-Tulsa College of Medicine; Dr. David Sholl, M.D., a prominent Tulsa family physician; Dr. Darwin Olson, M.D., graduate from the Cetec University Medical School Santa Domingo; and Dr. Michael Newnam, M.D., a specialist in sleep medicine and graduate of the University of Oklahoma College of Medicine.

In 2009, Dr. Valerie Ritter, D.O., started the pediatrics section, which quickly grew to include Dr. Kathleen Boyls, M.D., and Dr. Janet Jones, M.D. In recent years, the practice welcomed Dr. Jeffrey Chasteen, D.O., who had been a faculty member of the family medicine residency program at Oklahoma State University; and Dr. Jonathan McGhee, M.D., a family physician with a sports medicine fellowship.

The Harvard Family Physicians moved its facility to its own building at 7912 E. 31st Court in 2009. The new location allowed for expanded services and additional physicians in obstetrics, gynecology, pediatrics and family medicine. It brought an opportunity for advanced, on-site technology including a laboratory, x-ray equipment and imaging services.

Other physicians who have joined the family medicine side of the practice are Dr. Lawrence Lieberman, M.D.; Dr. Jess T. Roy, D.O.; Dr. Patrick VanSchoyck, M.D.; Dr. Larissa Guiliano, M.D.; Dr. W. Hugh Nesbit, M.D.; and Patrice D. Wagner, D.O.

The obstetrics and gynecology physicians are Dr. Angela Christy-Owens, D.O.; Dr. Shelley Shoun, M.D.; and Dr. Jon Calvert, M.D. Chiropractic services are performed by David M. Collins.

Harvard Family Physicians is the only independent primary care group in Tulsa and has grown into one of the largest in the state. It has retained patients from its founding and continues to add new individuals and families into its system of care.

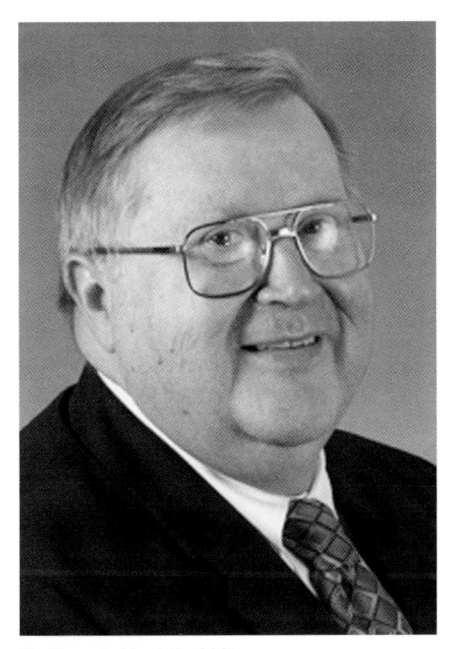

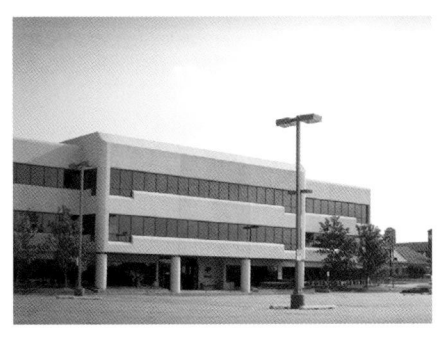

Dr. Kenneth Muckala, M.D.

C. Wallace Hooser, M.D.

Dr. C. Wallace "Wally" Hooser, a Tulsa radiologist and nuclear medicine specialist, gave the boost and foundation for the Tulsa County Medical Society's permanent home and led a 10-year campaign to open membership to osteopathic physicians.

Raised by a single mother in a poor Dallas neighborhood, Dr. Hooser attended the University of Texas in Austin, where he met and married his wife, Bobbie Jean, in 1965. He graduated from the Baylor College of Medicine in 1971, completing a residency at the University of Texas Southwestern Medical School in Dallas and fellowship at the University of California in San Diego. After becoming a doctor, he enlisted in the U.S. Army Medical Corp, serving two years at the Tripler Medical Center, which is called the "Walter Reed of the West." He retired as a captain.

Dr. Hooser arrived in Tulsa in 1977 to join the private group, Radiology Consultants of Tulsa, for 25 years. The group practiced at Saint Francis Hospital. In the late 80s, he became active with the Tulsa County Medical Society, where he became president in 1999. For 12 years, he served on the board for the Oklahoma State Medical Association. He was also a member of the Radiology Society of North American, Oklahoma State Radiology Association, Association of University Radiologists and Oklahoma State Medical Association.

An ongoing advocacy for Dr. Hooser was opening medical association memberships to osteopaths. The divide between allopath and osteopath education was narrowed in the 1970s as osteopathic schools embraced scientific methods. Dr. Hooser taught in the radiology rotations to medical residents at Saint Francis Hospital and the Oklahoma Osteopathic Hospital.

"I didn't see a dime's worth of difference in the equality, interest, learning capacity and dedication of students," Dr. Hooser, May 2016.

With assistance from TCMS Executive Director Paul Patton, TCMS welcomed osteopaths into its membership despite the state association's refusal.

"It wasn't just Paul and I, but a contingent of people. Tulsa County has always been a laboratory for innovation. We were the first county medical society to do this in the United States, and it made the state medical association change. We pushed for this for years and led to a domino effect around the country. It was a 10-year fight," Dr. Hooser, May 2016.

For the 95-year medical society's history, it had rented space for its offices. In 1996, the rent was being raised, and the board felt it was time to invest in its own facility. As a trustee in his family's foundation, the M.R. and Evelyn Hudson Foundation, Dr. Hooser challenged the membership to a 2-1 match in a fundraising drive. The effort raised a total of about $1.2 million. The facility was built and paid off at 5315 S. Lewis Ave. in 2007.

"The Tulsa County Medical Society is really about innovation. It attracts people who realize change is inevitable and want to promote the good change and stand against the bad change. It is in the greatest spirit of America, and I was just happy to be part of it," Dr. Hooser, May 2016.

Dr. Hooser retired in February 2002 and moved to Texas to be closer to the operations of the family foundation. He taught full-time at the University of Texas Southwestern Medical School from 2003 to 2012 and part-time through 2015. He and his wife have two children and three grandchildren. ∎

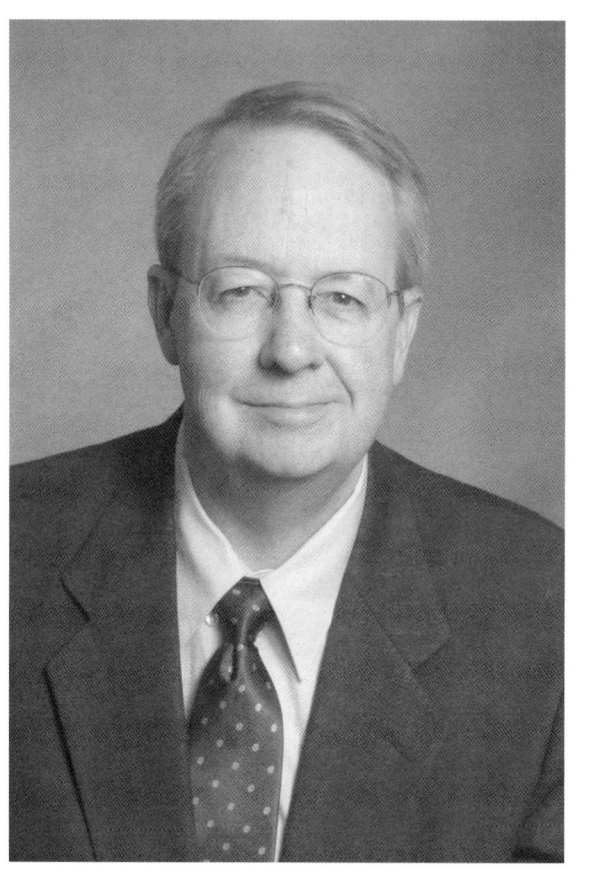

Bruce Hudkins, M.D.

Always with an interest toward invention and prevention, Bruce Hudkins, M.D., pioneered treatments and performed the first of several types of procedures in otolaryngology in Oklahoma.

An Indiana native, Dr. Hudkins earned his undergraduate degree from the University of Tulsa in biology in 1987. He spent a year at the University of Missouri School of Medicine before transferring to the University of Oklahoma College of Medicine, where he obtained his degree in 1990 and completed clinical training in 1992.

Dr. Hudkins discovered an interest in otolaryngology and finished his post-graduate education in 1997 at Rush-Presbyterian-St. Luke's Medical Center in Chicago. He served as an adjunct attending physician and continues to be affiliated with Rush Medical College as an instructor. The attraction to the specialty came from the mix of cases — patients needing consistent, ongoing care and those requiring one-time surgeries.

After moving back to Tulsa, Dr. Hudkins has spent his career in an individual private practice. He performed the first balloon eustachian tuboplasty, first radio frequency repair of nasal vestibular stenosis and first endoscopic dacryocystorhinostomy in the state.

In 2008, he completed the first balloon sinuplasty at Guy's Hospital in London while serving in a temporary appointment to the National Institutes of Health staff in Great Britain. Dr. Hudkins developed a cauterized therapy using sprays to stave off surgeries for patients with chronic sinusitis.

Dr. Hudkins has obtained three patents, the most known being No Bleed. It is an isoflavone cream sold over-the-counter that decreases persistent nose bleeds by at least 80 percent. He has been working on research in the bioluminescence of plants, using cellular structure to create light for detecting stress. That work is being licensed to a developer. The other patent is a collapsible gas can, which was inspired by seeing the large amount of space required at a convenience store for the item.

His other research in medicine has involved vocal fold paralysis treatments and electromagnetic frequency focusing probes. Among his publications are several topics in "Common Surgical Disease: A Handbook for Rounds and On-Call Problems" including epistaxis, thyroid nodule, laryngeal cancer, parotid mass, stridor, cervical lymphadenopathy, oral carcinomas and management of the difficult airway.

In 2002, Dr. Hudkins joined other Tulsa physicians in formed the Tulsa Spine and Specialty Hospital, 6901 S. Olympia Ave. He has served on the board since its opening. The hospital received a top ranking by the Centers for Medicare and Medicaid Services in 2015, only nine Oklahoma hospitals and three in Tulsa were given this rating.

Dr. Hudkins is a member of the American Academy of Otolaryngology-Head & Neck Surgery; American Auditory Society; American College of Surgeons (candidate group); American Academy of Otolaryngology Allergy; Chicago Laryngological and Otological Society and the Triological Society as a resident member.

He is married to Lisbeth Hudkins, and the couple has three children — son, Eric, and two daughters, Greer and Avery.

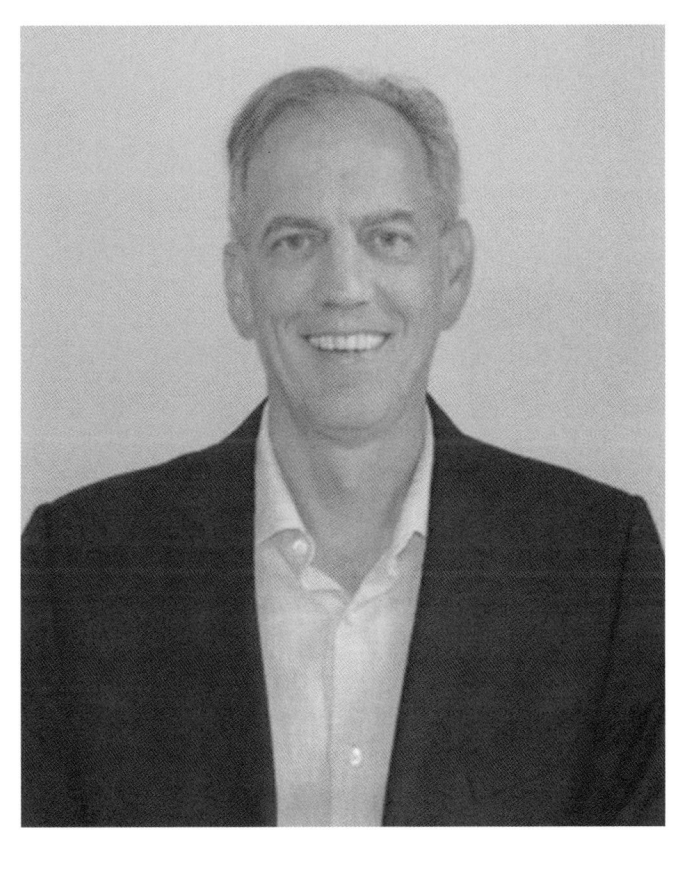

FUTURE LEGACIES

Charles Kemper Harmon, M.D., F.A.C.S.

"Go west, young man," was a slogan encouraging enterprising Americans to migrate westward. This call was heeded by Dr. Harmon's grandfathers. Although neither men were native to the state, they established their medical practices in Oklahoma in the early 1900s, just as Oklahoma herself was becoming a state.

Kemper Colley, his maternal grandfather, established a medical practice in Bigheart, Oklahoma — known later as Barnsdall — a city named after Osage Indian Chief James Bigheart.

His paternal grandfather, Thomas Franklin Harmon, a southern Illinois native, established a dental practice in Sallisaw, Oklahoma. His only child, Thomas Frederick Harmon, was born in Sallisaw in 1912.

He continued the Oklahoma medical legacy by graduating from the University of Oklahoma's medical school in Oklahoma City, but moved to Springfield, Illinois to join his father's fraternal twin, Charles Frederick Harmon, in a primary care medical practice. Thomas, who had surgical experience during World War II, took surgical courses and performed minor surgical cases in general surgery, OB/GYN, and orthopedics — back then, you didn't need to serve a surgical residency to have hospital privileges to perform certain surgeries.

It was in Springfield where Dr. Charles Harmon — named after his great-uncle — was born in 1940. Just like great Uncle Charles, he graduated from Washington University Medical School in St. Louis. (Washington University Dental School was his paternal grandfather's alma mater.) Influenced by Dr. Carl Moyer, the chief of surgery at the university, Dr. Harmon pursued a surgical specialty.

Just out of medical school, instead of going west, Dr. Harmon traveled east, serving an internship in Philadelphia, but he explored options outside Philadelphia for his residency in general surgery. He settled on the University of Florida in Gainesville. On the alternative Berry Plan, he spent one year in residency there before being shipped out to Shaw Air Force base in Sumter, South Carolina for two years of active duty during the Vietnam War.

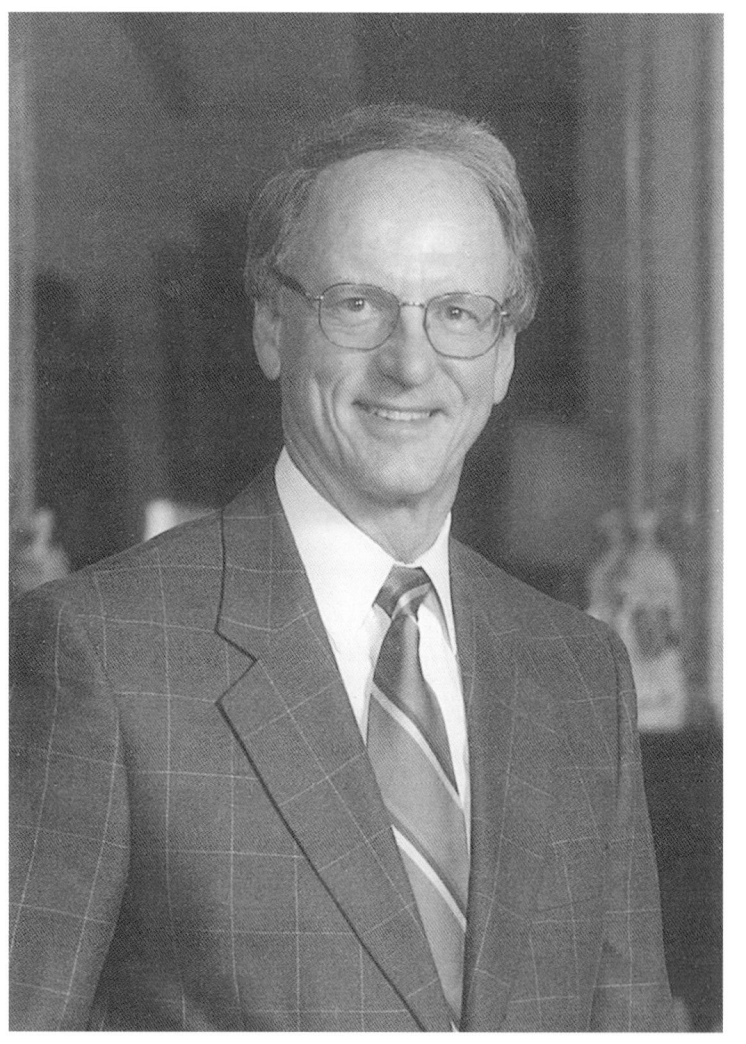

The university kept a slot open for him to finish his residency. He stayed in Florida, joining a surgical practice in Sanford, a small town north of Orlando.

A few years later, he decided that Florida wasn't where he wanted to practice and raise his family.

Exploring options, he contacted his cousin Kemper Lain, a cardiovascular surgeon in Tulsa. Growing up, their lives seemed to run parallel: his cousin was only one month older and both were surgeons and Vietnam War vets. Since Dr. Lain was older, he inherited their mutual maternal grandfather's Christian name.

After visiting the city, Dr. Harmon moved his family to Tulsa in 1977. Following in the pioneering spirit of his grandparents, he opened a solo practice in general surgery at the former Utica Square Medical Center. Since the Tulsa County Medical Society had their offices in this building, he established great connections. He thrived here, able to work at three major hospitals: Hillcrest, St. John, and Saint Francis. Later, he moved to South Harvard Medical Building.

Keeping in the spirit of a pioneer, in 1984, he afterward decided to join a multi-specialty group, Medical Care Associates of Tulsa (MCAT), as their first general surgeon. "I believed that the whole country was moving towards managed care," he explains.

During this phase of his career, Dr. Harmon made time for engaging in medical leadership activities. These included chairmanships of the departments of general surgery at Hillcrest Medical Center and Saint Francis Hospital as well as presidencies of the Tulsa County Medical Society, Tulsa Surgical Society, and Oklahoma Surgical Society.

In the late 1990's, the large health insurance companies were discontinuing their exclusive relationships with single, large multi-specialty groups. Warren Clinic, the physician part of the Saint Francis Health System, acquired MCAT. This began a long association of Dr. Harmon with Saint Francis Hospital.

Then in 2002, Dr. Harmon left the MCAT division of the Warren Clinic and joined Surgical Associates, a large private practice group of general surgeons serving Saint Francis Hospital. For a senior general surgeon, this association would turn out to be a perfect fit. Dr. Harmon describes this association as an enjoyable and rewarding way to wind down his career. He admits that he looked forward to retiring from the active practice of general surgery in 2007, but was lured back into doing some committee work at Saint Francis Hospital for a short time then into staffing the Saint Francis general surgery trauma group out-patient clinic on a part-time basis from 2010 to 2014.

He now has permanently retired, but has no regrets about returning to Oklahoma to continue the legacy in medical practice established by his father and his grandfathers. ■

Michael J. Haugh, M.D.

Dr. Michael Haugh has accomplished more than most neurologists during the course of his lengthy career. After graduating from Will Rogers High School, he attended Westminster College in Fulton, Missouri from 1955 to 1959 where he served as freshmen class vice president, junior class president, and student body president in his senior year before graduating with a bachelor's of arts degree. He then moved on to Saint Louis University Medical School where he received his medical degree in 1963.

Ben Taub General Hospital in Houston, Texas was the site of his internship from July 1, 1963 to June 30, 1964. In 1964, Haugh took a residency in Neurology at Baylor University Affiliated Hospitals. He later completed his residency at Barnes Hospital at Washington University in Saint Louis, Missouri.

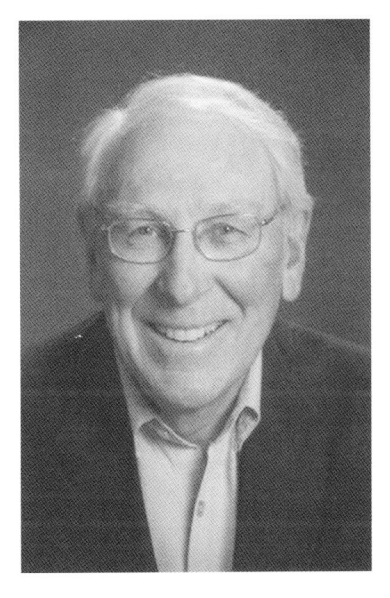

Between 1967 and 1969, Haugh served as a LCD in the Navy at the U.S. Naval Hospital in Oakland, California where he became chief of their neurology department. As soon as his military service was over, he went into private practice in Tulsa, Oklahoma where he remained until his retirement in 2001.

Don't think that Haugh has sat back and relaxed in retirement. He has maintained volunteer positions with the Medical Reserve Corps of Oklahoma and OK-1 DMAT where he has helped an impressive amount of people in times of tremendous disaster.

Haugh says, "I received a note left for me by a patient when I was volunteering during Hurricane Katrina. She wrote, 'All of you and doctor, thank you so much for being here.' It was so simple, but was the best compliment I ever received." ■

Edward W. Jenkins, M.D., F.A.C.S.

Edward Jenkins, M.D., a retired cardiothoracic surgeon, looks back fondly on his forty-four-year career. He began his college years with a full scholarship to Syracuse University's School of Journalism. Within a year, the U.S. Navy selected him for V-12 officers' training program. He was sent to Middlebury and Bates colleges. After serving almost four years as a Naval Officer, he returned home to Vermont and graduated from the University of Vermont (UVM). He entered UVM's College of Medicine and spent a year of internship there. Then he completed a four-year general surgery residency at Dartmouth Medical School in Hanover, New Hampshire. After a year at Boston University's Westfield Sanatorium performing cancer surgeries, he completed a thoracic surgery residency at the University Of Michigan.

Dr. Jenkins practiced in Springfield, Massachusetts for a year then joined Dr. Joe Burge in Tulsa. Since they were the area's only trained open heart surgeons at that time, they performed the first bypass operations in 1960. An interesting case was of a woman with a congenital cardiac defect that she passed onto her five children. Each child had a different father. This story made *TIME* magazine.

Another case that made national news, was of a woman brought to the hospital DOA. A single heartbeat was heard and Dr. Jenkins was called to the ER. Using all the methods of body warming, the woman survived. It was estimated her body temperature was in the 60's. Survival was thought to be due somewhat to the alcohol she had consumed on a freezing January night.

Upon arriving in Tulsa, Dr. Jenkins was surprised to be told he was the half-owner of a newly-purchased Beechcraft Bonanza. Both surgeons learned to fly, covering many cases in three surrounding states.

At that time, thoracic surgery included bronchoscopy, esophagoscopy, insertion of pacemakers, angiography, transthoracic biopsy, vascular bypass, aneurysm resection, and endarterectomies. Stenting had not yet been developed. Now, many of these procedures are performed by other specialties, making thoracic surgery a less desirable endeavor.

At one time, it was very difficult to enter a cardiothoracic surgery residency. Now the programs are having difficulty filling quotas.

As a pioneer in cardiothoracic surgery, Dr. Jenkins served in various leadership positions including starting a section of thoracic surgery in all the hospitals. He served as chief of thoracic surgery at Hillcrest and Saint Francis hospitals and chief of staff of Doctors' Hospital (once very busy). He was vice president and Board of Directors member of the Tulsa County Medical Society, and president of the Oklahoma chapter of the American College of Surgeons and Oklahoma Surgical Society. He served as associate professor at OU-TU's College of Medicine, clinical professor at Oral Roberts Medical School (now closed), and vice president and regent of the International College of Surgeons.

He and Mrs. Jenkins have participated in twenty-one medical missions around the world including in Uganda and the source of the Amazon in eastern Peru. Four of their five children serve in the medical field: master's-degree nutritionist, podiatrist, family medicine physician, and a vascular technician. Their fifth child is a landscape architect.

"Back then, physicians and surgeons wore suits and ties when they made rounds, and spent considerably more time with the patient and even visited them at home if warranted," notes Dr. Jenkins regarding changes in the profession since he started practice.

Editor's Note: Dr. Jenkins passed away on September 17, 2016 after the interview was conducted and the article was written.

FUTURE LEGACIES

George H. Kamp, M.D., F.A.C.R.

George Kamp, M.D.'s love for medicine began as a teenager, accompanying a doctor on house calls in Arkansas. He graduated from Hendrix College in Arkansas, received his medical degree at the University of Arkansas School of Medicine after spending part of his third year at Columbia-Presbyterian in New York City. He performed his residency in Arkansas in radiology. "I was always fascinated with intellectual and visual challenges…and found technology fascinating," he says about specializing in radiology. "I could contribute to patient diagnosis and care."

He came to Tulsa in 1966, joining Tulsa Radiology Associates serving St. John and Saint Francis, then one of only two radiology practices in Tulsa. When the group amicably split — one serving St. John — he joined the group serving Saint Francis renamed Radiology Consultants of Tulsa.

Dr. Kamp has witnessed many changes in radiology, especially transitioning from film-based to an all digital specialty, describing this as "probably the biggest change in radiology itself during my professional career." He helped lead the change, serving on the Board of Chancellors of the American College of Radiology and chairing their Government Relations Committee in Washington D.C.

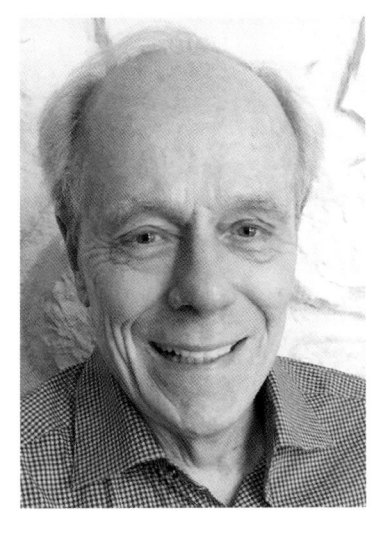

He served as president of many associations from the Tulsa County Medical Society in 1978 — a pivotal year of the development of the City of Faith Hospital — the medical staff at Saint Francis, and Oklahoma State Medical Association.

Dr. Kamp retired in 2005 but is active in conservation and birding; he and his wife have traveled to six continents together. Still a resident of Tulsa, he considers this city, "a great community and I'd choose it over again."

Grace Kennedy, D.O.

Pulmonology and Critical Care is the ideal specialty for Grace Kennedy, D.O. who enjoys the challenges of critical care medicine and seeing patients get better.

A native Oklahoman, she received her undergraduate degree in Zoology at the University of Oklahoma (OU) in Norman, OK. She attended medical school at the Oklahoma State University College of Osteopathic Medicine, and then completed her Internal Medicine residency at OU-TU Branch of Internal Medicine.

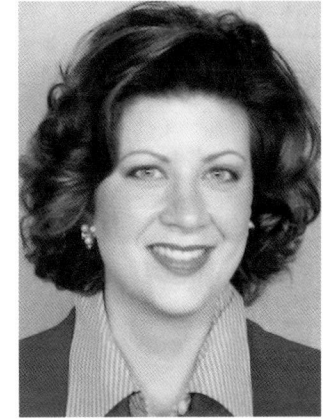

She completed a three-year fellowship at the University of Texas Southwestern Medical Center in Dallas. After starting her practice in Dallas, she returned to Oklahoma to practice with Pulmonary Medicine Associates in Tulsa.

In 2014, she opened a private practice at 73rd and Yale. Here she continues her office visits and procedures while still seeing inpatients at Saint Francis Hospital.

Having practiced for over twenty years in pulmonary medicine, she appreciates the breakthroughs in medicine that allow treatment for the previously untreatable conditions such as pulmonary fibrosis and some autoimmune disorders, as well as changes in technology such as the Endobronchial ultrasound. She cites many interventional developments that have emerged since 2007, allowing more options in treatment of diseases such as lung cancer and chronic obstructive lung disease.

These advances can help extend patients' lives. She states she always wants to tell her patients, "I've tried everything I can possibly think of to help you, and know in my heart, I've done everything I could for you."

The most rewarding aspect of her career is getting patients through their illness and home to their families. She knows this happens through a combination of knowledge, energy, and God's presence in her practice.

FUTURE LEGACIES

Merlin Kilbury, M.D.

Merlin Kilbury grew up in Little Rock, Arkansas. A third-generation physician, he followed in the footsteps of two men who forever changed his life — his grandfather, a pathologist, and his father, a surgeon. He went to college at Vanderbilt University in Nashville, Tennessee and then returned to Little Rock to attend the University of Arkansas medical school. After medical school, he began an internship at St. John's Hospital in Tulsa, OK after receiving advice from a colleague from medical school.

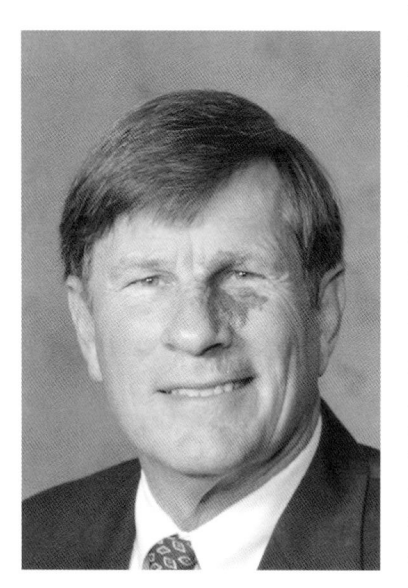

Dr. Kilbury enjoyed being in the operating room. He concentrated his internship on surgery entering the Tulsa Surgical Trust, a surgery residency that was in place before the University of Oklahoma took over the program. He completed four years of surgery residency in Tulsa before moving on to a peripheral vascular surgery fellowship at Baylor University in Dallas, Texas.

Once finished with his fellowship in Texas, Kilbury returned to Tulsa when the Tulsa Surgical Trust transitioned into the OU Tulsa Surgery Residency. Dr. Kilbury was taken into a partnership at the OU School of Medicine that involved a teaching position for residents and medical students. He did this for 15 years after returning to Tulsa.

During Kilbury's residency and teaching, he worked with some of the great Tulsa surgeons, including Robert Shepard and Harold White at St. John Hospital, C.T. Thompson at Saint Francis Hospital, and Frank Clingan at Hillcrest Medical Center.

He says, "They were wonderful surgeons and mentors. Not only were they a huge influence on me personally, but they are an integral part of Tulsa's surgical history."

For the past 10 years, Kilbury has driven the 180-mile round-trip from Tulsa, Oklahoma to Integris Baptist Regional Health Center in Miami, Oklahoma as part of his emergency room medicine practice. Although impressive, he believes his dedication to those suffering from alcoholism and substance abuse takes precedent.

In 1989, Dr. Kilbury recognized personal substance abuse and addiction. Since then, he has worked continually in recovery and has been the associate director of the Oklahoma Health Professional Program for 10 years. The program works with health professionals who have substance abuse and alcohol problems and tries to get them back to work.

He says, "My major interest now is helping others achieve sobriety and recovery. The Oklahoma Health Professional Program has helped more than 1,000 physicians in its 35 years and currently monitors and advocates for more than 200 health professionals."

He is also on the board of directors for the HOW Foundation, a local non-profit organization that houses 80-100 men who work full time and pursue their sobriety.

"One of my proudest moments this year was receiving my 21-year sobriety chip. I hope that my work in sobriety and recovery will serve as my legacy as a Tulsa physician," says Kilbury.

Described as a type-A nonconformist, Kilbury finds many ways to keep himself busy outside the field of medicine. A former national champion handball player, rugby player and avid golfer, he enjoys activities that keep him physically active. He loves to talk about his sons and daughters, many of whom are pursuing careers in medicine and how he married his high school sweetheart, Corinne, after 40 years of being apart.

The life that Kilbury lives is much like the atmosphere in an emergency room, exciting and dramatic.

Three generations of physicians; Dr. Kilbury Sr. and Dr. Kilbury Jr. at Merlin Kilbury's graduation.

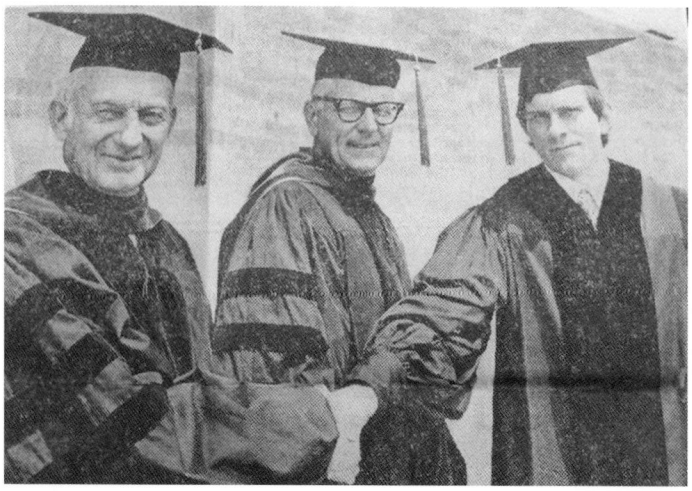

Lora J. Larson, M.D.

Lora Larson, M.D.'s career is a composite of mentors investing into her life during a time when female physicians were a minority. When she came to Tulsa in 1979 as a third-year medical student, Tulsa had very few female physicians in practice. "At the time, women accounted for approximately one quarter of the medical school classes and that has increased to over 50%," she shares.

Her first inspiration came from her piano teacher telling her she was smart and could be a brain surgeon. Ten years later, Dr. Larson attended the University of Oklahoma for her undergrad degree, studied at their medical school in Oklahoma City for two years, then finished at their Tulsa campus.

She specialized in Obstetrics and Gynecology — the variety this field provided from family practice, delivering babies, surgery, and psychiatry appealed to her. "In January 1980, I delivered my first baby and it was amazing. I thought, I could do this." Yet, Drs. Linda Nassif and Parvati Mittapali were the only female OB/GYNs practicing in Tulsa when Dr. Larson was a third-year medical student. Once practicing, Dr. Larson and Dr. Kathleen Glaze were the first female OB/GYNs on staff at St. John.

During her third year of medical school, she helped launch Women in Medicine, a social group associated with the Tulsa County Medical Society (TCMS). Dr. June Holmes, a doctor of education for Tulsa Medical College, Dr. Myra Peters, an orthopedic surgeon and first female president of TCMS, and Dr. Barbara Hastings, a neurologist and second female president of TCMS, were three of many physicians in the group. They mentored and networked with female medical students, sharing their experiences of running a practice and struggles such as managing the work-life balance. Dr. Larson connected with them and other mentors in the group including Dr. Linda Goldenstern, an internist, and Dr. Miriam Mills, a pediatrician, and called them for advice once she was practicing.

Dr. Larson performed her residency in Tulsa, rotating to different hospitals, then joined Dr. Glenn Haswell, a maternal-fetal medicine specialist — another pivotal mentor — in his private practice that later became known as Associated Women's Specialists. The practice expanded to cover Hillcrest, St. John, Saint Francis South, and Southcrest as more medical professionals joined.

After twenty-five years of private practice, she now works as an OB/GYN hospitalist at Saint Francis, a position with fixed hours and less stress. As a hospitalist, her primary purpose is safety where she's available for emergencies. She works closely with the nursing staff and trains them on drills and simulations. She assists on C-sections and makes rounds seeing patients.

Following in her mentor's footsteps, she gives back through serving as an associate professor. She enjoys teaching a new generation of residents and even gives them her phone number as a resource.

She's a member of the Tulsa County Medical Society, Oklahoma State Medical Association, and American College of Obstetrics and Gynecology. She served as president of the Tulsa County Obstetrical and Gynecological Society.

Dr. Larson's grateful for her opportunities provided by members of the medical community who've shaped her career. "Medicine is truly an apprenticeship in which the wisdom and experience of others is shared freely with the younger members of the profession; it is a fellowship and there is a camaraderie that I found both comforting and enriching."

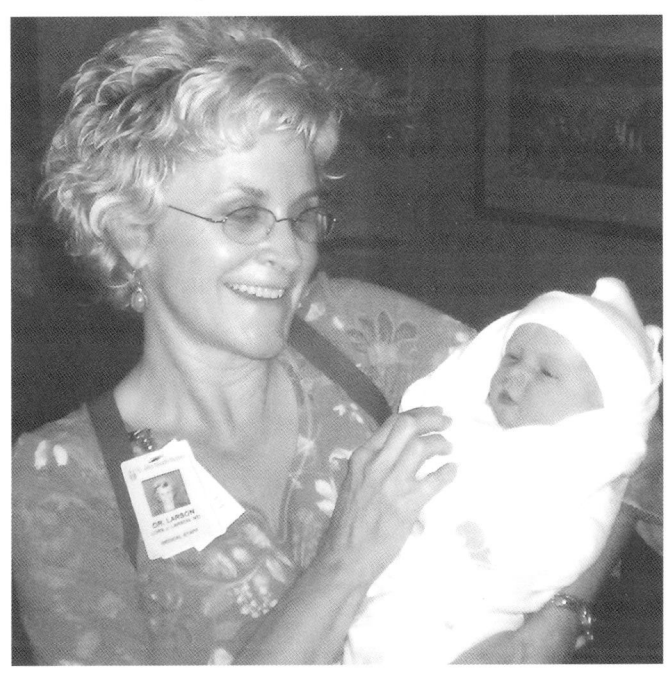

Dr. Larson holding a baby she delivered.

FUTURE LEGACIES

D. Price Kraft, M.D.

D. Price Kraft is a Family Physician, Geriatrician, Multi-Organizational Medical Director and former New York City taxicab driver. A son of an ascetic electrical engineer and an aesthetic artist, Price's early life exposures include an Appalachia country doctor granddad of southwestern Pennsylvania coal country.

"Granddad was a character — schnozzola, portly, well-padded frame, suit with tie formality, and president of the County Medical Society, the Board of Health and the Board of Education. A 'big fish in a small pond', routinely blasting impending 'socialized medicine', he more than made do receiving patients in his at home office and as medical director of numbers of coal mines. The grandkids rode along with him on rounds or death calls, and some became doctors."

That pre-1965, before Medicare, framed a preadolescent perspective of needs not so met.

Knowing himself as generalist, not proceduralist, Price completed his undergraduate degree at Washington University in St. Louis, preceding a 6-year M.D., J.D. program at Missouri-Columbia Medical School and Rutgers Law School. He completed the University of Oklahoma Family Medicine Residency in Tulsa by 1981 and centered on careers in emergency, hospital, family and geriatrics care.

Preparation intersected transitions to extended lifetimes with research and legislated lifelines, and to shifts of post-acute care from hospitals to nursing facilities in the early 21st century. Skilled nursing units enhance nursing facility quality and cut costs. SNUs are more the hands-on rehabilitation and time to heal of nursing facilities — post more the high tech procedures of acute/sub-acute hospitals. Post-acute care is

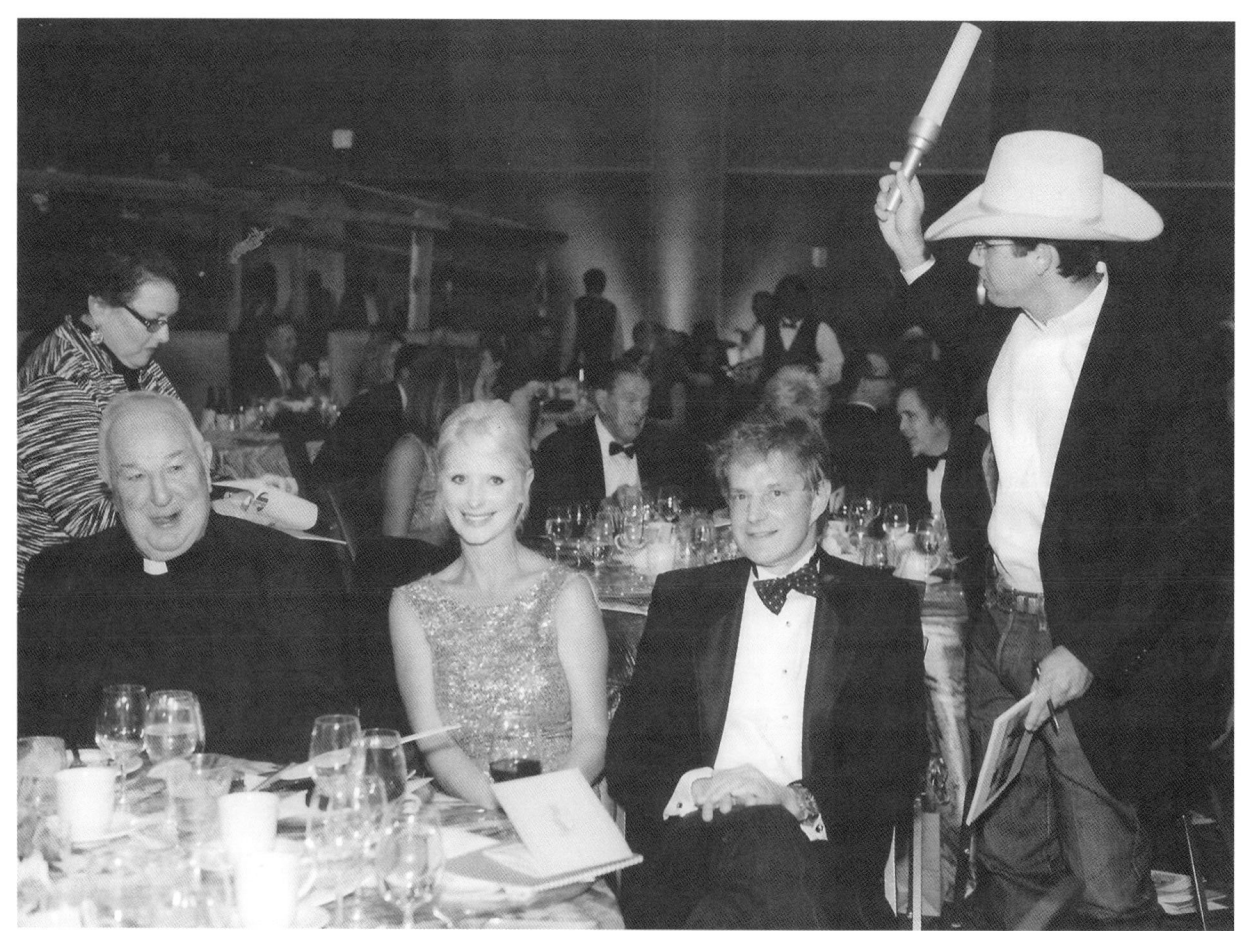

The 2012 Painted Pony Ball benefiting The Children's Hospital at Saint Francis — for a charitable ransom — on to the Kentucky Derby!

now second to hospitals in Medicare outlays.

The practice works with all Tulsa hospitals and the Saint Francis Health System for 35 years plus. The practice has included medical directorship of nursing homes, home health and hospice organizations, and a Tulsa hospital.

As "Snuist" — less supported with the infrastructure and medical staff of 'Hospitalists' — the practice shares professional relationships and insights with interested colleagues. The practice bedded lives have at times exceeded Oklahoma's largest hospital, an unlikely prospect with no ownership and no marketing.

"In the mix of transition is risk, not alone the predictable cast of med mal and regulatory menaces from without. Be it pretenders, the 'good guys' ceding the integrity of privileged relationships, or appreciation differentials — have mercy and know when to walk — street fighters are not much admired in our profession of medicine.

Nursing homes are highly regulated, may draw unwarranted fire, and can be tumultuous. Certainly, nursing homes are misunderstood. In the context of teamwork — righting distressed facilities with organization, documentation, and credibility, or gaining and retaining facilities' 5-star (highest) ratings — that is the practice."

Not of the Bar or a 'hired gun', Price shares his professional background — be it Tulsa County Public Defender's Office, government interests, attorneys with at times not so pretty clients, healthcare organizations, fellow physicians, and patients. Service always gratis to help the defense is its own reward.

"To cut a career path means mentors and support: an extended family, all teachers, a med school administrator implementing cross education (ouch), a hospital's founding family, a senior Wall Street executive who headed the legal department of the world's largest company by geography — special thanks to John L. Farrell, Jr., nursing facility owners and administrators and nurses, many physicians — 'no doubt brighter than myself', virtually all patients - and, yes, even some lawyers."

As the current Tulsa County Medical Society's only geriatrics listed physician in an organization of more than 1,100 members, he observes.

"Respect the aged. And, be grateful for those employed in nursing homes. They bear strenuous physical and emotional loads to help the helpless and families stricken with grief of the inevitability of loss, however expressed. A thank you is always welcome." ■

Bernard J. Maguire, Jr., M.D.

Bernard Maguire was inspired to pursue medicine by a family physician. He graduated from the University of Kansas undergraduate and medical school, served a one-year internship in Wichita, Kansas, then served on active duty for two years with the United States Coast Guard as a physician. During this time, he was stationed in New London, Connecticut; part of his duties here were directing the pediatric clinic.

After his military service, he spent two years at the University of Oklahoma training to be a pediatrician. He then accepted an opportunity in 1965 to join Doctors Richard Russell and Robert Endres in a pediatric practice at Springer Clinic in Tulsa.

After ten years at Springer, they left and established The Children's Clinic of Tulsa in the Kelly Building on the Saint Francis Campus where they practiced for twenty-five years.

A pioneer in the pediatric community in Tulsa, Dr. Maguire served in several leadership positions. At Saint Francis Hospital, he served as a member of the Board of Directors, Chief of Pediatrics, and President of the Medical Staff. Giving service to the Tulsa community, he also served on the Boards of Blue Cross Blue Shield, the Ronald McDonald House, and the Children's Medical Center. He is a past president of the Oklahoma chapter of the American Academy of Pediatrics and a retired Clinical Professor in the Department of Pediatrics, Tulsa. He has also served on the Admissions Board of the University of Oklahoma College of Medicine.

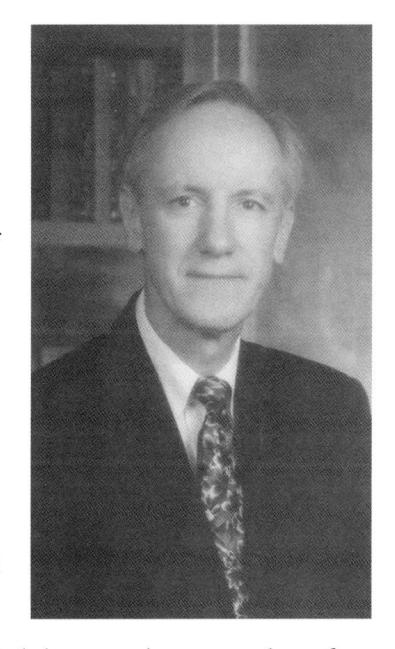

Dr. Maguire retired July 2006. He and his beautiful wife, DeEtta, have three grown children and seven grandchildren! ■

Thomas A. Marberry, M.D.

Thomas Marberry, M.D., knew as a young boy he would become a physician. As a teenage athlete having suffered various extremity injuries and multiple shoulder dislocations, he wanted to specialize in Orthopaedic Surgery.

He attended Vanderbilt University for undergrad, then returned to his native state to attend medical school at the University of Oklahoma Health Sciences Center. He stayed in Oklahoma City for a rotating surgical internship at St. Anthony Hospital, then an Orthopaedic Surgery Residency through the O'Donoghue program. At that time Dr. O'Donoghue was considered the leading sports Orthopaedic surgeon.

Desiring to specialize in shoulders, (maybe because he had several shoulder dislocations and shoulder surgery himself), he was accepted into a six month Visiting Fellowship at Columbia Presbyterian Medical Center in New York City, studying under Dr. Charles S. Neer, M.D. – considered the father of shoulder surgery. As part of his fellowship, he prepared a paper on "The Disadvantages of Radical Acromionectomy" presented at the American Academy of Orthopaedic Surgeons annual meeting (1981).

Dr. Neer was the first president of the American Shoulder and Elbow Surgeons Society, and Dr. Marberry attended the inaugural meeting of surgeons who then formulated the society. He became a member and enjoyed the meetings and fellowship with colleagues also specializing in shoulders.

In 1980, Dr. Marberry opened his solo practice in Tulsa, having privileges at St. John and Hillcrest, until he evolved solely to St. John. Initially, as a general Orthopod, he performed all musculoskeletal surgeries except spine surgery. He thanks predecessors, Doctors John Vosburgh, Jerry Sisler, Worth Gross, and Norman Dunitz for their advice and expertise.

As medical malpractice premium rates skyrocketed in the 80's and reimbursements started declining in the 90's, Dr. Marberry saw the need to form a group to share overhead and provide services a solo doc couldn't afford to undertake. Doctors at an initial meeting seemed enthusiastic about such a grouping, but nothing was formed until the late 90's. He's proud to have been a co-founder of Tulsa Bone & Joint Associates that's flourished into a comprehensive center, facilitating treatment for virtually all musculoskeletal issues.

Another reason Dr. Marberry chose Orthopaedic Surgery was: "this specialty has the most variety of problems, and treatment options than any other specialty. There's not only a huge surgical practice ability, but a non-operative office-type practice as well — an important part of this specialty." Furthermore, he states, "Orthopaedics is always a leader and on the forefront of technological advances and innovation." He relished the challenging environment of constant innovation; yet, with the magnitude of different pathologies, fractures, and treatment options, it was virtually impossible to become and stay proficient in every aspect of Orthopaedics. Having completed his ER on-call rotation requirement (2001), he could focus more on his love of shoulder problems. He credits colleagues for "helping me to specialize in shoulders by providing those kinds of referrals. I felt grateful and humbled that my fellow physicians trusted me to do shoulder surgeries, allowing me to gradually phase out of other areas."

He retired full-time in January 2015. He's enjoying traveling with his wife, visiting grandchildren, playing golf, going fly fishing, doing charity work with Helping Hands and Community Food Bank of Eastern Oklahoma, and being available as a Red Cross volunteer — just a few interests keeping Dr. Marberry busy.

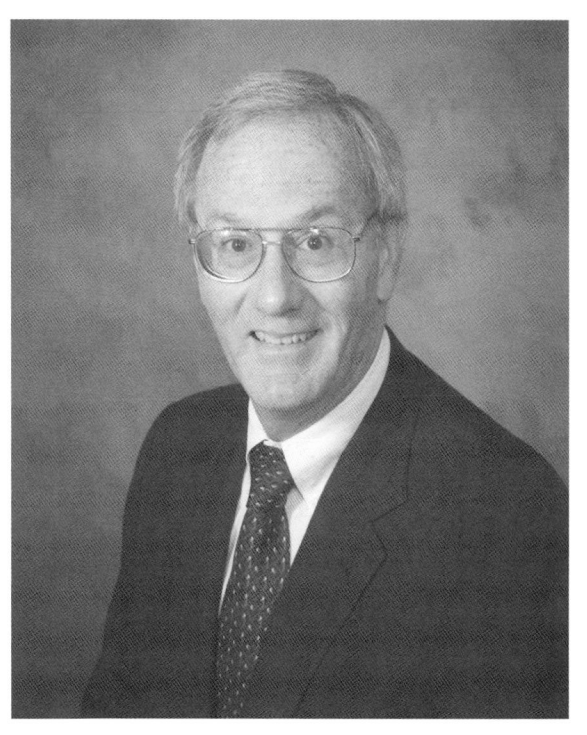

Fred R. Martin, M.D., F.A.C.S.

Fred Martin, M.D is a pioneer in plastic surgery in Tulsa. When he came here, he became only the third plastic surgeon practicing in Tulsa. His predecessors were Drs. James Kelly, semi-retired, and Herbert Forest, who had a well-established practice.

A native Oklahoman, he attended the University of Oklahoma (in Norman) for his bachelors and medical degree (in Oklahoma City). He completed his internship training at Detroit Receiving Hospital — arguably the busiest trauma hospital in the US.

Then on the Barry Plan, he served in the Air Force for three years stationed at Altus Airfare Force Base, only nine miles from his hometown. But the genesis of his plastic surgery career started in Dallas during his general surgery residency. Here, he was inspired by a couple of plastic surgeons who excelled in their field.

He went to St. Louis University for plastic surgery training and became trained in treating burn patients at the Cardinal Glennon Children's Hospital. He received training in head and neck surgery on cancer patients at the VA hospital, performing destructive surgery to remove all or part of the tongue and jaw, along with performing neck resection. "You're giving people life who would, otherwise, not be alive for very long."

Then he came to Tulsa, opening an office near St. John Hospital; thus, he conducted most of his elective practice there. Three years later, Dr. John Clark, a colleague during his general and plastic surgery training, joined him. They opened a second office near Saint Francis and were partners for several years. By this time, Drs. Kelly and Forest had retired, so the partners were only two of three plastic surgeons in the city. With this shortage, the surgeons were on call every night in the hospitals' ER rooms. (When Dr. Leonard Brown came to Tulsa, the plastic surgeons were able to rotate nights in the ER.) Later, the practice added two more partners but eventually, the partnership split, leaving Dr. Martin in a solo practice.

A highlight of his career was serving on the twelve-man committee to establish a burn center (all the members had experience in burn management). Modeled after the well-established Dallas Burn Center, the Tulsa Burn Center, (now the Alexander Burn Center at Hillcrest) became a hub for physicians in treating burn patients. Back then, all the hospitals could send doctors here even if they weren't on staff with Hillcrest.

In his specialty, he performed various procedures from cosmetic surgery, hand, head and neck surgery, breast augmentations, breast reductions, and congenital problems. Finding it rewarding to see children's quality of life improved, treating pediatric patients with congenital problems was a favorite of his, especially those with cleft lip and palates. "Having been trained well in St. Louis, I continued to do that as much as possible."

He was a member of various associations including the American Burn Association, Cleft Palate Association, American College of Surgeons, Plastic and Reconstructive Surgery Association, and the Tulsa County Medical Society.

After practicing for thirty-two years, he happily retired in 1998. So, what is his sage wisdom to young physicians deciding where to practice? The same advice Dr. Kelly gave him years ago: "Go wherever you want to live and if you do good work, you'll have plenty of work to do."

He and his wife, Norma, have been married for over sixty-one years. She practiced nursing prior to their move to Tulsa, then in Tulsa, she volunteered with helping in child abuse cases. Eventually she worked as a Sexual Assault Nurse Examiner. They have four kids, three of them are in the medical field, and five grandchildren, and two great-grandchildren.

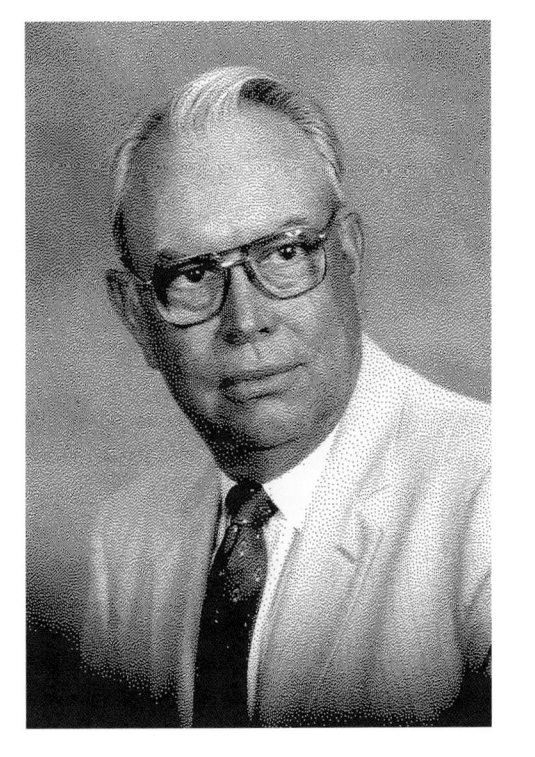

Bill P. Loughridge, M.D., F.A.C.C.

Dr. Loughridge was one of Tulsa's first cardiovascular surgeons.

"I have loved every minute of it," he said. "I love our doctors. They are still trying to do the right things for patients."

Dr. Loughridge has a long family history in Oklahoma with many of his ancestors moving from Georgia to Oklahoma's Indian Territory. One of the most prominent was the Rev. Robert McGill Loughridge, a Presbyterian minister who published the first English-Muscogee (Creek) dictionary. Camp Loughridge, a summer day camp for underprivileged youth in southwest Tulsa, is named for him.

Both of Dr. Loughridge's parents — William Floyd and Elizabeth (Shorter) — only completed school through the eighth grade. Dr. Loughridge and his older sister, Floydena, were the first high school graduates in their immediate family when they earned diplomas from Ardmore High School.

Always interested in sports, Dr. Loughridge was an active athlete in school through football, boxing and as an amateur bull rider. For his 40th birthday, he rode in his final rodeo, riding a bull for six seconds.

After graduating high school, he went to the University of Oklahoma with the intention of becoming a physician. In an unusual move, he majored in sociology as an undergraduate due to an interest in social issues and how medicine is connected to the larger society. He also had minors in chemistry and zoology.

While at OU, he joined the Sigma Chi fraternity and was honored about 40 years later as a "Significant Sig" for his lifetime achievements.

After graduating in 1957, he entered the OU School of Medicine in Oklahoma City. He paid his way with loans from the Kellogg Foundation, washing glassware at night at the Oklahoma Medical Research Foundation and as an exterminator for a pest control company. He was instantly drawn to the specialty of heart and cardiovascular health.

"It is the most exciting field and constantly changing. I was immediately sold," he said.

Dr. Loughridge graduated medical school in 1961 and then completed an internship at the University of Texas Medical Center in Galveston. Then, he spent four years as a general surgical resident at the Oklahoma Medical Center in Oklahoma City. In 1964, while still a resident, he received a fellowship from the National Institute of Health to conduct cardiovascular research. The research was pioneering work on the development of artificial tissue valves in heart surgery, and the findings were published in 1965 in the "Surgical Forum." He was the co-author of three other published scholarly articles during his residency.

In 1966, Dr. Loughridge was awarded a Fulbright Scholarship to study at the Sahlgrenska

Dr. Bill and Linda Loughridge.

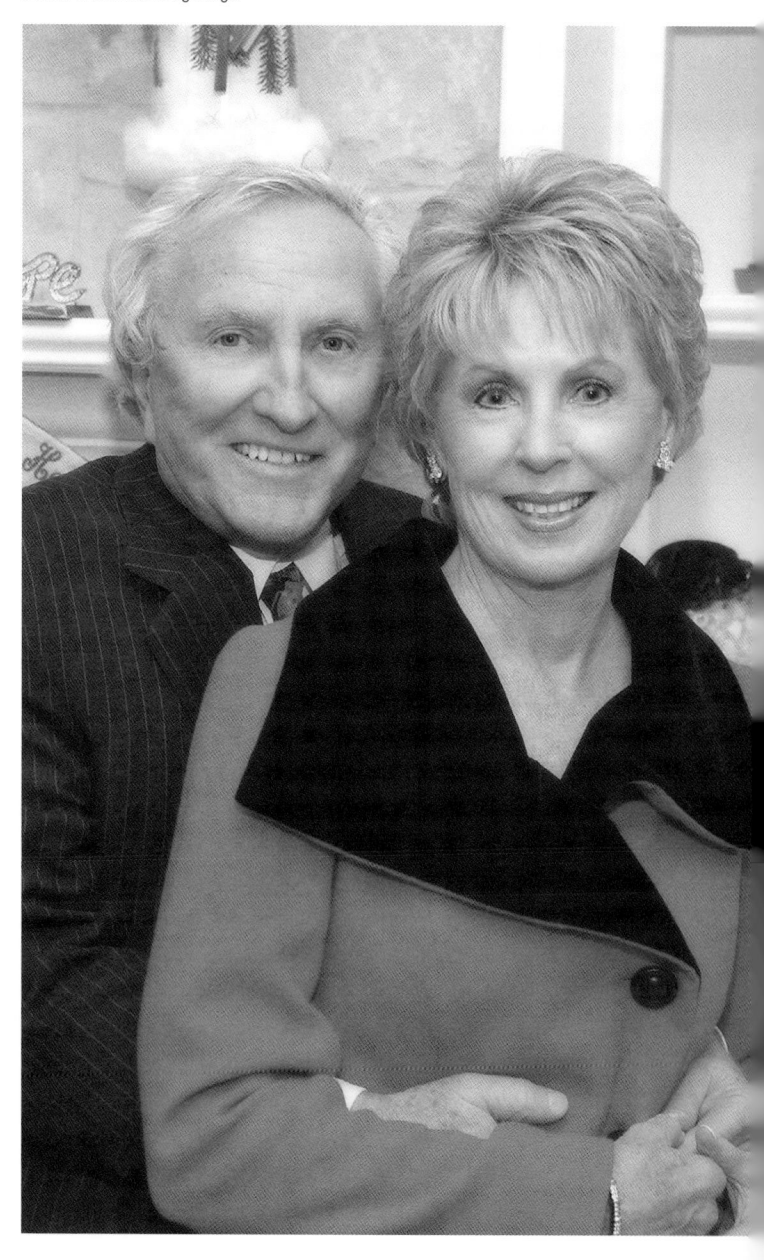

University in Göteberg, Sweden. While in Sweden, he did research on liver transplant techniques with Dr. Steg Bengmark, who became a world renowned expert on liver surgery and founder of the World Association of HPB. Results from his Fulbright research demonstrated a person could survive with the removal of up to 95 percent of the liver and that the liver would regenerate to its original size. The Swedish team also developed techniques for killing cancer cells by cutting off the arterial blood supply to the liver. It remains the basis of modern surgical treatment for liver cancer.

In 1967, Dr. Loughridge returned to Oklahoma and settled in Tulsa to join the Cardiovascular Surgery Inc., founded by Dr. Albert Lauck Shirkey (1933-2009). The two joined to perform the first heart-valve replacement surgeries in eastern Oklahoma and worked on creating an artificial heart with the Byron Jackson Pump Company, but the patent process proved too lengthy and laborious.

Dr. Loughridge enlisted in the U.S. Air Force Reserves and served as a medical officer from 1968 to 1971, reaching the rank of major. He moved to Syracuse, New York, in 1971 to work as the senior resident in thoracic surgery at the State University of New York Upstate Medical University.

In 1972, he returned to Tulsa and founded the Thoracic and Cardiovascular Surgery Inc., which he led until shortly before his retirement in 1998. While in practice, he performed more than 10,000 surgeries and specialized in heart, chest and vascular systems.

"I loved going to work. I couldn't wait to get to the hospital," he said. "The people I worked with were fantastic, fun and exciting. We enjoyed the early opening on a patient and closing. During the procedure, it was serious. In the end, we know we made this patient better."

In 1974, the American College of Cardiology elected Dr. Loughridge as a fellow. Two years later, he served as president of the Tulsa chapter of the American Heart Association. While in practice, he taught as a professor of surgery at the Tulsa campus of the OU School of Medicine and at Oral Roberts University School of Medicine.

"Tulsa is a great community and has been very good to us. If we needed some type of equipment, hospitals would get it. We were all partners — doctors and hospitals."

Dr. Loughridge was chief of thoracic surgery at St. John Medical Center and Saint Francis Hospital. He continued to present research and summaries of his work at various medical conventions.

Shortly before retiring from surgical practice, he was approached by an attorney to evaluate the evidence involved in a medical-related civil case. That led to nearly 15 years as an expert witness in legal cases dealing with health issues.

"To be a good expert witness, you have to spend a lot of time studying the case and studying the case records," he said. "A lot of busy practitioners do not have the time." The shift from the operating room to the courtroom proved to be fulfilling.

"It's fun. The deposing lawyers tried to discredit me on what I know versus what he knew. So, good luck," he said. "The idea is to keep a cool head, and the jury will trust you. Tell the truth. Juries know who is telling the truth. It also allowed me to keep up to speed with advancements in the field. I enjoy learning, a lot."

Among his many scholarly publications are books meant for the public to understand more about health and nutrition: *The Cardiac Surgeon's Diet and Health Design* (2000), *Every Breath You Take* (2002) and *Ticker: A User Guide for Everyone with a Heart* (2011).

"People don't know anything about their cardiovascular system or anatomy," he said. "I made it simple and written for Joe Six-Pack to understand. People are used to turning it all over to their doctors. This teaches you about anatomy and how the body works."

An equal partner was his wife of 51 years, Linda Faye Harrell. She was an active volunteer for many organizations. In 1974, she turned the American Heart Association's Heart Ball fundraiser into one of Tulsa's premiere charity events. In 1983, she held the Blass & Burgers event for St. John Medical Center to raise $1.5 million. She died in 2012 at age 72 from cancer.

Dr. Loughridge volunteered for the American Heart Association, Philbrook Museum of Art, Camp Loughridge and served on the ORU board of trustees. He provided primary medical care on a volunteer basis for indigent patients through Catholic Charities.

In 2010, he was appointed to the board of directors of the Oklahoma Medical Research Foundation. This position brought his life full circle, considering this was where he worked as a glassware washer to get through medical school.

He and his wife had three daughters and five grandchildren. In retirement, Dr. Loughridge spends his time traveling, visiting family, fishing and golfing. He continues to keep a current medical license. ■

Meyer C. and Ida Miller Hospice

Culturally sensitive, comprehensive, and compassionate describe the service Miller Hospice provides. Founded in 2008, by Bruce and Brenda Magoon in memory of their parents, Meyer C. and Ida Miller. Miller Hospice is an extension of the Tulsa Jewish Retirement and Healthcare Center and shares the same CEO, Jim Jakubovitz. Sherry Crockett, a certified nurse with eighteen years of hospice experience, serves as the Administrator.

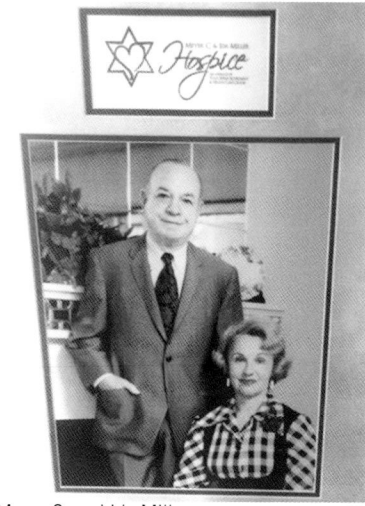

Miller Hospice works hard to demonstrate sensitivity to patients' cultural needs. The not-for-profit hospice formed to provide services sensitive to the Jewish community — the only hospice in Oklahoma trained by requirement annually (as part of the Tulsa Jewish Healthcare System) on Jewish culture.

Yet, Miller services all people within a fifty-mile radius of their South Tulsa office. With a majority of their patients not affiliated with Tulsa's Jewish community, Miller applies sensitivity to patients from other cultures — made easier by a staff representing a broad spectrum of cultural, religious, and ethnic backgrounds.

The comprehensive, holistic services they provide include the full range of services required as a State Licensed and Medicare-Certified Hospice provider (nurses and physicians for example). Miller also provides thirteen-month bereavement services for loved ones of patients who've passed on, helping them through the grieving process. They have access to a compounding pharmacy essential for palliative treatment. They're available twenty-four seven with an on-call nurse accessible after hours. Once a patient makes a call, the nurse makes a visit — their motto is "we look for a reason to make a visit."

Miller's passionate about providing the best possible service for their patients. They're constantly refining the quality assurance program, using previous experiences from patients to help current patients with similar problems.

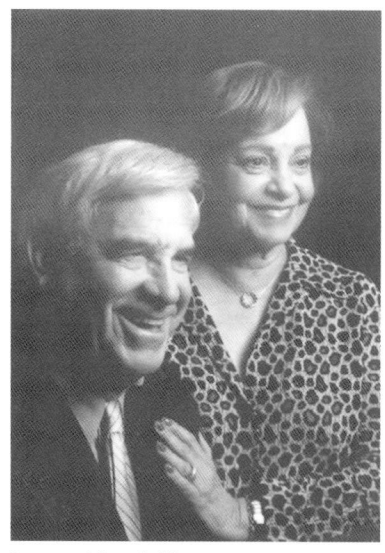

Miller seeks out feedback from referring physicians, the staff, facilities, and patients and their loved ones. Miller's Board of Directors, composed of prominent members of the community, help guide their service: "Each board member understands the regulatory scrutiny hospice is placed under. They actively help us monitor and avoid unnecessary difficulties," Administrator Crockett shares.

Compassion drives Miller Hospice. "We treat each patient as if they were our own loved one," Crockett shares of Miller's vigilance in customer care. "We try to always place the patient's needs first and at the same time 'figure out how to make the impossible, possible.' We are the hospice with highly skilled, trained nurses willing to provide high-tech care that few providers can match."

Miller has an excellent relationship with Clarehouse, a facility providing beautiful, caring, quiet, and comfortable homelike environment for families that prefer the end to not happen in the home. When someone is near the last 30 days of life in Miller's assessment, they facilitate care provision with Clarehouse, and Miller continues to be a very active part of the patient's care.

At Miller, their goal is 100% customer satisfaction when it's reasonably possible. They take every opportunity to implement new or update processes based on patient/family feedback and current care practices. "We understand there is no way to make up for less than perfect care in our industry. The care we give has to be on target, the first time, every time. The care we provide is how we choose to honor the memory of Meyer C. and Ida Miller as well as every person we serve."

FUTURE LEGACIES

Archibald S. Miller III, M.D., F.A.C.S., F.A.A.P.

Arch Miller, M.D. started his career following in his father's footsteps as a soldier. His father, a Scottish immigrant, retired as a lieutenant colonel after thirty years of service. Dr. Miller graduated from The Citadel Military College, then served as a U.S. Army artillery officer, and was airborne ranger qualified.

The direction of his life changed after his infant daughter died from acute myelocytic leukemia; later, his newborn son died at birth. "I changed completely. I became a different man," shares Dr. Miller about the tragedy. "My life became dedicated to wanting to be somebody that helped."

Motivated by his children, he received his masters' in Immunochemistry at the University of Texas (UT) in Austin. He taught at UT in Galveston while working on his doctorate. At the recommendation of Dr. Truman Blocker — president of the University of Texas Medical Branch (Galveston) and chairman of the plastics program — Dr. Miller enrolled in UT's medical school. He spent his general surgery residency and plastic surgery fellowship at Bowman Grey Medical Center at Wake Forest University.

He specialized in plastic surgery and was attracted to the reconstructive aspect of his new career: "I began writing papers and publishing in the area of trauma and burns."

He came to Tulsa in 1985 to join Dr. Palmer Ramey, Dr. John Clark, and Dr. Fred Martin at Plastic Surgery Associates. In 1990, he started an independent practice, now known as Tulsa Plastic Surgery. During his private practice, he has published in peer reviewed journals on many diverse subjects.

He now performs a variety of surgical procedures such as breast augmentations, breast lifts, tummy tucks, face lifts, thigh lifts, arm lifts, and liposuction. He also does extensive breast and chest wall reconstruction procedures. He and his staff at Tulsa Plastic Surgery pride themselves on providing a caring, loving environment for their patients, many of whom have or had cancer.

He enjoys giving back. He helped Barbara Schwartz, co-founder of Tulsa Project Women, coordinate with hospitals and surgeons to provide free breast reconstruction surgery for low-income cancer survivors. He performs surgeries for children through the Shriners, an organization in which he participated. (He's a Master Mason.)

He's a member of several medical societies such as the Tulsa County Medical Society, served as president of the Oklahoma Plastic Surgery Society, and serves on the board of the National Breast Cancer Reconstruction Committee. He is a professor in surgery for OU-TU and OSU medical schools. He's been repeatedly honored as an Outstanding Plastic Surgeon in Oklahoma for many years.

He initially invented and patented the chambered and shaped breast implant, now a common device in breast surgery. He invented the Sternal Talon, a patented device that holds the sternum together and stabilizes it. Using the device, he helps patients with sternal nonunion injuries. He's the COO of Maverick, the company promoting the Talon. He designs and uses original surgical instruments.

Dr. Miller explains about the advances in plastic surgery: "In addition to improved skills, the techniques we use now, provide superior form and function for tissue and bone. Every surgical procedure that we do now is better because of the improvements in equipment, making it more efficient, making the job quicker, and in many instances — like the Talon — stronger." Utilizing another advance in medicine, he uses mesenchymal stem cells — non-embryonic — to help with reconstruction including rebuilding ribs, sternums, and in breast reconstruction procedures.

He and his wife, Margo, have two grown children and six grandchildren, all of whom are active in the Tulsa community.

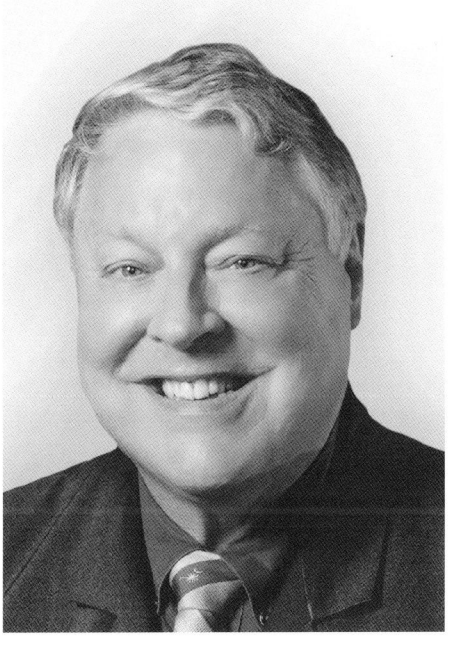

John D. Mowry, M.D.

Dr. John D. Mowry, M.D., grew up in Iowa, graduated Phi Beta Kappa from Drake University in 1974 and from the University of Nebraska College of Medicine in 1977. His internship was in general surgery at the University of Nebraska and his residency completed at the University of Texas Health Science Center at San Antonio in general surgery and in the specialty of otolaryngology - head and neck surgery.

Dr. Mowry arrived in Tulsa in 1982 to work in the private practice of Associated Ear, Nose and Throat of Tulsa, Inc., which later became Ear, Nose and Throat Specialists. Throughout his career, he has been involved in various medical organizations including serving as president of the Oklahoma Academy of Otolaryngology, president of the Tulsa Surgical Society, president of the St. John Medical Staff, delegate to the Oklahoma State Medical Association, chairman of the otolaryngology section of St. John Medical Center and a physician reviewer for the Otolaryngology-Head and Neck Surgery Journal.

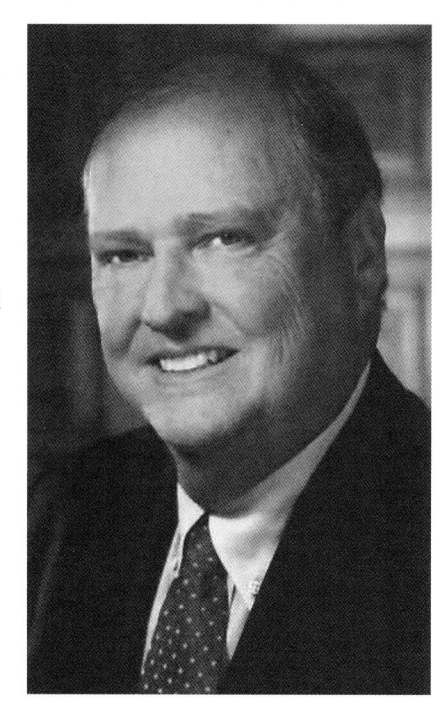

In 2000, he was awarded the presidential citation from the American Academy of Otolaryngology — Head and Neck Surgery.

Dr. Mowry volunteered on the cleft palate clinic team at the Children's Medical Center and for the nonprofit Neighbor for Neighbor clinic. He is married to Kathleen Mowry and the couple has two daughters and three grandchildren. He retired in January 2016.

Victor Neal, M.D.

Dr. Victor Neal was the first physician to administer anesthesia on a patient at Saint Francis Hospital after he join the newly formed Associated Anesthesiologists in 1960. It was an uncomplicated Caesarian section.

The native of Wanette, Oklahoma knew in high school he wanted to be a physician. After graduating in 1950, he majored in pre-med at East Central University in Ada. He entered the University of Oklahoma College of Medicine, completing his degree in 1957 followed by an internship and residency at OU.

In 1960, he joined Associated Anesthesiologists, a private practice in Tulsa founded by Dr. Howard A. Bennett, M.D., and Dr. Theodore R. Wenger, M.D. He remembers the service for anesthesia for a tonsillectomy cost $20 and $35 for a hernia.

On New Year's Eve in 1966, Dr. Neal, who was a 34-year-old with a wife and five sons, received a draft notice. He was inducted into the Army as a captain in the Medical Corps on Jan. 23, 1967, and sent to Saigon to serve in the Vietnam War. After one year, he was sent Fort Carson near Colorado Springs, Colorado, as its chief of anesthesiology, serving 40,000 troops and their families.

In 1969, Dr. Neal returned to Tulsa and worked at the practice as a partner until his retirement in 1993. He served as president of the Oklahoma Society of Anesthesiologists.

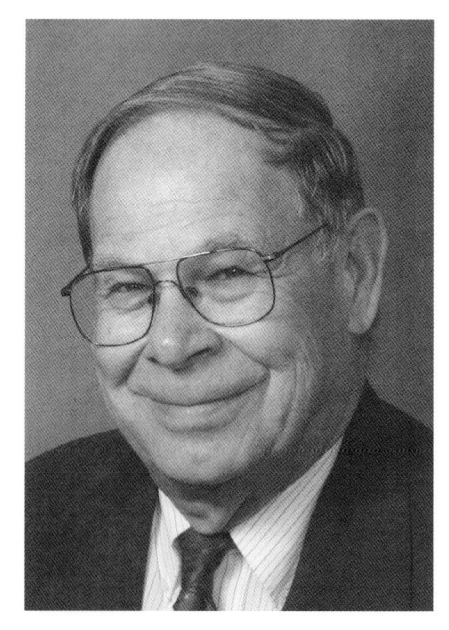

In retirement, he travelled and worked on a farm in Okmulgee with his wife, Mary, until her death in 2011. He is a member of the New Haven Methodist Church. The couple also has 10 grandchildren and many great-grandchildren and great-great-grandchildren.

Don G. Nelson, M.D.

Dr. Don G. Nelson spent 30 years practicing internal medicine and pulmonary diseases at Springer Clinic and then another five years at the Muskogee Veterans Administration Clinic.

Born in 1937, a native of Moline, Illinois, he attended the University of Illinois starting out in electrical engineering. During his junior year, he switched to pre-med because he felt helping people would be a more fulfilling life. He was accepted and eventually graduated from the University of Illinois Medical School, where he completed his internship. He was elected into the Alpha Omega Alpha Honor Medical Society during his junior year. One summer, he obtained a three-month research project at the National Institutes of Health in Bethesda, Maryland, studying protein metabolism of the parasite that causes Chagas' Disease.

After serving his military obligation in the Public Health Service, he went to the University of Cincinnati Medical Center for three years of internal medicine residency with one of those years serving as chief resident and faculty instructor. Then, Dr. Nelson spent two years in a pulmonary fellowship. During that time, he had two papers published in the "American Review of Respiratory Diseases," one on tuberculosis treatment and another on sarcoidosis.

Dr. Nelson arrived in Tulsa to practice medicine at Springer Clinic, which was a multi-specialty clinic that had two other pulmonary specialists on staff. Also, he was involved with the University of Oklahoma Tulsa Medical College as an instructor and later as an assistant clinical professor. He became the part-time medical director of Saint Francis Hospital Respiratory Department and Pulmonary Function Lab. For many years, he volunteered as the medical advisor to Oklahoma Lung Association and Oklahoma Respiratory Therapy Society. He was a member of the AMA, OSMA, American College of Physicians, American Respiratory Society and was a Fellow in the American College of Chest Physicians.

During his career, Dr. Nelson witnessed dramatic changes in medicine. When he entered the profession, 20 to 30 patient beds would be located to a single ward. The design was later made to single or double beds to a room. Early on, few antibiotics, antihypertensives or effective diuretics were available for treatment. The ventilators were primitive with no blood gas machines to monitor effectiveness. He recalls a time when tuberculosis was a major disease, and that has now been virtually eliminated in the U.S.

Dr. Nelson conducted the first fiberoptic bronchoscopy at Saint Francis Hospital. Previously, the primary instruments were rigid bronchoscopes.

He met his wife on a blind date while he was in medical school and she was attending nursing school. They were married on June 13, 1964. They have three children and three grandchildren. Nancy is a nurse with a masters degree in health education and has worked in various health fields and with organizations including the American Red Cross. She is currently employed with the Tulsa City County Health Department as the training coordinator for a program called Children First.

His avocation has always been participating in sports, particularly triathlons. He has competed in about 275 races including all 33 Tulsa Triathlons, which began in 1982. He has qualified for the USA Triathlon age group team and competed in 18 ITU World Championships events, finishing as high as 6th place several times. In retirement, he continues to train and race in swimming, running, and triathlon events. He also enjoys auditing college courses in a large variety of subjects at The University of Tulsa.

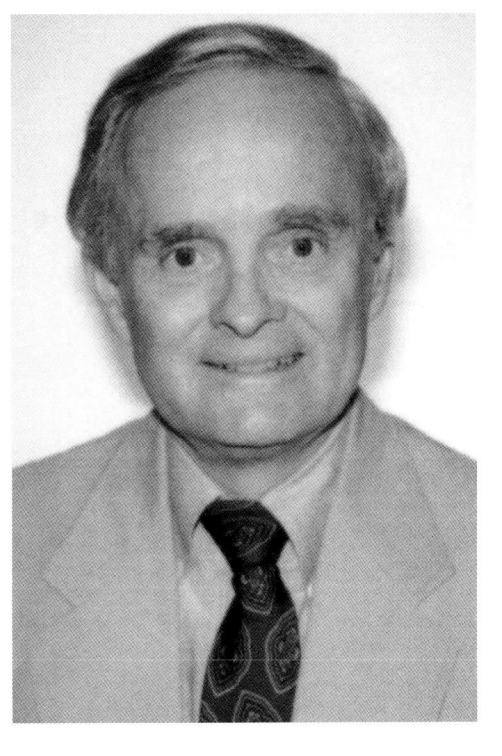

John B. Nettles, M.D.

An interest in obstetrics and gynecology and participation in medical research and health organization led John B. Nettles, M.D., to a life dedicated to community medicine and women's health.

With more than 40 years teaching at the University of Oklahoma College of Medicine and 71 years practicing medicine, Dr. Nettles has influenced generations of doctors and helped to lead the Tulsa systems into creating community medicine.

Born in Dover, North Carolina, to a Methodist minister, the family moved when he was a boy to South Carolina, where he graduated from the Medical University of South Carolina in 1944.

While a medical student, he was placed in the Army Specialized Training Program then promoted to first lieutenant after graduation. While on inactive status to finish his internship, the Navy needed more officers due to losses in the Pacific theater. At the urging of the War Department, Dr. Nettles transferred into the Navy as an active duty medical officer.

Due to his early interest in obstetrics and gynecology, Dr. Nettles took part in the early studies of identifying cervical cancer by using the Pap smear. In 1947, he began his residency at the University of Illinois in Chicago. While there, his research focus centered on kidney impairments associated with pregnancy.

Dr. Nettles always kept a foot in academia and in practice. From 1951-1957, he was an assistant professor at the University of Illinois College of Medicine in OB/GYN. He moved in 1957 to Little Rock, Arkansas, for a position as assistant professor at the University of Arkansas School of Medicine. While there, he served as the interim chairman of the OB/GYN department and began examining systems of health care delivery.

Dr. Nettles and other physicians saw a need for a more cooperative approach with the hospitals and schools working together. This model formed the basis of community medicine.

In 1969, Dr. Nettles brought this philosophy to Tulsa when he took a position with the OU School of Medicine in the Department of Obstetrics and Gynecology and was simultaneously the director of graduate education at Hillcrest Medical Center.

Under his service and leadership, residency programs were expanded at Hillcrest Medical Center, Saint Francis Health System and St. John Health System, and medical students were accepted there for the required clerkship in OB/GYN.

"By the physicians, hospitals and medical schools coming together, it provided for a better education, patient care and research," he said. "Tulsa is a leader in community medicine in the United States."

Though retiring at age 89, he continues to be active in issues of health care at 94 years of age.

He has held leadership positions in many organizations including the American College of Obstetricians and Gynecologists (ACOG) in which he served on the executive board and as its delegate in the American Medical Association House of Delegates, and on the American College of Surgeons Board of Governors. He is a life member of the Tulsa County Medical Society and the Oklahoma State Medical Society. He was president of the Oklahoma Division of the American Cancer Society.

In 2008, OU created the John Barnwell Nettles Award in Obstetrics and Gynecology to be given to a medical student for outstanding performance. When the university bestowed him the title of professor emeritus, it named the OU-Tulsa women's health center the "J.B. Nettles Women's Health Center."

As a supporter of many local health and human service organizations, Dr. Nettles was a founding member of the Margaret Hudson Program, which is a nonprofit supporting teenage mothers.

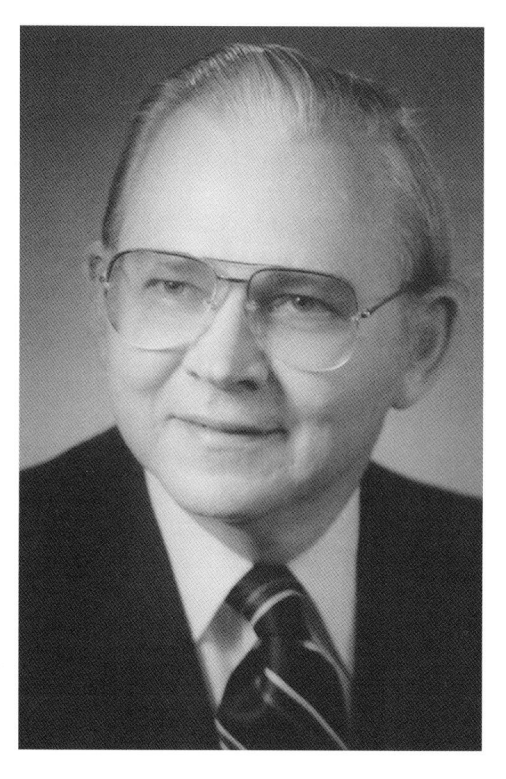

Oklahoma Pain and Wellness Center

Oklahoma Pain and Wellness Center promotes a holistic approach to chronic pain management, coordinating a complete pain management service with injection therapy and pharmacologic therapies. The center provides guidance in chiropractic therapies, acupuncture, massage therapy, and psychological counseling.

Oklahoma Pain and Wellness Center is a modern, all green facility designed to ensure patients have a pleasant and comfortable experience. Environmentally focused, the center is located in a formerly unused carpet warehouse building. Upon purchasing the iconic structure, owner Dr. Jayen Patel remodeled the building with an upscale industrial-chic design reminiscent of Tulsa's celebrated Art Deco period. The facility is heated and cooled by an in-ground geothermal well field deep below the parking lot. No fossil fuels are used on site and all equipment and products are purchased locally or in America. The facility makes every effort to be environmentally responsible. Oklahoma Pain and Wellness Center utilizes paperless records and promotes the use of renewable energy by supplying electrical vehicle plug-ins to staff.

Dr. Patel began his professional career at Boston University where he earned a bachelor of arts degree in Biology —Summa Cum Laude. For his research in mammalian neuroendocrinology, he was awarded the distinguished Howard Hughes fellowship award for independent research which led to a senior thesis concerning the hormonal effects of the brain that predict behavior. That research awarded Dr. Patel a distinction in Biological Sciences by Boston University and he was named class speaker. In his final year, he expanded his clinical activities to include medical missions in Kenya and Peru. Dr. Patel graduated from Boston University, School of Medicine. He was awarded his M.D. after completing his pre-clinical education with the faculty of Boston University and clinical rotations at Boston Medical Center.

Following his graduation from Boston University, Dr. Patel continued his training at Mount Sinai School of Medicine in Manhattan, New York where he completed a year of general surgery training. He furthered his specialization in anesthesiology at New York University and is board certified in anesthesiology through the American Board of Anesthesiology. Dr. Patel's specific interests lie in ultrasound guided nerve blocks, pain management, neuromodulation, and headache treatments.

Oklahoma Pain and Wellness Center is dedicated to reducing prescription drug abuse in the community. Rather than focusing on a traditional one-size-fits-all solution for patients, the center uses a holistic pain approach.

"We uphold the highest standards in preventing drug diversion and abuse by personalizing medicine," says Dr. Patel. "We are interested in long-term wellness, not just a temporary fix."

The vision of the Oklahoma Pain and Wellness Center is one that is focused on taking care of everyone. From the moment patients walk through the door, they are shepherded through a comprehensive assessment to determine an appropriate diagnosis.

The practice offers many services, including celiac plexus block, discogram, epidural injections, facet injections, hypogastric plexus block, joint injections, lumbar sympathetic block, occipital nerve block, peripheral nerve stimulation, radio frequency ablation, sacroiliac injections, spinal cord stimulation, stellate ganglion block, transforaminal injection, and vertebral fracture repair.

Oklahoma Pain and Wellness Center accepts worker's compensation, all motor vehicle insurance, personal injury cases, and is able to work with most insurance plans. ■

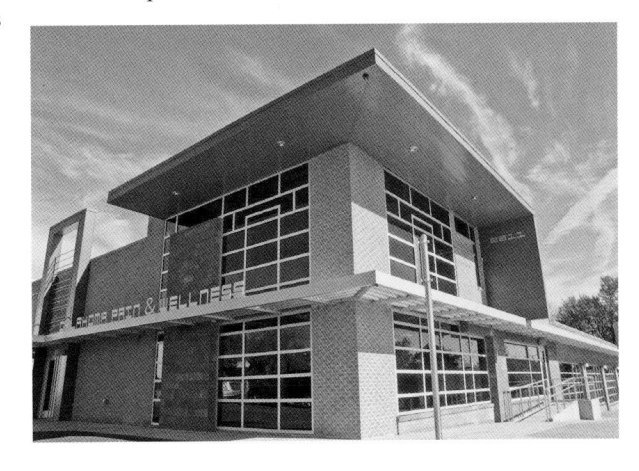

Jayen Patel, M.D.

Neurosurgery Specialists

In 1973, a young neurosurgeon, fresh out of residency from Baylor College of Medicine in Houston, arrived in Tulsa and became the original founder of Neurological Surgery Inc.

Dr. Anthony Billings completed medical school from the University of Oregon Health Sciences Center in 1966. Dr. Billings was known to travel from town to town, building relationships with outlying communities. In those days, there were very few neurosurgeons in Tulsa. In general, medicine and, in particular neurosurgery, was very different from present day. CT scanning was invented in 1972 and widely used by 1980. Early technology for MRIs had been invented, but wide-spread usage came later than CT imaging. Neurosurgeons, by today's standards, had a much more limited array of diagnostic studies available to them. As an aside, all studies had to be viewed at the hospital. It wasn't until the mid-1990s that car phones were becoming common place. Conversely, today, care providers can pull up images at their offices, homes or mobile devices. With these advancements, among many others, Tulsa experienced a rapidly growing need for neurosurgeons.

In 1975, Dr. Billings recruited his junior resident, Dr. David Fell to join him in Tulsa. Dr. Fell graduated from Yale University in 1966 with a degree in psychology. He attended Baylor College of Medicine and completed his neurosurgery residency in 1975. He enthusiastically served the Tulsa community until his retirement in December 2014.

Working longer and longer hours, Drs. Billings and Fell recruited Dr. Fell's junior resident, Dr. Benjamin Benner in 1978. Dr. Benner graduated with distinction from Dartmouth College in 1969 with a degree in psychology and completed his neurosurgery residency in 1978 from Baylor College of Medicine. While the physicians of this group have cared for patients of all ages, Dr. Benner had a particular calling for pediatric patients. In 2015, Dr. Benner transitioned to a non-surgical practice and is pursuing his interest in hospital design and construction. He has been instrumentally involved in the renovation of the Saint Francis Hospital surgical facilities and patient care units.

In 1989, Dr. Karl Detwiler joined the group of three. There had not been a new neurosurgeon in Tulsa for roughly 10 years. Dr. Detwiler graduated from Oklahoma State University in 1979 with a degree in chemistry. While he had a promised position with Phillips Petroleum, Dr. Detwiler chose to attend the University of Oklahoma Health Sciences Center and later a neurosurgery residency at the University of Iowa. After 22 years of service, he sadly passed away in 2011 at age 55.

In 1995, Dr. Billings retired from the group to pursue other interests, most notably art. In January 1996, Drs. Allen Fielding, James Rodgers and David Kosmoski of Tulsa Neursurgery Inc. joined the group. The name of the group officially changed to Neurosurgery Specialists. That relationship continued until 2000 when the latter three pursued separate interests. But, the name of this group remains.

In 2004, Dr. Doug Koontz joined Neurosurgery Specialists. In 1977, Dr. Koontz graduated with distinction from the University of Oklahoma with a degree in microbiology. He received his medical degree from the University of Oklahoma Health Sciences Center and completed his neurosurgery residency there in 1987. In 2015, Dr. Koontz retired from private practice and currently provides neurosurgical coverage in several regions of the United States.

In 2006, Dr. Daniel

Dr. Benjamin Benner, Dr. David Fell, Dr. Karl Detwiler, Dr. Anthony Billings (1994)

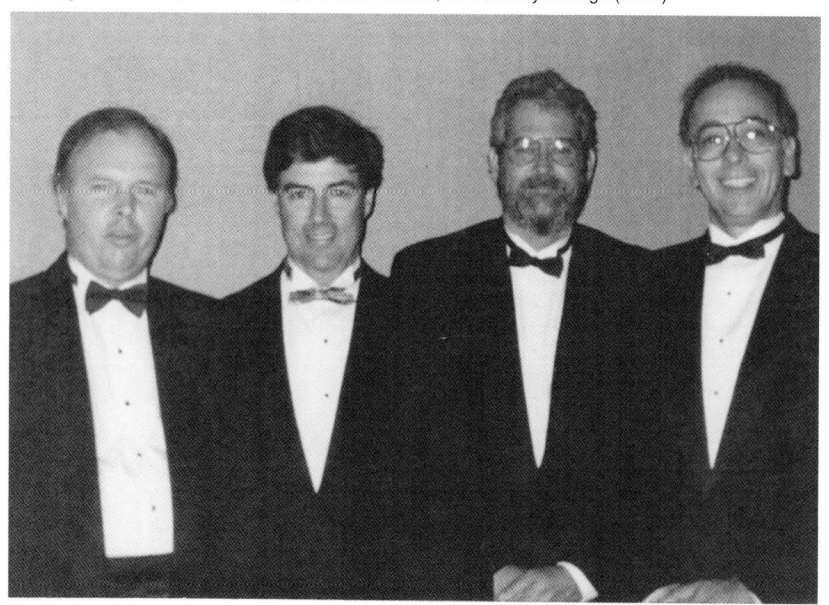

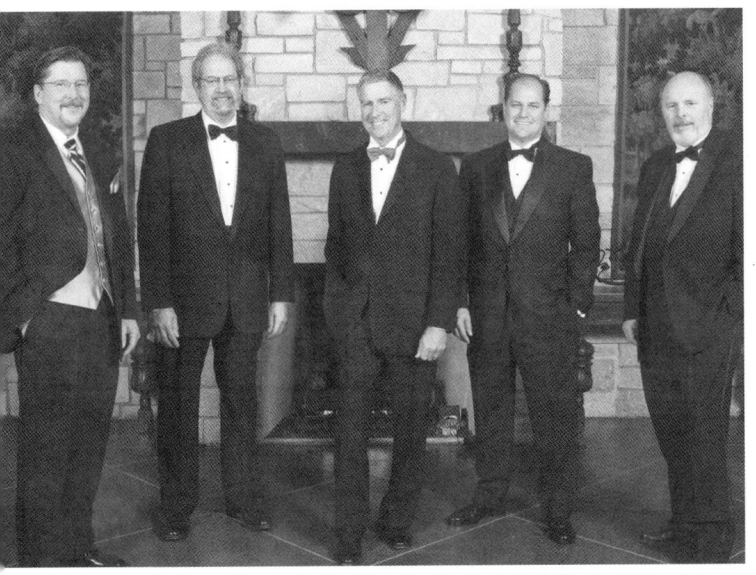

Dr. Doug Koontz, Dr. Karl Detwiler, Dr. David Fell, Dr. Daniel Boedeker, and Dr. Benjamin Benner (October 2009)

Boedeker joined Neurosurgery Specialists. He was raised in Tulsa and graduated with distinction in 1996 from the University of Oklahoma with a degree in zoology. He attended the University of Oklahoma Health Sciences Center for his medical degree and completed his neurosurgery residency in 2006 at the Baylor College of Medicine in Houston. Interestingly, several of the professors who trained Dr. Boedeker were peers in training with Drs. Billings, Fell and Benner.

In 2011, Dr. Ryan Rahhal joined Neurosurgery Specialists. Dr. Rahhal is a Tulsa native who graduated with distinction in 1999 from the University of Oklahoma, earning degrees in both chemistry and biochemistry. He earned his medical degree in 2004 from the University of Oklahoma Health Sciences Center and completed his neurosurgery residency there in 2011.

In 2006, Neurosurgery Specialists included its first physician assistant, Theresa Rogers. Theresa graduated with a degree in biology from Northeastern State University in Tahlequah, Oklahoma. In 2000, Theresa completed with distinction the Masters of Health Sciences, Physician Assistant program from the University of Oklahoma Health Sciences Center.

In early 2015, Neurosurgery Specialists hired its latest physician assistant, Meredith Jenkins. Meredith graduated with a degree in biology from Missouri Southern State University in Joplin, Missouri. In 2014, Meredith completed the Masters of Health Sciences, Physician Assistant program from the University of Oklahoma Health Sciences Center.

In August 2016, the practice added Dr. Shihao Zhang to its medical team. Dr. Zhang graduated with distinction from Louisiana State University with a degree in biochemistry. He attended medical school at LSU and completed his neurosurgery residency in 2016 from LSU Health Sciences Center.

While the neurosurgeons at Neurosurgery Specialists have areas of particular interest, they are expertly trained in all areas of neurosurgery including brain tumors, cranial vascular problems, spinal tumors, mechanical spinal disorders and peripheral nerve issues. This is particularly important in a community-based practice such as Tulsa.

During the past 40 years, Neurosurgery Specialists has grown from a one-doctor practice into a regional presence. In addition to the Tulsa location at 6767 S. Yale Ave., the practice has clinics in Vinita and Stillwater. The professionals of this group are highly dedicated individuals who have cared for Tulsans and surrounding Green Country

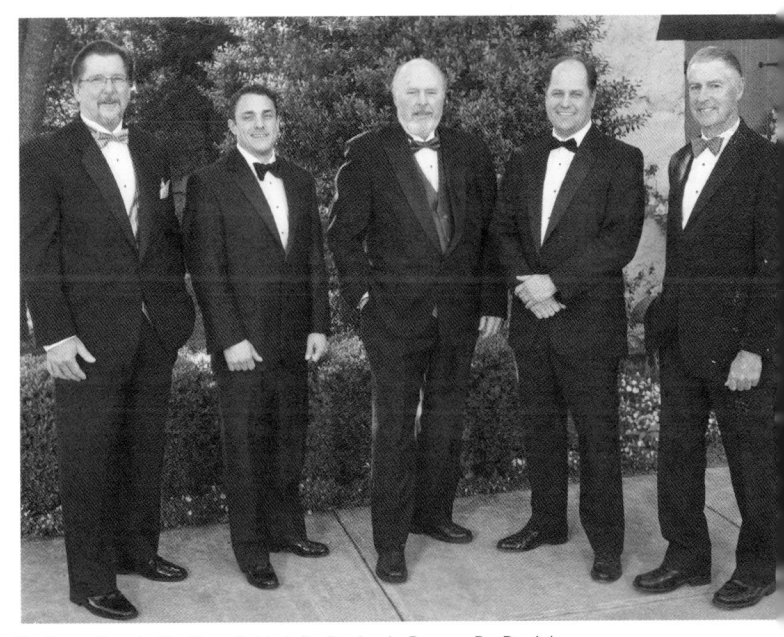

Dr. Doug Koontz, Dr. Ryan Rahhal, Dr. Benjamin Benner, Dr. Daniel Boedeker, and Dr. David Fell. (April 2012)

for multiple decades. These providers gave support to other Tulsa medical programs and practices. Drs. Fell and Detwiler were on the ground floor of developing local physician-owned hospitals including the Tulsa Spine and Specialty Hospital and Oklahoma Surgical Hospital. Drs. Koontz, Boedeker and Rahhal have continued their efforts. It is with great pride and a sense of a "job well done" that we reflect on the birth and growth of our practice and eagerly look forward to our future.

Oklahoma Surgical Hospital

In 2001, a group of quality conscious physicians came together with a combined vision to create a new hospital-delivery system dedicated to the achievement of nationally recognized clinical excellence in a patient-centered environment. This development was the result of several years of planning by its original 22-physician founders, which included local and highly respected orthopedic surgeons from Central States Orthopedic Specialists and Eastern Oklahoma Orthopedic Center, neurosurgeons (Drs. John Marouk and Karl Detwiler) and anesthesiologists from Associated Anesthesiologists, Inc. With their input into the hospital's overall operations, the founders wanted to place a high commitment on patients receiving outstanding medical care in a highly personalized manner. This commitment also included patients having access to the latest surgical techniques and medical technology as well as outstanding specialized nursing care. The site selected was the former Oral Roberts University City of Faith Hospital in the CityPlex Towers because of its available medical infrastructure. What started as Orthopedic Hospital of Oklahoma in 2001 has evolved 15 years later to the present-day Oklahoma Surgical Hospital.

Initially operating as Orthopedic Hospital of Oklahoma, the hospital experienced sustained growth through its specialization in orthopedic care and focus on high patient satisfaction. As more patients experienced the high level of care provided, the hospital increasingly received requests to expand the types of surgical procedures performed at OSH. In the fall of 2006, the first step of expanding medical and surgical offerings occurred with the addition of 10 general surgeons from Surgical Associates, Inc., one of the oldest general surgery group practices located in south Tulsa. In March 2007, the hospital changed its name to Oklahoma Surgical Hospital to better reflect the diversity and scope of services.

In January 2008, another larger group of surgical specialists, Urologic Specialists of Oklahoma, joined OSH. This allowed the hospital to expand further. Today, the hospital provides inpatient and outpatient services for most surgical procedures including orthopedics, neurosurgery, general surgery, colorectal, breast, gynecological, urology, ENT and plastic surgery. The hospital operates the Institute for Robotic

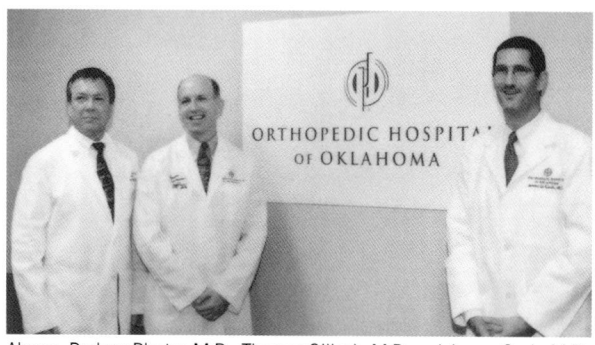

Above: Rodney Plaster, M.D., Thomas Gillock, M.D. and James Cash, M.D.

Below: Brad Boone, M.D.

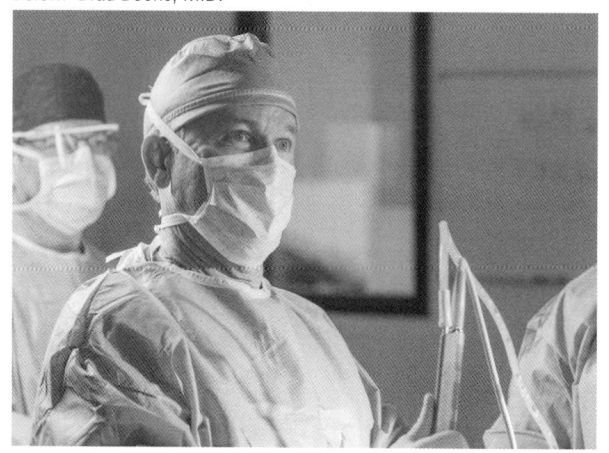

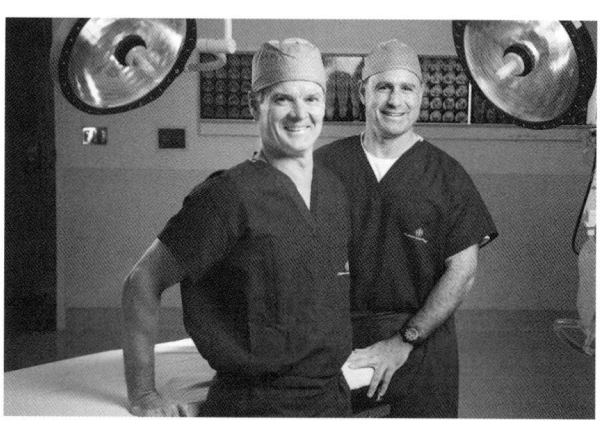

Above: Craig Johnson, M.D. and Scott Rahhal, M.D.

Below: Clio Robertson, M.D.

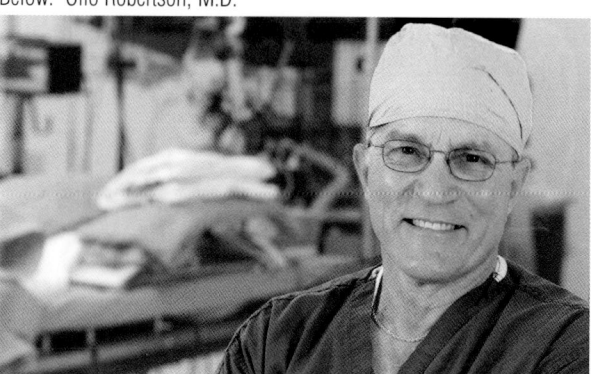

FUTURE LEGACIES

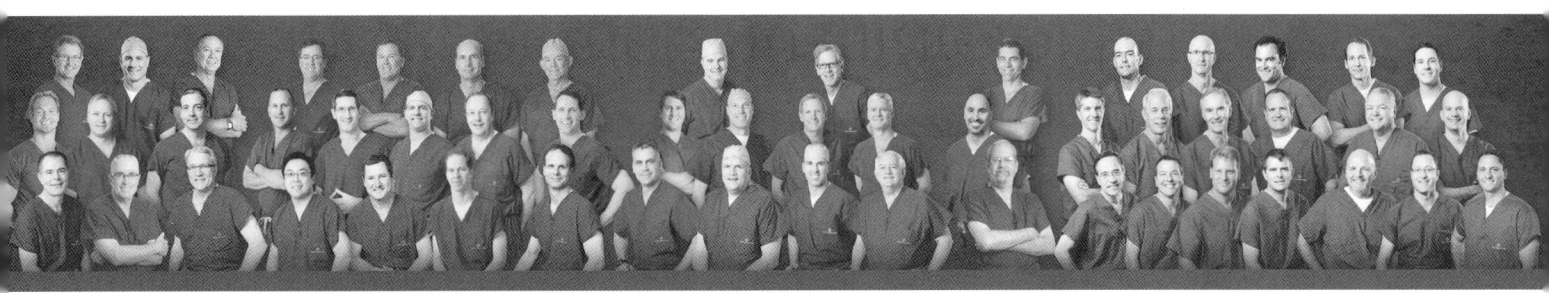

Pictured are the physician owners of OSH at the time of the hospital's 10-year anniversary

Surgery, Pain Management Center, Imaging Center, Endoscopy Center and Physical Therapy Center.

In 2009, the hospital enhanced its surgical technological commitment with the acquisition of the da Vinci Robotic system and the development of the Institute for Robotic Surgery at Oklahoma Surgical Hospital. This allows surgeons to perform detailed procedures using computerized robotics with minimal tissue injury and blood loss, which results in faster patient recovery. It is often used for prostate, kidney, gynecologic and upper and lower abdominal surgery procedures. OSH is designated as the main EpiCenter Training Site for colorectal procedures for the da Vinci Robotic system. In 2012, the hospital acquired the MAKOplasty robotic surgical system. It allows orthopedic surgeons to perform partial knee resurfacing with the advanced precision of robotic technology. OSH has become one of the largest and most surgically diversified robotics programs in Oklahoma.

Through the years, OSH has been honored by several national organizations. OSH received recognition from HealthGrades, a large national hospital ratings firm that analyzes more than 5,000 hospitals in 50 states on clinical outcomes and quality. Its ratings are based on information received from the U.S. Centers for Medicare and Medicaid Services. OSH has been named one of America's 100 Best Hospital's for Joint Replacement for 2014, 2015, 2016 and 2017. It has received Five-Star Ratings for both its Total Knee and Total Hip Replacement programs. It also received Five-Star ratings for Spinal Fusion Surgery. OSH was also named one of America's 100 Best Hospitals for Prostate Surgery. Additionally, it has been given the Outstanding Patient Experience and Patient Safety Excellence ratings by HealthGrades.

CareChex, a hospital rankings organization, evaluates the quality of inpatient care based on seven peer-reviewed methods. These include patient safety indicators, inpatient quality indicators, mortality rates, complication rates, readmission rates, core process measures and patient satisfaction. By 2016, CareChex ranked OSH 19th in the nation for overall surgical care, 12th for major orthopedic surgery and 11th for joint replacement. OSH was also ranked in the Top 100 Hospitals for patient safety.

As OSH continued to care for patients, it also continued to be recognized for the quality provided to those patients. In 2013, a report by *Consumer Reports Magazine* called "Your Safer-Surgery Survival Guide" ranked OSH the highest-ranking hospital in Tulsa. For three years in a row, OSH received the Press Ganey Guardian Award for Patient Satisfaction, an award honoring health-care organizations achieving and sustaining a score of 95 percent or above in patient satisfaction. In 2016, OSH was rated 1st out of 91 hospitals in Oklahoma for the lowest complication/highest patient safety measures for surgical patients by the U.S. Centers for Medicaid and Medicare Services. They were also rated 1st out of 48 hospitals in the state for the lowest complication rate following total hip and total knee surgery. OSH was also rated 2nd in the nation out of 2,771 hospitals for their low re-admission rate after hip and knee surgery. In 2016, OSH was one of 102 hospitals nationally (out of 4,746) and the only hospital in Tulsa, to receive a 5-Star Rating based on 64 quality measures for overall hospital care from Medicare.

"From day one, our focus has been on providing the best possible care for our patients. We believe our model, which allows physicians to participate in the operational aspects of the hospital, ensures that our patients and the care they receive remain our number one priority. This, along with our focus on specialization of surgical procedures and our outstanding nursing care, has allowed us to attain national recognition," according to Rick Ferguson, Oklahoma Surgical Hospital Chief Executive Officer.

More than 200 OSH physicians have provided care to hundreds of thousands of patients. It has been quite an accomplishment for its original founding physicians to see their vision develop into reality. Many of these physicians have experienced a variety of changes along with the evolution in the complexity of health-care today. However, the No. 1 priority at OSH remains consistent and is simple - to stay focused on taking care of patients.

University of Oklahoma Health Sciences Center

The University of Oklahoma has a long history of providing healthcare in the Tulsa community. In the late 1960s, the Tulsa County Medical Society partnered with the Metropolitan Tulsa Chamber of Commerce and local hospitals to hire a national consulting firm to determine the viability of a medical college for the Tulsa area.

The report showed that the Tulsa community supported a medical school being in Tulsa. The chamber lobbied the University of Oklahoma to bring an extension of the Health Sciences Center from Oklahoma City to Tulsa. In 1972, the State Legislature passed Senate Bill 453 that created the University of Oklahoma Tulsa Medical College.

As community leaders worked together, they formed the Tulsa Medical Education Foundation (TMEF). The TMEF was integral in the development of medical education in Tulsa. This group brought hospital leaders and OU administrators together to support medical education in Tulsa. At this time, the hospitals were running their own residency programs. In 1976, through relationships developed through TMEF, the hospitals turned over the administration and management of those residency programs to the University of Oklahoma Tulsa Medical College. These residents trained at local hospitals under the educational direction of the University of Oklahoma Tulsa Medical College faculty. Dean James M. Herman, M.D., MSPH credits the work of these early pioneers with the continued growth and success of medical education programs.

"Without their leadership and vision, we would

Dr. James Herman, Dean of the OU-TU School of Community Medicine, visits with medical students. The OU-TU School of Community Medicine is among the nation's leaders in the growing field of community medicine, which focuses on population-based health outcomes.

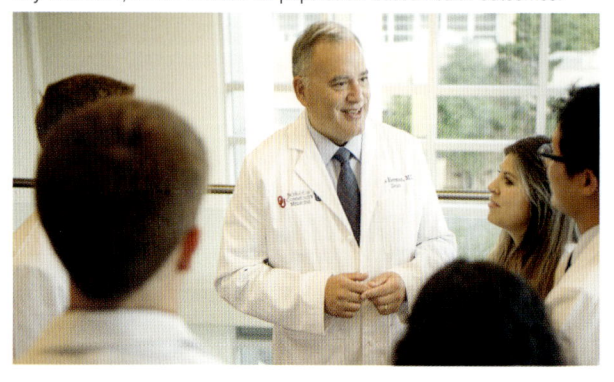

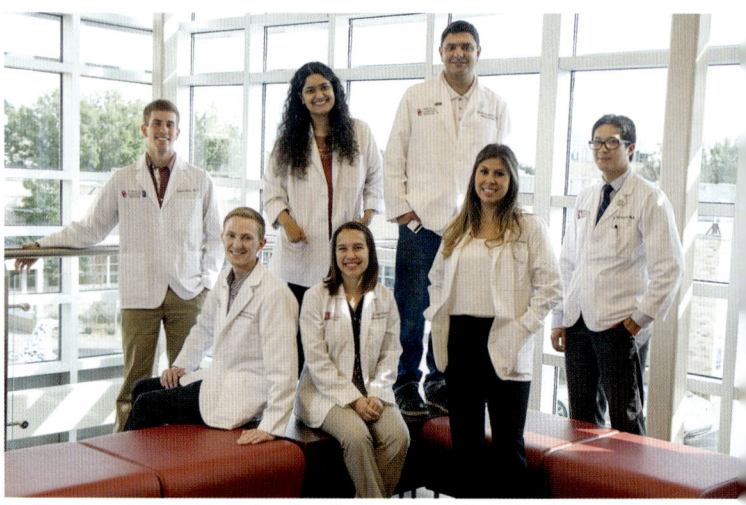

For more than 40 years, The University of Oklahoma's medical education programs have made a difference in Oklahoma through excellence in medical education. Over the past decade, the school has evolved further, with an unwavering commitment to improve the health of entire communities.

not be here today. For more than 40 years, OU has had a strong presence in medical education in Tulsa and that presence has grown and changed to meet community needs."

The first offices of the University of Oklahoma Tulsa Medical College were at 31st and Harvard in the Ranch Acres Medical Building. Leeland Alexander was the first employee of the University of Oklahoma Tulsa Medical College and he is still employed by the University of Oklahoma-Tulsa as an associate vice president. He remembers converting an old X-ray lab into office space for the new Dean and himself. In July of 1974, 17 third-year medical students arrived from the University of Oklahoma Health Sciences Center to begin their clinical rotations in Tulsa.

In 1980, the medical school moved to 28th and South Sheridan Road, where it remained for 20 years. The growth of the college was monumental, establishing eight clinics in Tulsa and Bartlesville and serving more than 100,000 patients annually in the 1980s.

In 1999, with financial support from the OU Foundation and a legacy gift to the University of Oklahoma from the Charles and Lynn Schusterman Family Foundation, the University of Oklahoma purchased the former BP Amoco 60-acre campus at 41st and South Yale Avenue.

"The campus was perfect for us. BP Amoco had

FUTURE LEGACIES

state-of-the-art testing labs and equipment, much of which was donated to the University of Oklahoma after we purchased the campus. This campus accommodated our growth and allowed us to bring all OU educational programs in Tulsa under one roof which was something that had never happened before," said Alexander.

Today, OU medical education programs in Tulsa have expanded from a clinical two-year campus for third-and fourth-year medical students to a four-year campus that welcomed its inaugural class of 27 first-year medical students in August of 2015. This new four year program is in collaboration with the University of Tulsa and is now named the OU-TU School of Community Medicine.

Herman says, "The OU-TU School of Community Medicine is a unique medical school. We feel it's important to not only educate our students and residents in the basics of medical education, but to educate our students and residents in the social determinants of health. There are many factors that determine a person's health in addition to medical care: socioeconomic factors, genetics, education and others. Our graduates have a firm understanding of these principles and utilize those determinants to help them provide care to their patients and the community."

The OU-TU School of Community Medicine provides students and residents with the knowledge and skills necessary to serve as well-rounded primary care or sub-specialty physicians, while learning a special skill set to reach out and improve the health of entire communities.

According to Herman, the OU-TU School of Community Medicine is an important part of the healthcare pipeline. "The United States spends more than any other western country on health care, approximately 18 percent of the GNP, but we remain at the bottom in many public health outcomes."

In Oklahoma, there are many areas that are underserved due to inadequate access to care. A medical school can make a huge impact by educating physicians in community medicine so they can graduate and practice where they can do the most good for the community.

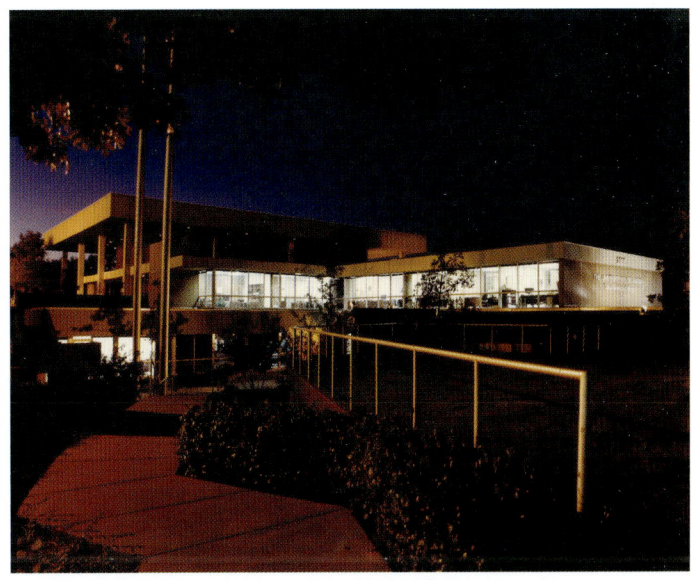

OU President David L. Boren and TU President Steadman Upham and first-year medical students at the dedication of the Tandy Simulation Center, which features the latest advances in medical simulation, training and feedback methods in which students practice in lifelike circumstances using models or virtual reality.

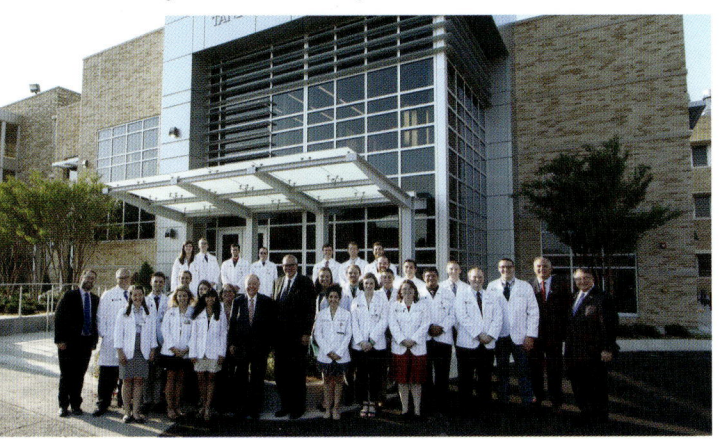

In 1980, the University of Oklahoma Tulsa Medical College moved to 28th and Sheridan Road, where it remained for 20 years.

Herman explains, "If everyone in the United States had a "medical home," a place where they get their care and where they are known and where they know their primary health care provider, then they would be more likely to get the basic care that makes a huge difference: flu shots, PAP smears, annual wellness exams, regular blood pressure monitoring- things we know that prevent disease."

The OU-TU School of Community Medicine has a history of programs that reach out and affect the social determinants of health. Moving forward, Herman sees the challenge of the future is to connect these programs to this emerging concept of population health.

He says, "We need to be using all our resources to care of our own population of patients. We would like to be a provider of choice for those people to get involved in these services. And as we do that, we will educate our medical students and residents to do the same, so when they graduate, they will be prepared to practice medicine as well as improve the health of entire communities."

Rollie Rhodes, M.D.

It was a four-year stint as a flight surgeon in the U.S. Navy and a medical internship that convinced Dr. Rollie Rhodes his future was in otorhinolaryngology.

His work led to co-founding the Eastern Oklahoma Ear, Nose and Throat Clinic, which has grown to be the largest ear, nose and throat clinic in Oklahoma specializing in pediatric and adult diseases. It has extensive experience in the treatment of head and neck cancer, ontological disorders and audiology and provides complete care for allergy and sinus problems.

Dr. Rhodes worked in private practice in Tulsa for 50 years.

"I loved the people. I loved what I did," Dr. Rhodes said. "It was dynamic and contributed to the community. After 20 years in practice, I started seeing the children of my patients. By the time I retired, I was seeing the grandchildren.

"This was the type of relationship I enjoyed. I knew all their histories. Each time someone came in, it was like seeing family."

A native of Kentucky, Dr. Rhodes graduated high school in 1949 and completed a bachelor's degree from the University of Louisville in 1953. He earned a medical degree in 1957 from the University of Louisville College of Medicine, and then served four years in the Navy as a lieutenant commander.

While in medical school, he became impressed by the work of an ENT team, and his military experience confirmed that interest. This was also a time of advancements in microscopes for better examination of the delicate bones of the ear. Eventually, X-rays, CT scans and MRI tests were developed for a better look at the head, neck and sinus areas.

"All of these things helped to evaluate and diagnose a patient," he said. "I saw this was a budding and growing specialty."

After leaving the Navy, he did a fellowship at the Mayo Clinic, earning a master's degree in otolaryngology in 1965. That year, he accepted a position in Tulsa at the Springer Clinic, where he worked for 10 years.

In 1975, he and an associate, Dr. Charles Heinberg, founded the Eastern Oklahoma Ear, Nose and Throat Clinic in the Kelly Medical Building near Saint Francis Hospital. In 1980, the practice built a facility at 5020 E. 68th St. It included a diagnostic clinic and an outpatient surgery center.

The approach to attracting and retaining staff was an equitable salary and collaborative work environment. Physician income was based on the amount of work performed, not seniority. Also, new doctors were given help establishing a patient base.

"It allowed everybody to work at the pace they wanted," Dr. Rhodes said. "We had a fair pay scale and always hired the best quality people we could find. A major factor in growth is quality employees. We provided good fringe benefits and better-than-average salaries."

Among his memorable moments were the opportunities to restore hearing.

"There is such emotion associated with suddenly being able to hear things they have never heard their entire lives or for the last 25 years or so," he said. "That is very satisfying both for the doctor and patient."

Dr. Rhodes married Sammie (Mason) on June 11, 1955. The couple had three daughters, eight grandchildren and one great-granddaughter. They were married for 55 years.

Dr. Rhodes retired on June 1, 2015, and has remained active as a volunteer, sitting on several boards including the First Oklahoma Bank of Tulsa, Tulsa Symphony Orchestra, Oklahoma Methodist Manor and Tulsa County Medical Society Foundation.

Among his certifications and memberships: American Board of Otolaryngology, American Medical Association, Tulsa County Medical Society, Oklahoma State Board of Medical Examiners, American Society of Otolaryngic Allergy, American College of Allergy and the American Association for Clinical Immunology and Allergy.

He served as president of the medical-dental staff and chairman of the department of otorhinolaryngology at Saint Francis Hospital. He served as a clinical professor and director of allergy education for the department of otolaryngology at the University of Oklahoma Health Sciences Center for 30 years.

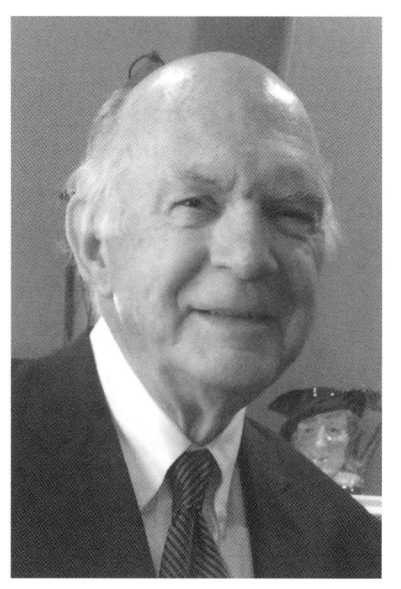

Anil K. Reddy, M.D., M.B.A.

Physiatrist Anil Reddy, son of a veterinarian surgeon, started his career as an orthopedic surgeon in India. He received a Bachelor of Medicine and Bachelor of Surgery and Masters of Surgery at Gandhi Medical College and residency training in Trauma and Orthopedic Surgery from the University of Health Sciences. He received advanced orthopedic surgical training at Neath General Hospital (Wales) and worked as a senior house officer in emergency medicine, accident, trauma, and orthopedics. He performed his residency at Metropolitan Hospital Center (NYC), receiving board certification in Physical Medicine and Rehabilitation and Electrodiagnostic Medicine through New York Medical College.

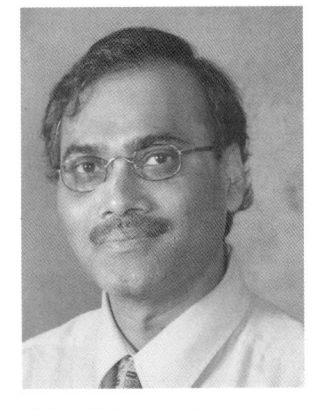

He settled in Tulsa in 2000, joining a group practice. In 2002, he joined Omega Practice Management, an outpatient clinic. "I do mainly musculoskeletal pain management by modalities, medications and injections, and also alternative medicine treatments. Physical medicine and rehab focuses on the muscle, bones, joints, and functional ability of the patient," he shares.

Utilizing a holistic approach, he encourages patients to adopt a lifestyle of a healthy diet, aerobic exercise, no smoking, and meditation — conventional advice among physicians — and yoga, his unconventional recommendation. "No other exercise in the world can stretch your muscles like yoga. A lot of musculoskeletal pain requires stretching exercises," shares Dr. Reddy.

He is a member of the Tulsa County Medical Society and American Association of Physical Medicine and Rehabilitation. He received an MBA in Health Care Management from the University of Texas.

Dr. Reddy follows the traditional approach in medicine by demonstrating compassion and spending quality time with patients. "I think medicine is a measure of art and science. The art is disappearing — the art of interviewing a patient and the art of dealing with the pain and resolving it. I still follow that tradition." ∎

Brian Ribak, M.D.

Born on the 4th of July in 1944, Brian Ribak, M.D. always knew from his earliest memories he wanted to become a doctor. All his schooling was in Albany, New York, including graduation from Albany Medical College in May 1970. While serving in a mixed surgical internship in Rochester, New York, he was drafted by the Army during the Vietnam War. During his two years at Fort Meade, Maryland, he was afforded the opportunity to train at Fort Rucker, Alabama to become an Aviation Medical Officer and receive flight time in helicopters.

Dr. Ribak was offered a surgical residency at Brooke Army Medical Center, San Antonio, Texas. During a rotation through anesthesia in his first six months of surgical residency, he got hooked by the specialty and switched to the anesthesia residency program. After completing his Army commitment in July 1977, he came to Tulsa that August, following his staff man from his third year of residency at Brooke.

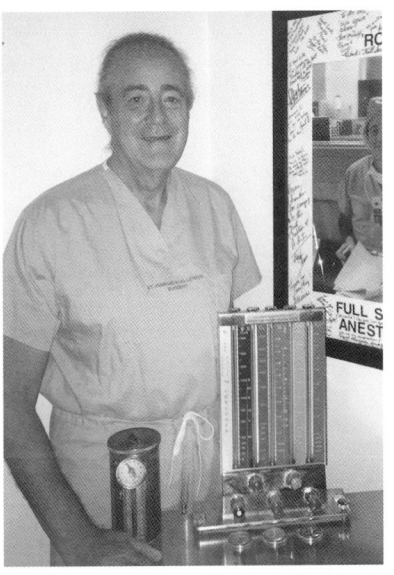

Dr. Ribak in front of an antique anesthesiology machine

They joined Anesthesia Associated, Inc. and worked at St. John Medical Center and its satellite facilities.

Dr. Ribak was instrumental in changing the group's practice from performing saddle blocks for women in labor to doing epidurals. "That's probably the one thing I started at St. John that I was the most proud of."

After Dr. Ribak endured a CABG in 1988, his compassion for patients grew. "I enjoyed doing anesthesia for open heart patients because I could relate better to them on both ends," he shares. "I think it made me a better anesthesiologist."

He retired in February 2010 to spend more time with his children, Deena, Adam, Elana, and Michelle, his grandchildren, and great-grandchildren. ∎

FUTURE LEGACIES

Oklahoma State University Center for Health Sciences
OSU Medical Center

For more than 40 years, the Oklahoma State University Medical Center has served as the teaching hospital for medical students training at OSU Center for Health Sciences (OSU-CHS), formerly called the Oklahoma College of Osteopathic Medicine and Surgery. During this time, OSU-CHS faculty has trained more than 3,000 physicians, many of whom practice in Oklahoma.

The mission of the OSU Medical Center and OSU-CHS is similar — to deliver high-quality health care services to Oklahomans with a particular interest in rural and underserved communities. The OSU Medical Center is one of the largest osteopathic teaching hospitals in the nation with more than 70,000 patient visits each year. In addition to student rotations, OSU Medical Center also offers 11 residency programs and nine fellowships in primary care and other specialties, training more than 150 residents each year.

The evolution of the relationship comes from shifts in needs and funding in Oklahoma. However, the history and tradition of osteopathic medicine runs deep in Tulsa.

Osteopathic practitioners have been in Tulsa before statehood. Because only allopathic doctors were granted hospital admission privileges, Dr. C.D. "Pop" Heasley founded the Tulsa Clinic Hospital in 1924 for osteopathic physicians and their patients. The 10-bed hospital quickly grew as the city's population grew. It operated under the regulations set forth by the Bureau of Hospitals of the American Osteopathic Association and eventually became the Oklahoma Osteopathic Hospital.

Through the early 20th century, the facility expanded to become one of the largest osteopathic hospitals in the nation and offered residencies and internships. The Oklahoma Osteopathic Association had successfully recruited medical students into the profession and had been proposing a state-supported college of osteopathic medicine since the 1950s.

The founding of the college came in 1972 after a legislative study indicated Oklahoma had a growing physician shortage. The problem was acute in all but Tulsa and Oklahoma counties. Gov. David Hall approved a bill to create two Tulsa medical schools - an allopathic branch for third- and fourth-year students offered by the University of Oklahoma and an osteopathic school developed with assistance from the Oklahoma Osteopathic Association through the Oklahoma State Regents for Higher Education. Originally called the Oklahoma College of Osteopathic Medicine and Surgery, it was the nation's first freestanding, public college of osteopathic medicine.

Classes were set to begin on Sept. 1, 1974.

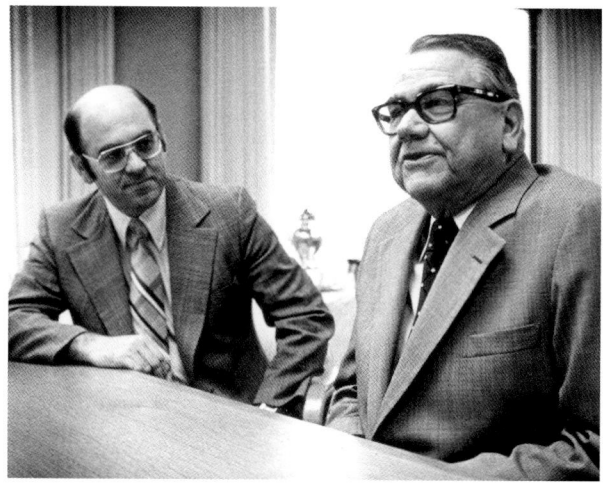

E.T. Dunlap (right), chancellor of the Oklahoma State Regents for Higher Education, was influential in recruiting Dr. John Barson (left) to lead the new Oklahoma College of Osteopathic Medicine.

A national search for a university president was launched by an advisory committee of the Oklahoma Osteopathic Association at the request of the state regents. Dr. John Barson was named the college's first president. He was an associate dean of the College of Osteopathic Medicine at Michigan State University.

Without a building, faculty, students or a budget, Dr. Barson faced significant challenges. After arriving in Tulsa, Dr. Edward Felmlee donated space in his office at 720 W. Seventh St. for the new president to begin planning.

The inaugural class of 36 students was selected from a pool of several hundred applicants. Of those, 32 were from Oklahoma. Coursework was offered in temporary classrooms.

FUTURE LEGACIES

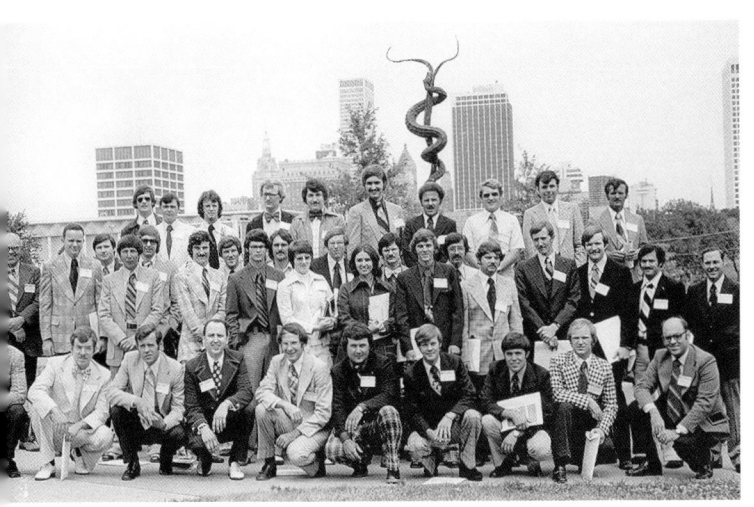

The inaugural class of 36 student graduates from the Oklahoma College of Osteopathic Medicine and Surgery.

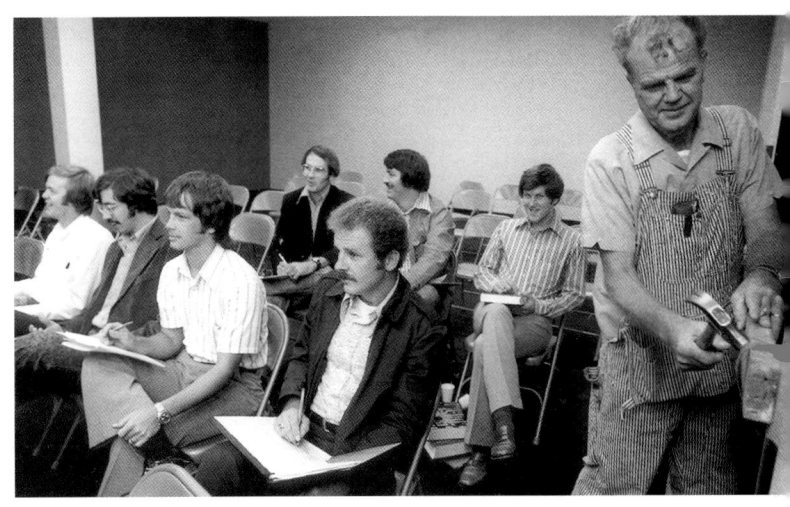

Early students attended classrooms while construction was ongoing. Pictured are (bottom left to right) James Campbell, Mike Mowdy, Paul Ruble and Gary Hoff. (Back row left to right) Bob Adams, Chris Hanson and Neal Templeton.

The faculty included Dr. Rodney Houlihan, associate dean for curriculum and professor of physiology; Dr. William G. Robertson, professor of physiology and chairman of the medical biology division; Dr. Robert S. Conrad, assistant professor of microbiology; Dr. Kirby L. Jarolim, assistant professor of anatomy; Dr. Clyde B. Jensen, assistant professor of pharmacology and physiology; Dr. Linda K. Massey, assistant professor of biochemistry; Dr. Theodore D. McClure, professor of anatomy; Dr. Paul D. Mooney, assistant professor of biochemistry; and Dr. Robert C. Ritter, associate professor of microbiology.

In November 1974, the college passed pre-accreditation by the American Osteopathic Association. However, a permanent facility was elusive until June 1975. The Tulsa Urban Renewal Authority sold 16.1 acres between the Arkansas River and West 17th Street for $125,000. The three-building complex cost about $5.9 million. A groundbreaking ceremony was held in December 1975, and it opened in December 1977.

Leadership History at the OSU Center of Health Sciences

1973: Dr. John Barson, president
1985: Dr. Rodney Houlihan, president
1987: Dr. Clyde Jensen, president
1991: Dr. Thomas W. Allen, provost and dean
2002: Dr. Paul P. Koro, interim dean
2003: Dr. John J. Fernandes, president and dean
2009: Dr. Stanley Grogg, interim president
2010: Howard Barnett, president
2013: Dr. Kayse M. Shrum, president and dean

During construction, the state regents hired Dr. J. Scott Heatherington as the dean of the Oklahoma College of Osteopathic Medicine and Surgery. He was well-known in the osteopathic community including service as the 1969 president of the American Osteopathic Association and several years as a member of the national association's board of trustees.

Because of the underserved rural areas, the college dedicated its first community-based health clinic in Vici, Oklahoma, located in Dewey County. The second clinic was announced in March 1977 and was in Helena, Oklahoma.

The official dedication of the new permanent facility was in the fall of 1978 with the administration building named the John Barson Administration Building.

In 1988, the Oklahoma College of Osteopathic Medicine and Surgery merged with Oklahoma State University and assumed a new name – the Oklahoma State University College of Osteopathic Medicine (OSU-COM). Under the umbrella of Oklahoma State University, a comprehensive land-grant university system, OSU-COM fortified its rural mission and experienced tremendous growth both in terms of program and capital expansion.

The OSU College of Osteopathic Medicine has been consistently ranked by U.S. News & World Report as one of the best medical schools in the country and as a leader in the training of primary care physicians. In 2012, the OSU College of Osteopathic Medicine was rated The Most Popular Medical School in the nation by the publication. In 2016, it was ranked #12 in the nation for producing primary care physicians by the same publication.

FUTURE LEGACIES

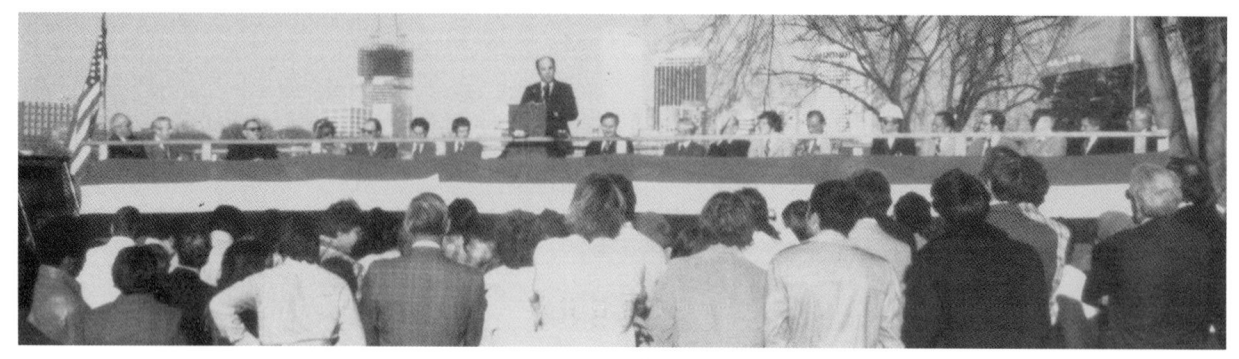

Above: President John Barson giving the keynote address during the Dec. 16, 1975, groundbreaking ceremonies for the new college.
Below: President Clyde B. Jensen wears an Oklahoma State University hat to welcome the cowboys after the college's merger with OSU.

The college has tracked the careers of its alumni and shows that more than 80 percent of its physicians continue practicing in Oklahoma. Nearly half who complete the residency program choose to work in primary-care settings, and nearly one in four moves to communities with a population of less than 10,000 people.

In 2012, OSU-COM increased enrollment to address a burgeoning physician shortage in Oklahoma. The medical school class size increased from 88 students in each class to 115 students per incoming class.

In addition to training physicians for Oklahoma, OSU Center for Health Sciences is a major provider of healthcare services in Oklahoma through its teaching hospital and network of clinics. OSU-CHS operates an extensive clinic system in Tulsa, the OSU Physicians Clinics, and partners with OSU Medical Center, its teaching hospital, to provide care for 240,000 patients annually.

The OSU Medical Center has served as the teaching hospital for OSU-COM since the college's inception. In the spring of 2006, OSU-COM signed a 50-year academic affiliation agreement with Tulsa Regional Medical Center for a permanent teaching hospital for the students. The Oklahoma Legislature appropriated $40 million in funding to improve the facility's technology and buildings. Among the renovations would be expansions to the intensive care unit and improvements to the women's health and neonatal care unit programs. On Nov. 2, 2006, the hospital was renamed the Oklahoma State University Medical Center. In 2013, the OSU Medical Center was formally transferred from the city of Tulsa to a state of Oklahoma trust, the OSU Medical Authority and Trust. In the fall of 2016, the OSU Medical Center entered into a long-term management agreement with Saint Francis Health System.

OSU-CHS has had a long and rich history of providing quality health care services to rural and underserved Oklahomans. In 1995, telemedicine was introduced by the college as a way to reach rural populations. It was created using a grant from Southwestern Bell and involves using two-way, audio-visual equipment connecting doctors and patients. In 2001, the OSU Center for Rural Health was created by the Oklahoma Legislature. The Center for Rural Health's mission is to support OSU-CHS and OSU-COM by seeking to improve healthcare in rural Oklahoma through 1) student education; 2) residency training; 3) research; 4) program applications; 5) advocacy; and 6) alliances with others who share its goals. In 2006, the Center for Rural Health championed the acquisition of a 39-foot, $450,000 bus equipped with satellite communication and other medical tools to provide specialty and general health care, screenings and procedures.

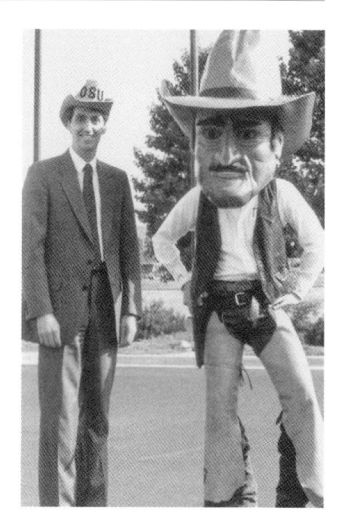

The Center for Rural Health also established the Rural Medical Track, a rural-focused medical curriculum in 2012, and played a pivotal role in the expansion of residency programs throughout rural Oklahoma. In June 2012, Gov. Mary Fallin signed the Oklahoma Hospital Residency Training Program Act, which provided $3.08 million for physician residency programs in rural and underserved areas of the state.

To recruit medical students, the OSU Center for Health Sciences started the Blue Coat to White Coat program in 2012 to encourage FFA students to consider careers in medicine. The next year, OSU-CHS established the Office for the Advancement of American Indians in Medicine and Science to

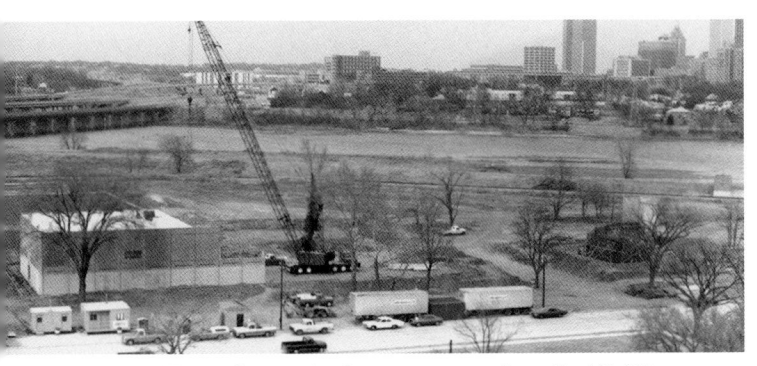

A Flintco Construction Company crane works on the 101,221-square foot Barson Building, which costs about $6.1 million and known for its energy-saving features.

encourage American Indian students to go into health care and jobs in science, technology, engineering and mathematics. Also, Operate Orange summer camps started to give rural high school students a chance to experience a day in the life of an OSU medical student.

In addition to the OSU College of Osteopathic Medicine, OSU Center for Health Sciences is also home to the School of Biomedical Sciences, School of Forensic Sciences, School of Health Care Administration and School of Allied Health. In 2001, Gov. Frank Keating signed a measure creating the OSU Center for Health Sciences in Tulsa to extend and expand OSU's reach and capabilities in the health sciences. In 2008, the college added the OSU School of Forensic Sciences after accreditation was granted. It also started offering an arson and explosives investigations option as part of the master's degree program. In 2012, the School of Health Care Administration was established to offer a Master of Science degree in health care administration. In 2015, OSU-CHS launched the OSU School of Allied Health through its Master of Athletic Training Program.

OSU Center for Health Sciences' campus has grown extensively over the years. The Center for Advanced Medical Education broke ground in 1995. It was bolstered by support from the Osteopathic Founders Foundation, the H.A. and Mary K. Chapman Charitable Trust, and the Merkel Family Foundation.

Groundbreaking on the Forensic Sciences and Biomedical Research Center occurred in 2009. When the facility opened in 2010, it housed the Tulsa Police Department Forensics Lab and Property Room. In 2014, the OSU Center for Health Sciences purchased a former Tulsa fire station near campus to create a crime scene investigations lab.

A groundbreaking in October 2015 launched a major project to build an 84,000-square-foot facility at the OSU Center for Health Sciences. The A.R. and Marylouise Tandy Foundation pledged $8 million toward construction of the $45 million four-story building. It is the largest private gift ever received by OSU Center for Health Sciences. The new facility was then named the A.R. and Marylouise Tandy Medical Academic Building in honor of the Tandy Foundation's generosity. The Tandy Medical Academic Building will include a hospital simulation training with a fully operational emergency room, operating room, intensive care unit, birthing suite and ambulance bay. Also, it will offer a clinic skills lab, osteopathic manipulative medicine lab, 18 exam rooms, lecture halls and office space to accommodate expected increased student enrollment.

The clinical skills and osteopathic manipulative medicine laboratories will be nearly double the square-footage of existing facilities on campus. The labs will include broadcast equipment enabling students to watch professors demonstrate clinical techniques.

"The Tandy Medical Academic Building will enable the College of Osteopathic Medicine to continue offering the best medical training in Tulsa. It will help us fulfill our land grant mission to train physicians to care for the citizens of Oklahoma," said OSU President Burns Hargis.

Other significant donors included the Anne and Henry Zarrow Foundation, Morningcrest Healthcare Foundation, Osteopathic Founders Foundation, U.S. District Judge Terence Kern and Jeanette Kern, Tim Headington, Blue Cross and Blue Shield of Oklahoma, Pedigo Products Inc., Dr. Gary and Jean Goodnight, Dr. Kevin and Glynda Conatser, Dr. Nabil and Penelope Srouji, the Class of 1988, and the Class of 1983. Opening of the new facility is expected in 2017. Dewberry designed the facility, and FlintoCo is the construction manager on the building.

"The OSU Center for Health Sciences and OSU College of Osteopathic Medicine have been a vital medical education training facility in Tulsa for more than 40 years. The Tandy Medical Academic Building will only further advance our outstanding reputation for training quality primary care physicians. Our students, residents and faculty physicians provide treatment for thousands of Tulsans every year through our clinic system and the OSU Medical Center. The state-of-the-art training that will be provided in the Tandy Medical Academic Building will help us utilize the best treatment and prevention options to combat the many health disparities that continue to plague our state," said OSU-CHS President Dr. Kayse Shrum. ■

FUTURE LEGACIES

Kristen R. Rice, M.D., F.A.A.D.

Kristen R. Rice, M.D., F.A.A.D. is a Board Certified Dermatologist, specializing in the treatment of diseases of the skin, hair, and nails for pediatric and adult patients. She received her bachelor's degree in Zoology – Biomedical Sciences at the University of Oklahoma, her M.D. from the University of Oklahoma College of Medicine, completed her intern year at the University of Tennessee Medical Center – Knoxville, and completed her dermatology residency at Duke University Medical Center.

Rice said her decision to select dermatology as her specialty came when she realized how life altering the treatments could be for her patients, many who suffered physically and emotionally as a result of their conditions. The outward changes her patients could experience rivaled any "extreme makeover" episode on reality television. Treatment can mark a new lease on life for many patients.

Rice, who was recently recognized by *Oklahoma Magazine* in their "40 under 40" edition, acts as a preceptor in her clinic for both medical students and residents. She is also active in the community service activities of her church, Asbury United Methodist Church in Tulsa. For Rice, the greatest compliments for her achievements come from patients who recognize her for her kindness and individual attention.

Rice serves her patients in the medical treatment of any number of cutaneous disorders, including psoriasis, eczema, acne, and skin cancer. She is trained in the surgical treatment of both benign and malignant skin lesions. Cosmetic treatments include injectables such as fillers and botulinum toxin, chemical peels, laser for hair reduction, rosacea, and dyspigmentation, and a variety of other state-of-the-art procedures.

Rice currently practices medical and surgical dermatology at Center for Dermatology, and cosmetic dermatology at Utica Square Skin Care, where she serves as Medical Director. She was born and raised in Tulsa, and feels blessed to be serving patients from the Tulsa community and the surrounding areas.

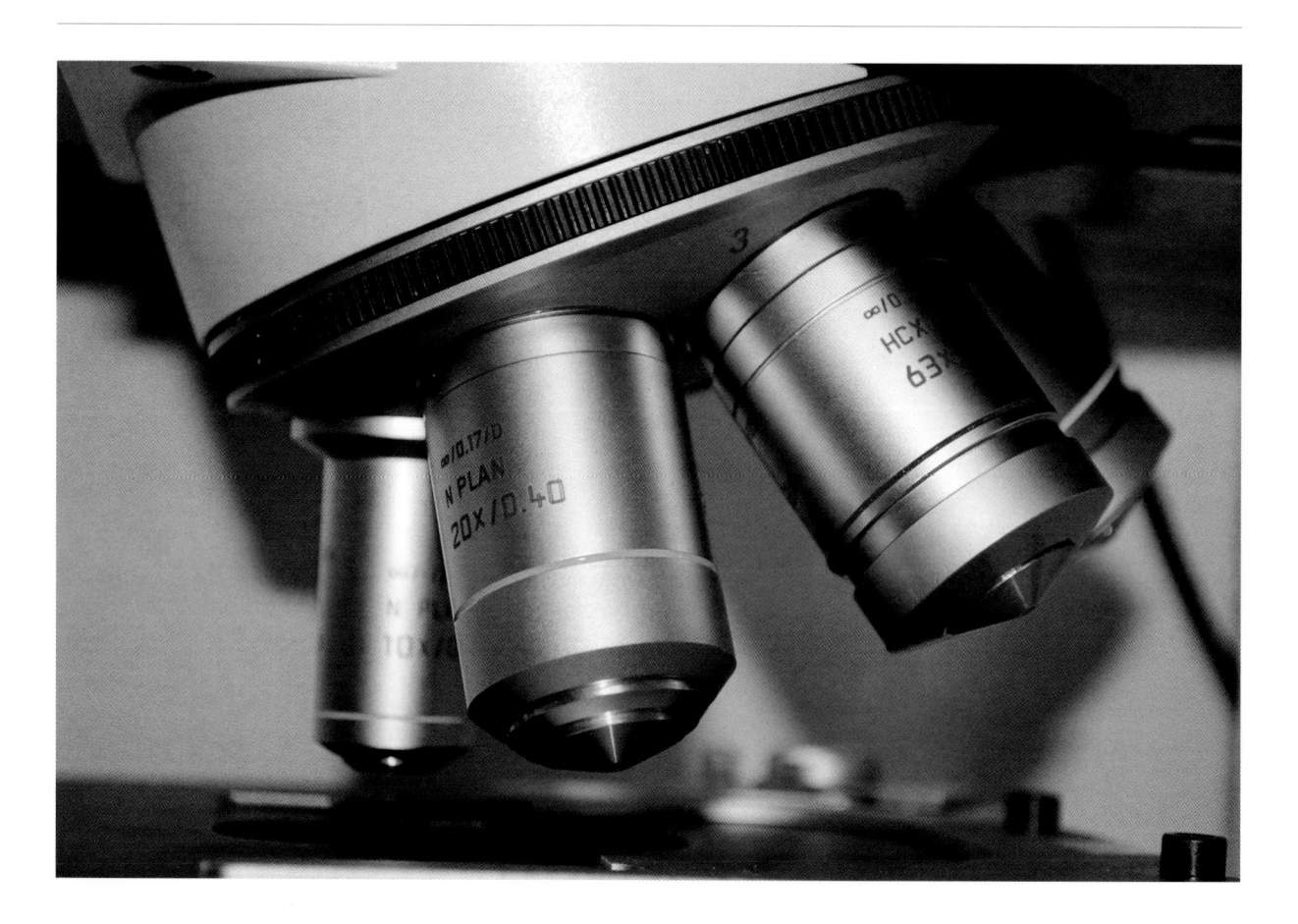

Lee Schoeffler, M.D.

Dr. Lee Schoeffler, ophthalmologist, and long time Tulsa resident, has helmed the Tulsa Eye Clinic in its more than 40-year history. Dr. Schoeffler received his medical degree from the University of Oklahoma College of Medicine and is on staff at multiple hospitals in the area, including Hillcrest Medical Center and Saint Francis Hospital.

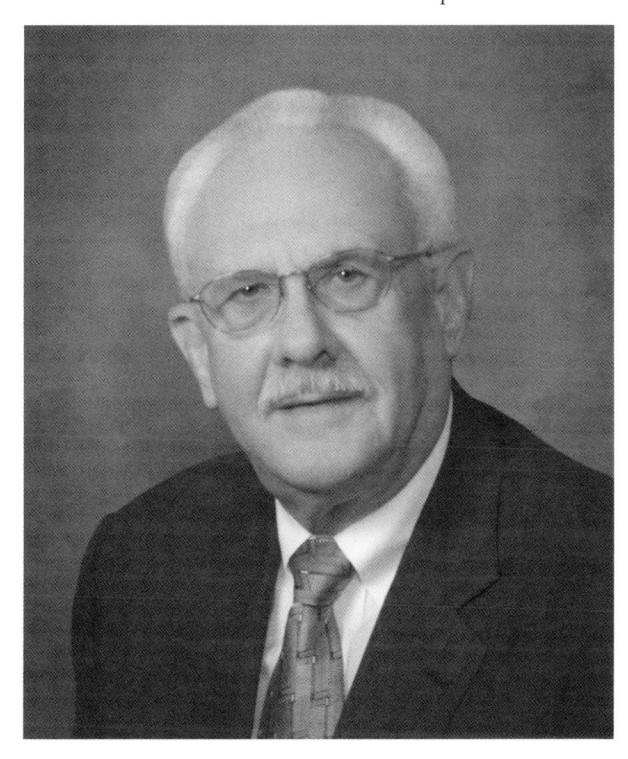

Asked why he chose the field of medicine, Dr. Scoeffler replied with one of his frequent quips, "I realized early on that I would never replace Mickey Mantle in center field for the New York Yankees."

In actuality, he knew becoming a doctor was his career choice from an early age. Prior to beginning his medical training, Dr. Schoeffler worked as a research chemist for an oil company but medicine has always been his first love. That love for medicine runs in the family as his son is a cardiologist in Oklahoma City and his brother is a dentist in Tulsa.

"I am in awe of how far ophthalmology has come since the early days of my career," says Schoeffler. "Success rates for complex ophthalmological procedures have skyrocketed since I graduated. The techniques that were used in ophthalmology in the 1970s were crude. They have been refined over the years to the point that every procedure is done with the utmost level of technical skill."

When not working in his medical career, he pursues his second passion: classical cars. At present, he is the proud owner of a 1964 356 Cabriolet Porsche and a 1970 914-6 Porsche. When discussing classic cars, it becomes very evident that his knowledge of automobiles is extensive.

"I recently acquired a 1937 Cord, a rare car that required me to jump through a number of hoops to obtain," he says.

Another side of Dr. Schoeffler is his active participation in the Oklahoma State Medical Society and his work with Physicians Liability Insurance Company. Interaction with those organizations has made him well-versed in medical laws and insurance legislation. Working with Physicians Liability and their board of directors, the company was able to recover from $142 million in the red to $64 million in the black within 11 years. According to Dr. Schoeffler, the company was recently sold to Warren Buffet for $83 million.

As someone who prefers to remain modest of his accomplishments and achievements, Dr. Schoeffler's accomplishments are numerous. Never one to promote himself, he sees those accomplishments as something he did of responsibility and dedication to his job as a doctor.

While pleased with his medical accomplishments, Dr. Schoeffler stated how the trust and confidence shown to him by his patients is a matter of pride.

He says, "To have patients place their health, sight, and life in your hands is the greatest honor that can be bestowed upon you."

Dr. Schoeffler's other passion is collecting classic cars including this rare 1937 Cord.

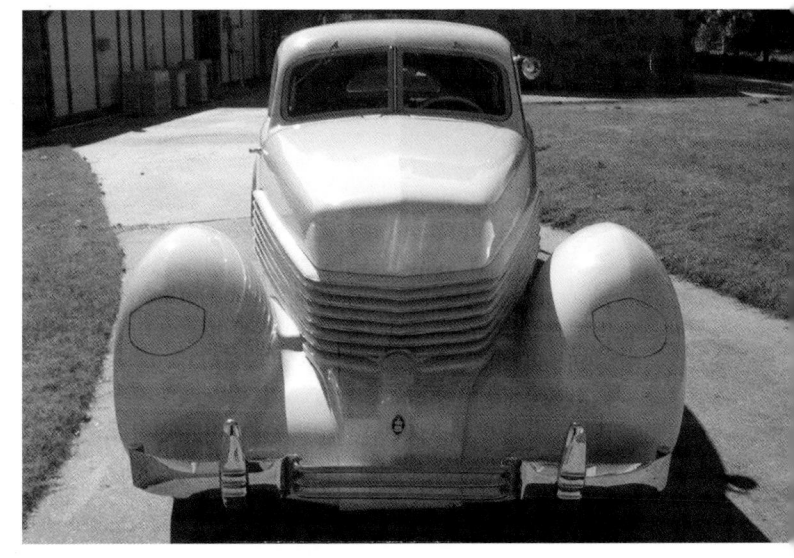

FUTURE LEGACIES

Charles William Simcoe, M.D.

Charles William (Bill) Simcoe was born in Stillwater, Oklahoma where he later attended college. When the Korean War broke out, he felt so strongly about serving his country that he enlisted in the United States Marine Corps for three years even though he had an academic deferment from the draft. He was deployed in front line combat for a year before being sent to Hawaii for the remainder of his enlistment. His time in the Marines, especially during combat for a year,

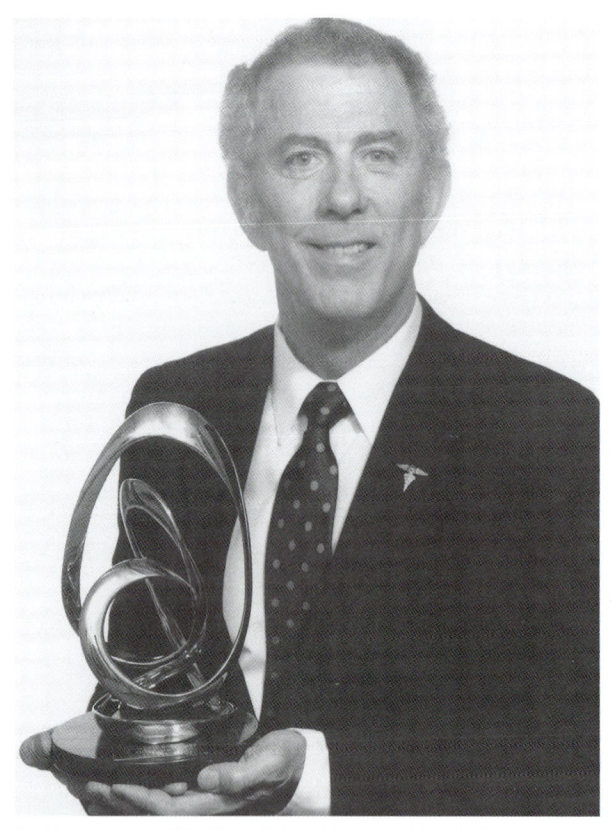

Dr. Simcoe received the Bennett Award in recognition of his contributions and innovative ideas.

shaped his desire to become a doctor-instead of taking lives, he wanted to give others a better life. When his enlistment ended, he returned to Oklahoma and attended the University of Oklahoma College of Medicine in Oklahoma City. After medical school, he interned at Gorgas Hospital in the Panama Canal Zone and did a three-year Ophthamology residency at the Hospital of the University of Pennsylvania (now the Scheie Eye Institute), before moving to Tulsa.

In the mid-1970s, California was taking steps to stop the manufacture and the use of intraocular lens because of problems that arose with the IOL touching the cornea. Dr. Simcoe developed a means of preventing intraocular lens-cornea touch during intraocular lens manipulation, penetrating keratoplasty, and following filtration surgery. Dr. Simcoe's innovations safely and effectively ensured corneal well-being following increasingly complex modern filtration and shunt procedures. His use of double armed 9-0 nylon suture or anterior chamber-bridging straight needles simplified safe placement of the intraocular lens.

One of his greatest accomplishments that made a significant impact on evolving modern cataract surgery and one that impacts most every person having cataract surgery today, was the introduction of a new, better, safer intraocular lens (IOL) design. Until the introduction of his "Simcoe open C loop," there were difficulties and hazards with the implantation and the contraption of the IOL — today's industry standard now known as the open C loop. Released in 1974, this compressible, ultra lightweight, open-loop posterior IOL design remains among the most widely used design concepts in cataract surgery worldwide. Each year there are over three million individuals in the U.S. alone that benefit from an IOL using the Simcoe open C loop design.

Another major accomplishment was the invention of a handheld surgical instrument, the Simcoe Canula which offered a distinct advantage in cataract surgery. It was a major improvement over other foot-powered instruments used to remove cataracts, with a design that enabled much greater efficiency and superior safety. The use of this instrument greatly reduced surgical complications and helped open up eye surgery in third-world countries. Its price tag was less that $20 and replaced machines that cost tens of thousands of dollars. With this instrument, Dr. Simcoe traveled

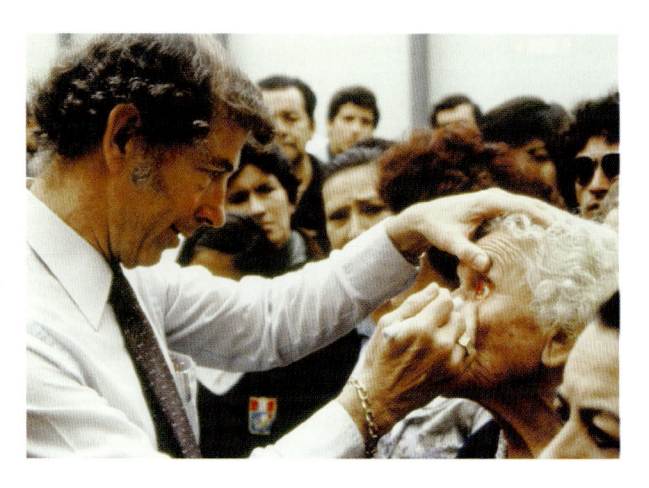

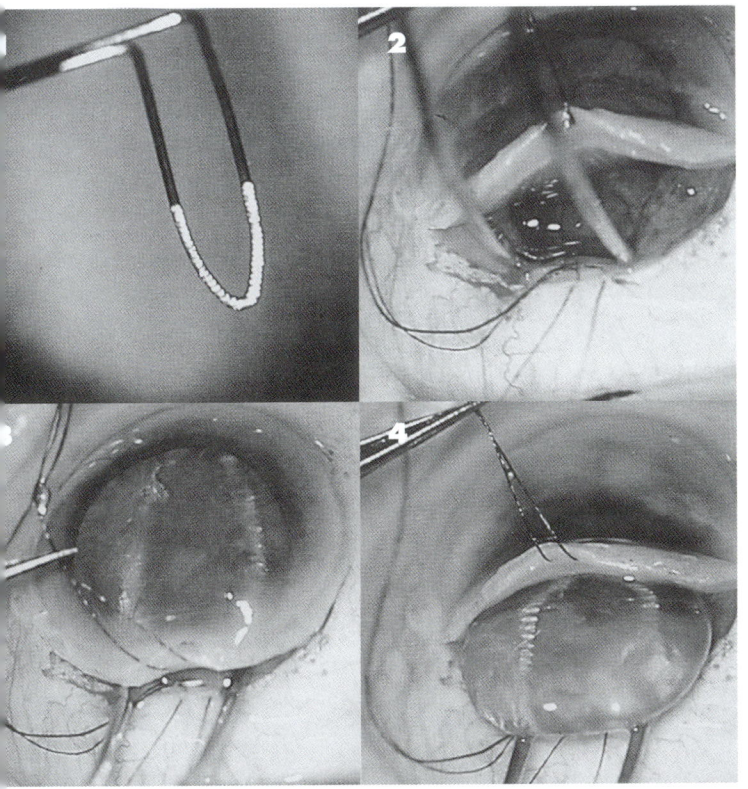

Removal of Nucleus using Simcoe Right-angled Nucleus Loop
Besides expression, vectis or an alternative instrument such as the Simcoe right-angled nucleus loop can be used to remove nucleus. They are useful in a soft eye where expression can be difficult.

around the world in a specially equipped plane, called "Project Orbis", teaching ophthalmologists how to do the safest and most cost effective cataract surgery possible.

Dr. Simcoe was on the board of directors for Project Orbis, the world's only flying eye hospital which was dedicated to saving sight worldwide. Inside, Orbis was a functional operating room where doctors from visiting countries could observe the surgeries in order to learn techniques. Dr. Simcoe went on teaching trips to many of the 92 countries that Project Orbis visited and performed many sight saving surgeries while on board. Notably, he was invited by Orbis International to the People's Republic of China for a three-week teaching tour. More than 250 Chinese surgeons watched video of the operations. During this time, the pro-democracy student uprising in Tiananmen Square took place. Dr. Simcoe has performed surgery in most American states and over 50 countries. His live surgery satellite telecasts have been seen all around the world.

While in private practice in Tulsa, Oklahoma, Dr. Simcoe was Chairman of the Ophthalmology Departments at St. John Hospital and Hillcrest Medical Center. Dr. Simcoe's techniques were in such wide demand that many doctors would come observe him during surgery which used only a few instruments, many of which he designed. When the operating room became too crowded, the hospital installed a camera on a microscope so that doctors could watch the procedure from an adjacent waiting room.

Dr. Simcoe has received numerous awards including a first prize medal for contributions to cataract surgery by the International Cataract Congress in Cannes, France in 1979. He was also honored on the 40th anniversary of Sir Harold Ridley's invention of the IOL with the American Society of Cataract and Refractive Surgery's Innovator Award in 1989 and the bronze Bennett sculpture entitled "Inspiration" in recognition of his contributions to the development of new and innovative ideas in the field of Ophthalmology. In 2010 Dr. Simcoe traveled to Hawaii where he received the Philip M. Corboy, M.D. Memorial Award for Distinguished Service to Ophthalmology.

During his career, he had the opportunity to meet many famous people including soccer great Pele and boxing legend Muhammad Ali. Ali told Simcoe, "Service to others is the rent you pay for your room here on Earth". This quote sums up the way Dr. Simcoe lives his life.

Removal of Cortex, Simcoe's Method
Simcoe uses a slightly different system. Aspiration is done with a large 20mm syringe in left hand and infused with a bulb held in right hand. The principle remains the same.

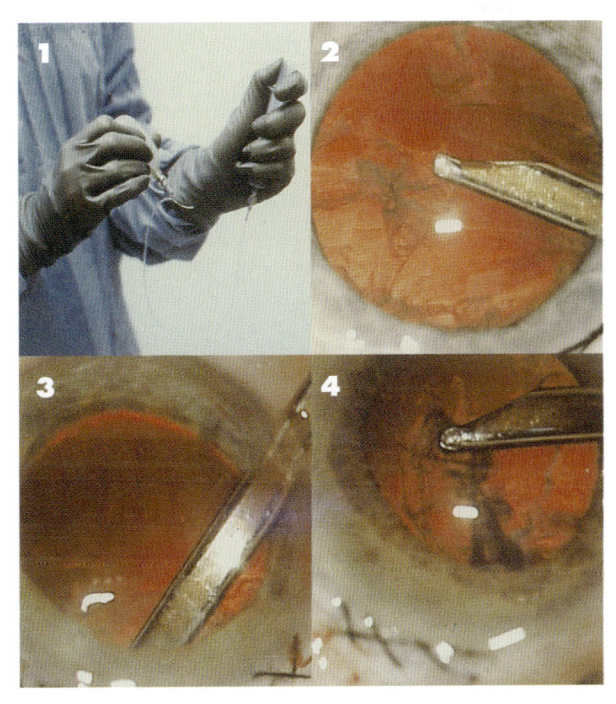

FUTURE LEGACIES

Saint Francis Health System

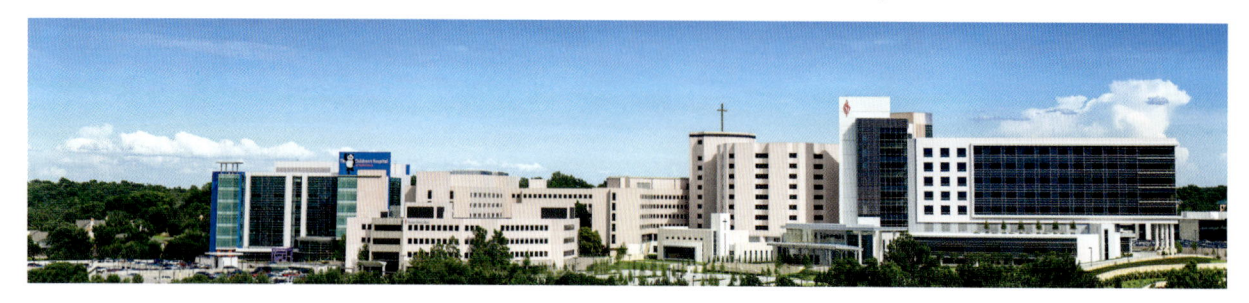

From the Beginning: Saint Francis Hospital

Created in 1945 by Natalie O. and William K. Warren, Sr., as a way to give back to the community that they called home, The William K. Warren Foundation set forth a goal of providing the finest possible medical care available in the Tulsa area. As a result, the Foundation planned and opened Saint Francis Hospital in 1960 and thus began the tradition of excellence that is now Saint Francis Health System.

In 1967, W.K. Warren, Sr. brought his son, W.K. Warren, Jr., into The William K. Warren Foundation as president. The Foundation expanded its mission of community service, and in 1994 the next generation joined the family legacy when W.K. Warren, Jr.'s son, John-Kelly, was recruited away from a financial career in Houston to head The William K. Warren Foundation. Today, W.K. Warren, Jr., serves as Chairman Emeritus, while John-Kelly Warren serves as Chief Executive Officer.

Throughout its existence, The William K. Warren Foundation has been guided by the belief that health education, medical research and quality healthcare services are essential components of a thriving community. This belief has led to many medical and scientific achievements in Tulsa that would not have been possible without the Foundation's support.

"During our lifetime and throughout eternity, if God ordains, our continuing interest shall remain in our prayers that life may be made more comfortable for all those people chosen by God who seek admittance here."
- Natalie O. and William K. Warren, Sr.

Today, Saint Francis Health System and medical research endeavors remain the primary recipients of the Foundation's grants. As a result of the generosity and vision cast by Mr. and Mrs. W.K. Warren, Sr., the Foundation remains focused on improving quality of life in the community by providing financial assistance to many non-profit organizations in support of worthy charitable, scientific, Catholic and health programs. In support of their charitable mission, the Foundation also established two research-based entities, The William K. Warren Medical Research Center in 1973 and in 2009, the Laureate Institute for Brain Research (LIBR) — the area's premier psychiatric and brain research center.

William Kelly Warren, Sr. made his name in petroleum, but his legacy is firmly rooted in a tradition of healthcare excellence and benevolence that was indivisible from his religious beliefs. Even the name of the hospital he founded, Saint Francis Hospital, was influenced by his Catholic spirituality. Warren was born on December 3 — the feast day of St. Francis Xavier. Throughout his life Warren had a special devotion to this saint and it was no surprise when he chose this saint as his hospital's namesake. The missionary spirit of St. Francis Xavier and the devout faith of W.K. Warren, Sr. are both integral to the present-day missions of The William K. Warren Foundation and Saint Francis Health System — Warren's most far-reaching act of charity.

William K. Warren, Sr. and Natalie O. Warren at the Saint Francis Hospital groundbreaking in 1958.

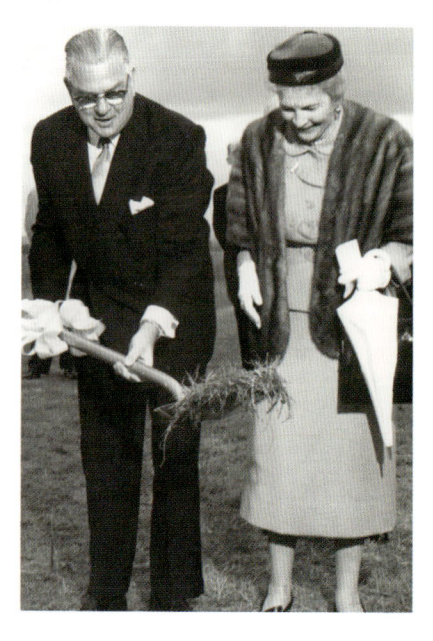

PIONEERS IN MEDICINE

As the summer of 1960 approached, construction on the hospital was nearing completion. With the state-of-the-art hospital finally a reality, active recruiting for a staff of physicians began.

By opening day on October 1, an accomplished staff of physicians was assembled and in place. After five years of planning and construction, the new hospital — Saint Francis — opened its doors with 275 beds.

The 260-acre site at 61st Street and Yale Avenue, was far from what was considered to be the city's center at the time. In fact, many Tulsans predicted the hospital's location would be its downfall. Yet, the pink hospital on the hill soon became a major health system, strategically anchored in the heart of Tulsa.

When Saint Francis Hospital first opened its doors, W.K. Warren, Sr. and his wife, Natalie, saw their dream to give back to the community come to life.

Saint Francis Hospital changed the face of medicine in eastern Oklahoma. Many practitioners — nearly all surgeons — were dedicated to making Saint Francis Hospital the hospital of the future. They began to form groups of specialists who wanted to commit to an institution — in the end, not only did this group of physicians devote their careers to the advancement of Saint Francis — the hospital leadership was devoted to the success and advancement of the physicians as well.

As the years passed and word of Saint Francis' excellence spread, its facilities continued to attract a number of highly qualified young physicians. As Tulsa expanded to the southeast, Saint Francis Hospital followed suit. By 1971, it was apparent Saint Francis was fulfilling the role of a regional medical center — soon to be health system.

CATHOLIC HERITAGE

From the very beginning, Saint Francis' Catholic roots have been core to the organization — visible within every entity, service line and program. The cross atop the hospital, crucifixes in each meeting room, patient care space and waiting area are a constant reminder of the hope intrinsic to Christianity.

The Prayer of Saint Francis Health System — prayed daily throughout the health system — points to the clear and uncompromising principles which guide and characterize the organization. For over 55 years, the mission of Catholic healthcare has provided the blueprint for the health system's patient-centered and service-oriented excellence in care.

WARREN CLINIC

With the goal of expanding the base of available primary care physicians in northeastern Oklahoma, The William K. Warren Foundation established the first Warren Clinic in Stillwater, Oklahoma, in January 1987.

Since then, Warren Clinic has expanded to over 80 practice locations with over 350 physicians and mid-level providers. As the clinic grew, so did the spectrum of services and specialties offered. What started as a small primary care office, now consists

Continued on following page.

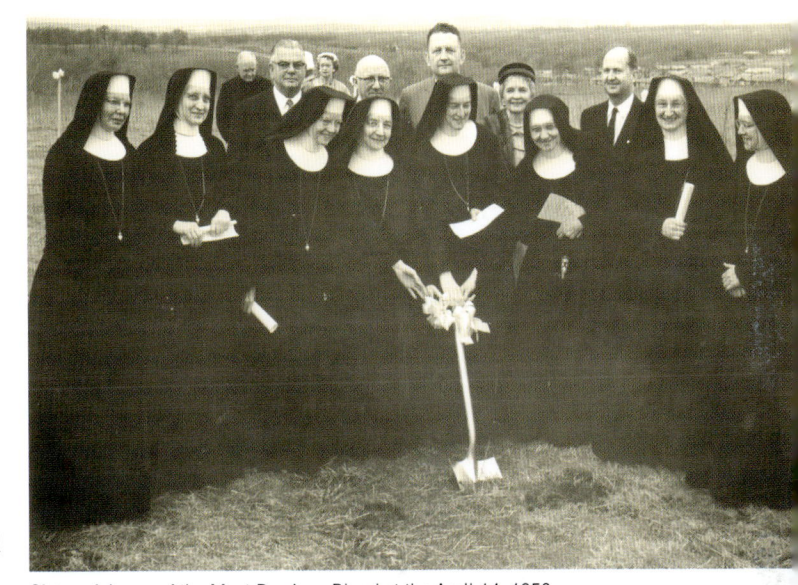

Sisters Adorers of the Most Precious Blood at the April 14, 1958 groundbreaking for Saint Francis Hospital.

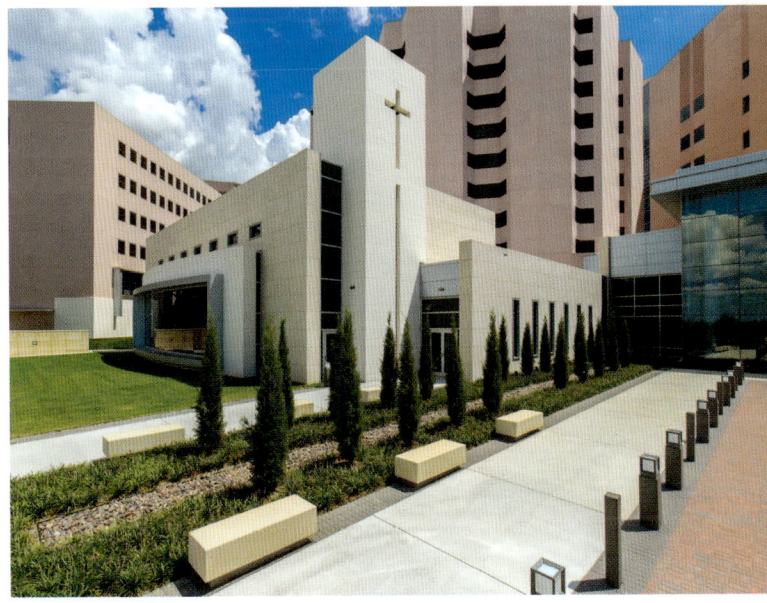

Saint Francis Hospital chapel, part of the 2014 Trauma Emergency Center renovation and expansion.

289

of 65 percent primary care physicians and 35 percent specialists and subspecialists. While the majority of Warren Clinic's office locations are found in Tulsa near the campuses of Saint Francis Hospital and Saint Francis Hospital South, other physician office locations can be found in communities that include Broken Arrow, Coweta, Ft. Gibson, Jenks, McAlester, Muskogee, Owasso, Pryor, Sand Springs, Tahlequah and Vinita.

Warren Clinic physicians offer a wide spectrum of primary care medical services from disease prevention to the management of patients with chronic medical conditions. A hallmark of Warren Clinic is professional excellence, combined with compassion and caring. For many patients and families, Warren Clinic doctors are their lifetime partners for health.

Warren Clinic South Memorial

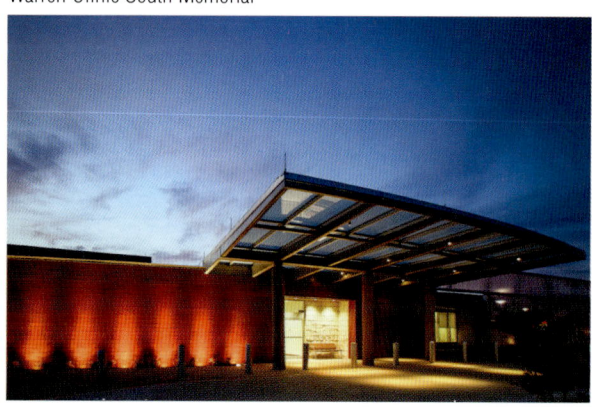

Laureate Psychiatric Clinic and Hospital

For some time, William K. Warren, Jr. had envisioned a place where those suffering from mental illness would be treated the same as patients having any other illness. That vision eventually became Laureate Psychiatric Clinic and Hospital which opened in 1989.

Designed as a residential setting, Laureate specializes in general psychiatry in the treatment of dementia, early onset Alzheimer's disease, stress, anger management, depression and grief. In addition to programs for children, adolescents and adults, Laureate also offers successful specialty programs for patients with chemical dependency and mood disorders. Laureate's Eating Disorders Program is nationally recognized for its outstanding treatment of anorexia, bulimia and compulsive overeating and patients travel from across the country to seek eating disorder treatment at Laureate.

From its earliest days, Laureate has been committed to research projects aimed at finding the most effective treatments for patients with mental illnesses. Particular emphasis has focused on three areas: schizophrenia — Laureate was the recipient of a World Health Organization sponsorship for the study of this disease — depression and eating disorders.

Laureate Institute for Brain Research

The Laureate Institute for Brain Research (LIBR) has only been in existence since 2009, yet the strides it has taken are impressive — and the impact it is making on public health far-reaching.

Despite the fact that LIBR is relatively new, the research it has been conducting is highly relevant to this community, as well as to mental healthcare as a whole. LIBR's collective efforts focus on various neuroscience approaches that hope to aid in early detection, better diagnoses and treatment for patients with mental illness.

Heart Hospital at Saint Francis

In an effort to address the urgent need for quality heart services in the area, Saint Francis Health System and area cardiologists partnered to open the Heart Hospital at Saint Francis in 2004.

Diagnostic heart disease capabilities offered at the Heart Hospital include electrocardiography, nuclear cardiology, echocardiography, cardiac computed tomography (CT) and magnetic resonance

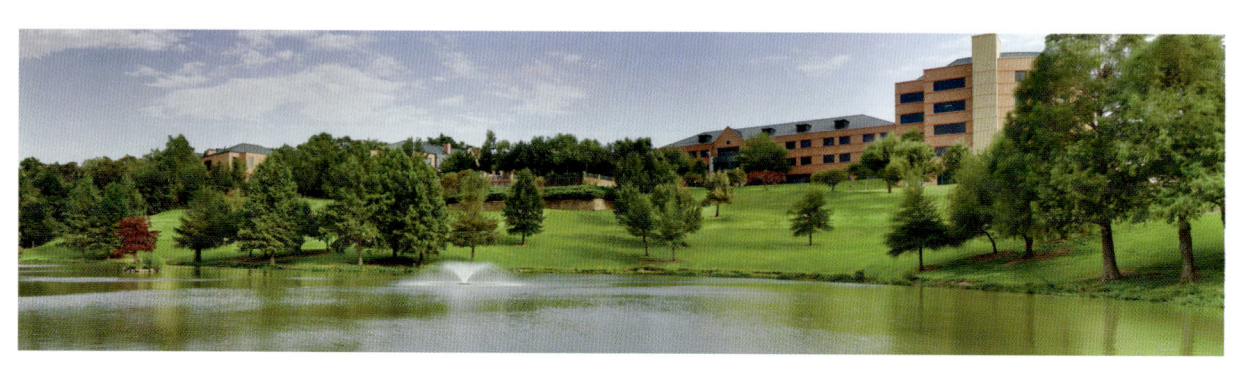

Laureate Psychiatric Clinic and Hospital

FUTURE LEGACIES

Saint Francis Hospital South

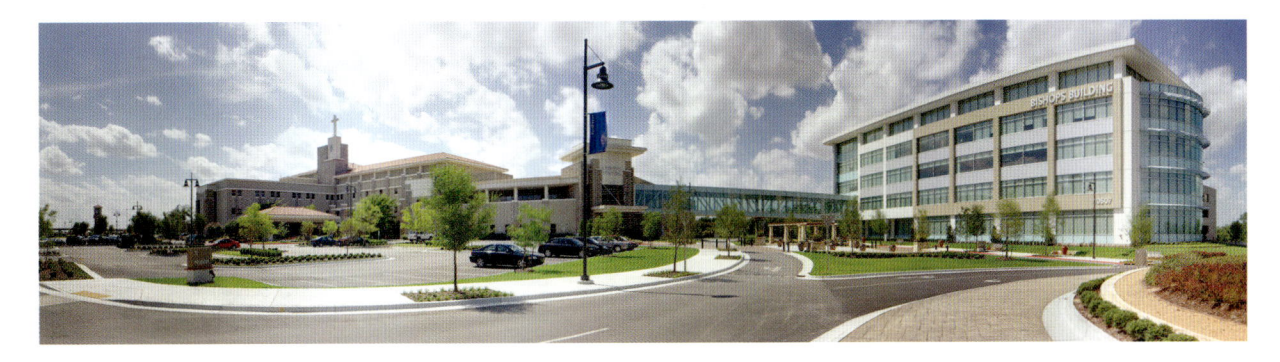

imaging (MRI). Cardiology specialists at the Heart Hospital at Saint Francis provide a broad spectrum of cardiovascular treatments, including angioplasty and stenting, catheter ablations and implanting pacemakers and defibrillators as well as the latest in cardiac care technology to help to reduce the risk for heart attack and stroke.

SAINT FRANCIS HOSPITAL SOUTH

First opening its doors in 2007, Saint Francis Hospital South is a 96-bed, not-for-profit community hospital that caters to the needs of residents in south Tulsa, Broken Arrow, Bixby and other neighboring communities. Saint Francis Hospital South offers general medical services, as well as many subspecialties generally reserved for larger city hospitals including a Level II Neonatal Intensive Care Unit (NICU), labor and delivery, orthopedics, pulmonology, expanded imaging services, cardiac catheterization lab, emergency services, urology and 24-hour, on-site anesthesia.

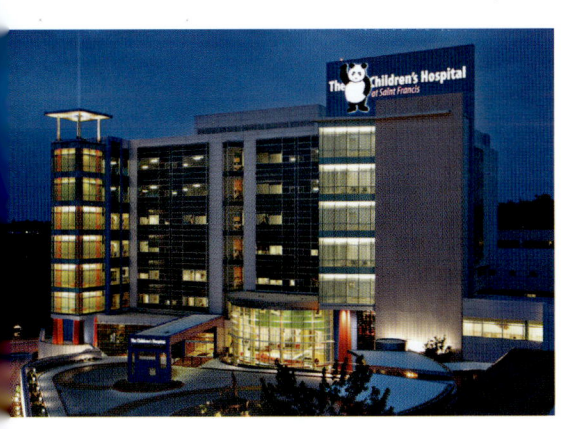

The Children's Hospital at Saint Francis.

THE CHILDREN'S HOSPITAL AT SAINT FRANCIS

Originally established as a special unit within Saint Francis Hospital in the mid-1990's, The Children's Hospital at Saint Francis opened as a new, 104-bed facility in 2008 and serves as the area's only hospital solely dedicated to pediatric healthcare. The Children's Hospital at Saint Francis' services includes general pediatrics, critical care medicine, pediatric surgery as well as numerous pediatric subspecialties such as neurology and neurosurgery, cardiology and cardiothoracic surgery, pulmonology, orthopedic surgery and much more within the Henry Zarrow Neonatal Intensive Care Unit — the area's only Level IV NICU — offering the most advanced care possible to premature babies or critically ill newborns in the region.

The hospital is also home of The St. Jude Affiliate Clinic at The Children's Hospital at Saint Francis. Opened in July 2016, it is the eighth such affiliate clinic in the United States and the only one in the state of Oklahoma. This affiliation allows the pediatric hematologists and oncologists at The Children's Hospital at Saint Francis access to St. Jude's treatment protocols and clinical research trials, all to provide the best available pediatric cancer care close to home.

To further support the children's hospital, The Children's Hospital Foundation at Saint Francis was established in 2005 to foster charitable giving. Since that time, the Foundation has continued to raise funds in support of the children's hospital, primarily through its flagship event, The Painted Pony Ball, and the hospital's affiliation with Children's Miracle Network Hospitals.

TRAUMA EMERGENCY CENTER AND PATIENT TOWER

When the new Trauma Emergency Center (TEC) and Patient Tower's services opened in September 2014, it was a signal of a new era in Saint Francis Health System's history. The eight-story, 500,000-square-foot patient tower and TEC is not only the newest facility, but also the largest expansion in Saint Francis Health System's history.

Features of the state-of-the-art facility include:
• expanded acute and critical care capacity;
• the ability to expand the emergency center to 114 clinical stations during mass casualty events;
• the ability to accommodate more than 120,000 emergency room patient visits each year;

Continued on following page.

- a new cardiac catheterization lab located within the TEC;
- 150 new acuity-adaptable private rooms (designed to be easily upgraded to an intensive care level); and
- two computed tomography (CT) suites within the TEC.

Giving Back to the Community

Since its beginning, the women and men of Saint Francis Health System have been influenced by two distinct, yet complementary, aspirations: to care for others as Christ would were He at the bedside and to carry forward the legacy of charity upon which Saint Francis Health System was founded. To this end, Saint Francis Health System has a long heritage of providing benefit to the community it serves. The women and men of Saint Francis have been skillfully and compassionately caring for others since Saint Francis opened its doors in 1960. They have nursed the sick back to health, helped bring babies into this world and provided comfort to those whose time on earth has come to an end.

As the region's largest private employer and leading provider of healthcare, Saint Francis is committed to ongoing charitable endeavors such as providing care to the uninsured and through supporting partnerships with community and faith-based organizations to foster education and collaborative initiatives that promote health and wellness. In Saint Francis' 2016 fiscal year over $50 million was provided in charity care and $19 million was provided in uncompensated care related to the treatment of Medicaid patients. Additionally, almost $5 million was donated to local nonprofits whose values are aligned with Saint Francis Health System; this number also includes payments made to organizations that provide assistance to persons seeking access to or enrollment

Saint Francis Health System Timeline

1954: Plans for Saint Francis Hospital announced publicly on December 3, the Feast Day of St. Francis Xavier

1958: Groundbreaking on the southeast corner of 61st Street and Yale Avenue

1960:
- September 24: Open house attended by 20,000 — Tulsa population at the time, 261,685
- First auxiliary planning committee attended by 22 prospective volunteers
- October 1: Saint Francis opens with 275-bed capacity

1962: Saint Francis opens city's first intensive care unit

1963: Medicall, the doctor paging system, installed

1964:
- First full capacity — 275 beds, 40 bassinets, 87% average occupancy
- Second wing announced in July — 350-bed total Saint Francis capacity

1966: Seven-story services wing planned as well as power plant

1967: Warren Professional Building opens — 10 stories, 70 suites, 120 doctors, 600 parking spaces

1969:
- Saint Francis Hospital expanded to 735 adult and pediatric beds and bassinets — expansion included a new "Y" section to match original structure and a seven-story specialty wing
- Tulsa's first dialysis machine installed

1970: Cardiac catheterization lab built

1975:
- Natalie Warren Bryant Cancer Center dedicated — one of the first centers where radiation therapy, chemotherapy services, laboratory and support services were grouped in a single location for the patient's convenience
- Kelly Building completed — 12 stories, 168,000 square feet, 100 offices

1977: West wing dedicated

1979:
- Tulsa Life Flight launched — the first helicopter service of its kind in the city
- Skilled nursing facility and a fetal maternal medicine unit added to services

1981: Oklahoma's first angioplasty performed at Saint Francis Hospital

1985: MRI (magnetic resonance imaging) scanner installed

1987:
- First bone marrow transplant performed
- The first Warren Clinic opens in Stillwater, Oklahoma

1989: Laureate Psychiatric Clinic and Hospital opens

1993: First heart transplant performed

2001: Xavier Medical Clinic opens

2005: The Children's Hospital Foundation at Saint Francis established

2008:
- Saint Francis Hospital South opens with 96 beds
- Relocation of the Heart Hospital at Saint Francis to the Yale campus
- Opening of The Children's Hospital at Saint Francis

2011: Newly remodeled Health Zone at Saint Francis opens

2014: Opening of new Trauma Emergency Center and Patient Tower

2016:
- The children's hospital oncology clinic becomes the nation's eighth St. Jude Affiliate Clinic
- Saint Francis acquires Craig General Hospital in Vinita, Oklahoma — now Saint Francis Hospital Vinita

2017: Saint Francis acquires EASTAR Hospital and clinics in Muskogee, Oklahoma, and Ft. Gibson, Oklahoma — now Saint Francis Hospital of Muskogee and Warren Clinic Muskogee

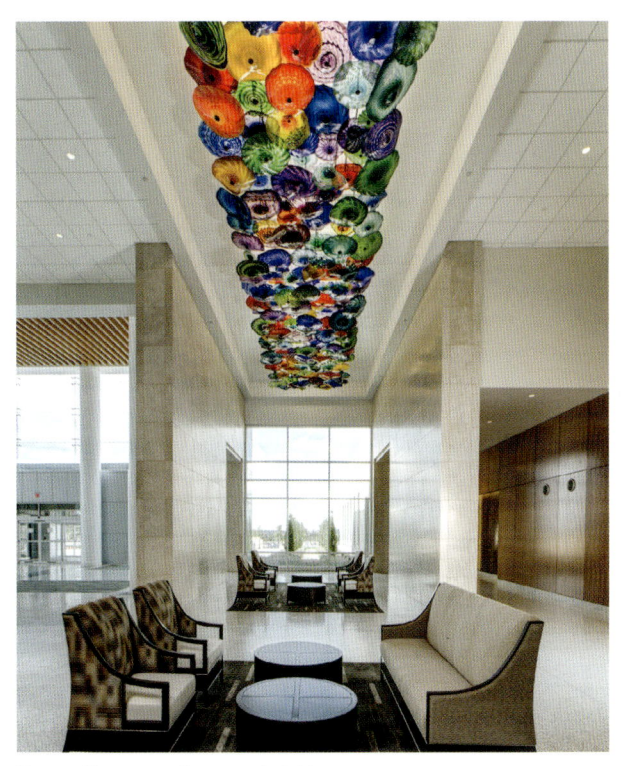

Trauma Emergency Center main lobby.

for healthcare benefits. Lastly, another $7 million was allocated to provide emergency services to the region — including the Saint Francis Trauma Institute — Tulsa's only trauma service that offers in-house, round the-clock coverage by surgical intensivists to meet the needs of the community.

Xavier Medical Clinic

Established by Saint Francis Health System in 2001, Xavier Medical Clinic has been serving the needs of those in the community, who are uninsured or do not have access to adequate healthcare. The free clinic offers the services of volunteer physicians, nurses and other health professionals. Xavier Medical Clinic provides limited outpatient primary healthcare services, facilitates referrals to specialists, teaches good health practices and increases access to traditional healthcare. Designed to reach women, children and men who are uninsured or underserved, Xavier Clinic exists to meet the needs of these vulnerable populations. Through its dedicated staff and volunteers, Xavier Clinic is able to reach a group that might otherwise avoid or have difficulties accessing basic healthcare services.

Medical Education

Saint Francis Health System is committed to building Tulsa's healthcare workforce. The future of care delivery in the region depends on a continued supply of well-educated and aptly prepared physicians, nurses, allied health professionals and researchers. Saint Francis Health System has been a long supporter and donor to local medical schools, nursing schools and allied health training providers.

To help assure the future of well-trained healthcare providers in the region, Saint Francis also works with local educational institutions to provide supervised clinical rotations for students in nursing, pharmacy, surgical and radiology technology and various allied health disciplines. Saint Francis' investment in medical education will have a positive impact on the region's economy, creating thousands of new jobs and providing greater access to care in the region.

An Enduring Legacy of Excellence

The twists and turns the healthcare industry has undergone over the past five decades may have changed the way Saint Francis operates from a logistical and pragmatic point of view, but they have not touched what the health system is at its core. Saint Francis Health System is — and always has been — a locally owned, locally operated, Catholic healthcare provider committed to serving the medical, psychological and spiritual needs of the Tulsa region.

As medical technology has continued to evolve, the dedication of the health system's physicians and staff members to the health and well-being of the people they serve has remained steady and consistent. Since its inception, Saint Francis' presence in the community has been of significant meaning and worth. With corporate acquisitions of other hospitals in Tulsa, Saint Francis Health System stands as Tulsa's only locally owned and operated health system.

"Being locally owned and operated adds a deep level of commitment as it relates to quality for our organization. Our vision drives us to be the leading integrated Catholic healthcare system providing high quality, comprehensive and innovative care across our regional continuum of services. This is our vision for healthcare; this is our commitment to Oklahoma."
- Jake Henry Jr., president and chief executive officer of Saint Francis Health System

For the last half-century, eastern Oklahomans have looked to Saint Francis in their time of need. They have come seeking medical care and spiritual support during some of the most intimate times in their lives. It is Saint Francis' privilege to serve the community in this way and it is a responsibility that the women and men of Saint Francis take seriously.

St. John Health System

Shortly before noon on February 11, 1920, Gen. John J. Pershing, leader of American forces during World War I, took a short-handled spade and broke ground for St. John's Hospital at the northeast corner of 21st Street and Utica Avenue in Tulsa, Oklahoma.

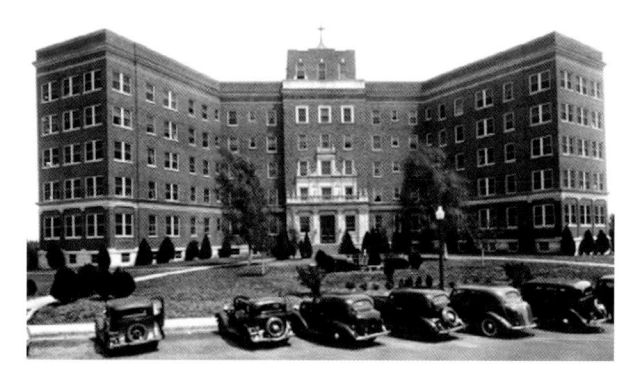

St. John Hospital as it appeared in 1929.

With that, St. John Health System began its journey to becoming one of northeast Oklahoma's most important medical service providers.

Three years before groundbreaking, the Sisters of the Sorrowful Mother, who had previously developed medical missions in Kansas, Wisconsin, and New Jersey, purchased 8 acres of farmland for $16,000 to build a freestanding hospital on what was then the outskirts of Tulsa. By 1920, the project was already in trouble. A fundraising campaign produced many pledges but little money. The hospital's original plans for 220 beds was reduced to an initial 50. By 1922, cash on hand was less than $6,000. Work stopped, and the partially constructed building stood vacant for nearly three years.

The sale of land owned by the Sisters in New Jersey and a much more successful fund drive allowed for renewed construction at St. John's throughout 1925. The hospital finally saw its official opening on February 22, 1926, with 20 patients admitted that day. To fulfill the city's need, St. John's had actually taken in a handful of patients days before, and saw Tulsa's newest citizen, a baby girl, born on Valentine's Day, eight days before the official opening.

Construction continued at St. John's through 1928 with the completion of the fifth floor as the new home for surgery, X-ray and the lab. To ensure quality patient care, the St. John's Hospital School of Nursing opened in the summer of 1926. By the time it closed 50 years later, it had graduated more than 1,400 nurses.

Once firmly established, St. John's began to expand its medical capabilities. By 1929, the hospital had its own electrocardiogram unit. In the mid-1930s, a $100,000 donation from oilman Waite Phillips, in memory of his late brother, Wiate, led to the construction of the Phillips Memorial Building, which housed a new 400-kilovolt deep therapy unit for cancer treatment.

After continued expansion, but with only 265 beds at its disposal, St. John's was overburdened by the mid-1940s. A six-story t-shaped extension was built on the south side of the hospital. Completed in 1948, it offered 125 new patient beds and a new home for surgery, radiology and pediatrics.

In 1953, St. John's admitted 21,807 patients. The hospital was out of space, again. Private patient rooms were converted to semi-private, waiting rooms — and at least one physician's lounge — were also converted to accommodate patients. In 1957, a $3.5-million addition to the hospital, this time on the west side, added more than 200 beds and became home to the emergency center, operating and delivery rooms, a psychiatric ward and a 25-bed unit for premature babies.

By then, St. John's was known as a regional leader in cardiovascular surgery. Tulsa's first pericardiotomy was performed there in 1953, and two years later the first valvulotomy, performed on a 4-year-old girl. Other firsts followed: the city's first successful installation of a pacemaker (1963), first coronary artery bypass (1969), the first replacement of a mitral valve with the heart valve of a pig (1976) and Oklahoma's first angioplasty (1979).

St. John's also led in other ways. In 1970, it became the first Tulsa hospital to operate a remote heart monitor network, linking the hospital with cardiac patients in nearby Claremore and Sapulpa. The state's first linear accelerator to treat cancer appeared the following year, as did the city's first neonatal intensive care unit.

By 1976, the hospital was completing its biggest renovation project to date. Gone to the wrecking ball were the original hospital building, the south wing and a chapel and convent, built for the Sisters in the 1930s. In their stead stood the $40 million, 14-story North Tower (now the J.A. Chapman Tower), the new home to nursing units, radiology and behavioral health. The hospital also saw the end of its old name and the adoption of a new one — St. John Medical Center.

FUTURE LEGACIES

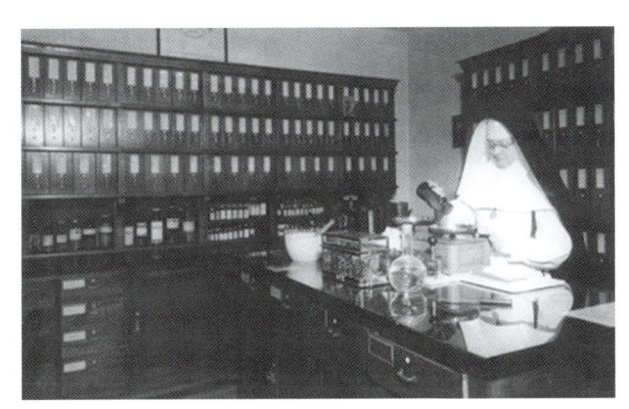

The Sisters of the Sorrowful Mother worked in many areas of St. John in its first decades, including the pharmacy.

The opening of the Chapman Tower and, in 1979, the opening of the Connecting Wing (now part of the Heyman Building), led to new vistas for St. John. The health system expanded to include residential care for seniors with the opening of Franciscan Villa in Broken Arrow, also in 1979. Four years later, Regional Medical Laboratory opened at St. John, and today performs more than 9 million tests a year across the U.S.

1989 brought three significant events: the founding of the Marian Health System, which enjoined the St. John Health System (as it was now known) with three other Catholic health systems: Via Christi Health System, Ministry Health Care and Via Caritas Health System; Wheeling Medical Group (later renamed OMNI Medical Group), was formed and, with several other physician groups, came under the umbrella of St. John Clinic in 2014, with physicians, advanced practice nurses and physician assistants throughout northeast Oklahoma and southern Kansas; and Jane Phillips Medical Center (soon to be a member of the St. John Health System) entered into an agreement with the Nowata (Okla.) General Hospital board of trustees to lease the hospital's facilities and convert it to Jane Phillips Nowata Health Center. Nine years later, Jane Phillips assumed ownership of the Nowata facility.

The 1990s saw St. John join in the development of its own health insurance company: CommunityCare, became operational in 1994, and is presently owned by St. John Health System and Saint Francis Health System, offering healthcare services to more than a half-million people. The '90s were also a time of acquisition and construction. In 1996, St. John entered into a co-sponsorship with Jane Phillips Medical Center in Bartlesville, and by 2002, Jane Phillips was fully sponsored by St. John. A year after its co-sponsorship with Jane Phillips, St. John acquired Bartlett Memorial Hospital in Sapulpa, renaming the facility St. John Sapulpa — the first hospital to carry the St. John name besides St. John Medical Center — in 2002.

Just before the turn of the millennium, St. John embarked on its most ambitious construction project. The 21st Street Project would change the landscape of St. John Medical Center as no other had, bringing an eight-story hospital expansion, an 11-story medical office building and an eight-floor parking garage.

It didn't stop there. By 2006, St. John had built its first new hospital in 80 years, St. John Owasso. Four years later, St. John built another new hospital in the state's fourth-largest city — St. John Broken Arrow.

This period of growth also brought a push for even more medical excellence. The St. John Medical Center Trauma Center, established in 1997, became 12 years later the only American College of Surgeons-verified Level II trauma center in northeast Oklahoma. Urgent care centers were established in Tulsa, Broken Arrow, Claremore and Sand Springs beginning in 2007, and the St. John Heyman Stroke Center, established in 2008, is the only Joint Commission-certified stroke center in eastern Oklahoma, and a multiple winner of Get With The Guidelines Gold Plus Performance awards from the American Heart Association/American Stroke Association. St. John Medical Center has earned Magnet® designation from the American Nurses Credentialing Center twice, once in 2010 and again in 2015.

Today, as a member of Ascension, the nation's largest non-profit and religious healthcare organization, St. John continues to expand its medical expertise through its telemedicine program, which will allow consultations between physicians at St. John Medical Center and those in outlying areas, and a new joint venture between St. John Health System and the Tulsa Cancer Institute. Called Oklahoma Cancer Specialists and Research Institute, it will provide comprehensive oncology services to eastern Oklahoma. ■

St. John Owasso, opened in 2006, was the St. John Health System's first new hospital in 80 years.

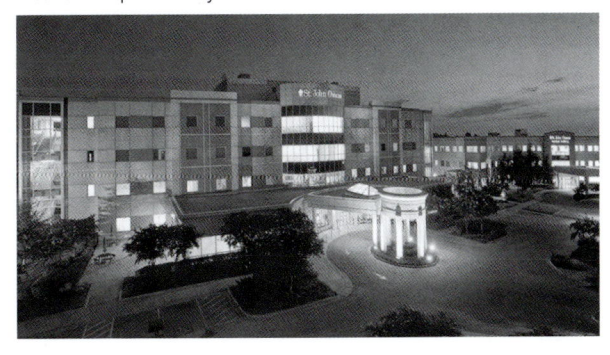

295

Donald R. Stout, M.D.

Donald Stout, M.D., was raised in Shattuck, Oklahoma, a small town serving as a medical mecca for surrounding areas — an ideal environment since he always wanted to be a physician.

He received his B.S. from the University of Oklahoma and his M.D. from Baylor University College of Medicine in Houston. He stayed in Houston for his internship. Wanting to pursue a surgical specialty, he opted out of an internal medicine Berry Plan deferment; thus, he was drafted into the Air Force during the Vietnam War. At Holloman AFB, New Mexico, he practiced Obstetrics and Gynecology for two years. Considering it a happy specialty with finite types of surgical procedures, he returned to Houston for an OB-GYN residency.

In 1970, he moved to Tulsa to join Dr. Eugene Cohen in private practice, primarily focused at St. John. The practice grew and was incorporated as Tulsa OB-GYN Associates — at one time becoming the largest OB-GYN practice in Tulsa.

Utilizing his residency training, Dr. Stout implemented many advancements at St. John including the Harvard Pump, a device providing constant rate of infusion for IV's. Before the pump, IV's were controlled manually using a clamp.

He recommended providing infant resuscitation equipment in labor rooms. "Eventually, all the labor rooms had an infant resuscitation table with positive pressure oxygen and all the necessities to start an IV and get the baby resuscitated if depressed at time of delivery," he shares.

He successfully advocated to the St. John Auxiliary to purchase electronic fetal monitors. Now, monitors are in every room and nursing station.

He and his partner were the first in Tulsa to provide diagnostic procedures laparoscopically, providing better visuals than culdoscopy. That was ten years before the first U.S. operative laparoscopic gallbladder was performed.

He worked with Dr. Richard Dixon providing infertility services before the emergence of IVF technology and infertility fellowships.

His interest extended to the community. He represented St. John as head of the OB-GYN department of the Tulsa Medical Education Foundation. Dr. Max Deardorff represented Saint Francis; Dr. Jack Nettles represented Hillcrest. Dr. Stout obtained a clinical professorship at OU-Tulsa Medical School.

In the '80's, when PPO's and HMO's were emerging, Dr. Stout and five other doctors formed Utica Physicians Association Limited (UPAL) a company providing business services to physicians. Originally, UPAL provided collective negotiation for physicians to obtain lower prices for medical and office supplies.

The company consulted with individual physicians negotiating contracts with insurance companies. Eventually, UPAL provided financial and retirement investment services totaling $210,000,000 for professionals.

Dr. Stout was president of UPAL from 1985-1999, board member from 1985-2004, and is currently on the financial management committee.

He retired in 2003, but stays active in the community. He's involved in the Drug Recycling Program through the Tulsa County Medical Society. He arranges speakers for the monthly luncheon for retired Tulsa physicians, held at St. John. He's been active in the OU Club in Tulsa since the '90's, having served as president and membership chairman. He received the OU Board of Regents Alumni award. And he sings in his church choir.

He married his wife, Judy, in 1964, and they have three children, Spencer, Jeffrey, and Kristin.

Having practiced during the "Golden Age" of medicine, Dr. Stout considered his time as a physician, "a good ride during an ideal time". ■

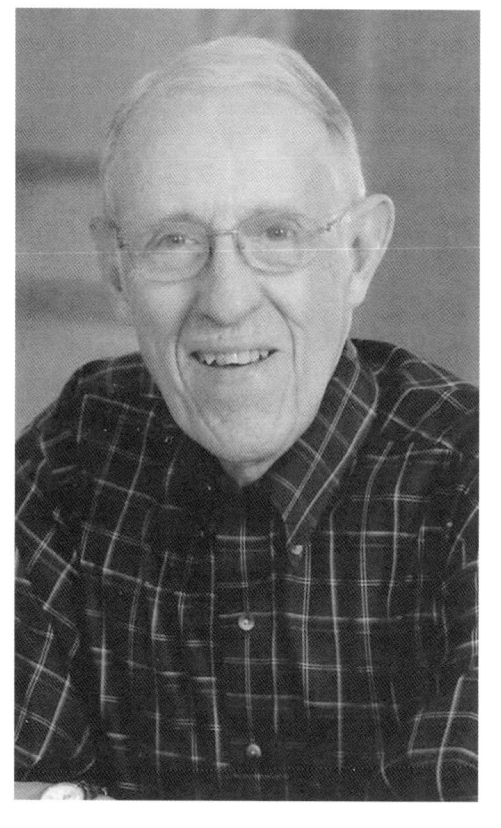

Donald Tredway, M.D., Ph.D.

After receiving his medical degree from the University of Illinois College of Medicine in 1966 and Ph.D. degree from the University of Southern California in 1974, Donald Tredway's medical career started with a bang. Dr. Tredway received his Ob/Gyn training in the U.S. Navy in 1971 and subspecialty training in reproductive endocrinology and infertility at the University of Southern California in 1974.

Tredway remains active in research and medical education with faculty appointments at the Loma Linda University, Oral Roberts University, University of Oklahoma, University of Chicago, University of California, and University of Southern California.

During his time at Loma Linda University and the University of Chicago, Tredway served as section chief of reproductive endocrinology. He also served as chairman of the departments of gynecology and obstetrics at King Fahd National Guard Hospital in Riyadh, Saudi Arabia, Tulsa Medical College of the University of Oklahoma, and Oral Roberts University.

In 2000, Tredway ended his clinical practicing career and joined Serono, Inc. as a Medical Director in the Clinical Development for Reproductive Health. This job lasted until 2006 when he was appointed Global Head of the Endocrinology and Reproductive Health Unit of Serono. Shortly after that time, Merck KGA acquired Serono, changing Tredway's role to Vice President and Global Head of the Fertility and Endocrinology CDU for EMD Serono.

In 2009, Tredway retired from EMD Serono to return to Broken Arrow, Oklahoma. Instead of getting on board with another company, he decided to open his own organization called Tredway Consulting, LLC. His business is responsible for providing experienced biotechnology and pharmaceutical consulting services in medical affairs, transitional medicine, business development, and clinical development.

He took the role of Chief Medical Officer of Repros Therapeutics in 2012 for six months. Tredway is a Clinical Professor at the University of Oklahoma-Tulsa School of Community Medicine, a full-time Assistant Professor at Tulsa Community College, and is on staff in the College of Counseling and Health Care at the University of the Nations, Kailua-Kona, Hawaii (YWAM).

Tredway served 20 years in the U.S. Navy in active and reserve status before retiring with the rank of Captain from the Naval Reserve in 1996. For two years, Dr. Tredway and his family served in a mission in Asia. The work Tredway does in the field continues with his responsibility with the College of Counseling and Health Care at the University of the Nations in Hawaii.

In the decades since Tredway graduated from University of Illinois College of Medicine, he has served in every possible role you could imagine.

Tredway says, "I want to be the one that does the hard work. Being a doctor is a remarkable opportunity to continually grow in the medical services profession."

Tredway's responsibilities in the present day include continuing his work with Tredway Consulting and being an assistant biology professor at Tulsa Community College.

The variety in his career gives him a special insight others might not possess. Between his military experience and medical expertise, Tredway has seen and done more than most people in the field of medicine.

He and his wife enjoy spending time with their family, working on their sprawling 100-acre ranch in Broken Arrow, and look forward to finally retiring.

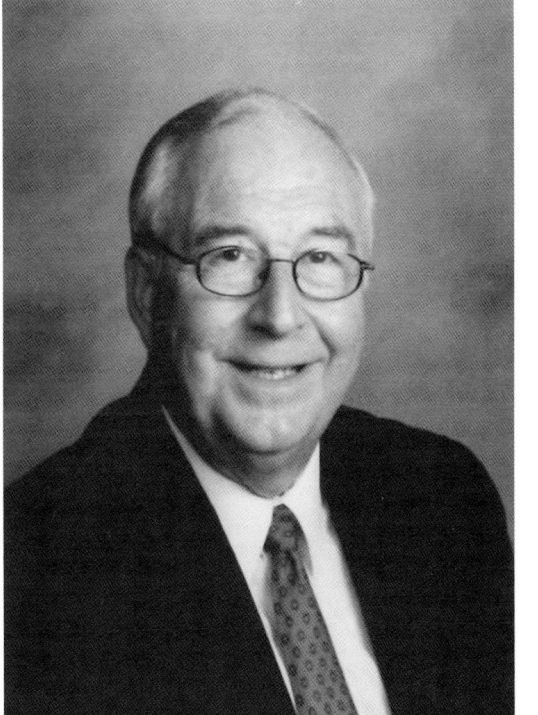

Surgical Associates

For 50 years, the board certified physicians of Surgical Associates have offered a range of treatment options in general surgery, while supporting the growth of the medical infrastructure of Tulsa and northeastern Oklahoma.

Starting with a handshake, four doctors founded Surgical Associates in 1966. The private practice was launched in Tulsa's Ranch Acres Medical Center by C.T. Thompson, M.D., W. Dean Hidy, M.D., Lowell Stokes, M.D. and Lester Nienhuis, M.D.

After its founding, the doctors decided to dedicate their energies and talents to Saint Francis Hospital, a small facility sitting alone on a hill in southeast Tulsa. In 1968, Surgical Associates became one of the first tenants in the Warren Professional Building, 6465 S. Yale Ave., where it remained for 46 years.

Through the decades, Surgical Associates was intertwined with the expansions of Saint Francis Hospital. In particular, Dr. Thompson offered significant contributions to the hospital's early mission - developing a top-notch acute care hospital with a regional and national presence.

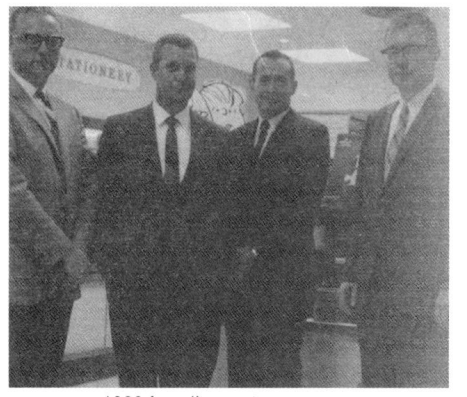

1966 founding partners

Many of Surgical Associates' physicians have served in the capacity of the hospital's chief of staff, chief of surgery and on its board of directors. As chairman of the hospital's cancer committee, James B. Lockhart, Jr., M.D., served as a co-principal investigator of cancer research at the Natalie Warren Bryant Cancer Center. In 2000, Dr. Lockhart was awarded the American Cancer Society's prestigious Lane Adams Quality of Life Award. The objective of this award is to recognize and reward individuals who are innovative and consistently provide excellent and compassionate skilled care, counsel, and/or service to persons with cancer.

During the 1970s, Dr. Thompson was a member of the National Trauma Committee of the American College of Surgeons. His efforts, along with those of Gerald E. Gustafson, M.D., led to trauma care becoming a special focus for Saint Francis and a cornerstone for the facility's reputation. The two physicians laid the foundation for the Saint Francis Trauma Emergency Center, which became the largest trauma center in the region. Dr. Gustafson led the expansion and redesign of the center several years later. Roger Siemens, M.D., contributed to the care of seriously injured patients and headed the American College of Surgeons Trauma Committee in Oklahoma.

In addition to the impact the physicians of Surgical Associates had on the development of Saint Francis, many doctors served the greater Tulsa community in other capacities.

When Dr. Thompson arrived in Tulsa, the city did not have an emergency medical system, with funeral homes providing ambulance service. He led an effort creating a professional ambulance service with trained personnel. He formed the Oklahoma Trauma Research Society to expand the training program statewide. In 1983, Dr. Thompson was presented with the American College of Surgeons highest honor, the Distinguished Service Award, for his trauma work.

Dr. Gustafson is credited with developing emergency medical systems in Tulsa and northeastern Oklahoma. He helped in the planning and delivery of the 911 emergency system, emergency helicopter services and programs for CPR and advanced cardiac life support.

In 2007, Surgical Associates changed its focus to partner with Oklahoma Surgical Hospital.

Oklahoma Surgical Hospital was established by local physicians who felt that hospital care should return to focusing on the needs of the patient. This vision created a hospital that provides outstanding medical quality in an environment of personalized service. This patient-doctor relationship is the cornerstone to delivering the best possible medical care.

Surgical Associates moved its office to Cityplex Towers at 2448 E. 81st St. in 2014, adjacent to Oklahoma Surgical Hospital. To this day, it remains a premier, independent, physician-owned practice.

As the practice celebrates its 50th year, the doctors continue to provide expert, state-of-the-art treatment in the areas of colorectal surgery, bariatric surgery, surgical oncology, benign and malignant skin lesions, breast care, esophageal and reflux surgery, hernia surgery, gallbladder surgery, minimally invasive/robotic surgery, thyroid and parathyroid surgery, trauma and critical care and varicose vein surgery.

FUTURE LEGACIES

SURGICAL ASSOCIATES' PHYSICIANS ARE:

Mark R. Meese, M.D., of Bartlesville, Dr. Meese earned his undergraduate degree from the University of Oklahoma and attended medical school at the OU Health Sciences Center. He has been in the practice of general surgery at Surgical Associates since 1990. He has extensive experience in minimally invasive procedures for hernia repair, gallbladder removal, solid organ removal and endocrine surgery. He has also used single-incision laparoscopy to minimize scarring and recovery time.

Craig S. Johnson, M.D., a native Oklahoman, graduated from OU and earned his medical degree from the OU Health Sciences Center. He completed a colorectal surgery fellowship at Louisiana State University in Shreveport. Dr. Johnson has specialized in colorectal surgery since 1992 and has practiced colorectal surgery at Surgical Associates since 1996. Since 2010, his practice has been focused on robotic colon and rectal surgery.

Steven B. Katsis, M.D., a native of Sioux City, Iowa, moved to Tulsa in 1984 to attend Oral Roberts University. He earned his medical degree in 1993 from the University of Nebraska College of Medicine. He joined Surgical Associates in 1999. Dr. Katsis is the past president of the Tulsa County Medical Society and the Oklahoma Chapter of the American College of Surgeons. Active in trauma and pediatric emergency surgery, and tactical medicine for law enforcement, he specializes in bariatric surgery.

Ronald Jackson, D.O., a native of Fort Worth, Texas, graduated from Stephen F. Austin State University in Nacogdoches, Texas, and earned his medical degree in 1978 from the Texas College of Osteopathic Medicine. Prior to joining Surgical Associates in 2001, Dr. Jackson had been in private practice in Tulsa since 1983. Among Dr. Jackson's special interests are laparoscopic-assisted surgery, surgical oncology and endocrine surgery.

Kevin T. Fisher, D.O., a Kansas native, graduated from Northwestern Oklahoma State University then earned a medical degree in 1993 from the OSU College of Osteopathic Medicine in Tulsa. He was in private practice in Woodward, Oklahoma, before joining Surgical Associates in February 2002. Dr Fisher's interests are in minimally invasive laparoscopic and robotic surgery and their application in treating diseases of the liver, pancreas and the digestive tract, as well as the surgical treatment of cancer.

Michael W. Griffin, D.O., a native Tulsan, graduated from William Jewell College in Liberty, Missouri, and earned his medical degree from the OSU College of Osteopathic Medicine in 1998. He joined Surgical Associates in 2004 and is active in all aspects of general surgery and has special interest in abdominal wall reconstruction and hernia surgery.

Christopher L. Cole, D.O., a native of Sallisaw, Oklahoma, graduated from Northeastern State University in Tahlequah, and earned his medical degree in 1993 from the OSU College of Osteopathic Medicine in Tulsa. He joined Surgical Associates in 2005. His special interests include laparoscopic, endocrine, breast and bariatric surgery and wound care.

Brandon D. Varnell, M.D., a Tulsa-area native, received his bachelor's degree from the University of Central Oklahoma in 1998 and his medical degree from the OU College of Medicine in 2002. Prior to joining Surgical Associates in 2008, he completed a fellowship at the University of Nebraska Medical Center in advanced laparoscopic and robotic surgery. His special interests are minimally invasive laparoscopic and robotic surgery in the treatment of hernia, GERD and bariatric surgery.

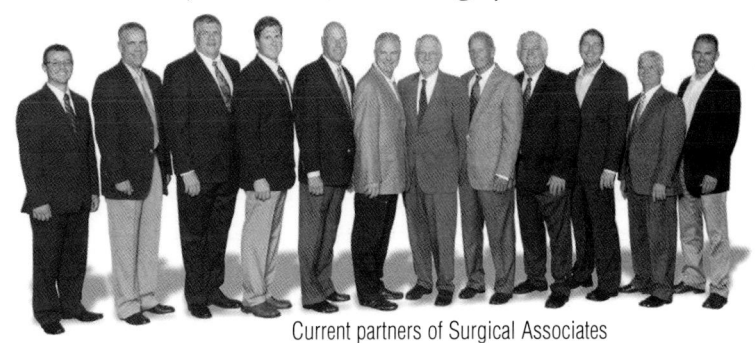

Current partners of Surgical Associates

W. Christopher Sutterfield, M.D., a native Tulsan, attended Tulsa Junior College and OU in Norman. He earned his medical degree in 1995 from the OU Health Sciences Center's Tulsa campus. Active in all aspects of general surgery at Surgical Associates from 2000 to 2003, Dr. Sutterfield spent six years practicing surgery in Dalton, Georgia, where he served as Hamilton Medical Center's trauma director. He returned to Surgical Associates in January 2009 and specializes in laparoscopic, robotic and access surgery for dialysis patients.

Bryce W. Murray, M.D., an Oklahoma native, graduated from Harding University in Searcy, Arkansas, then earned a medical degree in 2004 from the University of Oklahoma College of Medicine in Tulsa. He completed a fellowship in colorectal surgery at the Colon and Rectal Clinic of Orlando. He joined Surgical Associates in August of 2014. His special interests are laparoscopic and robotic surgery and their application in the treatment of inflammatory bowel disease and colon and rectal cancer. ■

Tulsa Coalition for Children's Health

It was over coffee one day when a group of pediatricians decided they could lead the way for better quality care by seeking a children's hospital in Tulsa.

Children's specialty care was fragmented across the city, determined by isolated efforts to recruit subspecialists. Children needing services had unequal access to care because of varying preferences among insurance companies.

"We thought this is a no-brainer. Why are we not vocal about needing a children's hospital? We knew it was time for Tulsa, but we needed buy in," said Dr. Dawn Mayberry.

The Tulsa Coalition for Children's Health was founded in 2000 out of that physician-led grassroots effort. Its mission: "To promote the health and well-being of children and their families through caregiving systems that are committed to excellence in providing healthcare to children."

With a primary focus on establishing an acute children's hospital, the group knew it needed to raise money for research to acquire backers and to determine a design.

The officers were Dr. Mayberry as president, Dr. Pat Hughes as vice president, Dr. David Siegler as treasurer and Claudia Jackson as secretary. Other board members were Drs. Don Zetik, Bill Geffen, Bill Jackson, Jere Cravens, Bob Block, David Jubelirer, Bill Kennedy and Dan Plunket. The group was assisted by attorney Tom Adelson.

The board represented all corners of the Tulsa pediatric community - hospital, private, academic and specialty practices. Of the city's nearly 100 pediatricians, most paid dues and all supported the coalition.

Officers made presentations to area civic groups and health-care institutions and decision-makers, established a mailing list for newsletters and sought grants.

An initial round of discussions with hospitals found encouragement for a children's hospital but lack of interest in taking on such an institution. In March 2003, the coalition was contacted by Saint Francis to have further discussions. At the same time, a $125,000 grant was obtained for a feasibility study, which was conducted by the Katz Consulting Group.

The six-month study found Tulsa's population could support a children's hospital and care would be more efficient and less costly if subspecialists were located in a single facility. Those results and the pediatrician unity shown by the coalition gave Saint Francis the incentive to build the hospital. The model would be a hospital within a hospital, with the facility on the northeast side of the medical center campus near 61st Street and Yale Avenue.

Agreements were made for pediatric residencies at the University of Oklahoma-Tulsa and Oklahoma State University Center for Health Sciences to be completed at the Saint Francis Children's Hospital.

In 2004, Dr. Mayberry stepped down as president, and Dr. David Siegler has been at the helm. The following year, Saint Francis broke ground on the $56 million children's hospital.

The existing pediatric subspecialties in Tulsa, were cardiology, neurology, oncology, endocrinology and child abuse. With the addition and rise of the Children's Hospital, the organization was able to recruit other greatly needed specialists, like orthopedics, infectious disease, pulmonology and pediatric neurosurgery. In 2016, Tennessee-based St. Jude Children's Research Hospital announced it would establish an affiliate clinic at the hospital.

"Our focus then went to how we can support the specialists," said Dr. Mayberry. "The coalition has remained and is working on other aspects of quality and access of children's care."

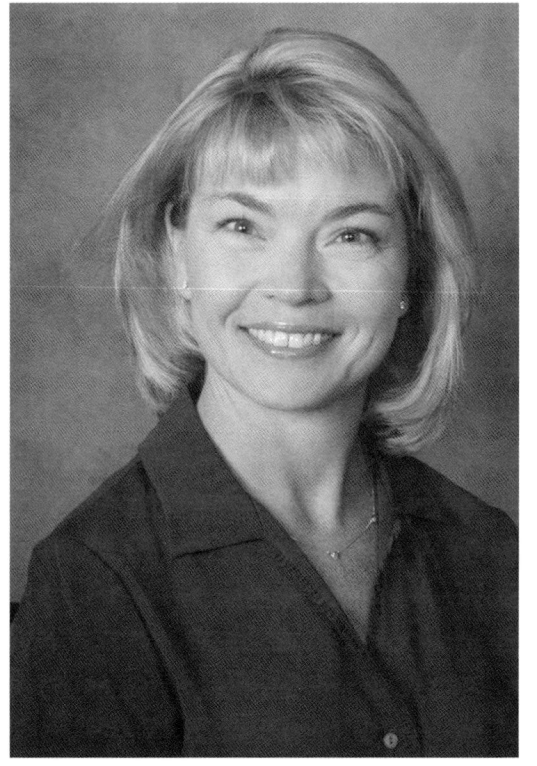

Dr. Dawn Mayberry, D.O., first president and founding member of the Tulsa Coalition for Children's Health

Robert Endres, M.D.

Dr. Endres planned on becoming a surgeon. He switched to a career in pediatrics after caring for orphans while serving as an Army physician in Korea.

"I just fell in love with those kids," said Dr. Endres.

He graduated from the University of Oklahoma Medical School in 1948 followed by an internship and general practice in Sallisaw. Then, he entered the military from 1951-53, serving in Korea and Japan. Upon return, he completed a pediatric residency and pediatric cardiology fellowship at St. Louis Children's Hospital.

In 1956, Dr. Endres moved to Tulsa and joined Dr. Dick Russell at Springer Clinic. Other physicians added were Drs. Albert Brownlee, B.J. Maguire, Del Gheen, Pat Hughes and James Lewis. In 1976, the pediatricians formed the Children's Clinic of Tulsa.

Dr. Endres led the pediatric section of the diabetes center at Saint Francis Hospital from 1980 to 1993 and was on the board of governors for 20 years. He also served as chairman of the Oklahoma chapter of the American Academy of Pediatrics (1967-1973).

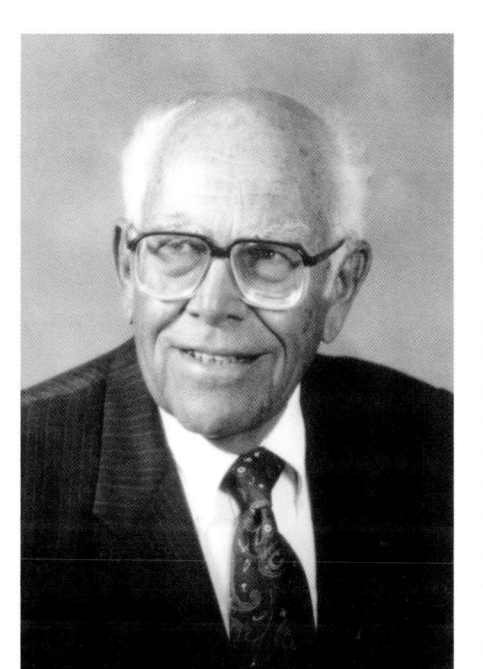

After 1993, he treated patients with endocrine disorders and diabetes, worked as a locum tenens and as an educator in the OU-Tulsa pediatric department. He retired in 2003 at age 80.

Dr. Endres and his wife Esther were married for more than 70 years, until her death in 2015. The couple has five children and five grandchildren.

James G. Coldwell, M.D.

In 1960, I was privileged to join the medical community where I was allowed to provide care for children. This followed medical school, a rotating internship and pediatric residency at the University of Oklahoma, University of Colorado and Washington University, St. Louis.

I was deferred from active medical service to attend medical school and then completed my residence through the Berry Plan. I went from inactive reserve to active duty, serving as the director of pediatric services at the 42nd Army Field Hospital in Verdun, France. This was an extremely rewarding experience, but I opted to terminate my service commitment after 13 years. My goal was to establish a pediatric practice, which came about after providing pediatric care at Children's Medical Center.

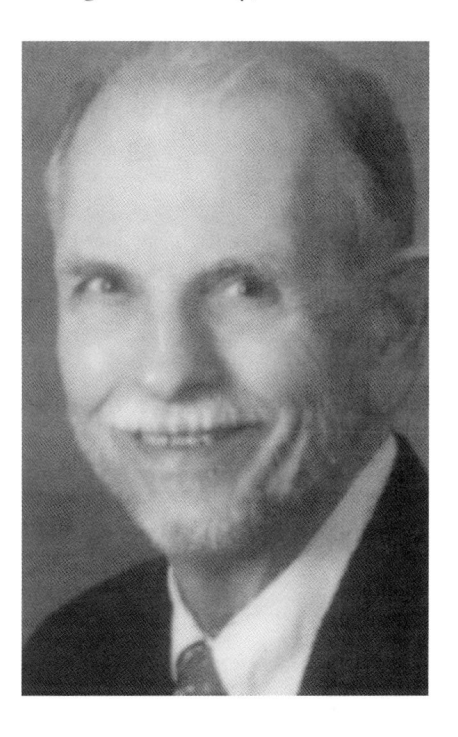

Later, I had the privilege to practice with superb pediatricians but found my niche with children with special health care needs. A fellowship at Johns Hopkins enabled me to become more competent to do so. I returned to Tulsa to direct pediatric services at Children's Medical Center, which expanded and added programs to become a catchment area for special needs children. Overall, traveling this road not commonly taken has been difficult but rewarding. The greatest difficulty was inadequate funding for quality care, which remains a persistent problem. Despite this, we were able to add research and education to our community service commitment.

The Women's Health Group (TWHG)

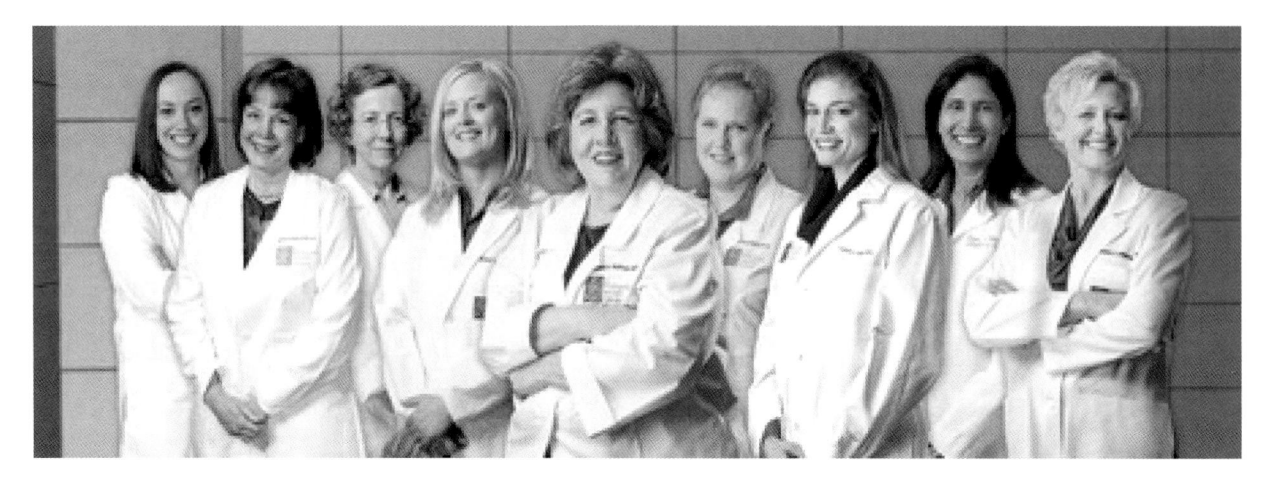

The Women's Health Group (TWHG) consists of eight exceptional female obstetricians and gynecologists and a quality support staff. Their growing practice strives to offer compassionate and respectful care. The physicians who have chosen to practice medicine at TWHG are Kathleen Heffron, M.D., FACOG; Tracey Lakin, M.D., FACOG; Stacy Noland, D.O., FACOG; Darla Lofgren, M.D., FACOG; Jennifer Gibbens, M.D., FACOG; Nirupama DeSilva, M.D., FACOG; Judith Blackwell, M.D., FACOG; and Jennifer Butler, M.D., FACOG.

Women deserve to receive care from physicians who understand their problems and with whom they are comfortable discussing their most personal issues. The physicians and staff at TWHG are dedicated to respecting the personal dignity of their patients and to maintaining the highest standards of care. The physicians and staff are guided by comfort, respect and quality medical care.

In the early 90's, there were very few female obstetricians and gynecologists practicing in Tulsa. In 1991, Dr. Heffron and four other female doctors realized that they could better meet the needs of their patients if they shared a practice and resources. Most of the doctors had young children at the time; therefore, sharing a practice and the accompanying resources afforded them the opportunity of a better work-life balance while still providing the best possible care for their patients.

TWHG's growing practice strives to offer compassionate, respectful, individualized care. The physicians are exceptional obstetricians and gynecologists and are supported by a dedicated and professional staff. TWHG provides a full range of pregnancy, gynecology, gynecological surgery, pediatric and adolescent gynecology and reproductive endocrinology services, as well as counseling regarding all women's issues.

The current doctors chose to work at TWHG because of the high standards and reputation of the group. The doctors and support staff know the necessity of teamwork, so they rely heavily on one another, have created a culture of trust, and are very unified in everything they do. The doctors know that whoever is on call will take care of their patients with the same care and dedication as they would.

TWHG takes pride in staying up-to-date on the latest surgery techniques and healthcare standards. The Women's Health Group currently has five doctors certified to perform da Vinci Robotic Surgery.

TWHG encompasses a broad spectrum of doctors as well as specialties. In addition to general obstetrics and gynecology, TWHG has one doctor who specializes in reproductive endocrinology (infertility) and one who specializes in pediatric and adolescent gynecology.

In 2013, TWHG moved to a larger facility in south Tulsa to better serve their patient population. The practice is located in the South Creek Medical Plaza at 91st Street and Highway 169. The new facility allows them to be more efficient and to offer more services.

The physicians of TWHG perform obstetrical deliveries, gynecologic treatment and surgery at Hillcrest Hospital South and St. John Medical Center. As of 2016, The Women's Health Group has eight talented physicians, trained at some of the nation's top medical centers, along with Physician Assistants and Registered Ultrasonographers.

Urologic Specialists

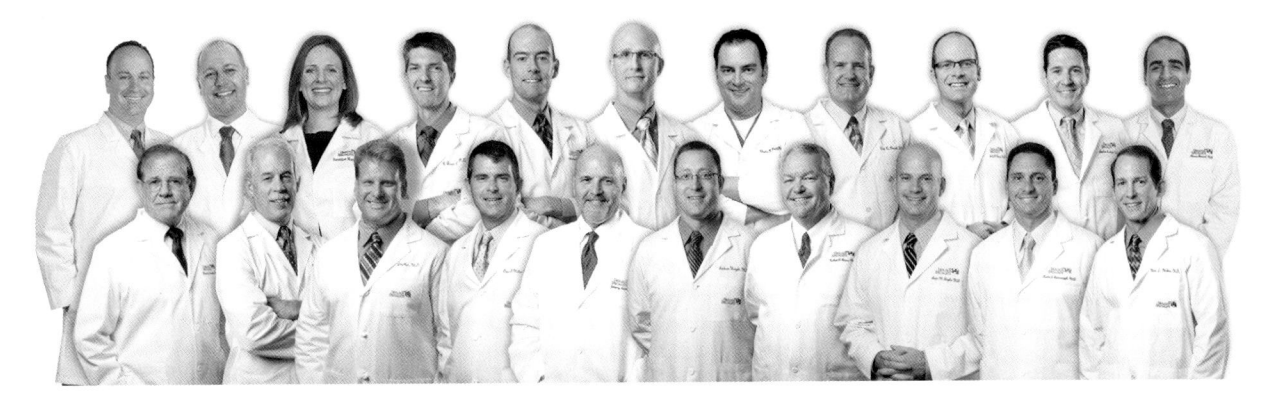

Since 1948, Urologic Specialists has offered exceptional and innovative urologic care for men, women, and children. The practice has 20 board-certified urologists including several subspecialists with additional training in urologic cancers, kidney transplantation, kidney stone disease, pediatric urology, female pelvic medicine, trauma and reconstructive surgery and male sexual health issues.

The practice prides itself on its extensively trained and experienced surgeons using the latest technology to deliver world class patient care.

Marc Milsten, M.D., founding member of Urologic Specialists, explains, "Our surgeons are pioneers in robotic surgery performing the area's first robotic prostatectomy in 2005. Since then we've continued to be on the cutting edge of minimally invasive surgery. Our surgeons performed the first robotic partial nephrectomy in 2009 and the first robotic cystectomy in 2010. Our physicians typically perform 10-14 robotic surgeries each week."

Why does this group breed such leadership? Founding member, David Harper, M.D., believes it stems from the original doctors who founded the group, and ultimately through subspecialization and diversification.

He says, "Among our group, we've had five Tulsa County Medical Society presidents and one Oklahoma State Medical Society president. There have been seven presidents of area hospital staffs including St. John, Saint Francis, and Hillcrest as well as three presidents of the South Central section of the American Urological Association and a president of the American Board of Urology."

Harper says, "One thing we felt was important in building urologic excellence was bringing in the best doctors from all over the United States with varying areas of expertise. Our urologists represent 17 different training programs."

Serving patients in Oklahoma, Arkansas, and Missouri, Urologic Specialists credits widespread contacts and a stellar reputation for allowing the practice to obtain the country's top talent.

Milsten says, "We have a network of people who know us and we know them. We have two physicians that we courted as early as medical school. We've built relationships over the years that have allowed us to expand the group in ways that benefit our patients."

Harper agrees, "We are known all over the country. Because of our high recruiting standards, we have physicians here as good or better than anyone in the country. We search for people who are training at the best programs across the country with ties to the Southwest or Midwest area. We have found over the years that having a local connection makes a doctor more likely to stay with the practice long term."

In 2004, Urologic Specialists centralized its five offices into one building located near intersecting highways allowing patients and staff quick access from anywhere in the city. The building's industrial style architecture and nod to Tulsa's Art Deco design period is pleasant and inviting with high ceilings, plenty of light, metal, and green spaces. Serving more than 400 patients a day, Urologic Specialists has a radiology department, full lab, and host of ancillary services offered within the walls of one building which reduces stress on patients and makes for a much more efficient practice.

The commitment to focusing not only on urology, but inspiring greatness in all facets of the business makes Urologic Specialists unique.

Milsten says, "It's very important to us to maintain this level of excellence. Many of us have worked in hospitals and taught at universities with budget constraints and other issues. Coming to a private practice such as ours allows our doctors to do anything they are trained to do and do it well."

The University of Tulsa College of Health Sciences

The University of Tulsa (TU) has its heritage in the Presbyterian School of Indian Girls, a small boarding school in Muskogee, Indian Territory. The school was founded in 1882 by Alice Mary Robertson, later Oklahoma's first female United States representative. In 1894, at the request of the Synod of Indian Territory, the Board of Home Missions of the Presbyterian Church elevated the academy's status and chartered it as Henry Kendall College, a name that honored the first general secretary of the Home Missions Board.

Financial difficulties prompted school officials to seek a new location. Successfully courted by the business and professional community of Tulsa, Henry Kendall College relocated to Tulsa in 1907. Years later, McFarlin College, named after oilman Robert M. McFarlin, was proposed for the city. The Henry Kendall College trustees proposed the two colleges affiliate under the common name, The University of Tulsa.

In 1928, the School of Petroleum Engineering opened, earning international recognition for its curriculum and faculty. The college of Business Administration was established in 1935. In 1943, the law school became part of the University. The University includes the Henry Kendall College of Arts and Sciences, the Collins College of Business, the College of Engineering and Natural Sciences, the College of Law, the Graduate School, and the Division of Continuing Education.

In 1968, after several years of extensive research by the university's administration and faculty, interested citizens, hospitals and medical centers, and local, state, and national nurses, the Board of Trustees decided to create the College of Nursing. The College of Nursing was approved by the Oklahoma Board of Nurse Registration and Nursing Education in 1970 and the first baccalaureate nursing class graduated in 1973. More than 1,400 nurses have received Bachelor of Science degrees in nursing.

In 1991, the Athletic Training Program became an offering within the School of Nursing. In 1998, the program implemented a new degree, Exercise and Sports Medicine, adding a teacher certification emphasis in 2003. The Physician Assistant Program was developed in 2008 in partnership with the University of Oklahoma.

In 2014, The University of Tulsa decided to create a new college of Health Sciences combining programs previously scattered in other parts of The University of Tulsa. The college supports TU's role in the Tulsa School of Community Medicine (TCSM), a joint four-year community medical education program formed with the University of Oklahoma to help address Oklahoma's low health status, low health systems performance, and physician shortage.

Gerard Clancy serves as the 20th President of The University of Tulsa. A strong advocate of community-based medicine, Clancy believes the medical college is an integral part of a continuing effort to improve the health of Tulsa and Oklahoma.

Gerard Clancy, M.D., President

He says, "Oklahoma is a hot-spot for hypertension, cardio-vascular disease, mental illness, and diabetes. We have some of the worst health outcomes in the entire nation, and these are made even worse by disparities in access to health care in our state."

Through this college, students have the ability to earn a Master's in Athletic Training or Doctor of Nursing Practice degree. Other degree options include Bachelors of Exercise and Sports Science, Athletic Training, and Speech Pathology. Students studying Speech Pathology can earn a Masters in Speech Pathology after graduation.

In 2015, TU started its M.D. program partnership with the University of Oklahoma and created the Mary K. and John T. Oxley College of Health Sciences. This name is a tribute to the Oxley Foundation's devotion to the university and its health science initiatives. The partnership between TU and OU is revolutionary among institutions of

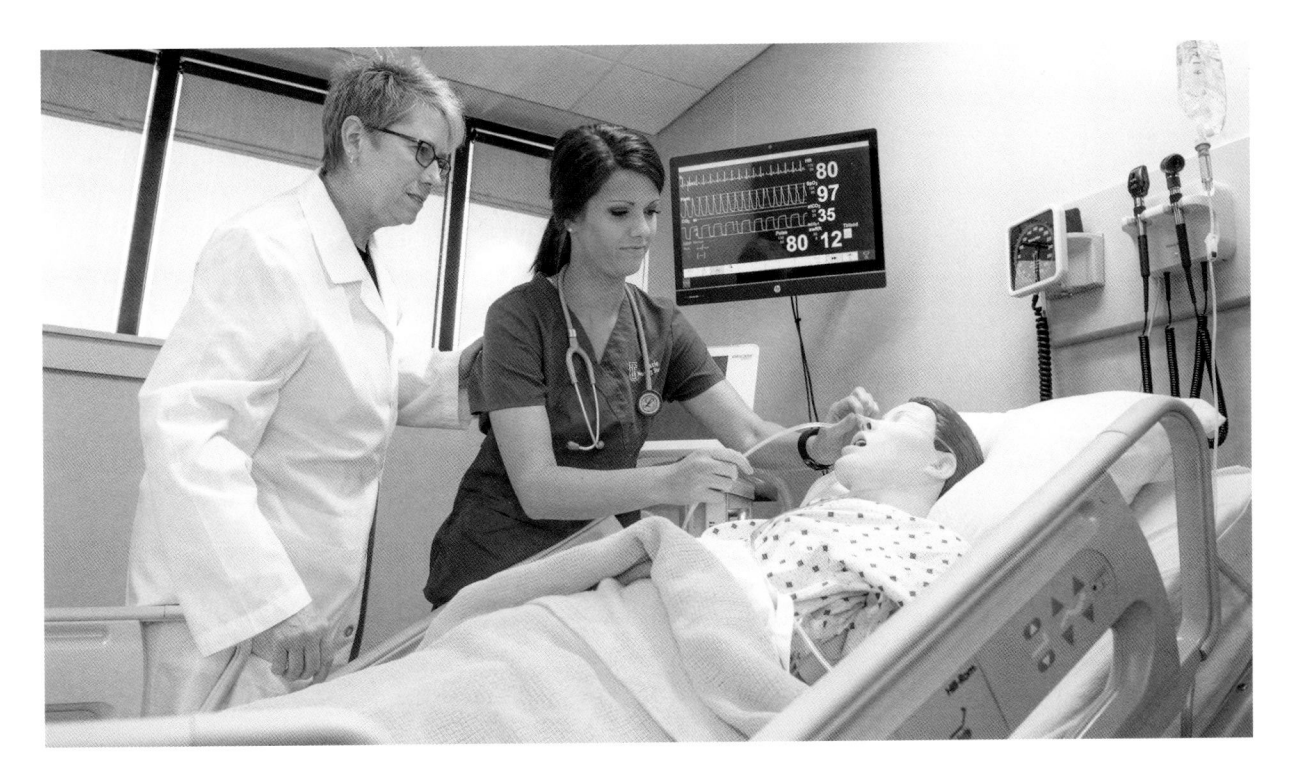

The college's state-of-the-art facilities feature advanced technology and simulators for experiential learning opportunities.

higher learning in the United States.

In early 2016 the college and all of its programs were relocated to the former Blue Cross Blue Shield building in downtown Tulsa. The new building offers TU the opportunity to use 50,000 square feet of space for classrooms and other state-of-the-art facilities for the college's community medicine, exercise and sports science, athletic training, and nursing programs.

Currently there are 350 students in the College of Health Sciences. With an expansion plan in place, the college expects to increase enrollment to at least 600 students. Clancy says the project is timely and provides a huge opportunity for The University of Tulsa.

A fully outfitted clinic open to university employees and the community is housed within the college.

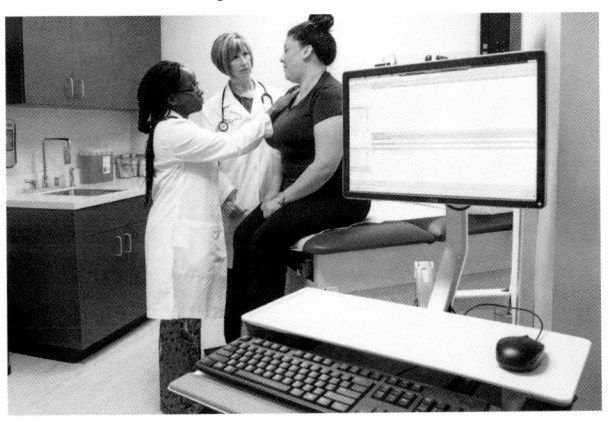

He says, "If you look at the job growth for health professions, physicians 5-year job growth is expected to be 20%, nurse practitioners is 34%, and physician assistants is 38%. So there's a huge growth in jobs. Our country is one million nurses short and one hundred thousand physicians short. And Oklahoma is behind the national averages. We want to be in the position to graduate students that have highly satisfying and well paying jobs."

In addition to the new facility, the College of Health Sciences provides faculty for the Laureate Institute for Brain Research through a sponsorship by the Warren Foundation, and is collaborating with Tulsa Public Schools through its Athletic Training Program.

"Interdisciplinary study is key to the College of Health Sciences, where students and faculty are encouraged to collaborate with other departments – and even other colleges – to find solutions. Health Sciences students can learn from their peers in engineering, law, psychology, computer science, and business," says Clancy.

Throughout the course of TU's history, they have remained dedicated to providing its students with the highest level of professional, graduate, and undergraduate education in applied health sciences, nursing, law, engineering, education, business, humanities, sciences, and arts. ■

FUTURE LEGACIES

Utica Women's Specialists

Utica Women's Specialists, an obstetrics and gynecology practice, has roots dating back seventy years. Founded in the 1940's by Dr. William F. Thomas, the practice has remained independent. Dr. McShane, Dr. Dennehy, and Dr. Lackey joined the practice through the years; in 1983, Dr. Lynn Frame joined and was fortunate to know Dr. Thomas.

The practice has incorporated and become Utica Women's Specialists with three doctors on staff: Lynn E. Frame, M.D., J.D.; Daran L. Parham, M.D.; and Melissa A. Dietz, M.D.

The overriding philosophy here is patients first. "We pay a great deal of attention to our patients," says Dr. Frame of their service emphasis. "All three of us answer our own phone calls, and we don't have nurses call them back. If someone has a lab test done, or mammogram, or X-ray, we call them and report the results immediately."

"We are patient advocates," Dr. Parham adds. "We really are there for our patients and try to do what we can. If we can't, then we try to figure out who can take care of them."

They're available to handle emergencies twenty-four, seven. "If somebody calls and says, 'I have an emergency,' we see them the same day," says Dr. Frame.

Dr. Frame received his undergraduate and medical degrees through the University of Oklahoma (OU), performed his residency in Tulsa, then served two years in the Army at Fort Leonard Wood. He returned to Tulsa in 1983. He has a law degree and has recently completed eighteen years of service on the Board of Physicians Liability Insurance Company of Oklahoma.

The three doctors together have delivered thousands of babies, and they describe their field as happy and rewarding, where they give people good news. They summarize their practice as a hybrid of surgical specialist and primary care. They perform a variety of female surgeries such as hysterectomies, laparoscopies, C-sections, pelvic support and repairs. "We do a lot of primary care for women, especially for birth control, endocrinology, pregnancy, and treatments for hormones, menopause issues, and osteoporosis," Dr. Frame expounds.

Dr. Parham joined Utica Women's Specialists in 2013. He received his undergraduate and medical degrees through OU and performed his residency at Hillcrest through OU. He worked at a private practice before joining Dr. Frame.

Dr. Dietz received her undergraduate degree from the University of Central Arkansas, received her medical degree from the University of Arkansas, and performed her residency at Hillcrest through OU. Then she practiced at a hospital in Grove, but eventually moved back to Tulsa, joining the same practice where Dr. Parham had worked. In 2015, she joined Utica Women's Specialist.

The doctors serve the medical community as well. Dr. Frame teaches at the OU-TU School of Community Medicine. He was president of the Tulsa County Medical Society, Tulsa County Obstetric and Gynecology Society, and Tulsa Surgical Society. He has served as chairman of the Obstetrics and Gynecology Committee at St. John. Dr. Parham served this department as secretary and chairman of the nurse liaison committee. Dr. Dietz served as a faculty physician at Oklahoma State University.

Although the trend is toward hospital-owned practices, the doctors at Utica Women's Specialists are proud of remaining independent for seventy years; thus, they can provide what Dr. Parham describes as "more personable attention."

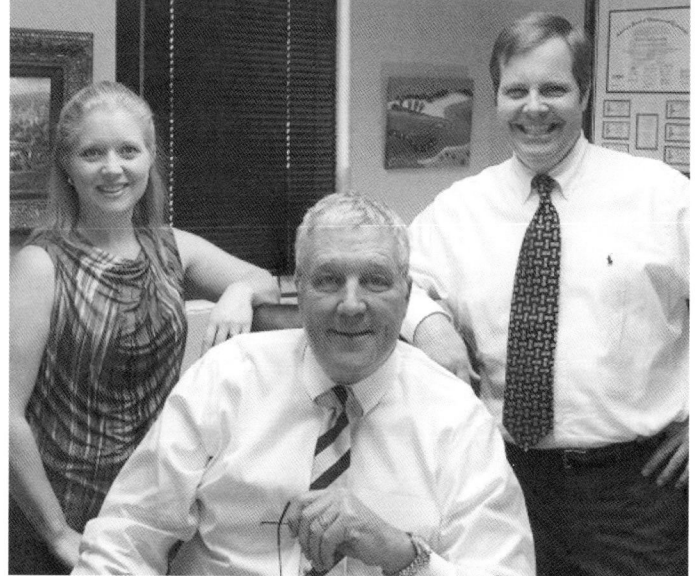

Lynn Frame, M.D. (seated), Melissa Dietz, M.D. (left), & Daran Parham, M.D. (right)

FUTURE LEGACIES

Lynn Wiens, M.D.

Past Tulsa County Medical Society (TCMS) president, Dr. Lynn Wiens, became involved with the medical society almost four years ago. He was searching for an opportunity to give back to the community and attended an annual TCMS meeting. He quickly recognized the importance of Leadership Medicine.

"What doctors really seem to need the most is either mentorship or support," says Wiens.

Doctors are pulled in multiple directions. They used to see each other during rounds, but today hospitalists carry out that task so doctors become isolated in their office, never connecting with colleagues who understand their daily struggles.

He says, "When we talk to doctors about mentorship or support, they just light up! So here are TCMS, we have implemented a mentorship and support program for physicians at every stage of their careers."

The mentoring program began by matching physicians willing to donate their time and energy with students and residents with similar attributes, needs, and styles of communication. If the model of matching doctors works for this age group, the medical society may apply it to a matching program for mid-career doctors.

Wiens stresses the importance of TCMS membership. He says, "You have no idea what goes on unless you are actively involved in the medical society. It's been quite a learning experience for me, especially in terms of the legislature. We take for granted the many things that happen that benefit the medical profession."

He urges members to get to know other doctors in the community. Whether the physicians get involved by volunteering for the mentoring program or simply attending a meeting, he believes providing support to each other can make a big difference.

"I think my passion is to invigorate other physicians to do what their passion is and be a connecting network where doctors feel like someone actually listens to them," says Wiens. "There's real value in becoming a TCMS member."

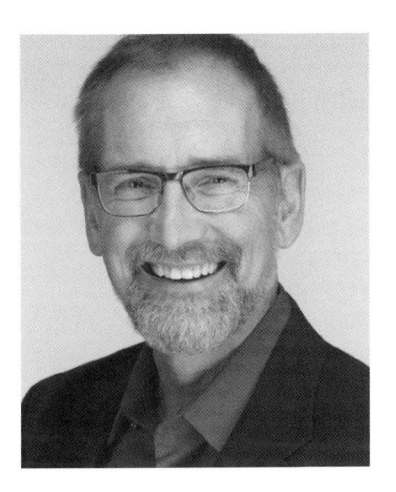

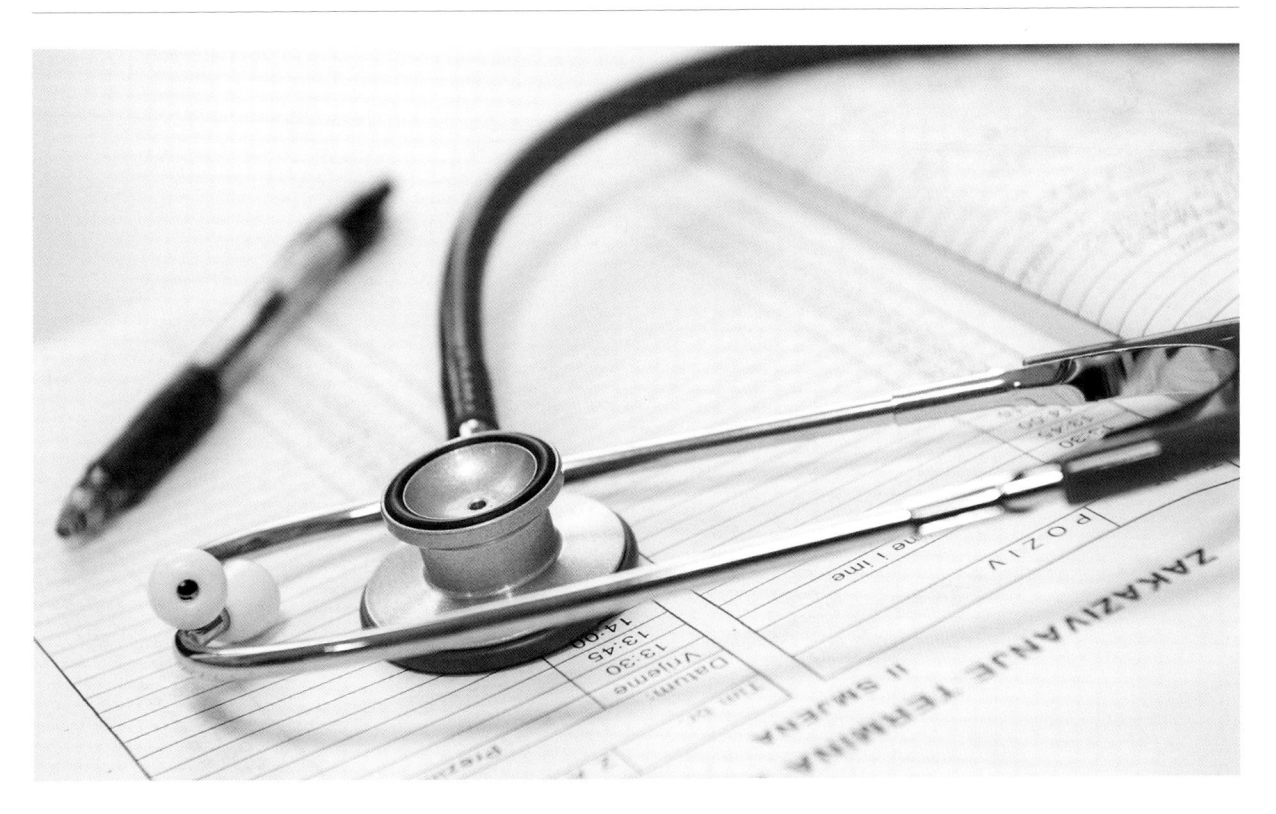

FUTURE LEGACIES

Gregory Patrick Williams, M.D.

Gregory Patrick Williams wanted to be a physician for as long as he can remember. His father, Pat Williams, M.D., was a small town family physician and Williams' role model.

"I remember going on hospital rounds and house calls with him as a youngster. The way he interacted with patients and colleagues became the standard in the way I practiced medicine for nearly 40 years," he says.

Williams graduated from the University of Oklahoma School of Medicine in 1974. During his internship at St. John Hospital in Tulsa, he was greatly influenced by Richard L. Winters, M.D., a family physician in Poteau, Oklahoma. He joined Dr. Winter's practice in 1975 where he stayed for the next five years. He chose to specialize in pathology and completed his residency at Baylor University Medical Center in Dallas, Texas in 1984. He joined the pathology group at Saint Francis Hospital that spring and remained there for 29 years.

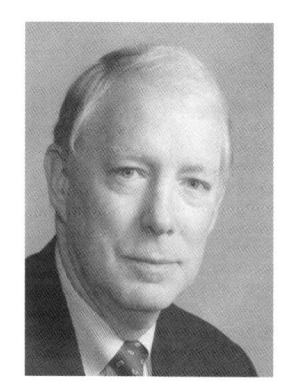

The group has provided pathology services to Saint Francis Hospital since 1965. Its private laboratory, South Tulsa Pathology, and later, Tulsa Medical Laboratory, provides pathology services to physicians on the Saint Francis campus and several smaller hospitals in the Tulsa area. He has seen many advancements and improved technologies that have changed the practice of pathology.

He says, "Major changes during my career include the development of immunohistochemistry to aid in more precise tissue diagnosis and more recently, the development of molecular pathology."

Retired since 2013, Dr. Williams enjoys golfing and spending time in the great outdoors at his vacation home in Durango, Colorado. But mostly, he enjoys spending time with his wife, Connie J. Williams, EdD, their children Ryan, Megan, and Sarah, and four grandchildren.

"It's been a fast 40 years," he says. "I am greatly indebted to my family for their continual support and to the Tulsa County Medical Society for including my story in their history."

Patrons

Linda Goldenstern, M.D.

Phyllis Lauinger, M.D.

David Nierenberg, M.D.

Dan Calhoun, M.D.

IN MEMORIAM

Remembering Those Who've Passed

REMEMBERING THOSE WHO'VE PASSED

In Memoriam
Terrell Covington, Jr., M.D.
(August 25, 1918 - April 13, 2014)

Terrell Covington, M.D. left a legacy in Tulsa's community. A modern thinker, he advocated medical advancement and new specialties, yet upheld tradition and decorum, instilled by parents from established Southern families in Pensacola.

A family man with seven children, thirteen grandchildren, and three great-grandchildren, he never missed school and extra-curricular activities. He was proud of their school accomplishments and involvement in sports and music.

Covington graduated from Washington University (St. Louis) in 1940 and their medical school in December 1943. Drafted during WWII, he served a rotating internship as Second Lieutenant in the Army in Paterson, New Jersey, where he met his first wife, Adriana Sisco, a registered nurse.

After officer's training at San Antonio, First Lieutenant Covington was transferred to Swannanoa, North Carolina where he was ward physician at a temporary hospital, treating soldiers from the Pacific theatre. He cared for many with tropical diseases; the experience was pivotal training for his career as an Internal Medicine-Diagnostician.

As Captain, Covington served at Fort Belvoir, Maryland, as Chief of Medicine. The opportunity to work with Dr. Jonas Salk was a highlight. Together, they administered Salk's flu vaccine to 1500 engineers going overseas. After the war, Covington went to Dallas for a residency program in Internal Medicine at Southwestern Medical School.

In 1950, Dr. Covington moved his family to Tulsa. He officed in the Court Arcade Building and tended patients at three hospitals until early 1970s when St. John Medical Center became his primary hospital. As an advocate of Tulsa's medical community, he served on the teaching staff at St. John and became Chief of Staff in 1971. That year, he married Nancy Findley.

Covington served as VP of the Tulsa County Medical Society; served the Tulsa City-County Board of Public Health for thirty years; was a founding member of the Moton Health Center and president of the Board of Directors. He was a board member of the Tulsa Educational Foundation, working for the development of learning impaired classes. He provided physicals for students in sports. He performed cardiology services for Vinita State Hospital and Hugh Perry Clinic. He ran a pediatric rheumatic heart clinic; and was involved in establishing the Tulsa American Heart Association, serving as president. At retirement, he taught OU-Tulsa medical students how to take patients' history and physicals.

In the 1960s, Covington was called to counsel Washington University on their direction for doctors. He and other internists, including C.S. Lewis, traveled to the nation's capital to meet with congressional leaders to discuss the formation of Medicare.

Dr. Covington was a member of John Knox and then Southminster Presbyterian Churches for fifty years. He taught Sunday school and served as Elder. "Terrell's faith was a big part of who he was. He lived it out by helping all peoples," Nancy shares.

Compassion and attention to every aspect of care were key to Covington's style of medicine. When the children were older, wife Nancy worked as the office's business manager. When asked how he knew why the patient was ill, he'd say, "If you listen, the patient will tell you what the problem is."

Dr. Covington's medical legacy continues through son Christopher, a Tulsa physician, granddaughter Andrea Covington, an internal medicine resident, and two granddaughters, Anna and Emily Moseley, medical students at their grandfather's alma mater, Washington University.

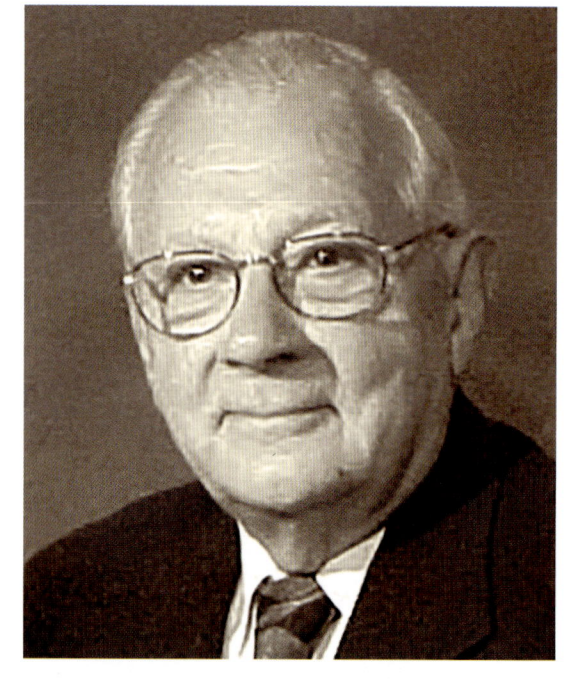

In Memoriam
Floyd F. Miller, M.D.
(March 15, 1930 - August 1, 2011)

"I went in to medicine to help people, not to make money." DR. MILLER

Anyone who knew Floyd Miller, M.D. would agree he served the medical community and his patients well. Yet, growing up he didn't sense a medical calling, but considered a liberal arts focus.

When he was a freshman sociology major at the University of Oklahoma (OU), his mother — who, as a young widow, raised him and his three older sisters alone — was diagnosed with cancer. After her death, he decided to pursue a medical career. He attended OU's medical school then trained at the University of Michigan's (U of M) internal medicine residency program. He was an intelligent and disciplined student — always at the top of his class: valedictorian in high school, in undergrad (a Phi Beta Kappa), and in medical school (an Alpha Omega Alpha).

During the first year of residency, he discovered a gift for treating asthmatics. After residency, he spent a year fellowship in Allergy and Immunology upon the invitation of U of M's chief of Allergy and Immunology.

He served two years at Lackland Air Force Base in San Antonio where he examined the seven Mercury astronauts including John Glenn and Alan Shepard.

During Dr. Miller's first year at Lackland, Dr. Manual Brown, an allergist in Tulsa, recruited him to join in private practice. Just before he was discharged from the Air Force, he was asked to head U of M's Allergy and Immunology service. Since Dr. Miller always kept his word, he declined the university's generous offer and joined Dr. Brown in Tulsa. The two physicians were partners for thirty-six years; when Dr. Brown retired, Dr. Miller remained in practice by himself.

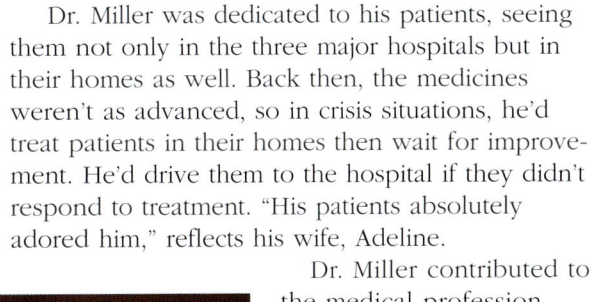

Dr. Miller was dedicated to his patients, seeing them not only in the three major hospitals but in their homes as well. Back then, the medicines weren't as advanced, so in crisis situations, he'd treat patients in their homes then wait for improvement. He'd drive them to the hospital if they didn't respond to treatment. "His patients absolutely adored him," reflects his wife, Adeline.

Dr. Miller contributed to the medical profession, serving as president of the Tulsa County Medical Society and Oklahoma State Medical Association. While president-elect of the state association, he was named to the board of Physicians Liability Insurance Company (PLICO) and served as chair from 1996-2000. He considered his involvement in the formation of PLICO as a great accomplishment in his medical service.

Dedicated to the community, he volunteered one morning a week to staff a free clinic at Hillcrest. His passion, medical contribution, and affable charisma are reflected in the many awards he had received such as the Regents Award through OU and Physician of the Year from the OU College of Medicine Alumni Association. In 2011, the Board of Directors of Tulsa's medical society selected him as their designee for the Oklahoma State Medical Association's Memorial Wall.

Reflecting on her husband's career, Adeline shared how he truly loved people from his patients, his staff, and fellow physicians: "He always had their respect."

He loved his family as well. He and Adeline were married fifty-eight years and were blessed with two sons Mike and his wife, Rainy, Steve and his wife, Lisa, five grandchildren, and four great-grandchildren. ■

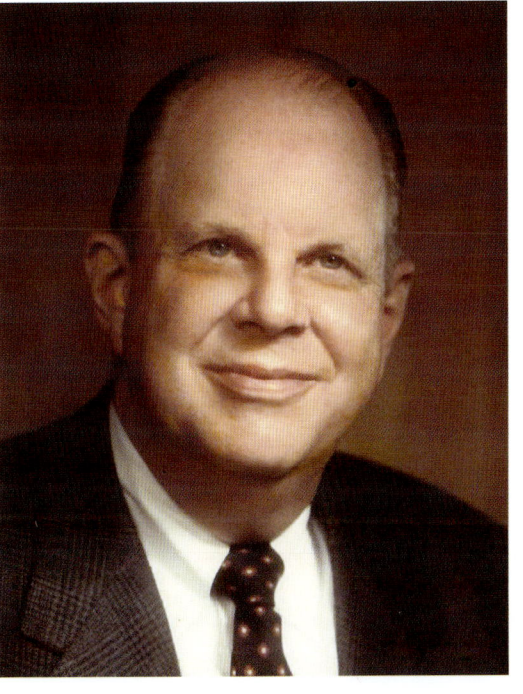

REMEMBERING THOSE WHO'VE PASSED

In Memoriam
Nicholas D Mamalis, M.D.
(September 13, 1952 - June 30, 2011)

Dr. Nicholas D. Mamalis arrived in Tulsa to start his practice in gastroenterology in 1982 at Saint Francis Hospital. He was an active member of the staff for 28 years and founded the Adult Gastroenterology Associates (AGA) and Tulsa Endoscopy Center (TEC), where he worked until his retirement in January 2010 due to health issues.

Dr. Mamalis was born in Knoxville, Tennessee, to the Rev. James and Janet Mamalis on Sept. 13, 1952. He graduated summa cum laude at Spring Hill College in Mobile, Alabama, when obtaining his bachelor's degree. After earning his medical degree from Emory University, Dr. Mamalis completed a residency at Truman Medical Center in Kansas City, Missouri, and fellowship at the University of Alabama-Birmingham. He belonged to several national medical associations and held numerous leadership positions.

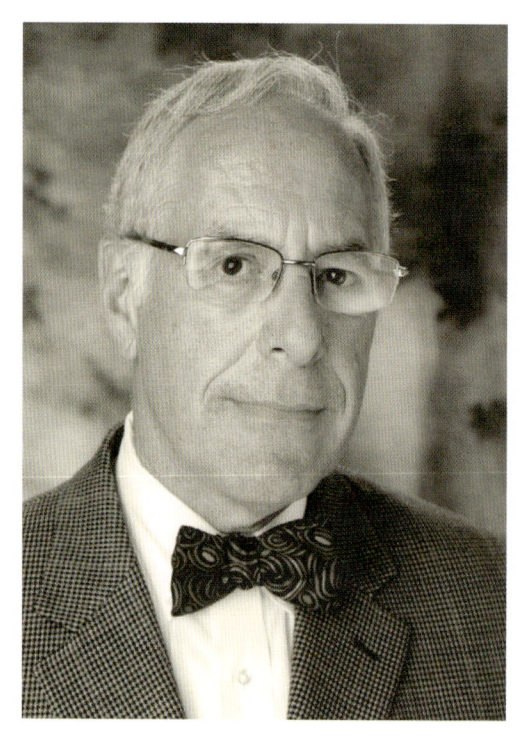

Dr. Mamalis was married to his wife, Carla, for 30 years, and the couple had two daughters, Christina and Stephanie Mamalis. He was an active member of the Holy Trinity Greek Orthodox Christian Church.

As a motorcycle enthusiast, he toured many regions of the U.S. with friends. He also traveled to 35 countries to teach or vacation with family.

Dr. Mamalis died on June 30, 2011. He will always be missed. ∎

We are grateful to these physicians who've passed for leaving an indelible legacy to the Tulsa medical community.

Bibliography

"A History of The Tulsa County Medical Society: An Account of Thirty-Seven Years of Medical Progress By The Physicians of Tulsa County." The Tulsa County Medical Society. 1945. tcmsok.org.

A History of Tulsa Hospitals - 1900-1965. Tulsa County Medical Society. August 1965. tcmsok.org.

"Abortion Agency Opens State Offices." United Press International. *Tulsa World*. Aug. 14, 1971.

"A pain worth bearing." *Tulsa Tribune*. Editorial. Aug. 11, 1988.

"Agency to provide AIDS unit." *Tulsa World*. Feb. 18, 1988.

"Air Ambulance Service Lawsuit Settled." *Tulsa World*. April 29, 1987.

Alzheimer's Association Oklahoma. www.alz.org

American College of Obstetricians and Gynecologists. www.acog.org

American Heart Association. www.heart.org

American Medical Association. www.ama-assn.org

AncestryLibrary.com - U.S. City Directories, 1821-1989. 1921, "Asylums, Hospitals and Homes."

"Ancient Egyptian Medicine," The History Learning Site. www.historylearningsite.co.uk.

Appel, Mary Ellen Ray Storts. Obituary. *Tulsa World*. Nov. 21, 2004.

Archer, Kim, "Center Seeks to Ease Transition." *Tulsa World*. Sept. 15, 1991.

Archer, Kim, "Needed in Health Care." *Tulsa World*. May 22, 2000.

Archer, Kim, "Oklahoma Heart Institute now a part of Hillcrest." *Tulsa World*. April 22, 2008.

Archer, Kim, "St. Francis Hospital closing its heart transplant program." *Tulsa World*. Feb. 22, 2008.

Archer, Kim,"Saint Francis Marks 50th Anniversary." *Tulsa World*. Oct. 1, 2010.

Archer, Kim, "Smokeout Trial Run For Policy." *Tulsa World*. Nov. 21, 1988.

"Arizona's Smoking Ban." *Lewiston Daily Sun*. Sept. 6, 1973.

Arsphenamine, Penicillin. Wikipedia, online. January 2016.

Asher, Gilbert, "Pastor realizes dream, far beyond expectations." *Tulsa World*. Sept. 8, 1949.

Aspinwall, Cary and Ziva Branstetter, "Fallin emails show debates on politics of health-care decisions." *Tulsa World*. Aug. 12, 2014.

"Astonishing revolution under say in U.S. attitude toward birth control." *Tulsa World*. July 6, 1965.

Atkinson, Pat, "Abortion - A Woman's Decision Complicated by Old Laws." *Tulsa World*. Feb. 6, 1972.

Atkinson, Pat, "Computer System, 3 Cities Figure in Kidney Transplant." *Tulsa World*. May 3, 1973.

Atkinson, Pat, "Dedication Ready at St. John's." *Tulsa World*. Feb. 21, 1976.

Atkinson, Pat, "First Phase of $40.3 Million Hospital Program Approved." *Tulsa World*. Jan. 2, 1972.

Atkinson, Pat, "Hillcrest Planning Big New Building." *Tulsa World*. May 5, 1974.

Atkinson, Pat, "Illegal Abortion Terrifying; Legislation Pending." *Tulsa World*. Feb. 7, 1972.

Atkinson, Pat, "Liberalized Abortion Law Seen in Next Legislature." *Tulsa World*. July 19, 1970.

Atkinson, Pat, "Moton Health Center Ready." *Tulsa World*. Feb. 6, 1969.

Atkinson, Pat, "Medicare Payments in Second Year Increase 37.5 Per Cent." *Tulsa World*. June 30, 1968.

Atkinson, Pat, "New Facility to Provide Children Medical Care." *Tulsa World*. Aug. 8, 1976.

Atkinson, Pat, "Number of Kidney Patients to Grow." *Tulsa World*. March 26, 1974.

Atkinson, Pat, "Price Controls Felt By Hillcrest Officials." *Tulsa World*. July 22, 1973.

Atkinson Pat, "Rare Smallpox Vaccine Disease Hits Tulsa Girl." *Tulsa World*. July 21, 1974.

Atkinson, Pat, "3 New Medical Schools Usher In New Tulsa Era." *Tulsa World*. Dec. 7, 1975.

Atkinson, Pat, "Transplanted Kidney Functions Well." *Tulsa World*. Jan. 11, 1973.

Atkinson, Pat, "Tulsa's Medical Students Welcomed." *Tulsa World*. Aug. 15, 1974.

Atkinson, Pat, "Tulsa Osteopathic Displays Historic State License." *Tulsa World*. Sept. 17, 1968.

Averill, Mike, "Life Expectancy gap between ZIP codes in Tulsa County narrows." *Tulsa World*. Step. 3, 2015.

Averill, Mike, "OSU Center for Health Sciences students studying obesity medicine." *Tulsa World*. Jan. 8, 2016.

Averill, Mike, "OSU Center for Health Sciences to begin psychiatric residency program." *Tulsa World*. March 14, 2016.

Averill, Mike, "Price of Alzheimer's, dementia: Physical, financial." *Tulsa World*. April 13, 2016.

Averill, Mike, "Tulsa Health Department to focus on social detriments of health in north Tulsa." *Tulsa World*. July 5, 2016.

Averill, Mike, "Tulsa School of Community Medicine welcomes first class of students." *Tulsa World*. Aug. 24, 2015.

Averill, Mike, "30 years later: After the lawsuit that shut down Hissom, families receiving assistance are thriving." *Tulsa World*. April 26, 2015.

Bachelor, Don, "Retired Woman Osteopathic Nearing 91, Recalls Long, Pleasant Tulsa Practice." *Tulsa World*. Feb. 1, 1958.

Barker, Tim, "Tulsan Gets New Heart at St. Francis." *Tulsa World*. Sept. 25, 1993.

"Bartlett Opens New Hissom Building." *Tulsa World*. June 11, 1968.

Bate, Charles Dr., Junior League of Tulsa historical preservation project. Interview. May 6, 1980. Online. Available through the Tulsa City-County Library, recording and transcribed interview.

"Bell Willing to Set Up '911' System." *Tulsa Tribune*. April 16, 1969.

"Bellmon signs AIDS education bill." *Tulsa Tribune*. April 25, 1987.

"Bellmon vetoes AIDS testing measure." *Tulsa Tribune*. June 3, 1987.

"Birth Control Move Passed." *Tulsa Tribune*. March 15, 1965.

"Birth Control Row Top Religious Story of '59." *Tulsa Tribune*. Dec. 19, 1959.

Blum, David, "Changing Face of Health Care Put Hospitals on Alert for 90s." *Tulsa World*. Jan. 21, 1990.

Blum, David, "Close-knit AIDS Network Growing," *Tulsa World*. Aug. 23, 1987.

Bond, Jo Ann, "Hospitals Await Medicare Impact." *Tulsa Tribune*. June 17, 1966.

Bradshaw, Anita, "Kidney Transplant Landmark Here." *Tulsa Tribune*. Jan. 10, 1973.

Bradshaw, Anita, "St. John's Tower Bid $32 Million," *Tulsa Tribune*. Jan. 25, 1973.

Brown, Wesley, "City's homeless linked to mental illness, drug abuse." *Tulsa World*. Jan 22, 1996.

Brown, Wesley, "TMM dedicates homeless shelter." *Tulsa World*. Oct. 30, 1994.

"Cagelike Cribs Taken to Prison." *Tulsa World*. Nov. 30, 1963.

"Cage-Type Hissom Cribs May Go." *Tulsa Tribune*. Nov. 8, 1963.

Capages, Cheryl, "Whooping Cough Kills Tot." *Tulsa World*. Aug. 1, 1976.

Cartledge, Paul, "Abortion Bill Passes in 26-20 Senate Vote." *Tulsa World*. April 12, 1973.

"Charity Care Report Given." *Tulsa Tribune*. Oct. 8, 1974.

Chase, Winnifred, "School's Best When You Can't Play Like Other Youngsters." *Tulsa World*. April 9, 1945.

"Children's Hospital Wing Dedication Set Sept. 19." *Tulsa Tribune*. July 12, 1953.

"City, County Health Tieup is Completed." *Tulsa Tribune*. February 1950.

"City Hospital Opening Intensive Care Unit." *Tulsa Tribune*. Aug. 2, 1962.

Clinton, Dr. Fred S., "The Indian Territory Medical Association." *Chronicles of Oklahoma*, volume 26.

Clinton, Dr. Fred S., "First Hospitals in Tulsa." *Chronicles of Oklahoma*, volume 22.

Clinton, Dr. Fred S., "Tulsa, Oklahoma." *Journal of the Oklahoma State Medical Association*. May 1910.

Colberg, Sonya, "Tulsa Couple Working To Free Refusenik." *Tulsa World*. Sept. 29, 1988.

"Coming: You May Dial 911 to Call for Help." *Tulsa Tribune*. Jan. 12, 1968.

Community Service Council. Website. www.csctulsa.org.

"County Birth Control Plan Proposed." *Tulsa Tribune*. March 11, 1965.

Cox, Lauren, "The Top Medical Advances of the Decade." ABC News Unit. Dec. 17, 2009. www.medpagetoday.com.

Cracraft, Mary, "Studies find ways to nip allergies in the bud." *Tulsa Tribune*. Nov. 7, 1987.

Curtis, Gene, "Only in Oklahoma: World brought hidden disease into light." *Tulsa World*. May 16, 2007

Curtis, Gene, "Only in Oklahoma: Oral vaccine conquers polio in 1960s." *Tulsa World*. March 11, 2007.

Daxon, Linda, "I suppose I can hold out." *Tulsa Tribune*. Dec. 22, 1976.

Daxon, Linda,"Mother's addiction often passed on." *Tulsa Tribune*. Oct. 31, 1975.

Daxon, Linda, "Pediatric center busy." *Tulsa Tribune*. Nov. 18, 1976.

Daxon, Linda, "Tulsa OU med school branch finds 'home.'" *Tulsa Tribune*. April 7, 1976.

"Dean Takes Psychiatry to the Streets." *OU Medicine*. A publication of the University of Oklahoma College of Medicine. Fall 2003.

Debo, Angie, "Jane Heard Clinton." *Chronicles of Oklahoma*, volume 24.

Deller, Martha, "911 system escapes rash of 'curiosity' calls." *Tulsa Tribune*. May 16, 1980.

Deller, Martha, "911 work goes on." *Tulsa Tribune*. March 2, 1981.

"Demise of smallpox celebrated." *Tulsa Tribune*. May 8, 1980.

"Dental Clinic Plans Drawn." *Tulsa Tribune*. May 1, 1951.

"Doctors' Hospital Co-Founder Dies." *Tulsa World*. June 7, 1996.

"Doctors' Hospital Facilities Please Physicians." *Tulsa Tribune*. July 12, 1966.

"Doctors' Hospital Here Is Purchased." *Tulsa Business Chronicle*. May 16, 1988.

Doenges, Brad, "Less Smoking: Business Smoking Policies Change." *Tulsa World*. Oct. 21, 1982.

"Does polio still exist? Is it curable?" World Health Organization. October 2015. Online, www.who.int.

Doucleff, Michaeleen, "IVF Baby Boom: Births from Fertility Procedures Hit New High." Feb. 18, 2014. National Public Radio.

Douglas, Clarence B., *History of Tulsa: City with a Personality*. Volume I-III. S.J. Clarke Publishing Company. 1921.

Dowd, Tim, "St. John's to Enter Atomic Medical Field." *Tulsa World*. Jan. 7, 1953.

"Drive Begins to Ban 'Doctored' Hamburger." *Tulsa Tribune*. June 3, 1950.

"Dr. Jackson and the Tulsa Riots." *Journal of the National Medical Association*. July-September edition, 1921.

"Dr. McPike at 91 Recalls Pioneer Practice Story." *Tulsa World*. June 27, 1959.

"Dr. McPike Rites Set; Veteran Osteopath." *Tulsa World*. Jan. 17, 1960.

Dunn, Nina, *Tulsa's Magic Roots*. Oklahoma Book Publishing Company. 1979.

"Each Year Brings Increase in Baby Crop at St. John's." *Tulsa World*. April 26, 1954.

Eaton, Kristi, "The da Vinci code." *Tulsa People*. May 2011.

"Emergency? One Number to Call Will be Costly." *Tulsa Tribune*. Feb. 17, 1966.

Endres, Dr. Robert Kendall, "A History of Pediatrics in Tulsa and Eastern Oklahoma." Tulsa County Medical Society. 2009.

Ervin, Chuck, "AIDS bill is vetoed by Bellmon." *Tulsa World*. June 3, 1987.

Ervin, Chuck, "State Bars Discrimination in New AIDS Policy." *Tulsa World*. May 28, 1987.

Erwin, Jane, "Hospital Fitness, Prevention Programs Growing Popular." *Tulsa Business Chronicle*. Nov. 21, 1983.

Everly-Douze, Susan, *Tulsa Times: A Pictorial History*. Photographs from the Beryl D. Ford Collection. World Publishing Company. 1986.

Fallis, Mary Margaret, "Old Mansion Designed for Gracious Living." *Tulsa World*. Sept. 30, 1964.

Fassihi, Theresa Simons, "Building the Perfect You." *Tulsa Tribune*. Jan. 8, 1987.

Fincher, Jack, "New Hospital Plans Bared for Hillcrest." *Tulsa World*. Nov. 12, 1955.

"First Clinic Held for Birth Control." *Tulsa World*. March 18, 1937.

"First St. Francis Baby Named." *Tulsa Tribune*. Oct. 3, 1960.

"$4.5 million in 'Quick Money' will prolong his life, Oral Roberts says." Associated Press. Jan. 10, 1987.

Ford, Brian, "State HIV Cases Must Be Reported." *Tulsa World*. Jan. 29, 1988.

Foresman, Bob, "GP Hospital Construction Planned." *Tulsa Tribune*. June 1, 1964.

Foresman, Bob, "300-Bed St. Francis Hospital Has Operated at a $90,000-a-Month Deficit." *Tulsa Tribune*. May 16, 1961.

Foresman, Bob, "Computers Make Medicare Possible." *Tulsa Tribune*. July 1, 1966.

Fox, Sam, "Physician Arrested in Abortion Raid." *Tulsa Tribune*. March 2, 1972.

Francis, Zoe, "Board Bans Student Smoking at All Tulsa Public Schools." *Tulsa World*. May 21, 1987.

Francis, Zoe, "Cleanup Kits Purchased As AIDS Safeguard." *Tulsa World*. Nov. 22, 1987.

Froeschle, Nora, "Orthopedic hospital coming soon." *Tulsa World*. May 30, 2001.

Gallery of Mayors. City of Tulsa website. www.cityoftulsa.org.

Gibbs, Rachel Dr. Interview. February 2016.

Gibson, Megan, "The Long, Strange History of Birth Control." *Time* magazine. June 2, 2015.

"Girl Recovers From Vaccine Reaction." *Tulsa Tribune*. Nov. 26, 1974.

Gold, Freda, "Hospital to Add New Six-Story, $2 Million Wing." *Tulsa World*. Dec. 29, 1952.

"Gone but not Forgetting." Oct. 15, 1963. *Tulsa World*. Photo and caption.

Graham, Ginnie, "Lawmakers hear of need for mental health parity." *Tulsa World*. March 31, 2007.

Graham, Ginnie, "Mental health crisis teams provide hospital without walls." *Tulsa World*. Aug. 30, 2015.

Graham, Ginnie, "Smokers' lives changed after surgeon general report." *Tulsa World*. Jan. 11, 2014.

Graham, Victoria, "Deadly Pill-Drink Combination on Rise." Associated Press. *Tulsa World*. Oct. 19, 1975.

Gravely, George, "Hissom Center Plans Okayed." *Tulsa Tribune*. April 11, 1961.

Gravely, George, "Hospital Loaded with Latest Gadgets." *Tulsa Tribune*. Sept. 23, 1960.

Gross, Worth M. Dr. and Dr. Harry E. Livingston, "Myra Peters, M.D." Interview for the Tulsa County Medical Society. July 31, 2002.

Habib, Nour, "11 fellows selected for Albert Schweitzer program." *Tulsa World*. March 12, 2016.

Hamilton, Arnold, "Elevator scuffle prompts challenge of smoking law." *Tulsa Tribune*. Dec. 8, 1979.

Hamilton, Arnold, "911 emergency telephone system to begin preparation." *Tulsa Tribune*. April 28, 1980.

Haniotis, Betty, "Gadget Board Aids Polio Victims." *Tulsa World*. June 19, 1953.

Harrison, Kevin, "911 woes: Non-emergencies, pranks tie up vital line." *Tulsa Tribune*. Sept. 29, 1982.

Hayden, Don, "Lawmen probe feasibility of statewide 911 system." *Tulsa Tribune*. July 31, 1980.

"Health Bill is Endorsed by Doctors." *Tulsa Tribune*. March 30, 1945.

"Health Board Approves Program at New School." *Tulsa World*. Jan. 11,1961.

"Health Group Asks $5,000 From Public." *Tulsa Tribune*. Feb. 11, 1947.

Henry, Larry, "Tulsa's 911 Emergency System Attacked in Research Report." *Tulsa World*. Jan. 15, 1982.

Hill-Burton Act of 1946. Wikipedia. Online.

"Hillcrest Board Elders Make Finances." *Tulsa Tribune*. Feb. 14, 1975

"Hillcrest Earns Magazine Honor." *Tulsa World*. Sept. 16, 1976.

"Hillcrest Has $30 Million Expansion Plan." *Tulsa World*. April 23, 1972.

"Hillcrest Medical Center Leader in Kidney Transplants." *Tulsa World*. Jan. 19, 1994.

"Hissom Center Work Under Way." *Tulsa Tribune*. Photo cutlines. Aug. 1, 1961.

"Historic Plan to Broaden Social Security Program Passes 68-12 in Senate." *Tulsa World*. July 10, 1965.

"History of Mental Health Treatment." DualDiagnosis.org. 2016.

"HIV/AIDS Surveillance." U.S. Centers for Disease Control and Prevention. January 1990. www.cdc.gov/hiv.

Hoberock, Barbara, "Oklahoma State Medical Association urges doctors to mull leaving Medicaid over 25 percent rate cut." *Tulsa World*. April 4, 2016.

Horowitz, Dr. Leon, "Let's prohibit another type of leaf burning - tobacco." *Tulsa Tribune*. Jan. 9, 1987.

Horowitz, Dr. Leon, "Think twice before you speak once." *Tulsa Tribune*. Oct. 5, 1987.

Horowitz, Dr. Leon, "Tulsan sees failures of Soviet system." *Tulsa Tribune*. Dec. 9, 1989.

"Hospital Expansion Plan Outlined for Lay Board." *Tulsa Tribune*. Feb. 12, 1953.

"Hospital Model Shows Hillcrest Growth Plan." *Tulsa World*. June 25, 1974.

"Hospital receives Boehm figurines." *Tulsa Tribune*. Oct. 15, 1979.

"Hospitals Anticipating Woes From Medicare." *Tulsa Tribune*. Aug. 2, 1965.

"Hospitals Up County Rate." *Tulsa Tribune*. June 9, 1952.

"Hospitals' suit over Life Flight is settled." *Tulsa Tribune*. April 28, 1987.

"House AIDS-test bill includes prostitutes, clients, inmates." *Tulsa Tribune*. May 28, 1987.

Hower, Bob, "Angels of Mercy." Compilation of memorabilia collection of Maurice Willows from the 1921 Tulsa Race Riot. Printed by Homestead Press. 1993.

"How Tulsa Aids Crippled Children," *Tulsa Tribune*. Oct. 30, 1927.

"Improving Vaccines." *Tulsa World*. Editorial. Nov. 10, 1986.

"Inoculation ordinance to be heard." *Tulsa Tribune*. March 28, 1878.

Jackson, Debbie, "Throwback Tulsa: '70s energy crisis brought gas rationing, 55 mph speed limit." *Tulsa World*. Jan. 14, 2016.

Jackson, Debbie and Hilary Pitman, "Throwback Tulsa: Riverside Drive's long, winding history of controversy." *Tulsa World*. July 16, 2015.

Jensen, Ron, "St. John: 60 years of healing." *Tulsa Tribune*. June 5, 1986.

Jensen, Ron, "Wagoner parents regret AIDS-virus candor." *Tulsa Tribune*. Oct. 28, 1987.

Johnson, Marla, "Test-tube twins best Christmas gift." *Tulsa Tribune*. Dec. 16, 1983.

Jones, Corey, "Saint Francis to house first Oklahoma affiliate clinic of St. Jude Children's Research Hospital." *Tulsa World*. May 20, 2016.

"Junior League Anniversary." *Tulsa World*. Editorial Aug. 24, 1961.

"Junior League Home on Way Up Monday." *Tulsa World*. Aug. 28,1927.

"Junior League Hospital Now is a Community Institution." *Tulsa Tribune*. Oct. 10, 1951.

"Junior League to Keep Home Open on Trial." *Tulsa Tribune*. June 24, 1949.

Junior League of Tulsa, "The Gusher, 40th Annual Anniversary Issue," February 1963.

Kelly, Nellie, "Hillcrest Healthcare System, Doctors Hospital to Close." *Tulsa World*. Nov. 17, 2000.

Kelly, Nellie, "Hillcrest sells tie to SouthCrest." *Tulsa World*. Jan. 2, 2001.

Kelly, Nellie, "Hospital almost finished." *Tulsa World*. Sept. 22, 2002.

"Kidney Stone Crusher OKd For St. John." *Tulsa World*. Oct. 25, 1984.

Killman, Curtis, "Riverside Mansion May Become Bed-and-Breakfast." *Tulsa World*. Sept. 22, 1996.

Kimbrell, Mike, "911 Emergency Line Officially Operating." *Tulsa World*. July 1, 1980.

King, Dennis, "Chronic Abuse Fuels Help Groups." *Tulsa World*. March 27, 1983.

King, Dennis, "Physician Group Wants Smaller Med School Classes." *Tulsa World*. Nov. 24, 1981.

Kita, Natalie, "History of Plastic Surgery." About Health website. www.plastic-surgery.about.com. Oct. 23, 2015.

Koontz, Pat, "Employee Assistance Programs Growing Popular." *Tulsa Business Chronicle*. Aug. 6, 1984.

Krehbiel, Randy and Barbara Hoberock, "Medicaid 'rebalancing' proposal is popular - in theory." *Tulsa World*. April 25, 2016.

Krehbiel, Randy, "Race Riots - The Questions that Remain." *Tulsa World*. Compilation of all coverage. Tulsaworld.com/app/race-riot/timeline.html.

Krehbiel, Randy, *Tulsa's Daily World: A Story of a Newspaper and Its Town*. World Publishing Company. 2007.

Krehbiel, Randy, "TU Names Gerry Clancy President." *Tulsa World*. May 5, 2016.

Lang, Rusty, "Doctors, Nurses Learn Ways to Curb Costs." *Tulsa World*. June 8, 1983.

Lang, Rusty, "Hospitals Plan Eating Disorder Programs." *Tulsa World*. June 21, 1984.

Lang, Rusty, "Hospital to Establish $23 Million Trust." *Tulsa World*. Sept. 25, 1983.

Lang, Rusty, "Kidney Transplants Now Common at Hillcrest Center." *Tulsa World*. July 2, 1984.

Lang, Rusty, "Officials Planning to Sell Doctors' Hospital to Chain." *Tulsa World*. May 25, 1983.

Lawrence, Jon, "Astronauts to 'Coach' Olympics at Hissom." *Tulsa World*. June 26, 1969.

Lawrence, Jon, "Cobalt Bomb and New X-Ray Add To St. John's Cancer-Battling Array." *Tulsa World*. Aug. 28, 1957.

Leaden, Cecil, and Stephen J. Love, "Hospitals to seek end of construction freeze." *Tulsa Tribune*. Feb. 14, 1979.

"League's Home is Permanent." *Tulsa Tribune*. May 19, 1950.

"League Names Home's Board." *Tulsa Tribune*. July 6, 1949.

"League Home's 'Test Period' Shows Gains." *Tulsa Tribune*. Feb. 24, 1950.

Lee, Mark, "AIDS Expert Calls Sooner Cases 'Tip of Iceberg.'" *Tulsa World*. Dec. 15, 1987.

Levine, Ghita, "Increased Medicare Costs to Help Oldsters Bring in New Year of Higher Living Expenses." *Tulsa World*. Dec. 14, 1975.

"Life insurers move toward lower rates for non-smokers." *Tulsa Tribune*. Oct. 22, 1979.

"Life Flight past infancy." *Tulsa Tribune*. Sept 12, 1980.

Litchfield, Yvonne, "Ward for Treatment of Mentally Ill Is Established at Hillcrest Hospital." *Tulsa World*. Nov. 6, 1949.

"Local Leaders Would Keep Smallpox Vaccine Program." *Tulsa World*. Nov. 16, 1969.

"Low-Nicotine Brands Failed To Lower Heart Attack Risks." *Tulsa World*. Feb. 24, 1983.

Lucas, J. Bob, "Medicare to Provide $76 Million in State." *Tulsa Tribune*. Aug. 3, 1965.

Lucas, J. Bob, "Uniform Emergency Call Urged." *Tulsa Tribune*. Oct. 2, 1967.

Lyon, Jared, "The G.I. Bill's Impact on the Past, Present and Future. " University of Syracuse Institute for Veterans and Military Families.

Lyons, Albert, "Medical History - The Seventeenth Century." Online. www.healthguidance.org.

Macklin, Beth, "Courts May Alter State Abortion Law." *Tulsa World*. Oct. 18, 1971.

Macklin, Beth, "Medals, Memories Tumble From St. John Cornerstone." *Tulsa World*. Aug. 31, 1978.

McMahan, Liz, "Parents of AIDS-Infected Boy Hail Favorable Ruling." *Tulsa World*. Nov. 7, 1987.

Marks, Kim Alyce, "All Oklahoma inmates tested for AIDS." *Tulsa Tribune*. Nov. 6, 1987.

Marler, Ralph, "More Rights for Mental Patients Urged by Judge." *Tulsa World*. March 14, 1976.

Matava, Mary Ellen, "Hillcrest, Tulsa Regional to Merge." *Tulsa World*. Oct. 20, 1994.

Martindale, Rob, "State Lags in Handling of AIDS Victims." *Tulsa World*. April 29, 1988.

Mayberry, Dawn Dr. Interview. July 2016.

McAfee, Melinda, "Nurse Uplifts Tulsa's Medical Face." *Tulsa World*. Oct. 26, 1970.

McCune, Arthur, "Playing it safe: Most health care workers opting for protection against AIDS." *Tulsa Tribune*. Aug. 10, 1987.

"Medical school plans second family center." *Tulsa Tribune*. April 18, 1977.

"Medicare Approval Seen for St. Francis After Check." *Tulsa Tribune*. May 17, 1966.

"Medicare Bill Passes House by Wide Edge." *Tulsa World*. April 9, 1965.

"Medicare Expenses Going Up." *Tulsa Tribune*. May 31, 1973.

"Medicare in State Shared by Firms." *Tulsa Tribune*. Feb. 10, 1966.

"Medicare's 1st Birthday Brings Mixed Reactions." *Tulsa World*. Aug. 10, 1967.

"Medicine and Health on the Lewis and Clark Expedition." University of Virginia, the Historical Collections at the Claude Moore Health Sciences Library. Online. exhibits.hsl.virginia.edu.

"Medicine and Health in the 1930s: Overview." DISCovering U.S. History. Student Resources in Context. Nov. 29, 2015.

"Men of Affairs and Representative Institutions of Oklahoma." World Publishing Company compilation. A newspaper reference guide. 1916.

Milam, Cathy and Nick Foltz, "AIDS-Positive Testees' Names to Be Reported." *Tulsa World*. March 17, 1988.

Milam, Cathy, "AIDS: Prevention Through Awareness." *Tulsa World*. Sept. 27, 1987.

Milam, Cathy, "Anonymous AIDS Testing Offered." *Tulsa World*. Feb. 24, 1987.

Milam, Cathy, "Birth of Frozen Embryo Historic." *Tulsa World*. May 15, 1987.

Milam, Cathy, "City Hospitals Cutting Budgets." *Tulsa World*. March 22, 1988.

Milam, Cathy, "Doctors Study New Drug for Stroke Victims." *Tulsa World*. Nov. 6, 1988.

Milam, Cathy, "Experts Urge Tulsa Firms to Develop AIDS Policies." *Tulsa World*. May 27, 1988.

Milam, Cathy, "Group Seeks Home for Local AIDS Victims." *Tulsa World*. Nov. 14, 1986.

Milam, Cathy, "Imager Gives Preview of Face Surgery." *Tulsa World*. Nov. 13, 1988.

Milam, Cathy, "Lasers Aid Hemorrhoidectomies." *Tulsa World*. Aug. 22, 1986.

Milam, Cathy, "Life Flight Suit Filed By Hillcrest." *Tulsa World*. April 2, 1987.

Milam, Cathy, "Many Tested for AIDS Don't Ask Results." *Tulsa World*. Aug. 28, 1987.

Milam, Cathy, "Protein Tested at St. Francis." *Tulsa World*. Dec. 8, 1988.

Milam, Cathy, "Red Cross, Health Department Swamped With AIDS Queries." *Tulsa World*. March 18, 1987.

Milam, Cathy, "Roberts Makes Plea for Med School Aid." *Tulsa World*. Nov. 5, 1985.

Milam, Cathy, "Roberts to Close Hospital, Medical School." *Tulsa World*. Sept. 14, 1989.

Milam, Cathy, "Roberts Raise $3.5 Million, Repeats Death Belief." *Tulsa World*. Jan. 6, 1987.

Milam, Cathy, "Smoking Ban Proponent Says He's No 'Zealot,' Want to Clear Air." *Tulsa World*. March 15, 1987.

Milam, Cathy, "St. Francis Agrees to Manage Okmulgee Memorial." *Tulsa World*. Feb. 21, 1986.

Milam, Cathy, "St. Francis Begins Tests of Drug That Attacks Blood Clot." *Tulsa World*. July 2, 1986.

Milam, Cathy, "Two Tulsa Hospitals to Get Raises in Medicaid Payments." *Tulsa World*. Nov. 10, 1988.

Milam, Cathy, "Weight Loss Reduces Disease Symptoms." *Tulsa World*. Dec. 2, 1987.

"More Than 12 Million Sign Up for Medicare." *Tulsa Tribune*. Feb. 4, 1966.

Morgan, Marjorie, "Polio Shot Neglect Cited Here." *Tulsa Tribune*. Oct. 29, 1974.

Morgan, Marjorie, "Through the 'Mill' with Policewoman." *Tulsa Tribune*. April 8, 1971.

Morgan, Rhett, "Tisdale health clinic has its official opening." *Tulsa World*. Dec. 3, 2013.

Morris, Virginia, "League Incorporates Children's Hospital." *Tulsa World*. June 13, 1961.

"Movie Man First Medicare Applicant," *Tulsa Tribune*. Sept. 2, 1965.

"Mrs. McNulty Dies: Co-Founded Hospital," *Tulsa World*. Feb. 23, 1972.

Muchmore, Shannon, "Access Denied: Oklahoman's Health Care Crisis." *Tulsa World*. Oct. 2, 2011.

Muchmore, Shannon, "Education center open at Wayman Tisdale Center." *Tulsa World*. Dec. 3, 2014.

Muchmore, Shannon, "Mid-level practitioners vital to sustain post-reform health care." *Tulsa World*. Oct. 3, 2011.

Muchmore, Shannon, "OSU Health Sciences Center adding simulation building to west Tulsa campus." *Tulsa World*. March 31, 2015.

Muchmore, Shannon, "Physician shortage contributes to looming health-care crisis." *Tulsa World*. Oct. 1, 2011.

Muchmore, Shannon, "Wayman Tisdale health clinic begins $1.8 million expansion in Tulsa." *Tulsa World*. March 13, 2014.

Myers, Jim, "Bellmon Signs Jail, Non-Smoking Bills." *Tulsa World*. June 25, 1987.

Nascenzi, Nicole, "Ardent cites progress after a year in Tulsa." *Tulsa World*. Aug. 14, 2005.

Nascenzi, Nicole, "St. Francis to build Children's Hospital." *Tulsa World*. Feb. 8, 2005.

"Natalie Warren Dies." *Tulsa World*. Sept. 4, 1996.

National Kidney Foundation. www.kidney.org. May 2016.

"New Station Wagon for Home." *Tulsa Tribune*. Jan. 31, 1946.

"New Technique Is 'Sound.'" *Tulsa Tribune*. Jan. 4, 1961.

"New Wing at St. John's Dedicated With Ceremony." *Tulsa World*. May 17, 1957.

"No Smoking Law Upheld 2-1 by Court." *Tulsa World*. Sept. 4, 1981.

"No surprises: Hospital begins 'pre-admission.'" *Tulsa Tribune*. March 19, 1986.

"90 percent of Tulsans Surveyed Back 911 Back Number." *Tulsa World*. March 19, 1978.

"Oklahoma's Abortion Laws Termed 'Tragic.'" *Tulsa World*. Oct. 27, 1972.

"Oklahoma Alzheimer's State Plan." Feb. 22, 2010. www.alz.org.

"Oklahoma Heart Institute Saves Lives." *Tulsa World*. Feb. 28, 2014.

"Opinion Strikes Down State's Abortion Law." *Tulsa World*. Feb. 1, 1973.

"Oral Roberts tells of talking to 900-foot Jesus." *Tulsa World*. Oct. 16, 1980.

"ORU Med, Law School Plan Questioned." *Tulsa Tribune*. April 29, 1975.

"ORU phasing out school of dentistry." *Tulsa World*. June 22, 1985.

"OU board okays rental for Tulsa med school." *Tulsa Tribune*. Jan. 15, 1976.

"OU Med School Man Scores Abortion Law." *Tulsa Tribune*. July 20, 1971.

"Our History." Morton Comprehensive Health Services. Online. www.morton-health.org. January 2016.

Overall, Michael, "Landmark study sheds light on alcohol abuse." *Tulsa World*. Sept. 23, 1999.

Overall, Michael, "Woman Marks 33rd year as a kidney transplant recipient." *Tulsa World*. Dec. 10, 2007

Painter, Irma, "Children's Hospital Patients Publish Paper, 'Tumbleweeds.'" *Tulsa World*. Feb. 8, 1952.

Parker, John, "AIDS video shown in Broken Arrow not state-approved." *Tulsa Tribune*. Dec. 3, 1987.

Parrott, Susan, "Polio Problem of 50s Shot Fear into Families; Disease Suppressed in the U.S., but Still Threat to the World." *Daily Oklahoman*. June 27, 2004.

Patrick, Imoene, "The Country Doctor." *Oklahoma Today*. July-August 1956.

Pearson, Janet, "Adult Clinic Joins Tulsa's List of Specialized Care Facilities." *Tulsa World*. Aug. 4, 1978.

Pearson, Janet, "Flying Out to Save Lives." *Tulsa World*. Sept. 9, 1979.

Pearson, Janet, "ORU Med School Wins Accreditation." *Tulsa World*. Feb. 17, 1979.

Pearson, Janet, "Return of the Family Doctor." *Tulsa World*. Sept. 4, 1977.

Pearson, Janet, "St. John Votes ORU Affiliation." *Tulsa World*. Sept. 29, 1978.

Pearson, Janet, "Taping of 'Today' Show Follows Hillcrest Program." *Tulsa World*. May 12, 1977.

Peterson, Joyce, "Cuts stymie mental health care." *Tulsa Tribune*. Nov. 18, 1986.

Peterson, Joyce, "Shrinking budgets slow shift away from hospitals." *Tulsa Tribune*. Nov. 18, 1986.

"Pioneering black physician Charles James Bate dies." *Tulsa World*. Feb. 11, 2004.

"Plan Revealed for $4 Million Hospital Here." *Tulsa World*. Dec. 3, 1955.

"Plans revealed for new air ambulance service." *Tulsa Tribune*. Dec. 18, 1986.

"Pollen Count Plan Initiated." *Tulsa World*. Feb. 28, 1975.

"Pre-school immunizations clinic set." *Tulsa Tribune*. July 21, 1977.

Prothro, George W., "Adults also need immunizations." *Tulsa Tribune*. Editorial. Feb. 15, 1984.

Prothro, George, Jr., "Daily room rates hiked at two Tulsa hospitals." *Tulsa Tribune*. Jan. 4, 1978.

Prothro, George, Jr., "Hillcrest won't train ORU med students." *Tulsa Tribune*. Dec. 22, 1977.

Prothro, George, M.D., "History of the Tulsa City-County Health Department (Tulsa Heath Department)." tcmsok.org.

Prothro, George, Jr., "Medicare, Medicaid blamed." *Tulsa Tribune*. May 17, 1978.

Prothro, George, Jr., "ORU dental school opens." *Tulsa Tribune*. Aug. 21, 1978.

Pruitt, Bernadette, "Anti-Smoking Campaign Breathing With Success." *Tulsa World*. Dec. 2, 1982.

Pruitt, Bernadette, "Cosmetic Surgery for Men: Coming Face to Face with Age." *Tulsa World*. July 15, 1984.

Pruitt, Bernadette, "Four Tulsa Hospitals Report Losses." *Tulsa World*. May 15, 1988.

Pruitt, Bernadette, "Girls' Smoking Rate Surges." *Tulsa World*. March 5, 1984.

"Radio series studies school drug abuse." *Tulsa Tribune*. July 21, 1979.

Randle, Judy, "911 Working for Tulsa." *Tulsa World*. March 7, 1982.

Reilly, Joe, "One of Most Modern Out-Patient Clinics In State Will Open at Hillcrest Monday." *Tulsa World*. July 27, 1952.

"Rescue Copters 5th Busiest in U.S." *Tulsa World*. Sept. 18, 1983.

"Retired Surgeon C.D. Beasley, 86, Dies." *Tulsa World*. Aug. 16, 1979.

"Review Team Looks at Moton Center," *Tulsa Tribune*. Aug. 22, 1969.

Ridenour, Windsor, "Hillcrest Fears It May Need to Cut Care." *Tulsa Tribune*. Jan. 28, 1974.

Ridenour, Windsor, "Other Hospitals 'Outbbuild' Hillcrest." *Tulsa Tribune*. Jan. 29, 1974.

Riedel, Dr. Stefan, "Edward Jenner and the History of Small Pox and Vaccination." Baylor University Medical Center, January 2005 newsletter.

"Rigid Check of City Meat is Proposed." *Tulsa Tribune*. June 7, 1950.

Roberts, Rebecca, "Psychiatric hospital gains support." *Tulsa Tribune*. Aug. 22, 1986.

Robson, Nate, "In Pursuit of Breakthroughs in State's Mental Health Coverage." *Oklahoma Watch*. Sept. 19, 2014.

Rolland, Megan, "Gov. Mary Fallin says Oklahoma will not develop health care exchange under Affordable Care Act." *Daily Oklahoman*. Nov. 19, 2012.

Rubinstein, Greg, "Cigarette Ignites Brawl in Elevator." *Tulsa World*. Aug. 3, 1979.

"St. Francis Gets Medicare Okay." *Tulsa Tribune*. June 16, 1966.

Saint Francis 40. The Saint Francis Health System. Published in commemoration of the 50th anniversary of the hospital. 2010.

"St. Francis Hospital raises room rates," *Tulsa Tribune*. July 1, 1975.

"St. Francis Hospital to End First Year Sunday." *Tulsa World*. Sept. 30, 1961.

Sanger, Janett, "Hillcrest Plans Big Physicians Building." *Tulsa World*. June 11, 1954.

"School AIDS policies passed." *Tulsa Tribune*. Sept. 2, 1987.

"School Board Not 'Merging' Health Work." *Tulsa Tribune*. Dec. 3, 1948.

Schriewer, Scott, "Tulsans Who Received a New Lease on Life Prepare for Games." *Tulsa World*. July 20, 1994.

"Sharp Verbal Clashes Erupt in Capital Abortion Hearing." *Tulsa World*. April 8, 1971.

Sheldon, Ruth, "Pitiful Tales Told at Birth Control Center." *Tulsa Tribune*. March 17, 1937.

Sherman, Bill, "Good Samaritan traveling clinic gets third medical truck." *Tulsa World*. Nov. 22, 2014.

Sherman, Bill, "In His Image roots goes back to ORU medical school." *Tulsa World*. July 11, 2015.

Silver, Shawn A., "Thanks, But No Thanks: How Denial of Osteopathic Service in World War I and World War II Shaped the Profession." *Journal of the American Osteopathic Association*. February 2012.

Showman, W.A. Dr. Junior League of Tulsa historical preservation project. Interview. Feb. 5, 1980. Online. Recorded interview available through the Tulsa City-County Library.

"Small Hospitals That Fail Medicare Test May Close Doors." *Tulsa Tribune*. April 14, 1966.

"Smallpox Vaccination Termed Still Needed." *Tulsa Tribune*. April 5, 1972.

"Smoke Stunts Kids' Lungs, Study Finds." *Tulsa World*. Sept. 22, 1983.

"Smokers catch flu more often." *Tulsa Tribune*. Oct. 21, 1982.

"Smoking is linked to specific cancers." *Tulsa Tribune*. Feb. 22, 1982.

"Smoking Says 'Passive Smoking' Harmful." *Tulsa World*. April 17, 1984.

Somersault, Lynne, "ORU Breaks Ground for Med School." *Tulsa World*. Jan. 25, 1976.

Stafford, Melvin R. Dr. "Tulsa Anesthesia: The founding, establishment, growth and progress of anesthesia in Tulsa, Oklahoma, 1927-2004." Self published.

Stanley, Tim, "Physician was a founder of Tulsa's Doctors Hospital." *Tulsa World*. Aug. 25, 2010.

"State AIDS guide backs abstinence." *Tulsa Tribune*. June 23, 1987.

"State May Boost 'Pill' Recipients." *Tulsa World*. Nov. 22, 1968.

"State Popular Target for Traffickers Seeking Pharmaceutical Drugs." *Tulsa World*. Feb. 15, 1988.

"State's first osteopathic doctor dies." *Tulsa Tribune*. Aug. 15, 1979.

Sterling, Dana, "Immunizations lacking." *Tulsa Tribune*. Aug. 9, 1988.

"Structure 'Topped Out.'" *Tulsa World*. Photo caption. July 8, 1978.

Stubler, Elizabeth, "Junior League Hospital Will Add Two Wings." *Tulsa World*. Oct. 11, 1950.

Stubler, Elizabeth, "Polio Gloom Chased at Day Camp." *Tulsa World*. June 27, 1950.

Stubler, Elizabeth, "They'll Have Company at League's Home." *Tulsa World*. Jan. 27,1948.

"Study of Women Smokers Finds High Heart Attack Risk." *Tulsa World*. Nov. 26, 1983.

Stueve, Tracy, "Panel Discussion On AIDS Seeks to Dispel Myths." *Tulsa World*. April 1, 1987.

"Surgery in Depot Recalled as Tulsa Hospitals Hold Open House." *Tulsa World*. May 16, 1963.

Sussman, Barry, "Drug Abuse: It's Still Popular." *Tulsa World*. June 23, 1985.

"Syphilis facts," U.S. Centers for Disease Control and Prevention. Online.

"10,000 for Life Flight." Editorial. *Tulsa World*. Jan. 5, 1987.

"3 Hospitals in Dire Need of Personnel." *Tulsa World*. June 2, 1960.

"350 Attend Dedication Of New Hillcrest Wing." *Tulsa Tribune*. Sept. 22, 1952.

"Tempting Luck." *Tulsa World*. Editorial. Aug. 10, 1988.

"The Pharmaceutical Century: Ten Decades of Drug Discovery," American Chemical Society. Online publication. 2000. www3.uah.es/farmamol.

"They Make Family Hospital a Reality." *Tulsa Tribune*. Aug. 26, 1966.

Timeline of HIV/AIDS. Wikipedia. May 2016.

"Tiny Beauty Salon Worth Weight in Gold at Children's Hospital." *Tulsa Tribune*. April 11,1953.

Tobacco Settlement Endowment Trust. History. Website. www/ok.gov/tset/About_Us/History/
http://ok.gov/tset/About_Us/History/

Troy, Frosty, "Birth Control Bill Given Senate Okay." *Tulsa Tribune.* Feb. 13, 1967.

True man, C.N., "Medicine And World War Two." The History Learning Site. Online. historylearningsite.co.uk. March 6, 2015, and Dec. 16, 2015.

Tulsa CARES. www.tulsacares.org.

Tulsa Day Center for the Homeless. Tulsadaycenter.org.

"Tulsa Doctor Arrested in Lake Abortion Raid." *Tulsa World.* March 26, 1972.

"Tulsa Health Unit is Given Federal Grant," *Tulsa Tribune.* Nov. 26, 1968.

Tulsa Life Flight. Pamphlet from the dedication ceremony. Oct. 7, 1979.

"Tulsa 911 Into Action Thursday." *Tulsa World.* April 20, 1980.

"Tulsans Again Seek Funds for Planned Birth." *Tulsa World.* Jan. 31, 1949.

"Tulsa's Regional Picks First Female Chief of Staff." *Tulsa World.* Jan. 27, 1994.

"Tulsa Solon Plans New Abortion Bill." *Tulsa Tribune.* Jan. 23, 1973.

Turk, Jay, "Health War Hot: The Faces of Moton." *Tulsa Tribune.* July 29, 1969.

Turk, Jay, "Moton Booming." *Tulsa Tribune.* April 7, 1969.

"Two new medical office buildings announced." *Tulsa World.* Dec. 15, 1999.

University of Oklahoma-Tulsa Schusterman Center, website, OU.edu.

Upton, Pat, "Oral Roberts Opens City of Faith." *Tulsa World.* Nov. 2, 1981.

"U.S. Says Immunization in Oklahoma Inadequate." *Tulsa Tribune.* Jan. 19, 1973.

Vance, Ray, "Health Care - It's also a Business." *Tulsa World.* Aug. 28, 1977.

Vance, Ray, "It's Complex, but Hillcrest Trades Old Bonds for New to Save Millions in Interest." *Tulsa World.* July 31, 1972.

Vietnam, Warren, "Q&A: What Obamacare Ruling Means for Oklahomans." *Oklahoma Watch.* June, 25, 2015.

"Venereal Disease and Treatment During World War II." U.S. Medical Research Center, World War II. Online, www.med-dept.com/articles. January 2016.

"Lloyd Verret." Obituary. *Tulsa World.* Dec. 26, 2007.

Ward, Steve, "Non-smoking jurors want isolation." *Tulsa World.* Sept. 3, 1981.

"Warning Issued About Smallpox." *Tulsa World.* April 11, 1973.

Watkins, Bob, "Tulsa's Health Is Better Than Other Cities in State." *Tulsa Tribune.* Dec. 25, 1957.

Watkins, Bob, "You Name It ... New Hospital Has It." *Tulsa Tribune.* March 26, 1960.

Wehrs, Roger, M.D., "The History of Otolaryngology in Tulsa, Oklahoma, 1950-1970." tcmsok.org.

Wesley, George, "Police Hit Suspected Tulsa Abortion Ring; Trio Detained in Jail." *Tulsa World.* Nov. 14, 1970.

Wheat, Chuck, "Machine to Ease Woes at Hospital." *Tulsa World.* Jan. 24, 1962.

Wheat, Chuck, "Medics Gear for Flood,Then Wade Into Trickle." *Tulsa World.* July 2, 1966.

Wheat, Chuck, "Project Starting In Fall To Double Hospital's Size." *Tulsa World.* July 12, 1964.

Wheat, Chuck, "Retarded Minds Can Work, Too." *Tulsa World.* May 3, 1962.

Wheat, Chuck, "Sonar 'Sounds' Skulls." *Tulsa World.* July, 30, 1964.

"Whooping cough immunization available." *Tulsa Tribune.* Aug. 2, 1976.

Wimer, Jack, "911 plan costly, 'slow,'" *Tulsa Tribune.* Oct. 27, 1978.

Wittkopp, Pear, "Abortion Fight Gets Push Here." *Tulsa Tribune.* Aug. 5, 1970.

"W.K. Warren, Philanthropist, Oilman Dies." *Tulsa World.* June 12, 1990.

Williams, Grant, "Brighter future seen for Roberts organization." *Tulsa Tribune.* Dec. 29, 1986.

Winslow, Laurie, "Breaking Ground." *Tulsa World.* Sept. 16, 1997.

Winslow, Laurie, "Doctors close door on past." *Tulsa World.* May 10, 1998.

Winslow, Laurie, "Focus: Finding new ways to treat Alzheimer's." *Tulsa World.* Sept. 27, 1999.

Winslow, Laurie, "Hospitable hospital." *Tulsa World.* Feb. 2, 1999.

Winslow, Laurie, "Jail Panel Discusses Mentally Ill Prisoners." *Tulsa World.* Sept. 8, 1995.

Winslow, Laurie, "More Men Turning to Plastic Surgery," *Tulsa World.* July 11, 1988.

Winslow, Laurie, "New Alzheimer's center dedicated." *Tulsa World.* Sept. 3, 1999.

Winslow, Laurie, "Oh, baby, it's open." *Tulsa World.* May 4, 1999.

Winslow, Laurie, "Oklahoma not a healthy place, report says." *Tulsa World.* March 4, 1999.

Winslow, Laurie, "Physician assistant field grows as health law adds to patient volume." *Tulsa World.* Feb. 2, 2014.

Winslow, Laurie, "Summers were a time of fear." *Tulsa World.* July 6, 1997.

Winslow, Laurie, "Tulsa health care sector provides massive economic impact." *Tulsa World.* Feb. 2, 2014.

Wiseman, Mary C., and Tom M. Campbell, "Dreams, Challenge and Change: A History of Oklahoma Osteopathic Hospital and Tulsa Regional Medical Center." A project by the public relations department of Tulsa Regional Medical Center. 1994.

Wolfe, Ron, "Lying, drug abuse go together, father learns." *Tulsa Tribune.* Aug. 28, 1981.

Wood, Tom, "Memory of Full Life in Pioneer Tulsa Strong for Osteopath as She Turns 90." *Tulsa World.* Feb. 4, 1958.

Wood, Tom, "Sunny Day Sets Tone of Heath Center Dedication." *Tulsa World.* April 28, 1969.

Wood, Tom, "Three Scoops From Earth Symbolize Start of City of Hope for Retarded." *Tulsa World.* July 2, 1961.

Wright, Muriel H., and Joseph B. Thoburn, *Oklahoma: A History of The State and Its People.* Lewis Historical Publishing Company, Inc. New York. 1929.

Wright, Muriel H., "A Brief Review of the Life of Doctor Eliphalet Nott Wright (1858-1932)." *Chronicles of Oklahoma,* volume 10.

"X-ray in the Round." *Tulsa Tribune.* Photo with caption. Oct. 6, 1961.

"Young Polio Patients Find Novel Gym Aid in Recovery." *Tulsa Tribune.* Feb. 23, 1953.

Zubeck, Pam, "Hillcrest closes unit as protest." *Tulsa Tribune.* Aug. 18, 1988.

Photo Credits

Sources used and the photo's page number (and identifying locations where appropriate) are as follows:

Abandoned OK.Com:
99

Allergy Clinic of Tulsa:
92, 93

American College of Osteopathic Surgeons:
35

Charles Bate's book, *It's Been A Long Time:*
57 (middle)

Children's Medical Charities Association:
81

Clarence B. Douglas's book, *History of Tulsa* **
61 (bottom)

Flickr:
7 by Tulsa Topics at https://flic.kr/p/69ahY,
9 (bottom) by JymPoiranges at https://flic.kr/p/s7r3CH,
87 by Zeiss Microscopy at https://flic.kr/p/bpYfH6,
124 by Scott & White HealthCare at https://flic.kr/p/nKoxRW,
160 by Wellcome Images at https://flic.kr/p/9RQsr9

Greenwood Cultural Center:
32

Hillcrest HealthCare System:
36 (all), 37 (all), 53, 70, 79, 132-133, 170, 171, 209 (all), 211

In His Image:
203, 218

Library of Congress:
6-7, 48, 59 (top), 86

National Archives Catalog:
51

National Institutes of Health:
59 (bottom), 87 (bottom. Flickr at https://flic.kr/p/MsLaBG), 89, 155, 177 (https://flic.kr/p/CAWSxQ), 181, 215 (Flickr at https://flic.kr/p/JzoLak)

Oklahoma Historical Society:
4

Oral Roberts University:
111, 112, 121, 122, 123, 141, 142, 143

Oklahoma State Department of Health:
156

OSU Medical Center & Library:
46, 47***, 64***, 65***, 76***, 78, 126 (top)***, 173

OSU Center for Health Sciences:
Dust Jacket Front (middle pic), 167, 200, 205, 206

OU-TU School of Community Medicine & Library:
Dust Jacket Front (top pic), 63, 96, 116, 117, 118, 119, 128, 182, 198, 199, 203

Saint Francis Health System:
91, 94, 95 (top), 107, 126 (bottom), 129, 130 (all), 150, 168-169, 174, 178-179, 191, 212, 213

Courtesy of Dr. Simcoe:
165

St. John Health System:
29 (all), 83, 114, 115, 139, 193, 210

Courtesy of Tulsa City-County Library, The Beryl Ford Collection:
8 (all), 9 (top), 10, 11, 12 (top), 14, 15, 16, 17, 18, 19, 21, 23, 26 (top), 27 (cover), 28, 33 (bottom), 38 (all), 40, 42-43, 44, 49 (top), 50, 52, 54, 58, 68 (all), 69 (all), 71, 73, 77, 84, 85, 90, 100, 101, 113

Courtesy of Tulsa City-County Library, The African American Resource Center Collection:
30, 31 (bottom)

Courtesy of Tulsa City-County Library, Developing Tulsa: The Austin Hellwig Collection:
140

Tulsa County Medical Society:
39 (all), 45 (bottom), 49 (bottom), 55, 56 (all), 57, 59 (middle), 61(top), 75, 95 (bottom), 103, 137, 151, 184

Tulsa Day Center for the Homeless:
180

Tulsa Historical Society:
5 (cover), 12 (bottom), 20, 22, 24-25, 26 (bottom), 31 (top), 33 (top),

University of Tulsa:
Dust Jacket Front (bottom pic),

Wikipedia:
2, 3 (all), 41 (cover), 45 (top right), 60, 62, 67, 88, 104-105, 108, 109, 134, 158, 163, 176, 195, 217, 218

Thank you for sharing your photos and helping Tulsa County's medical history come alive!

NOTES:
* Full credit for the book *It's Been a Long Time*:
Bate, Charles James. *It's Been a Long Time (and We've Come a Long Way): a History of the Oklahoma Black Medical Providers, the Black Healers.* Tulsa, Oklahoma: Acorn Printing Press, 1986.

**Full credit for the book *History of Tulsa* in Bibliography

***Full credit for the book *Dreams, Challenge and Change* in Bibliography

Index

*Bold entries denotes photos

911 phone system, 146, 147, 148

A

Abbey, Paul, 207
Abbott, Matthew, 199
Abortion, 135, 136, 137, 138
Adcock, David, 135
Adelson, Tom, 300
Aesthetic Surgery Institute of America, 227, **227**
Aetna, 102
Affordable Care Act, 194, 195, 196, 197, 202, 208
AIDS/HIV, 140, 152, 153, 154, 155
Aikman, Robert Dr., 251
Albert, Erick, 11
Albert Schweitzer Fellowship, 206
Alexander, Leeland, 276, 277
Allen, Thomas W. Dr., 281
Allergy Clinic of Tulsa, 92, 93, **93**, 230, **230**, 231, **231**, 232, 233, **233**
Alzheimer's Center of Tulsa, 177
American Academy of Pediatrics, Oklahoma chapter, 216
American Association of Railroad Surgeons, 15
American College of Osteopathic Hospital Administrators, 78
American College of Osteopathic Surgeons, 35
American Dental Association, 72, 122
American Hospital Association, 45
American Medical Association, 3, 9, 14, 44, 48, 63, 66, 72, 85, 104, 136
American Osteopathic Association, 45, 63
American Red Cross, 23, 31, **31**, 33, 34, 65, 172
Anderson, Lloyd Dr., 242
Andrews, Mason Dr., 236
Anesthesia Services, 45
Apffel, Richard Dr., 70
Appel, Mary Ellen Storts, 148
Apple Orchard Hospital, 11
Aran, Peter Dr., 225
Archer, Robert L. Dr., 117
Ardent, 171, 173
Armstrong, Max Dr., 73
Arnold, Karen, **230**
Ashcroft, Thomas L. Dr., 110
Askins, Jari Lt. Gov., **220**
Associated Anesthesiologists, 110, 210, 274
Atchley, R.Q., 97
Atkins, Jack O. Dr, 55
Atkins, Walter Dr., 100
Ayoub, Catherine, 133

B

Bailey Medical Center, 170, 171, 208, **209**
Bailey, Claude, 73
Baldwin, Howard C. Dr, 63, **64**
Banner, William Dr., 214
Barnett, Howard, 281
Barnum, Mike and Paul, 169
Barson, John Dr., 280, **280**, 281, **282**
Bass, Haskell H. Dr, 166
Bate, Charles Dr., 57, 57
Bauer, Louis H. Dr., 85
Baxter, L.C., 64, **64**, 69, **69**, 76, **76**, 77, 78
Baxter, Michael Dr., 185

Beal, Jeffrey A. Dr., 154
Beaman, Jason Dr., 201
Beasley, Joli (Farmer), 243, 244, **245**
Beasley, Todd Dr., 243, **244**
Bell, William H., 133
Benign, Paul F. Dr., 63
Benner, Benjamin Dr., 272, **272**, 273, **273**
Bennett, Howard Dr., 110, 268
Berger, Edwin Dr., 169
Bernier, Ralph Dell, 119
Berry, Charles Dr., 191
Besser, Mr. and Mrs. James T. and Robert, 8, **8**
Billings, Anthony Dr., 272, **272**, 273
Binstock, Marcel Dr., 228, **228**
Birnie, Sallie, 12
Birth Control, 48, 49
Biscup, Walter, 60
Black Wall Street, 25, 30
Blackburn, George, 161
Blackwell, Judith Dr., 302, **302**
Bland, Wayne Dr., 157
Blankenship, Robert Dr., 110
Block, Robert "Bob" Dr., 119, 157, 158, **184**, 184, 185, 228, 238, 300
Blue Cross Blue Shield, 45, 54, 78, 102, 104
Boedeker, Daniel Dr., 272, 273, **273**
Booker, W.P. Dr., 7
Boone, Brad Dr., **274**
Boren, David L., **277**
Bowyer, Frank Dr., 122, 123
Boyer, Jenny Dr., 225
Boyls, Kathleen Dr., 251
Braesfield, John, 97
Brannin, Dan Dr., 189
Bridgewater, R.T. Dr, 31, 32
Brockman, Todd Dr., 225, 229, **229**
Brooks, Harold, 169
Brown, Kathryn Dr., **230**, 231, 232, 233
Brown, Leonard Dr., 263
Brown, Manual Dr., 311
Brown, Paul Maj. Dr., 31
Brownlee, Albert Dr., 229, **229**, 301
Brownlee, Stephen Dr., 240
Brownson, Richard Dr., 125
Bruce, Robert, 19
Brunton, Mimi, 124
Bundren, J. Clark Dr., 159, 236, **236**, 237, **237**
Burge, Joe Dr., 256
Burman, Don, 210, 211
Burnett, Glenn, 156
Burton, Carney A., 102
Butler, G.H. Dr., 25
Butler, Jennifer Dr., 302, **302**

C

Calabrese, Kenneth Dr., 169
Caldwell, George Dr., 127, 218, **220**, 234, **234**
Calhoon, Ed Dr., 136
Calhoun, Dan Dr., 308
Calvert, Jon Dr., 251
Campbell, John Dr., 125
Cancer Treatment Centers of America, 210
Capehart, John, 97
Cardiovascular Surgery Inc., 126, 265
Carney, Andre B. Dr., **69**

Carney, Michael P. Dr., 169
Carr, John and Ord, 8
Cash, James, Dr., **274**
Central States Orthopedic Specialists, 210
Chasteen, Jeffrey Dr., 251
Childers, Emil Dr., 251
Children's Advocacy Center, **182**
Children's Medical Center, 34, 62, **63**, 82, 168, 169, 216
   Saint Francis, **212**, 216,
Choctaw Nation, tribal board, 4
Christy-Owens, Angela Dr., 251
Clancy, Gerald "Gerry" Dr., 199, 204, 207, 304, **304**
Clark, John Dr., 203, 267
Clayton, Charles, 119
Clifton, Curtis Dr., 97, 251
Clingan, Rodney L. Dr., 235, **235**
Clinton, Fred Dr., 8, 9, 10, 11, 12, 13, 14, **14**, 15, 16, 20, 21, 22, 24
Clinton, Jane, 15, **15**, 16
Cloud, William Robert, 137
Coates, Chase, 243, **243**
Coates, Sarah, **244**
Coburn, Zachary Dr., 235
Cohen, Fredrick (Rick) Dr., 238, **238**
Cohlma, George Dr., 110
Coldwell, James G. Dr., 216, 218, 301, **301**
Cole, Christopher L. Dr., 299, **299**
Cole, Kali (Farmer) Dr., 243, **244**, 245
Cole, Scott Dr., 243, **244**
Coleman, Todd, **230**
Collins, David M. Dr., 251
Columbia HCA/Healthcare, 171, 172
Compton, Paul Dr., 235
Condrin, William R. Dr., 235, **235**
Conrad, Robert S. Dr., 281
Convalescent Home for Crippled Children, 80, 81, **81**
Conway, W.Q., 25
Cook, Albert W. Mrs., 80, 222
Cooper, Charlie Dr., 238
Cooper, Donald L. Dr., 137
Cotham, Phyllis, 169
Cottrill, Eric Dr., 225
Council of Hospitals, 15
Covington, Terrell Dr., 310, **310**
Cowan, Jane, 230
Cox, Doug Dr., 127, 128, 196
Cravens, Jere Dr., 300
Crockett, Sherry, 266
Crouch, John Dr., **204**, 246, 247, **247**

D

Daley, Patrick Dr., 241, **241**
Dargatz, Jan Dr., 143
Dart, Bruce, 207
Davidson, G.W., 151
Davis, Nathan Dr., 3, **3**
Day, Charles Dr., 37
Deardorff, Max Dr., 136, 239, **239**
Deckert, Gordon Dr., 192
DeSilva, Nirupama Dr., 302, **302**
Denniston, Joseph Dr., 99
Detwiler, Karl Dr., 210, 272, **272**, 273, 274
Dickson, Warren Dr., 183, 186
Dietz, Melissa Dr., 306, **306**

Dixon, Richard Dr., 160, 296
Doctors' Hospital, 96, **96**, 97, 110, 129,144, 146, 168, 170, 171, 172, 182
Dodson, Thomas Dr., 125, 163
Doss, Nannie, 85, 86
Douglass, Clarence, 21, 22
Drug abuse, 157, 158, 159
Duffy, Daniel F. Dr., 121
Duininck, Mitch Dr., 203, 217, **218**, 247
Dunlap, E.T., 280, **280**

E

Eastern Oklahoma Ear, Nose and Throat (EOENT), 240, **240**, 278
Eastern Oklahoma Orthopedic Center, 210
Eimen, Michael Dr., 169
Elgin, Donald, 119
Endres, Robert "Bob" Dr., 56, 216, 261, 301, **301**
England, John, 119
Ensley, Douglas Dr., 191
Estill, Paul, 65
Ewell, William, 97

F

Fallin, Mary Gov., 177, 189, 194, 195, 197, **222**
Family Medical Care of Tulsa, 217, 246, **246**, 247, **247**
Farmer, Chad Dr., 243, 244, **244**, **245**
Farmer, Charles (Bo) Dr., 242, **242**, 243, **243**, 244, **244**, 245, **245**
Farmer, Sheri, 242, 243, **243**, 244, **244**, 245, **245**
Fell, David Dr., 211, 217, 272, **272**, 273, **273**
Ferguson, Rick, 275
Fernandes, John J. Dr., 281
Fetter, Charles D., 137, 138
Fieker, Dan Dr., 154, 225
Fielding, Allen Dr., 272
Finley, Roy, 97
First babies, 8
First incorporated hospital, 11
First licensed osteopathic physician in Oklahoma, 35
First nurses, 12
First post office, 7, **8**
Fisher, Kevin T. Dr., 299, **299**
Follansbee, Charles, 69
Fore, Frank Dr., 110
Forest, Herbert Dr., 263
Fortner, Benjamin F. Dr., 8, 9, 10
Foster, Michael Dr., 251
Foulks, Charles Dr., 208
Founders of Doctors' Hospital, 172
Frame, Lynn Dr., 221, 225, 239, 306, **306**
Freeman, Richard, 125
Freewill, L.J., **69**
Fried, Mark, 178
Frissell Memorial Hospital, **24**, **25**, 31
Fugate, Colony, 201
Fuller, Munson, 125
Fuquay, Maurice, 124

G

Galen, Claudius, 2, 3
Galles, Jeffrey Dr., 222, 225, 248, **248**
Gallo, Robert C. Dr., **104**, **105**
Galusha, Harley Dr., 125, 126, **126**
Garber, Bradley Dr., **221**, 241, **241**
Garcia, Vanessa, 206
Garrett, Robert Dr., 110, 249, **249**
Gary, Walter, Dr., 235
Gates, Allen, 158

Gates, William, 65
Geffen, William Dr., 176, **221**, 225, 300
Gennis, M.H. Dr., **69**
Gheen, Del Dr., 301
Giant, Zach, 207
Gibbens, Jennifer Dr., 302, **302**
Gibbs, Rachel, Dr., 217, 250, **250**
Gillock, Gail, **221**
Gillock, Thomas Dr., **274**
Glaze, Kathleen Dr., 259
Glenn, John, 311
Gold, Rachel, 206
Goldenstern, Linda Dr., 259, 308
Goldthorpe, John C., 145, 168, 169
Good Samaritan Health Services, 203, 204, **204**, 218
Graham, Hugh Dr., 39, **39**
Graham, Hugh, Jr. Dr., 39, **39**
Great Depression, 42, 43
Greenberg, Martin Dr., 157
Grewe, Terry Dr., 169
Griffin, Michael W. Dr., 299, **299**
Griffiths, David Dr., 251
Grogg, Stanley Dr., 281
Grosshart, Ross Dr., 22, **22**, 25, 40
Grosshart Sanitarium, 22, 25, **26**
Group Hospital Service of Oklahoma, 54
Guiliano, Larissa Dr., 251
Gustafson, Gerald Dr., 95, **95**, **221**, 225, 298
Gwartney, Warren, 97, 251

H

Hagar, Kenneth, 150
Haglund, Roger V. Dr., 124, 250, **250**
Hall, Charles H. Dr., 37
Hall, David Dr., 240
Hall, H.C. and J.M., 7, 8
Halladay, James Dr., **64**
Halliday, John E. Dr., 63
Hamilton, Carl Dr., 122
Hamilton, Frank Dr., 247
Hammans, Carol, 59
Hampton, Carl Dr., 123
Hancock, Taylor Naomi, 171
Haney, T. Paul Dr., 70, 72
Hargis, Burns, 283
Harmon, Charles Kemper Dr., 254, **254**, 255
Harper, David Dr., 303
Harris, David Dr., **222**, 225
Hart, M.O. Dr., 97
Harth, C.P. Dr., 63, **64**
Harvard Family Physicians, 218, 251, **251**
Harvey, James, 84, 123, 129, 132, 151
Harwell, Bill, 125
Hastings, Barbara Dr., 103, 259
Haswell, Glenn Dr., 259
Haugh, Michael J. Dr., 225, 255, **255**
Hawley, S.D. Dr., 25
Hays, Anna "Luverne" Dr., 55, **55**
Health disparities, 202, 203, 204, 205, 206, 207
Heart transplants, 191, 192
Heasley, C.D. "Pop" Dr., 34, 35, **35**, 45, 46, 63, **69**, 280
Heatherington, J. Scott Dr., 281
Hedrick, Paul, 65
Heffron, Kathleen Dr., 302, **302**
Heinberg, Charles, 125, 240, 278
Helmerich, Walter H., 133, 151
Henrie, W.J. Bryan Dr., 137

Henry, Jake Jr., 213, 214, 293
Henthorn, Randall, 119
Henthorn, Sharon Manor, 119
Herman, James Dr., 199, 276, **276**, 277
Hershey, Lynn, 204
Hess, James, 198
Hidy, Dean Dr., 298
Hill, Gary, 119
Hillcrest Infertility Center, 159, 160
Hillcrest Medical Center, 1, 22, 23, 36, 39, 56, 58, **58**, 59, **70**, 73, 76, **79**, 82, 84, **84**, 85, 94, 97, 102, 103, 104, 110, 119, 122, 123, 124, 125, 129, 131, 132, 133, 137, 145, 146, 150, 151, 156, 158, 160, 161, 163, 168, 169, 170, **170**, 171, 172, 173, 208, 210
Hillcrest Pregnancy Center, 206
Hillcrest South, **171**
Hillcrest Specialty Clinic, 210
Hippocrates, 2, 3
Hissom Memorial Center for the Mentally Retarded, 98, 99, **99**
Holley, Leroy and Mrs., 94
Holmes, Dan P., 65
Holmes, June Dr., 259
Homeward Bound, 99
Hooser, Wallace C., 225, 252, **252**
Horowitz, Betsy, 92, 93
Horowitz, Leon Dr., 56, 92, **92**, 93, 230, 231, 232, 233
Houlihan, Rodney Dr., 281
Howard, Paul Dr., 162, 163
Howell, Joseph W. Rev., 151
Hubbard, Charles, 23, 24, 25
Hubbard, Charlotte Moton, 101
Hubner, John Dr., 225
Hudkins, Bruce Dr., 253, **253**
Hudson, David V. Dr., 70, 74, 75
Hudson, Margaret Dr., 70, 74, 75, **75**
Hudson, Robert Dr., 160
Hughes, Pat Dr., 300, 301
Hum, Margaret Dr., **213**
Humphrey, Bill, 128, 129
Humphreys, Buel Dr., 97
Hurewitz, David Dr., 230, **230,** 231, 232, 233

I

Imphotep, 2
Inbody, Donald Dr., 161
Indian Territory, 6, 7, 11
Indian Territory Medical Association, 8, 14, 220
Influenza outbreak of 1918, 21, 23, 24
In His Image, 217, 218, 246, **246**, 247, **247**
Insurance programs, 43, 44, 45, 194, 195, 196, 197
Ivey, Reggie, 207

J

Jackson, Andrew C. Dr., 32, **32**
Jackson, Bill Dr., 200
Jackson, Claudia, 300
Jackson, Ronald Dr., 299, **299**
Jakubovitz, Jim, 266
James, J. Frank, 179
Jarolim, Kirby I. Dr., 281
Jenkins, Edward W. Dr., 256, **256**
Jenkins, Meredith, 273
Jenkins, Woody Dr., 196
Jennings, Hal B. Dr., **163**
Jensen, Clyde B. Dr., 281, **282**
Jewell, Maggie, 133

Jobe, Virgil Dr., 138
John Hope Franklin Reconciliation Center, 34
Johnson, Craig S. Dr., **274**, 299, **299**
Johnson, E.S. Jr., **69**
Johnson, Lyndon President, **89**, 101
Johnson, Paul I., 65
Johnson, Robert, 119
Jones, Craig, 197
Jones, Georgia Lloyd, 49, 94
Jones, Howard W. Jr Dr., 236
Jones, Janet Dr., 251
Jones, Janice, **33**
Jubelirer, Bill Dr., 300
Junior League Convalescent Hospital, 34, 81
Junior League of Tulsa, 29, 34, 62, 80, 81, 82

K
Kamp, George H. Dr., 257, **257**
Katsis, Steven B., 225, 299, **299**
Keller, Alan Dr., 166
Kelly, James Dr., 263
Kennedy, Bill Dr., 300
Kennedy, Grace Dr., 257, **257**
Kennedy, S.G. Dr., 5, 13
Keown, John Dr., 251
Kerekes, Ernest S. Dr., **69**
Kidney transplants, 124, 125, 163, 164
Kiefer, Mark, Dr., 235
Kilbury, Merlin Dr., 258, **258**
Kim, Insung Dr., 177
King, James, 119
Kirkpatrick, Ben O., 69
Kirkpatrick, Gregory Dr., **213**
Knight, Jon Dr., 118
Knowles, Doyal, 58
Koberling, Joseph, 64
Koontz, Doug Dr., 272, **273**
Koro, Paul P. Dr., 281
Kosmoski, David Dr., 272
Kraft, D. Price Dr., 260, **260**, 261
Kramer, John C. Dr., 56, **56**
Krautter, Paul M. Dr., 251
Kruse, Missy, 133

L
Lakin, Tracey Dr., 302, **302**
Larrabee, Walter Dr., 49, **49**
Larson, Lora J. Dr., 259, **259**
Lauinger, Phyllis Dr., 308
Laureate Psychiatric Clinic, **178**, **179**, 182, 290, **290**
Lavendusky, William Dr., 118
Lawrence, Archie, 151
Lawson, Robert Dr., 169
Lee, Laura Dr., 235
Leibovitz, Martin, 97
Leimbach, Wayne Dr., 209, 210
Lewis, C.S. Dr., 110, 310
Lewis, James Dr., 301
Lewis and Clark expedition, 6
Lieberman, Lawrence Dr., 251
Life Flight, 150,**150**, 151, 156
Lilly, Charles, 97
Lister, Joseph Dr., 3
Lockhart, James B. Dr., 298
Loehr, Anthony Dr., 240
Lofgren, Darla Dr., 302, **302**
Lohr, Anthony Dr., 125
Longacre, Jackie, 137
Lorack, Donald A., 170
Loughridge Bill P. Dr., 110, 126, 264, **264**, 265
Love, James Dr., **230**, 231, 232, 233
Lucas, LaTasha, 207
Luce, Tanya, 225, 226, **226**
Lundy, Michael, 119
Lusk, Earl, 97
Lyda, Van and Deborah, 159

M
MacCallum, James, 169
MacKenzie, Ian Dr., 59, **59**
Madson, Walter, 72, 73
Magoon, Bruce and Brenda, 266, **266**
Maguire, Bernard J. Jr. Dr., 261, **261**, 301
Mahaffey, Robert Dr., 251
Mahone, James Kelly, 119
Mamalis, Nicholas Dr., 312, **312**
Marberry, Thomas A. Dr., 262, **262**
March of Dimes, 59
Margaret Hudson Program, 75
Marouk, John Dr., 210, 274
Marrs, Richard Dr., 160
Marshall, James, Dr., 169
Marshall, Thurgood, **86**
Martin, Fred R. Dr., 263, **263**, 267
Mason, D., **69**
Massey, Linda K. Dr., 281
Mathis, Beverly Dr., 175
Maxwell, Myrta, 24
Maurice Willows Hospital, **33**, 62
Mayberry, Dawn, Dr., 212, 213, 216, 217, 300, **300**
McAlliester, Etta, 12, 13
McBeath, Shannon, 206
McBirney, Sam, 11
McCarter, Jack, 65
McClure, C.W. Dr., 164
McClure, Theodore D. Dr., 281
McCullough, Robert D. Dr., 63, 64, **64**, 169
McDonnell, Glenver, 72
McEntee, Charles, 119
McEntee, William C. Dr., 165, 192
McGhee, Jonathan Dr., 251
McKay, Bernice Tibbens, 81
McLaurin, George W., 86, 87
McNulty, Dolly (Brown), 23, 25, 35, 36, **36**, **37**
McNulty, M.J., 23
McPike, Mary S. Dr., 46, 47, **47**
Medagoda, Rumali Dr. **230**, 231, 232
Medical Arts Building, **38**, 50, 55, 90
Medical Credit Bureau, 55
Medicare/Medicaid, 100, 101, 102, 104, 105, 128, 129, 131, 144, 145, 168, 192, 194
Medlock, Thomas R., Dr., 124
Meese, Mark R. Dr., 299, **299**
Meisenheimer, William O., 124
Mental health, 178, 179, 180, 181, 182, 183, 201, 202
Mental Health Association of Tulsa, 180, 181
Mercy Hospital, 102, 169
Merifield, David Dr., 125
Merrill, James A., 136
Meyer C. and Ida Miller Hospice, 266, **266**
Meyers, G.H. Dr., 63
Miller, Archibald, 267, **267**
Miller, Floyd F. Dr., 311, **311**
Miller, Meyer C. and Ida, 266, **266**
Mills, Miriam Dr., 259
Mills, Richard Dr., 126
Milsten, Marc Dr., 225, 303
Minielly, John Dr., **221**, 225
Mishler, Don Dr., 125
Mittapali, Parvati Dr., 259
Mohamed, Ashraf Dr., **213**
Monroe, Shelley, 119
Mooney, Paul D. Dr., 281
Moore, Evan Dr., 240
Moore, William, Dr., 110
Morningside Hospital, 23, 25, 35, 36, **36**
  School of Nursing, **37**
Moro, Paul Dr., 117
Morton Comprehensive Health Services, 196, 206
Moton, Robert Russo, 62, **62**
Moton, William, T. Dr., 45
Moton Memorial Hospital, 62, 88, 100, **100**, **101**
Mourad, Ahmad Dr., 231, **231**
Mounger, Patrice, 155
Mount Zion Baptist Church, **30**
Mowry, John D. Dr., 268, **268**
Muckala, Kenneth Dr., 218, 251, **251**
Murray, Bryce W. Dr., 299, **299**

N
Naimeh, Lodie Dr., **230**, 231, 232, 233
Nassif, Linda Dr., 259
National Guard, **31**
National Medical Association, 32
Neal, James H. Dr., 70
Neal, Victor Dr., 110, 268, **268**
Neal, Wayne R. Dr., 110
Nebergall, Robert Dr., 169
Neinhuis, Lester Dr., 298
Nelson, Arnold G. Dr., 122
Nelson, David Dr., 192
Nelson, Don G. Dr., 269, **269**
Nelson, Robert Dr., 125, 240
Nesbit, Hugh Dr., 251
Nettles, John B. Dr., 270, **270**
Neurosurgery Specialists, 217, 272, **272**, 273, **273**
Newman, Michael Dr., 251
New York Stock Exchange, **41**
Nicholas, Hugh, 97
Nickel, Timothy Dr., **230**, 231, 232
Nierenberg, David Dr., **221**, 308
Nissen, Tim, 206
Noland, Stacy Dr., 302, **302**

O
Obama, Barack President, 194, **195**
O'Brien, L.A. Dr., 13
Oklahoma College of Osteopathic Medicine and Surgery, 116, 117, 140, 176, 280, **281**, 282
Oklahoma Department of Health, 72, 135, 156
Oklahoma Department of Mental Health, 179
Oklahoma Department of Mental Health and Substance Abuse, 183, 201
Oklahoma Health Care Authority, 169
Oklahoma Heart Institute, 208, 209, **209**, 210
Oklahoma Hospital, 21, **21**
Oklahoma Hospital Association, 197
Oklahoma Kidney Foundation, 124
Oklahoma Pain and Wellness Center, 271, **271**
Oklahoma Organ Sharing Network, 191
Oklahoma Osteopathic Hospital, **27**, **46**, 63, **65**, 76, 77, **77**,78, **78**, 102, 116, 125, 126, 129, 145, 151, 172, 175
Oklahoma State Board of Mental Health, 98
Oklahoma State Hospital Association, 15
Oklahoma State Medical Association, 10, 20, 40, 60, 192, 222

323

Oklahoma State Nurses Association, 13
Oklahoma State University Center for Health Sciences, 117, **167**, 173, 198, 200, **200**, 201, 203, **205**, **217**, 280, **280**, 281, **281**, 282, **282**, 283, **283**
Oklahoma State University College of Osteopathic Medicine, 1, 34
Oklahoma State University Medical Authority, 173
Oklahoma State University Medical Center, 1, 34, 173, **173**
Oklahoma State University Telemedicine Bus, 203, **206**
Oklahoma Surgical Hospital, 211, 274, **274**
Oklahoma Territory, 6, 7
Olpin, Jack, 168
Olson, Darwin Dr., 251
Oor, Herbert, 97
Oral Roberts University, 112, 116, 120, 121, 122, 123, 126, 140, 141, 143, 210
   City of Faith, 116, 120, 121, 123, **123**, 140, 141, **141**, **142**, 143, **143**, 146
   Mabee Center, 112, **112**, 140
   Medical School and Family Practice Center, **111**, 116, 120, 121, 122, **122**, 123, 126, 203
Orman, John W. Dr., 63, **64**
Orthopedic Hospital of Oklahoma, 210
Osborn, George Dr., 60, **61**
Osteopathic Hospital Founders Association, 63

P
Page, Charles, 13
Parham, Daran Dr., 306, **306**
Parker, Danny, 124
Parker, Joseph L., 123
Pascucci, Lucien Dr., 88, 137, **137**
Passmore, Sarah Dr., 185
Patel, Jayen Dr., 271, **271**
Patel, Nicole Dr., 227, **227**
Paton, Alistair Dr., 163
Patrick, Joe, 8
Patton, Paul, 176, 222, 224, **224**, 225, 226, 252
Pearl Harbor, **51**, 52
Perryman, Legust Hon., 7
Pershing, John J. Gen., **29**, 294
Peters, Myra Dr., 103, **103**, 259
Pfeifer, Donald Dr., 133
Phillips, Robert Jr. Dr., 191
Physicians and Surgeons Hospital, 25, **26**
Physician shortage, 197, 198
Pickering, Ernest Dr., 117, 169
Pigford, Jack Dr., **69**
Planned Parenthood, 49, 137
Plaster, Rodney Dr., **274**
Plunket, Dan Dr., 228, 238, 300
Polio, 58, 59, 62, 103, 108, 109
Port of Catoosa, **113**
Preston, Jack Dr., 125
Prothro, George W. Dr., 134, 135
Public Health Association, **42**, **43**, **44**, 70
Purdie, Jack, 146, 151
Purser, Jane Dr., **230**, 231, 233

R
Rahhal, Ryan Dr., 273, **273**, **274**
Ramey, Palmer Dr., 162, 163, 267
Ramsey, Jenks, 11
Ray, Arlis Garel, 119
Reagan, Nancy, 157, **158**
Reddy, Anil Dr., 279, **279**
Reed, A.G. Dr., 34, 63, **64**, **69**

Reeder, C.L. Dr., 12, **12**
Reiter, L.A. Dr., 63
Rhodes, Rollie Dr., 125, **221**, 225, 240, 278, **278**
Ribak, Brian Dr., 279, **279**
Rice, Kristen Dr., 284
Richards, Irene, 12
Ritter, Robert C. Dr., 281
Ritter, Valerie Dr., 251
Ritz Theater, 90, **90**, 102
Robards, Victor L. Dr., **124**, 225
Roberts, Oral, 116, 120, 121, **121**, 122, 123, 141, 143
Roberts, Richard, 143
Robertson, William Dr. 281
Rogers, James Dr., 272
Rogers, Theresa, 273
Roller, Don Dr., 127
Roman, John W. Dr., 63
Roth, Jack E., 133
Rothlein, Jerry, 168, 171
Rouleau - Florence, Rose and Victoria, 25
Routsong, James F., 64
Roy, Jess Dr., 251
Rubin, Herschel J. Dr., 56, **56**
Russell, Dick Dr., 216, 261, 301
Rylander, Edward Dr., 247

S
Sabin, Albert Dr., 59, **104-105**, 105,
Sacra, John Dr., 166
Saint Francis Medical Center (also listed as St. Francis in some archived stories), 1, 90, 91, **91**, 94, **94**, 95, 96, 102, 104, 106, 107, 110, **120**, 122, 125, 126, 129, **129**, 130, 131, 132, 145, 150, 151, 156, 161, 164, 165, 166, 169, 173, 174, 175, 182, 185, 191, 192, 205, 210, 213, 214, 288, **288**, 289, **289**, 290, **290**, 291, **291**, 292, 293, **293**
   Cancer Center at 51/Garnett, **126**
   Children's Hospital, 212, **212**, 213, **213**, 214, 291, **291**
   Heart Hospital, 191, **191**, 290, 291
   Laureate Institute for Brain Research, 290
   Laureate Psychiatric Clinic, **178**, **179**, 182, 290, **290**
   Life Flight, 150, **150**, 151, 156
   Natalie Medical Building, **174**
   Natalie Bryant Cancer Center, 126
   South, 168, 169, 291, **291**
   Trauma Emergency Center and Patient Tower, 291, 292, **293**
   Xavier Medical Center, 293
   Warren Clinic, 289, **289**, 290
St. Anthony, 169
St. John Hospital/Medical Center, 1, 28, **28**, 29, **40**, 45, 59, 73, **73**, 76, 79, 80, 83, **83**, 87, 88, 94, 100, 101, 103, 104, 110, 114, **114**, 115, **115**, 119, 123, 124, 125, 126, 129, 134, **139**, 145, 146, 148, 151, 158, 160, 164, 166, 168, 169, 182, **193**, 210, 294, **294**, 295, **295**
   School of Nursing, 29, **29**
   Broken Arrow, **210**
   Air Evac, **139**, 151
St. Jude Children's Research Hospital, 214
Salamy, Joseph Dr., 97, 251
Salk, Jonas Dr., 59, **59**, 88, 195, 310
Sanger, Margaret, 48, **48**
Satterwhite, J.W., 65
Sawyer, William II Dr., 240
Schlezinger, Ira, 145

Schoeffler, Lee Dr., 285, **285**
School, James, 206
Scott, Kate, 12
Serota, Scott, 161
Sethney, Walter F. Dr., 56, **56**
Shadid, Olivia, 207
Shannon, Misti (Farmer), 243, **244**, **245**
Sharp, Paul, 118, 119
Shea, Louis M. Dr., 63
Shepard, Alan, 311
Shepherd, R.M. Dr., **69**
Shirkey, Albert, Dr., 110, 126, 265
Sholl, David Dr., 251
Shoun, Shelley Dr., 251
Showman, W.A. Dr., 60, 61, **61**
Shrum, Kayse Dr., **167**, 200, 281, 283
Siddiqui, James Dr., 225, 229
Siegler, David Dr., 225, 300
Siemens, Christopher Dr., 240
Siemens, Roger Dr., 298, 300
Silva, John, 196
Simcoe, William C. Dr., 164, 286, **286**, 287, **287**
Simms, Fred Dr., 72
Sims, Katie, **230**
Sippel, Mary Edna Dr., **69**
Sister M. Therese Gottschalk, 115, **115**, 242, 249
Sister Mary Agatha, 83
Sister Mary Alfreda, 29
Sister Mary Blandine Fleming, 96, 130, **130**, 131, 151
Sisters Adorers of the Most Precious Blood, 95, 106, 289, **289**
Sisters of the Charity of the Incarnate Word, 96, 130, 131
Sisters of the Sorrowful Mother, 28, 116, 295, **295**
Sister Sylvia Schmidt, 180
Smallpox, 133, 134, 135
Smith, D.O. Dr., **69**
Smith, Elizabeth, 25
Smith, H.B. Dr., 9
Smith, Jim, 191
Smoking, 186, 187, 188, 189, 190
Soulek, Erin, 230
Southcrest Hospital, 170, 171, 172, 208
Spann, Logan Dr., 5, 97
Spears, Jack Dr., 222, 223, **223**, 226
Stalnaker, Eugene, 119
Start, Armond Dr., 135
Stewart, Harry Boyd Dr., 45, **45**, 54
Stokes, Lowell Dr., 298
Stewart, Doug Dr., 225
Stokes, Elmer Malcolm Dr., 138
Stokes, Lowell Dr., 298
Stone, Lloyd, 222
Storts, Daniel Dr., 148
Stout, Donald R. Dr., 296, **296**
Street, Daron Dr., **220**
Sulzycki, Mike, 150, 151
Sunny Side Hospital, 25, 35, 36
Surgical Associates, 95, 298, **298**, 299, **299**
Sutterfield, W. Christopher Dr., 299, **299**
Sutton, Michael, 207
Swanson, Gerald D, 186
Syphilis, 60, 61

T
Taliaferro, Paul E. 133
Thaxton, Gene, 151
The Women's Health Group, 302, **302**

Thomas, Harlan Dr., 97
Thomas, Williams F. Dr., 306
Thompson, C.T. Dr., 95, **95**, 96, 298
Thurman, William G. Dr., 119
Tobacco Settlement Endowment Trust, 190
Tompkins, Robert G., 151, **151**
Tredway, Donald Dr., 297, **297**
Triad, 170, 171, 172
Tulsa Children's Clinic, 216
Tulsa Clinic Hospital, 34
Tulsa Coalition for Children's Health, 212, 213, 216, 300
Tulsa County Medical Society, 29, 31, 34, 37, 38, 40, 43, 44, 45, 49, 50, 54, 55, 57, 59, 68, 74, 75, 88, 103, 105, 140, 141, 147, 148, 176, 218, 220, **220**, 221, **221**, 222, **222**, 223, 224, 225
Tulsa County Medical Society Auxiliary, 147, 148
Tulsa Day Center for the Homeless, 180, **180**
Tulsa Eye Clinic, 285
Tulsa General Hospital, 49, **49**
Tulsa Health Department (city-county), 18, 19, 20, 69, **69**, 70, 71, 74, 75, 88, 100, 134, 135, 154, 155, 189, 206
Tulsa Hospital, **10-11**, 12, 13, 14, 15, 20
Tulsa Hospital Association, 12, 15
Tulsa Municipal Hospital No. 2, 62
Tulsa Orthopedic Society, 103
Tulsa Osteopathic Hospital, 45, 46, 47
Tulsa Otolaryngology Society, 125
Tulsa Public Health Association, **42-43**, **44**, 69
Tulsa Race Riot, 30, 31, 32, 33, 34
Tulsa Regional Medical Center, 34, 82, 171, 172, 175, 182, 200
Tulsa Spine and Specialty Hospital, 211, **211**
Twitty, Bryce, 84, 85, **85**

U

University of Oklahoma Medical School, College of Medicine (OU Health Sciences Center), 66, 86, 116, 118, 122, 136, 169, 276, 277
University of Oklahoma-Tulsa Medical College, 116, **116**, 118, **118**, 119, 121, 126, 127, 140, 172, 276
University of Oklahoma-University of Tulsa School of Community Medicine, 1, 185, 199, **199**, 201, 206, 276, **276**, 277, **277**
University of Oklahoma-University of Tulsa Medical Center and Family Medical Center, 119, **119**, **128**, 276
University of Tulsa College of Health Sciences, 304, **304**, 305, **305**
Upham, Steadman, **277**
Urologic Specialists, 303, **303**
Utica Square, 68, **68**, 83, 85
Utica Women's Specialists, 306, **306**

V

Vaidya, Atul Dr., 240
Vanderlip, Erik Dr., 202
VanSchoyck, Patrick Dr., 251
Varnell, Brandon D. Dr., 299, **299**
Vaumen, Adolpt Dr., 136, 137
Verret, Lloyd, 96, 130, **130**, 131
Vesalius, Andreas, 3

W

Waddell, R.S. and Ora, 12
Wagner, Patrick Dr., 251
Wagner, R.S. Dr., 25
Wall, William L. Dr., 73
Wallace, Arthur Jr. Dr., 169
Wallace, Kenneth, 73, 76, 83, 101
Walls, Lesley Dr., 127
Walsh, John, 182
Warren, John-Kelly, 213, 288
Warren, Natalie, 91, 94, 106, 107, **107**, **288**
Warren, William K., 90, 91, 94, 106, 107, **107**, 288, **288**, 289,
Warren, W.K. Jr., 90, 91, 107, 288, 290
Washington University, Children's Hospital, 216
Wayman Tisdale Specialty Clinic, **203**, 204, 205, 206
Weeks, Willliam, 174, 175
Wehrs, Roger Dr., 125
Weisz, Michael Dr., 225
Wenger, Theodore R. Dr., 110, 268
White, David Dr., 240
Whiteneck, James Dr., 191
Whitmire, Mona, 222, 225, **225**
Whitten, Mindy, 208
Wiens, Lynn Dr., 225, 307, **307**
Wilbanks, Charles, 97
Wiley, A. Ray Dr., 85
Wiley, C. Zenas, Dr., 12, **12**
Williams, Gregory Patrick Dr., 308, **308**
Williams, Theodore, 97
Willows, Maurice, 31, 33
Wilsey, Doug Dr., 127
Winslow, James Dr., 141
Wolff, Eugene Dr., 45
Woodson, Fred Dr., 97, 110
Wooley, Ralph Dr., 154
Wortham, J.W. Edward Jr. Ph.D., 159, 236
Wright, Eliphalet Nott (E.N.) Dr., 4, **4**, 9, 10
Wright, Muriel, 4
Wright, W.E. Dr., 18
Wyatt, Meredith, 207

Y

Young, Anthony, 171, 172

Z

Zanotti, Danielle, 206
Zarrow, Henry, 151
Zetik, Don Dr., 300
Zhang, Shihao Dr., 273
Ziegler, Henrietta C.C., 12, 21
Zollinger, William Dr., 125